Language Disorders in Children
A Multicultural and Case Perspective

Celeste Roseberry-McKibbin
California State University, Sacramento

13

PEARSON

Boston   New York   San Francisco
Mexico City   Montreal   Toronto   London
Madrid   Munich   Paris
Hong Kong   Singapore   Tokyo   Cape Town   Sydney

Executive Editor and Publisher: *Stephen D. Dragin*
Editorial Assistant: *Katie Heimsoth*
Senior Marketing Manager: *Kris Ellis-Levy*
Production Editor: *Janet Domingo*
Editorial Production Service: *Nesbitt Graphics, Inc.*
Composition Buyer: *Linda Cox*
Manufacturing Buyer: *Linda Morris*
Electronic Composition: *Nesbitt Graphics, Inc.*
Interior Design: *Nesbitt Graphics, Inc.*
Photo Researchers: *Annie Pickert and Naomi Rudov*
Cover Administrator: *Kristina Mose-Libon*

For related titles and support materials, visit our online catalog at www.ablongman.com.

Between the time website information is gathered and then published, it is not unusual for some sites to have closed. Also, the transcription of URLs can result in typographical errors. The publisher would appreciate notification where these errors occur so that they may be corrected in subsequent editions.

Library of Congress Cataloging-in-Publication Data

Roseberry-McKibbin, Celeste.
Language disorders in children : a multicultural and case perspective / Celeste Roseberry-McKibbin.
p. cm.
Includes bibliographical references (p.   ).
ISBN 0-205-39340-3
1. Language disorders in children. 2. Language and culture. 3. Multicultural education. 4. Education, Bilingual. I. Title.

RJ496.L35R67 2007
618.92'855--dc22

2006050061

Printed in the United States of America

10 9 8 7 6 5 4 3 2 1   **RRD-VA**   10 09 08 07 06

Photo Credits: 1, Robert Harbison;15, Robert Harbison; 34, Robert Harbison; 46, Frank Siteman; 67, Frank Siteman; 87, Image 100; 102, Chuck Savage; 134, Robert Harbison, 138, Ellen B. Senisi/The Image Works; 159, Robert Brenner/PhotoEdit; 183, Lindfors Photography; 205, Lindfors Photography; 224, Frank Siteman; 241, Frank Siteman; 268, Frank Siteman; 288, Pierre Tremblay/Masterfile; 305, Ellen Senisi/The Image Works; 318, Myrleen Ferguson Cate/PhotoEdit; 347, Joseph Sohm/ChromoSohm/Bettmann/Corbis; 372, Stockbyte/Getty Images; 395, Robin Sachs/PhotoEdit; 415, Bill Aron/PhotoEdit; 439, Lindfors Photography; 445, David Mager/Pearson Learning Photo Studio.

To my precious son Mark
Thank you for teaching me firsthand about child language
And so much more

With all my love

CONTENTS

3   The Impact of Second Language Acquisition and Bilingualism on Children's Developing Language   67

4 Factors Impacting Language Development in Culturally and Linguistically Diverse Children   102

5 Assessment of Children with Language Impairments: Basic Principles   138

8 Language in School-Age Students and Adolescents with Learning Disabilities   268

10 The Impact of Environmental Factors on Language Development   349

11 Language Impairment in Special Populations   397

12 School Language and Classroom Programs for Children with Language Impairment: Collaborating with Parents and School Personnel   441

Alejandro E. Brice and Roanne G. Brice

As I was turning six years old, my family of two parents and four little girls sailed to the Philippines, where my parents would serve as Baptist missionaries for the next ten years. I lived in the Philippines from ages six to seventeen years. I think it would be fair to say that my sisters and I were culturally and linguistically diverse (CLD). Filipino children from a local school would come to gaze at our pale blonde hair, light eyes, and white skin. They would pinch our cheeks and stroke our arms in wonder. As we walked by nipa huts on our tiny island of Tablas, mothers would hold up crying babies as we passed. The babies would stop mid-wail and gape in wonder; they had never seen a white person before. We were such a novelty that we even stopped babies from crying!

At home, we spoke Mainstream American English. With our Filipino friends in the neighborhood, which for several years was a coconut grove by the ocean, we spoke pidgin English and Odionganon—the language of the little town of Odiongan. In school, we learned Tagalog (the Filipino national language); church services were conducted in Hiligaynon. In the elementary schools I attended in third and fourth grade (two different islands; we moved), I was the only white child and native English speaker in the entire school. At a young age, I developed great empathy for children who are diverse; children whose language and culture are different from those of the majority; children who have linguistic and cultural challenges to deal with.

I was seventeen years old and a college freshman when my family and I returned to the United States. I was fortunate to do well in college, because schools in Southeast Asia are very rigorous. But though I was now "mainstream," I still felt different from everyone else. I had never heard of *Leave it to Beaver* or *Father Knows Best*. I couldn't get over the fact that houses in the United States had carpets and hot running water! And it seemed that everyone had a car; in the Philippines, probably 10 to 20 percent of the families have cars, especially in rural areas like those where we lived. It took many years for me to fit in here in the United States; to this day, I still am not too hip sometimes. A colleague recently said something about *One Flew Over the Cuckoo's Nest*. After I opened my mouth to ask what that was, I shut it quickly. Over the years, with Americans, I had become accustomed to "the look"; the one that says, "Where did you grow up, in a cave somewhere?" I have actually heard those words more than once! Most of my life in the United States has comprised experiences of being "different"; if not in looks, at least in background knowledge and cultural know-how. Let me put it this way: you don't want me as a partner in Trivial Pursuit. I continue to have empathy for students and their families who work hard to fit in and succeed in US culture.

As a twenty-three-year-old beginning clinician right out of my master's degree program at a California university, I got a job in a low-income district with many children who came from non-English-speaking homes. Although I had a great deal of personal empathy for these children, at that time, there were no university textbooks or courses that prepared me for dealing with all this diversity. They say that when all you have is a hammer, everything looks like a nail. Well, to assess for the possible presence of language impairment in CLD children, all I had were standardized English tests; mysteriously, all the children were diagnosed with language impairments and subsequently placed on my ever-burgeoning caseload. Sadly, it was one or two years before I put two and two together—but eventually I learned.

I am so thankful that things are different today. I want to thank Steve Dragin of Allyn & Bacon, who asked me to write this book and who encouraged (and prodded!) me along the way. Steve, you are the best; thank you for all your patience as my life circumstances have sometimes slowed down my progress. It is a joy and privilege to work with you. Meaghan Minnick has been most helpful and supportive: Meaghan, thank you! Additional thanks to the reviewers: Jacqueline Bauman-Waengler, Clarion University; Lynn S. Bliss, University of Houston; Thalia J. Coleman, Appalachian State University; Priscilla Nellum Davis, University of Alabama; Vera F. Gutierrez-Clellen, San Diego State University; Heidi M. Harbers, Illinois State University; Karla McGregor, University of Iowa; Michael McKaig, Stephen F. Austin State University; Anne van Kleeck, University of Georgia; and Janice M. Wright, Ohio University.

As I have been a university instructor over the years, I have taught courses in child language development and disorders. I have used some excellent textbooks, and some that were not so excellent. Through this, I have learned many of the things that students are looking for in a textbook, and I have tried to incorporate students' ideas here. I have actively sought feedback from my students about what they are looking for in a basic child language disorders textbook; the students have given me honest (sometimes brutally honest!) feedback about what they like and do not like. I have used this feedback to guide me in the writing of this book; I thank my current and former students so much for their input over the years.

The purpose of this text is to be an introduction—to give students a foundation upon which to build in future coursework. Many concepts are introduced in a basic, straightforward way with the assumption that these concepts will be built upon and extended in future courses. I have supported my information with research as much as possible. Though this is a beginning textbook for an audience with no prior background, I still believe it is important for information to be grounded in research. Evidence-based practice is a current and important emphasis in our profession, and it is important for any claims or information to be based on research. However, one danger of describing many studies in detail is that beginning students in the major become turned off. They lose the forest for the trees. As I have talked with my students over the years, they have acknowledged the importance of research but have told me that, often, textbooks that describe a great deal of research confuse them and obfuscate the information the author is trying to convey.

In light of this situation, I have done my best to create a balance in this book: citing some research and describing a few key studies. I have also used a pedagogical device called *Connect and Extend* to help students immediately know where they can go for more information about certain topics. I have especially recommended primary sources of research in this way so that 1) students can read the research on their own, and 2) instructors can choose to assign these research articles as readings that supplement the text. Again, I am assuming that this book is an introduction to child language disorders; the goal is to give students a firm foundation for future, more advanced coursework in this area.

In addition to *Connect and Extend,* I have used a number of other pedagogical devices to help beginning students comprehend, remember, interact with, and integrate the material. Each chapter begins with a case study to engage the reader and pique her interest in the chapter's contents—to put "life" into the chapter. Throughout each chapter, there are *Points to Ponder* and *Cases to Consider*. The goal of these pedagogical devices is to help students interact with and think about the material, and to engage in the learning process actively instead of just passively taking in information. I have been somewhat redundant in this book, because I have found over the years that students are really helped by hearing important concepts more than once. If I use a term in Chapter 11 that was defined in Chapter 2, the reader may have forgotten what the term meant. Thus, some of the information is deliberately repetitious in order to help the beginning reader retain and truly understand the information. I have tried to relate the contents of each chapter to other chapters in the book. I have put a summary at the end of each chapter section for quick review. *Chapter Highlights* are included at the end of each chapter for additional review.

At the end of each chapter, there are study and review questions. Students learn differently, and thus I have asked questions in three different formats: essay, fill-in-the-blank, and multiple choice. The multiple choice questions are designed to be very similar to the questions asked on the PRAXIS in order to give beginning students practice for taking the PRAXIS in the future. The PRAXIS contains many very long, "case study"–type questions, and I have tried to put some similar questions in this book. Answers to study and review questions are listed in an appendix at the end of the book..

In addition to being a university professor, I work part time as an itinerant speech-language pathologist in the public school system (I do drink a lot of coffee). The majority of the cases in this book come from my direct experience. It is my great hope that through the case studies, I have brought the information in this book to life for beginning students in the major. I remember when I was a nineteen-year-old junior beginning in speech-language pathology; I had little experience with children and found myself reading books and memorizing information for exams—but I didn't realize how this information actually applied to children. Over the years, I have come to see that many of my students are in a similar situation.

I have written this book with four goals: 1) present accurate information, 2) present current information, 3) present research-based information as much as possible (with an emphasis on evidence-based practice), and 4) give "heart" to the information to help students begin to truly care about the children they will eventually be serving. Throughout this book, I have tried to bring facts alive to students and to help them genuinely care about the information that they will eventually be using to change children's lives. And I've even dared to have a little fun now and then. I've definitely given myself free rein (perhaps too free) to share stories of children from my clinical experience. I have often found, when I encounter my former students after they have graduated, that what they remember most from my classes is the stories about actual children.

I have chosen to write this book in first person. My tone is informal and conversational. I have also chosen to alternate the pronouns "he" and "she" because this is much less awkward than she/he and even than the plural "children." In addition, I've integrated information about CLD children into the main text as much as possible. In many textbooks, cultural and linguistic diversity information is contained in one discrete chapter while the other chapters deal exclusively with issues related to monolingual English-speaking children. This book does have several chapters dealing primarily with CLD issues; however, CLD issues are integrated into each chapter as well. My goal has been to avoid the artificiality of separating CLD issues from "mainstream" issues. I believe we can no longer afford to do that in our profession. Far from being tucked away in a separate chapter or section, CLD issues need to become part of the fabric of mainstream thinking.

This book has been a labor of love. As I continue to practice part-time as a public school clinician in California's fastest-growing school district whose students represent more than 80 different languages, I am constantly confronted with the great needs of these students. I see their faces, talk to them, and interact with their families. Just the other week, I met with an immigrant Chinese mother who could not stop crying for the better part of an hour. She was distraught about her son's first-grade performance, about her lack of English facility, about the family's finances, and about their future in general. I sat there handing her Kleenex, thinking about her overwhelming needs, and wishing I could do even more for her son and for her. For me, writing this book has not just been an esoteric exercise. As I have written, I have remembered the faces and heard the voices of so many of my children and their families over the years. In this book, I have tried to do them justice and to help readers care as I do.

We as speech-language pathologists are crucial to the success of our CLD children—our nation's future. It is for these children that I have written this book—and I feel deep gratitude for the opportunity to make this contribution to our field. I hope that readers will enjoy the book, learn a lot—and become competent, knowledgeable, compassionate clinicians who truly make a difference in the lives of others.

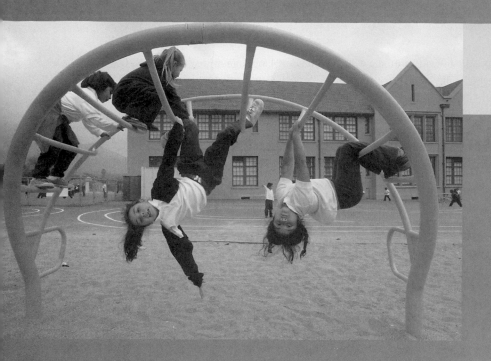

Introduction to Language and Language Disorders

CASE STUDY

Crystal S. was a recent graduate from a speech-language pathology program in the Midwest. She was beginning her new job in New York, where her husband had recently been offered a job. Crystal felt that she had received a good education and was eager to begin as an itinerant public school speech-language pathologist (SLP). Within Crystal's first month of employment, she found that she was receiving referrals of children from many culturally and linguistically diverse (CLD) backgrounds. Crystal had grown up in a state where most residents were from European American backgrounds and spoke only English. In her clinical practicum during graduate school, Crystal had served primarily Anglo European American, monolingual English-speaking children.

Suddenly she found herself confronted with the need to evaluate the language skills of children who spoke languages like Tagalog, Farsi, Uzbeki, Urdu, Khmer, Spanish, Vietnamese, and Russian. Her program director told her that in the district, children represented more than eighty different languages. Crystal realized, belatedly, that she had no idea about the normal language parameters of these kinds of children; nor did she have the skills and knowledge to decide if they had language differences due to the influence of their first language or actual **specific language impairment (SLI)**. She decided to get out her college textbooks and brush up on components of language as well as characteristics of children with SLI. She realized that she needed to supplement this information with some research and exploration into the aspects of CLD children's language development and what consituted a language impairment in these children. Without this information, she was sure to mislabel them as being language impaired when they really were not; she also did not want to deny services to these children if they truly needed it.

INTRODUCTION

Cultural and Linguistic Diversity

In the twenty-first century, the United States is becoming increasingly culturally and linguistically diverse. SLPs now have the privilege of serving children from all over the world. Some of these children are born in the United States into CLD homes; others immigrate from other countries with their families. I was raised in the Philippines from ages six to seventeen years by Baptist missionary parents and believe that the increasing diversity in the United States is an enriching and exciting phenomenon. Because we are serving so many more **culturally and linguistically diverse** (CLD) students than ever before, we as SLPs have the opportunity to constantly learn and grow.

For example, in the Sacramento area of California where I live, the primary CLD populations used to be Hispanic and Southeast Asian. In the late 1990s, there was a large influx of immigrants from the former Union of Soviet Socialist Republics (USSR). In 2004, there were over 100,000 individuals from the former USSR living in Sacramento. Now in Sacramento schools, students speak Uzbeki, Armenian, Ukrainian, and Russian in addition to Spanish, Vietnamese, Chinese, Hmong, and many, many other languages. It has been a rich and exciting experience (not to mention humbling) for me and my colleagues to learn about all the different languages and cultures of these students from the former USSR!

> The increasing numbers of CLD children in American public schools provide SLPs opportunities to continually learn new things and grow professionally.

Because I work part time as a public school itinerant SLP in addition to being a university professor, I am privileged to be constantly learning new information so I can effectively provide services to a very diverse group of children. In my school district, children from more than ninety different language groups are represented. Because of the increasing cultural and linguistic diversity not only in Sacramento but everywhere in the United States, we as SLPs are provided with constant opportunities to continue to expand our skills and knowledge so we can effectively serve children from many different backgrounds.

> The population growth in the United States is predominantly occurring among CLD populations.

The US Bureau of the Census (2000) reported that in the 1990s, racial and ethnic minorities accounted for up to 80 percent of the nation's population growth. Over the past twenty years (1980–2000), the non-Hispanic White population grew by 7.6 percent while the population of individuals from minority groups increased by more than 90 percent. During the decade of the 1990s, in contrast with the growth of 7.6 percent by the White non-Hispanic population, the Hispanic population increased by 58 percent, the Asian population increased by 48 percent, the Native American/Alaska Native population increased by 26 percent, and the African American population increased by 16 percent. The number of immigrants to the United States has more than tripled from 9.6 million in 1970 to 28.4 million in 2000.

Various terms have been used in descriptions of persons from CLD backgrounds. The term **race** refers to a category of persons who share biologically transmitted traits considered socially significant (e.g., hair and skin color). There are no biologically pure races; *race* is a label that people apply to themselves and to others based on physical appearance. The term **ethnicity** refers to groups characterized by a common language, culture, or nationality (Betancourt & Lopez, 1993). A friend of mine who was born and raised in Hong Kong says that in terms of *race*, he is Asian; in terms of *ethnicity*, he is Chinese.

Sometimes sociologists and other professionals use the term **minority group** (e.g., as I did in a previous paragraph when referring to statistics from the US Bureau of the Census) to label a group of people who are discriminated against or treated with lack of equality. However, usually people use the term *minority group* to refer to a numerical minority compared to the total population (Woolfolk, 2004). Some professionals don't use the term *minority group* because it is often inaccurate.

For example, in California, Whites are a minority group because California has such a large population of Hispanics, Asians, and African Americans. In the public elementary school where I work part-time, a classroom might have two White children and twenty-eight children from CLD groups. Thus, throughout this book, I will use the term CLD rather than "minority group." Crowley (2003, p. 2) defines the term CLD in detail:

> [The term] *culturally diverse* describes an individual or group that is exposed to, and/or immersed in, more than one set of cultural beliefs, values, and attitudes. [The term] *linguistically diverse* describes an individual or group that is exposed to, and/or immersed in, more than one language or dialect.

Because of the increasing cultural and linguistic diversity in the United States, SLPs have received an increasing number of referrals of culturally and linguistically diverse children with communication disorders. Many of these children are referred for SLI. In fact, Roseberry-McKibbin, Brice, and O'Hanlon (2005) found in a large national survey that of the CLD students on public school clinicians' caseloads, more than 80 percent of these children had been diagnosed with language impairments. However, the results of the survey also indicated that many of the respondents had not had coursework regarding service delivery to bilingual children. One wonders how, without information and coursework, clinicians were able to make appropriate decisions about whether or not the children on their caseloads truly had SLI.

It is crucial for us as SLPs to understand typical parameters of language as well as SLI in not only monolingual children but in CLD children as well. Accordingly, in this chapter we will look together at common language terms, approaches to language disorders, characteristics of children with SLI, and considerations in working with CLD children who have SLI.

CONNECT & EXTEND

The results of a survey of SLPs' practices with CLD children across the United States are described in Roseberry-McKibbin, C., Brice, A., & O'Hanlon, L. (2005). Serving English language learners in public school settings: A national survey. *Language, Speech, and Hearing Services in Schools, 36,* 48–61.

Evidence-Based Practice

In this chapter and throughout this book, we will also be referring to the concept of **evidence-based practice**. When providing services for any population (children with language impairments in this book), SLPs must always operate from the framework of evidence-based practice. Peach (2002) defined evidence-based practice as asking focused questions about treatment for specific clinical problems and seeking answers in high-quality evidence from the published literature. The American Speech-Language-Hearing Association (ASHA, 2005) stated that the goal of evidence-based practice is to integrate clinical expertise, best current evidence, and client values to provide high-quality services to the clients whom we serve. A further description is found in Roseberry-McKibbin & Hegde (2006, p. 615):

> Evidence-based practice ensures that the clients receive services that are known to be based on reliable and valid research and sound clinical judgment. . . . Most experts consider efficacy for treatment procedures to be a significant part of evidence-based practice. It is unethical to use treatment procedures that have not been supported by experimental research. . . . Evidence-based practice requires an integration of best research evidence for clinical methods with clinical expertise and sound judgment. Evidence-based practice is always client-centered. . . . In selecting assessment and treatment procedures, the clinician takes into consideration not only the research evidence, but also what is best for an individual patient and his or her preference.

CONNECT & EXTEND

The American Speech-Language-Hearing Association has developed formal statements regarding evidence-based practice. To access these statements, go to www.asha.org.

Thus, it is the goal of this book to discuss only those concepts, materials, and strategies for service delivery that are supported by research and that emphasize the individual child's best interests. The language taxonomies described below are based on evidence-based practice.

DEFINITIONS AND TERMINOLOGY

Nelson (1998) states that a variety of systems may be used to categorize language. Two distinct but compatible taxonomies are used by most specialists. The first taxonomy uses the linguistic categories of semantics, morphology, syntax, pragmatics, and phonology. The second taxonomy defines content (semantics), form (syntax, morphology, and phonology) and use (pragmatics) (Bloom & Lahey, 1978). Figure 1.1 pictures the relationship between these two taxonomies. This section defines and describes semantics, morphology, syntax, pragmatics, and phonology.

Semantics

Semantics is the study of word *meaning* in a language. The semantic component refers to the meaning conveyed by words, phrases, and sentences. Semantics also refers to the rules governing meaning relations among words and sentences. Semantics involves a person's

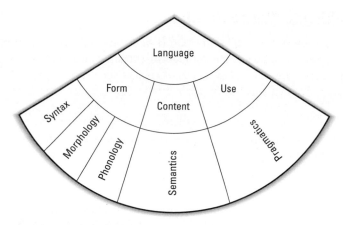

FIGURE 1.1 Components of Language

From Robert E. Owens Jr. *Language Development: An Introduction*, 6e. Published by Allyn & Bacon, Boston, MA. Copyright © 2005 by Pearson Education. Reprinted by permission of the publisher.

vocabulary or lexicon. Vocabulary development depends heavily upon environmental exposure, cultural experiences, and the individual capacity each child brings to the learning situation. As a child grows, she not only learns more new words; she also develops new ways to use the words and refines the meanings of words she already knows (Hulit & Howard, 2002).

For example, a small child may learn that a glass of ice water is *cool* to the touch. When she goes to elementary school, there is a **vertical** expansion of her definition of the word *cool*. She learns that *cool* has various meanings; for example, it is not *cool* to wear a TeleTubbies shirt; however, it is extremely *cool* to wear a Dora the Explorer shirt. She will also undergo **horizontal** expansion of the definition of "cool" as she adds more semantic features to her understanding of the word (e.g., that an air-conditioned room feels cool, that she is cool on the playground without her sweater in November, etc.).

> Semantics is the study of meaning; it refers to a child's vocabulary development.

A child's vocabulary is inextricably intertwined with her linguistic and cultural background. For example, in the Carolinian language in one area of the Pacific Islands, there are more than ten words that depict the various stages of the growth of a coconut. In the Philippines, a country known for its strong emphasis on good interpersonal relationships, the word *pakikisama* indicates smooth and harmonious relationships between people, especially in a group. In some Western countries such as the United States, where there is more emphasis on individualism, there is no equivalent expression. When a CLD student's vocabulary is being evaluated, it is critical to consider the influences of environment, culture, and language background as well as word and world knowledge.

Important phenomena to consider in a child's language development are *word knowledge* and *world knowledge*. **World knowledge** involves a child's experiential and autobiographical memory and understanding of particular events. **Word knowledge** is

POINTS TO PONDER How does a child's environment, including his cultural and linguistic background, affect semantic development?

_____

_____

_____

> Important aspects of a child's semantic growth include development of both word and world knowledge.

primarily verbal and involves word and symbol definitions. A child's word knowledge depends heavily upon his or her world knowledge. For example, a child from the Philippines who has grown up on beaches but never seen snow (world knowledge) might have difficulty understanding and using the word *snow* (word knowledge).

Important aspects of a child's semantic development include knowledge of **antonyms**, or opposites (e.g., *hot-cold*), and **synonyms**, or words that mean similar things (e.g., *clear-transparent, attractive-pretty*). Another important aspect of semantic development is understanding and use of words with multiple meanings (e.g., *rock, pound*).

Part of a child's semantic development also involves comprehension and use of **deictic words**, or words whose referents change depending upon who is speaking (e.g., *come, go, this, here, that*). Deictic words are very challenging for many CLD children who are learning English as another language because they are abstract and, as stated, change depending upon the speaker's perspective. Another important aspect of semantic development is the use of **semantic categories**, which are used to sort words. Examples of a few of these categories are **recurrence** (concept of *more*), **rejection** (*no*), and **causality** (*cause-and-effect*).

> Important aspects of a child's semantic development include knowledge and use of deictic words, semantic categories, recurrence, rejection, and causality.

An important concept emphasized today in semantics is **quick incidental learning** or **fast mapping**. This refers to a child's ability to learn a new word after just a few exposures to it. Children who are developing in a typical manner use fast mapping to rapidly expand their vocabularies. For example, it is estimated that the average typically developing (TD) preschooler learns to understand up to nine new words a day (McLaughlin, 2006).

Another important semantic aspect of children's language development is developing **categorization**, or the ability to categorize words. For example, children must learn that *chair, table, couch, bed* fall under the category of *furniture*. The use of categories helps bring order to the child's experiences. The child who is not successful at categorizing treats each experience as a totally new one (Reed, 2005). It is as if the child's brain is a file cabinet with no drawers. She needs drawers (categories) so she can organize incoming information. If the child has normal ability to

> Categorization is a very important semantic skill for children to develop.

categorize words, then new experiences may be "filed" under preexisting categories or the child's mental constructs that allow her to group similar items together.

As children grow, they also develop semantically in the ability to use **humor** (e.g., jokes, puns, riddles) and figurative language. **Figurative language** includes proverbs, metaphors, and idioms. A **proverb** is a wise saying or statement of truth (e.g., An ounce of prevention is worth a pound of cure). An **idiom** is an expression that is unique to a certain language or group of people (e.g., She made money *hand over fist*). A **metaphor** is a figure of speech that uses a likeness to stand for an idea, word, or referent (e.g., That guy has a heart of gold) (Bernstein & Levey, 2002).

> Development of figurative language includes knowledge and use of proverbs, idioms, and metaphors.

The use of figurative language depends heavily on a child's cultural and linguistic background. Many CLD students will not know various structures present in American figurative language. For example, if a student immigrated from Japan and was new to the United States, it would be inappropriate to expect him to understand figures of speech such as *It's raining cats and dogs* or *A penny saved is a penny earned*. Other cultures have their own figurative language structures, and it can be very interesting to see how these figurative language structures reflect the culture of the student. For example, in Japan, modesty and humility are highly valued. A person's goal is to blend harmoniously into the group and not draw attention to himself. The Japanese have a saying that "The nail that sticks up gets hammered down." Here in the United States, people talk about "tooting your own horn."

CASES TO CONSIDER

Rupinder Singh (not his real name) was a five-year-old kindergartener from a Punjabi-speaking home. His parents had immigrated from India, and Mrs. Singh had worked inside the home for the first five years of Rupinder's life caring for him and his younger sister. When Rupinder came to kindergarten at the elementary school where I work part-time, he was referred for a speech-language assessment. Rupinder's teacher said that he "didn't know words in English." Rupinder had failed the kindergarten screening, where he was asked to label shapes, colors, letters, and numbers in English. Additionally, Rupinder was extremely shy and would not make eye contact or engage with unfamiliar adults. The school team wondered if Rupinder had a language learning problem and needed speech-language therapy. As part of my evaluation, I talked with Mrs. Singh extensively and found out that Rupinder had been raised solely in a Punjabi-speaking environment for the first five years of his life. He had never been to preschool. The family did not attend church or temple. Mrs. Singh shared that she felt it was very important for Rupinder to never be away from her in the company of strangers. Do you think that Rupinder's vocabulary "problems" could be explained by his environmental history?

_____

_____

_____

Morphology

Morphology involves the study of *word structure* and describes how words are formed out of more basic elements of language, called morphemes. **Morphemes** are the smallest meaningful unit of a language; they are considered minimal because if they are subdivided any further, they become meaningless (McLaughlin, 2006). Morphemes are used to form words. Each morpheme is different from the others because each signals a distinct meaning.

> There are two kinds of morphemes: bound and free morphemes.

Free, **base**, or **root** morphemes are words that have meaning, cannot be broken down into smaller parts, and can have other morphemes added to them. Examples of free morphemes are: *table, tree, hair, pool.* All these words mean something, can stand by themselves, and cannot be broken down into smaller parts. These words can have other morphemes added to them. **Bound** or **grammatic morphemes** must be joined with free morphemes in order to have meaning. They cannot convey meaning by themselves. In the following examples, the free morphemes are underlined; the bound morphemes are in capital letters:

picnicS   DISappear   establishMENT   colorFUL   UNbutton

Common bound or grammatic morphemes include the following:

- *ing*   The present progressive (cook*ing*, writ*ing*)
- *s*   The regular plural morpheme (cat*s*, basket*s*)
- *s*   The possessive inflection (man's, lady's)
- *ed*   The regular past tense (comb*ed*, wash*ed*)

Bound morphemes can be divided into the subcategories of prefixes and suffixes. A **prefix** is added at the beginning of a base morpheme; a *suffix* is added at the end of a base morpheme. For example:

Whole Word	Prefix	Base Word	Suffix
indoctrinate	in	doctrine	ate
disappointing	dis	appoint	ing
miscommunication	mis	communicate	ion

Allomorphs are variations of morphemes and, as such, do not alter the original meaning of the morpheme. Allomorphs often are spelled the same but pronounced differently. For example, the plural morpheme can be denoted by the following allomorphs: fox*es* (ez), loave*s* (z), hut*s* (s). Although these are both written as "s," they are pronounced differently. The past tense morpheme is usually written as *-ed*, but it is pronounced differently depending upon its root word. For example, in most words that end in sounds that are not voiced, the speaker will say the *-ed* morpheme as /t/ (e.g., cook*ed*, cough*ed*, kiss*ed*). However, in most words that end in voiced sounds, the speaker will say the past tense *-ed* morpheme as a /d/ (e.g., mov*ed*, vacuum*ed*, clean*ed*).

> Prefixes and suffixes can be added to free morphemes to change the meaning of a word.

CONNECT & EXTEND

Children who speak African American English and have SLI have unique morphological characteristics as described by Oetting, J.B., & McDonald, J.L. (2001). Nonmainstream dialect use and specific language impairment. *Journal of Speech-Language-Hearing Research, 44*(1), 207–223.

Allomorphs are variations of morphemes that do not alter the original meaning of the morpheme—for example, the plural allomorphs are *-s, -z, -ez.*

Morphemes are a means of modifying word structures to change meaning. The morphology of a given language describes the rules of such modifications. It describes what kinds of morphemic combinations are permissible in a given language. Languages vary greatly in their uses of morphemes. For example, in Japanese, the suffix *san* is used as a term of politeness. Thus, the secretary of an executive named Mr. Nakahara might refer to him as Nakahara-san. There is also no plural morpheme; *hon* means both *book* and *books* (Cheng, 1991).

A TD child who speaks African American English might delete possessive *-s* and/or copula *-s*, saying, for example, "That Antoine book" instead of "That's Antoine's book." When evaluating a child who speaks a language other than Mainstream American English, it is extremely important to take the child's primary language into account when assessing morphological development.

Morphology is heavily interrelated with *syntax.* Speakers arrange morphemes so that they can change the meaning of a sentence. For example, one can change "She walk*s* to the store" to "She walk*ed* to the store." Through adding the past tense *-ed* morpheme and omitting the third person singular *-s*, the speaker changes sentence meaning.

Syntax

The basic meaning of the word **syntax** is to join, to put together. In language, syntax is one of the two parts of grammar; the other part of grammar, as previously noted, is morphology.

McLaughlin (2006) states that in the study of language, syntax involves

- word order and overall structure of a sentence
- the arrangement of words to form meaningful sentences
- a collection of rules that specify the ways and order in which words may be combined to form sentences in a particular language

Syntax involves word order and the arrangement of words to form meaningful sentences.

Languages have different syntactic structures. In English, the basic syntactic structure is the subject + verb + object sequence (He eats popcorn). This structure, usually called the **kernel sentence**, can also be called the *phrase structure* or *base structure*. The syntactic rules of languages differ from one another. For example, in English, one might use the phrase "*the new house.*" In Spanish, one might say "*una casa nueva*" ("the house new"). The language of Cantonese has little grammatical morphology and is primarily a subject-verb-object language with only a few regular deviations such as object-subject-verb. Thus, a Cantonese-speaking child may say, "*Today food I already buy*" instead of "*I've already bought food for today*" (Fung & Roseberry-McKibbin, 1999).

All languages are creative, and children can generate an infinite variety of structures. These structures, however, are governed by rules of syntax. A TD child does not produce structures with random and meaningless word order. For example, an English speaker could say, *She told me she'd feed the cat, but she didn't.* Due to syntactic rules, this same speaker could not say, *Told she'd me she the cat feed didn't she but.* A child who speaks a language other than English needs to be evaluated in his first language (L1) to ascertain if he is following the syntactic rules of that language. (A child's first language, or L1, is the language she was exposed to earliest in life—the language she was exposed to beginning in infancy.) All children can be evaluated in a variety of ways, including through analysis of the types of sentences they produce.

> The base syntactic structure of English is called the kernel sentence, which is subject-verb-object.

Sentences can be classified according to their types or functions. For example:

- **declaratives**, which make statements ("*I love reading this great book.*")
- **imperatives**, which involve commands or requests ("*Give me the book.*")
- **exclamatory** sentences, which involve strong feeling ("*I'll keep this book forever!*")
- **interrogatives** or questions ("*Can you believe how interesting this book is?*")
- **active** sentences, where the subject performs the actions of the verb (*The student read the book.*)
- **passive** sentences, where the subject receives the action of the verb (*The book was read by the student.*)

It is important to remember that different languages may emphasize certain sentence types more than others. For example, in Japan, adults and especially children might avoid imperatives because they would be viewed as rude and imperious. In American English, imperatives are accepted because Americans value directness and forthrightness in communication.

> There are six types of sentences: declarative, imperative, exclamatory, interrogative, active, and passive.

Regardless of their cultural and linguistic background, all children eventually begin to use *compound* and *complex* sentences. A **compound sentence** has two or more *independent clauses* joined by a comma and a conjunction or with a semicolon. A **clause** contains a subject and predicate. An **independent** or **main clause** has a subject and predicate and can stand alone. There are no subordinate clauses in a compound sentence. For example:

The dog started barking,	and	the mailman backed off.
(independent clause)	*(conjunction)*	*(independent clause)*
The baby cooed in her crib;		later she began to fuss.
(independent clause + semicolon)		*(independent clause)*

A **complex sentence** contains one independent clause and one or more **dependent/subordinate clauses**. A dependent or subordinate clause has a subject and predicate but cannot stand alone. For example:

> **POINTS TO PONDER** Define *morphology* and *syntax*. Give several examples of how other languages differ from English in the areas of morphology and syntax.
>
> _____
>
> _____
>
> _____

I will pick you up at school *(independent clause)*	if you are ready to go. *(dependent clause)*
You can watch a video *(independent clause)*	after you brush your teeth. *(dependent clause)*

Pragmatics

Pragmatics involves the study of rules that govern of language use in social situations. In pragmatics, one focuses on how a child uses language in context. Pragmatics places greater emphasis on *functions*, or uses of language, than on structure. Functions of language include **commenting** (describing or identifying objects; e.g., "That's a kitty."); **labeling** (naming something; e.g., a child is playing with a doll and says, "Barbie") and **protesting** (objecting to something; e.g., my son's favorite, "Stop combing my hair!"). Chapter 2 and Chapter 7 describe children's development of pragmatic language skills in greater depth.

> As they mature in language development, children begin to use complex and compound sentences.

Pragmatics can be viewed as the dimension of language that considers the **function** of the utterance (e.g., the purpose or goal) as well as the **context** of the utterance (e.g., the situation, the listener-speaker relationship). Language context involves where the utterance takes place, to whom the utterance is directed, and what and who are present at the time. As they get older, children with effective pragmatics skills distinguish between and appropriately use **direct** and **indirect speech acts**. Indirect speech acts are used to convey politeness.

> Pragmatics studies rules that govern language use in a social context.

For example, as a direct speech act, a child could say, "Bring me the ball." To say this indirectly and more politely, the child could say, "Will you bring the ball over to me?" The use of direct and indirect speech acts is heavily influenced by culture. For example, in Japanese society, indirect speech acts are believed to convey speaker sophistication and sensitivity. In American culture, people who use many indirect speech acts may be viewed as weak, unassertive, and unsure of themselves (Tannen, 1990).

> As children develop pragmatics skills, they gain facility with appropriately using direct and indirect speech acts.

In addition to appropriately using direct and indirect speech acts, a child needs to develop other aspects of appropriate pragmatics skills. One of these aspects involves providing listeners with adequate information without being too redundant. Two days ago, I assessed a thirteen-year-old boy with Asperger syndrome (described more fully in Chapter 9). I asked him a polite question about karate, thinking I'd get a three- to four-sentence answer. Brian talked enthusiastically for at least ten minutes about karate, detailing all the levels one could go through and talking about the historical origins of karate. He repeated much of the information several times. I was provided with more than adequate information! Even when I tried to change the subject, Brian didn't take the hint. It was as if I wasn't even in the room. Students with difficulties in the area of providing adequate information without being too redundant need to learn to consider their listener's interest level and involvement with the topic.

Another aspect of pragmatics involves the ability to maintain coherence of sequential statements (order in which statements are logically presented). Children must also learn to repair communication breakdowns as well as to maintain a topic with one or more conversational partners. In addition, children need to develop adequate turn-taking skills in order to keep a conversation moving forward.

> Turn-taking is an important skill to develop; rules of turn-taking are heavily determined by culture.

Turn-taking is highly dependent on a child's cultural and linguistic background. For example, children from African American families may not observe traditional turn-taking during conversations; speaking is often highly competitive, and interruptions are permitted and expected. Thus, children who speak African American English might be misjudged as having a clinically significant problem with the pragmatics skill of turn-taking when, in reality, they are behaving within the norms of their linguistic community (Roseberry-McKibbin, 2008; van Keulen, Weddington, & DeBose, 1998; Wyatt, 2002).

Pragmatics skills also involve the appropriate knowledge and use of discourse, or the connected flow of language. **Discourse** refers to how utterances are related. Discourse can involve a monologue, a dialogue between two people, or even conversational exchange in a small group. **Narratives** are a form of discourse where the speaker tells a story or talks about a logical sequence of events. This sequence can involve an actual episode from the speaker's life, such as a family gathering at Christmastime; it can also involve a story about an event (such as a fairy tale or movie) that did not happen to the speaker directly.

> Discourse refers to how utterances are related; narratives are a form of discourse where a speaker tells a story.

Narrative structure is very heavily influenced by culture, and CLD children's storytelling styles may differ from mainstream expectations. These differences can lead to incorrect judgments about the pragmatics skills of children who speak African American English, for example (Terrell & Jackson, 2002; van Keulen et al., 1998). When they tell stories, African American students often used a topic-associating style characterized by presupposition of shared knowledge between speaker and listener, lack of consideration for detail, and structured discourse on several linked topics. African American students may show a preference for lengthy narratives and may embellish a story with jokes, metaphors, slang, and exaggeration (Champion & Mainess, 2003).

On the other hand, Japanese children may tell stories in a style that is "exceptionally succinct" (compared to African American and European American children) because Japanese

CASES TO CONSIDER

Satsuki H., a Japanese kindergartener from a Japanese-speaking home, was referred for a speech-language screening by her teacher, Mrs. Brown. She said that although Satsuki was a sweet girl who appeared to be learning some English, Satsuki was always "very quiet" and told stories that were "extremely brief" during story time. She said that Satsuki did not maintain a topic initiated by an adult. For example, if the adult talked about a field trip, Satsuki nodded and smiled politely but did not add comments or questions of her own. What would you tell Mrs. Brown about how Satsuki's cultural background might be affecting her pragmatics skills in the classroom setting?

_____

_____

_____

> Phonology is the study of how sounds are put together to form words and other linguistic units.

CONNECT & EXTEND

Several excellent sources for more information about phonology include 1) Peña-Brooks, A., & Hegde, M.N. (2007) *Assessment and treatment of articulation and phonological disorders in children.* Austin, TX: Pro-Ed; 2) Bernthal, J., & Bankson, N. (2004). *Articulation and phonological disorders* (5th ed.). Boston, MA: Allyn & Bacon; and 3) Bauman-Waengler, J. (2004). *Articulatory and phonological impairments: A clinical focus* (2nd ed.). Boston, MA: Allyn & Bacon.

value discourse that is implicit and relies heavily on the empathy of the listener (Gutierrez-Clellen & Quinn, 1993). Spanish-speaking American children may deemphasize sequencing of events when they tell stories and may focus more on descriptive information related to personal relationships and family (Mahecha, 2003; McCabe, 1997). When language development in the pragmatics realm is evaluated, a child's linguistic and cultural background must always be taken into account.

Phonology

The term **phonology** has been a conceptual entity for linguists since the beginning of the twentieth century; however, it is only within the last few decades that SLPs have begun to widely use the term. Phonology is the study of how sounds are put together to form words and other linguistic units such as phrases (Bernthal & Bankson, 2004). Phonology is concerned with the relationships among speech sounds of a language. Berko Gleason (2005) further defines phonology as including all the important sounds, the rules for combining these sounds to make words, and other parameters such as intonation and stress patterns that accompany these sounds and words.

Phonology is intricately related to other aspects of language development. Baumann-Waengler (2004, p. 6) stated that

> Phonology is closely related to other constituents of the language system, such as morphology, syntax, semantics, and pragmatics. A child's phonological system, therefore, can never be regarded as functionally separate from other aspects of the child's language growth. Recent studies. . . . have documented that delayed phonological

development occurs concurrently with delayed lexical and grammatical development. Although the direct relationship between phonological and grammatical acquisition remains unclear, interdependencies certainly exist between these areas.

 SUMMARY

- Language can be analyzed according to five components: morphology, syntax, semantics, pragmatics, and phonology.
- Semantics involves word meanings and vocabulary or lexicon.
- Morphology involves the study of word structure, and syntax includes rules for word order and rules for combining words into sentences.
- Pragmatics refers to the social skills of language—how language is used, where, when, and with whom.
- Phonology is the study of how sounds are put together to form words and other linguistic units such as phrases. Phonology is concerned with the relationships among speech sounds of a language.
- Children from CLD backgrounds develop in each of these areas as monolingual English-speaking American children do, but different cultures and languages have different rules that must be taken into account when evaluating a child's developing language skills. SLPs must be especially careful to take CLD children's first languages (L1s) into account.

Add your own summary points here:

_____

_____

_____

APPROACHES TO LANGUAGE DISORDERS

Models of Language Disorders

Two major models of child language disorders are the categorical or etiological model and the descriptive-developmental model (Bernstein, 2002; Bliss, 2002; Paul, 2001). The **categorical-etiological** model represents a medical model that attempts to identify specific causes of language problems. Bernstein (2002) summarized McCormick and Schiefelbusch's (1984) classification of five etiological categories of language disorders: language and communication disorders associated with 1) motor disorders (e.g., cerebral palsy) 2) sensory deficits (e.g., visual or hearing impairment); 3) central nervous system damage; 4) severe emotional-social dysfunctions such as autism; and 5) cognitive disorders (e.g., mental retardation).

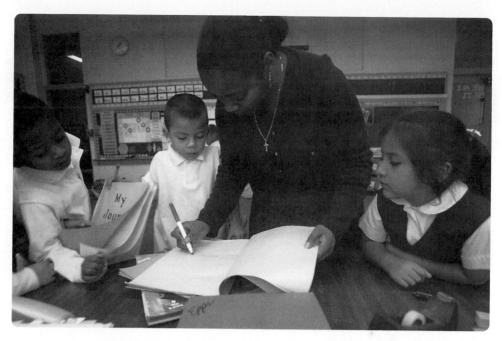

When we work with CLD children, we must account for the unique cultural and linguistic characteristics they bring to tasks.

An advantage of this model is that a diagnostic label can be very useful in helping children obtain services and educational placements through such agencies as the public schools. A disadvantage of this model is that it is often not possible to identify a single cause of a language problem; language problems can have multiple causes. In addition, Bliss (2002) points out that etiology is not the sole determinant of language behavior; language behavior is also influenced by cultural, emotional, social, and motivational factors. Lastly, a danger in categorizing children is that clinicians may take a "one size fits all" approach to treatment without individualizing to the extent necessary for each child.

> Two major models used to describe language disorders are the categorical-etiological model and the descriptive-developmental model.

The **descriptive-developmental** model does not focus on the etiology or cause of the language disorder. Rather, the child's behavioral strengths and weaknesses are described in detail. In addition, the child's language behaviors are compared with developmental norms; where is the child in the sequence of typically developing language? Does the six-year-old with SLI use the syntactic skills of a TD three-year-old? Advantages of this model are that the clinician does not have to find a cause of the language impairment; also, the detailed description in the assessment of the child's language skills leads to specific directions for intervention.

Disadvantages to the descriptive-developmental model are that describing a child's language behavior in detail can be very time consuming. In addition, children with language

CASES TO CONSIDER

I worked with Ganesha H., a sixth-grade student who appeared to the school team (speech pathologist, resource specialist, psychologist, and teacher) to have PDD (pervasive developmental disorder, a form of autism). Ganesha's mother did not live in the home, so her father came to all the meetings. He refused to accept the diagnostic label of PDD, but the resource specialist and I were able to enroll Ganesha for needed services anyway without this diagnosis. However, as Ganesha was finishing sixth grade, we encountered a dilemma: in junior high school, Ganesha would not receive comprehensive services unless she had the label of PDD. How would you handle this type of situation in a sensitive yet honest way? How could you use elements of both the categorical-etiological and descriptive-developmental approaches to help Ganesha get the services she needs in junior high school?

_____

_____

_____

impairments may not receive services if they are not classified or labeled in a way that makes sense to educators, medical personnel, and others. If a child has not been assigned an etiological label (e.g., "autistic"), she may not receive intervention. Because I work part-time as a public school itinerant SLP, I can personally vouch for the fact that labels are necessary for children to receive services. The case of Ganesha H. (above) illustrates this point.

Terminology

Sometimes a child has difficulty with his language development. Several terms have been used to describe the set of problems experienced by children who have difficulty with language. These terms include **language learning disability (LLD), specific language impairment (SLI), language disorder**, and others.

Law, Garrett, and Nye (2004, p. 924) state that

> Speech and language delay/disorder may present either as a *primary* condition, where it cannot be accounted for by any known etiology . . . or as a *secondary* condition, where it can be accounted for by another primary condition such as autism, hearing impairment, general developmental difficulties, behavioral or emotional difficulties, or neurological impairment. The term *specific language impairment* is sometimes used, but exactly how specific such a condition is remains debatable given the reported comorbidity. . . .

Specific language impairment, or SLI, is defined as language impairment that exists in the absence of other clearly identifiable problems such as hearing impairment, autism, or intellectual disability. On the surface, a child with SLI appears to be normal, except for his language acquisition, which does not match that of his peers (Reed, 2005).

Children with SLI are heterogeneous, and researchers have identified subtypes of SLI. For example, one child might have better ability to understand language (listening or **comprehension**) than to express herself through talking (**expression**); another child might appear to have age-appropriate expression, but his comprehension is poor. A third child with SLI might have equal difficulty with both comprehension and expression. Generally, children with SLI have a combination of both expressive and receptive language problems. These can be oral, written, or both. Children with SLI can have difficulty with talking, listening, reading, and writing; these language problems are described in more detail below.

General Characteristics of Children with SLI

In subsequent chapters, we shall be considering language impairments (as described above by Law et al. 2004) that are secondary to some condition such as autism, mental retardation, and others. In this chapter, we will consider a description of SLI. We previously stated that children with SLI are a heterogeneous group and that children with SLI have a variety of profiles (Dollaghan, 2004). However, there are certain general characteristics that describe children with SLI as a group.

1. *Children with SLI manifest an impairment that is specific to language.* As previously stated, the impairment in language skills is not related to sensory deficits or developmental disabilities such as mental retardation or autism. Children with SLI generally have normal hearing, although they may have had episodes of otitis media that have impacted their language development. Their nonverbal intelligence is within or even above the normal range (Rice, Tomblin, Hoffman, Richman, & Marquis, 2004). Laws and Bishop (2003, p. 1325) state that

> A diagnosis of SLI is applied to children developing otherwise normally but with language difficulties that cannot be explained by psychiatric or neurological conditions, by sensory loss, or by inadequate language environments . . . SLI is not a homogeneous condition, and a number of subtypes of the disorder have been identified. . . .

CONNECT & EXTEND

SLI is described fully by Laws, G., & Bishop, D.V.M. (2003). A comparison of language abilities in adolescents with Down syndrome and children with specific language impairment. *Journal of Speech, Language, and Hearing Research, 46(6),* 1324–1339.

2. *Children with SLI are slow to develop language.* They are often late in starting to talk. For example, the TD child generally says her first word at around twelve months of age; the child with SLI might not say her first word until she is almost two years old. TD children will usually begin to put two words together at around eighteen months of age; some children with SLI may not combine words until they are almost three years old. TD children have a great vocabulary spurt between eighteen and twenty-four months of age; SLI children usually do not show this spurt.

3. *Children with SLI generally do not outgrow it.* They usually continue to face challenges into adulthood. Researchers have conducted

> Children with SLI manifest an impairment specific to language. This impairment is not outgrown and is related to genetic abnormalities in brain structure and function.

longitudinal studies, where they have followed the same SLI children over a period of years (e.g., Aram & Nation, 1980; Tomblin, Zhang, Buckwalter, & O'Brien, 2003). The results of all these studies have indicated that children with SLI continue to have difficulties throughout their later years. For example, in a follow-up study of children identified with SLI at five years of age, it was found that 71 percent of these children exhibited clinically depressed language skills at eighteen years of age (Johnson, Beitchman, Young, Escobar, Atkinson, Wilson et al., 1999).

4. Research shows that there is a genetic component to SLI and that this is related to abnormalities in brain structure and function. A number of studies have used magnetic resonance imaging (MRI) to show that children with SLI have the same brain structure and function deficits as other people in their families. Hugdahl, Gundersen, Brekke, Thomsen, Rimol, Ersland, & Niemi (2004) studied Finnish family members with SLI in comparison to a matched group without SLI. Like American researchers, they concluded that individuals with SLI showed reduced activation in areas of the brain that are critical for phonological awareness and speech processing. Other researchers have also described a genetic component to SLI (e.g., Bishop, Price, Dale, & Plomin, 2003; Flax et al., 2004; Gilger & Wise, 2004; Tomblin & Buckwalter, 1998).

Ellis Weismer, Plante, Jones, and Tomblin (2005) conducted a study using behavioral and neuroimaging techniques to examine the claim that processing capacity limitations underlie SLI. They used functional magnetic resonance imaging (fMRI) to look at verbal working memory in adolescents with SLI and matched TD peers. fMRI results showed that during certain tasks, the adolescents with SLI had reduced brain activity (hypoactivation) in areas of the brain associated with language processing. The adolescents with SLI exhibited atypical coordination of activation across brain regions during certain tasks. Ellis Weismer et al. concluded that their findings supported the idea that persons with SLI do have limitations in processing capacity.

 SUMMARY

- Various terms describe children who do not develop language normally.
- The categorical-etiological model of language disorders attempts to identify the causes of language disorders.
- In the descriptive-developmental model, one does not look for a cause. Rather, one describes the child's language behaviors in detail and compares these language behaviors to developmental norms.
- Specific language impairment (SLI) is a common term used to describe children who have difficulty with language.
- Children with SLI show certain common characteristics such as an impairment that is specific to language (no identifiable cause or associated problem such as autism),

slowness in developing language, not outgrowing the language problem, and possibly having abnormalities in brain structure and function that are genetically related.

Add your own summary points here:

_____

_____

_____

LINGUISTIC CHARACTERISTICS OF CHILDREN WITH SLI

Traditionally, clinicians and researchers have described the **linguistic** or **language** problems of children with SLI—for example, problems with morphology, syntax, and pragmatics. Current research suggests that children with SLI also have **processing** problems (Conti-Ramsden, 2003; Hoffman & Gillam, 2004; Windsor & Kohnert, 2004). Deevy and Leonard (2004, p. 802) state that "Current theories of . . . SLI in children fall into two general classes: those that attribute SLI to processing limitations and those that attribute the disorder to deficits in grammatical knowledge." The American Speech-Language-Hearing Association (ASHA) defined SLI or language disorders as follows (1980, pp. 317–318):

> A language disorder is the abnormal acquisition, comprehension, or expression of spoken or written language. The disorder may involve all, one, or some of the phonologic, morphologic, semantic, syntactic, or pragmatic components of the linguistic system. Individuals with language disorders frequently have problems in sentence processing or in abstracting information meaningfully for storage and retrieval from short and long term memory.

Thus, ASHA supports the notion that children with SLI have difficulty in two primary areas as stated above: 1) linguistic skills and 2) processing skills. In this section, the linguistic skills of children with SLI are described.

Researchers and clinicians have delineated a set of linguistic characteristics that are common in children with SLI. The extent and pattern of these characteristics vary from individual to individual; however, most children with SLI have difficulties in each language area. The information below is adapted from the following sources: Bernstein, 2002; Bernstein Ratner, 2005; Gilger & Wise, 2004; Gray, 2003; Hegde, 2001a; Nation, Clarke, Marshall, & Durand, 2004; Nelson, 1998; Owens, 2004; Paul, 2001; Roseberry-McKibbin & Hegde, 2006.

Children with SLI generally have difficulties in two major areas: linguistic skills and processing skills.

Semantics

Children with SLI demonstrate a number of semantic difficulties (Gray, 2004; Nash & Donaldson, 2005). They have difficulty learning new words and storing and organizing words they already know. Children with SLI usually have small, reduced vocabularies as compared to TD peers. They also have trouble with abstract language, and will generally use concrete rather than abstract words to express themselves. An SLI child would have a lot more difficulty than a TD child with learning to appropriately use a saying like "There is a fork in the road." For the SLI child, this fork is literal; she pictures a piece of silverware lying in a road. The TD child understands that this saying means that two different directions can be taken.

Studies have shown that SLI children particularly have trouble learning new action words, or verbs (Alt, Plante, & Creusere, 2004; Brackenbury & Pye, 2005; Eyer, Leonard, Bedore, McGregor, Anderson, & Viescas, 2002). This presents difficulty for them because verbs play such central roles in even the most basic of sentences. As SLI children grow older, they also experience difficulty with words with multiple meanings.

> Children with SLI have difficulties with semantic skills in that they tend to have smaller, more concrete vocabularies than TD children.

For example, if one asked a TD child to "tell me all the things the word *rock* could mean," the TD child would say something like "There is a kind of rock that is like a stone, or you can rock a baby, or there is a kind of music called rock." The SLI child might say, "I can think of a rock that you find on the ground, like a stone"; but she would not be able to think of any other meanings of the word *rock*.

Fast mapping, or the ability to learn a word based on one or two exposures to it, is also a challenge for SLI children. Gray (2003) found that some children with SLI, in order to learn new words, may require twice the practice opportunities and exposures that their TD peers do. Again, SLI children typically take longer to learn new words than TD children do, and they need to be exposed to the words more often to truly learn them.

Children with SLI commonly have **word finding** or **word retrieval** problems. They know the word; they just can't think of it when they need it. You can probably remember times when a word was on the tip of your tongue; you just couldn't remember it in the particular situation. This occurs very commonly for SLI children.

POINTS TO PONDER   Describe two semantic, syntactic, and morphological characteristics of children with SLI.

_____

_____

_____

Syntax

It is a widely accepted fact the SLI children use shorter, simpler sentences than those used by their peers. SLI children's speech is often **telegraphic**; the sentence has the content words and omits the function words—the smaller grammatical elements are left out. For example, a TD six-year-old might say, "Today we went on a field trip to Apple Hill and ate lunch with our friends." An SLI six-year-old might say, "We goed on field trip to Apple Hill, ate lunch." SLI children use compound and complex sentences as well as transformations less frequently than TD peers. Many SLI children use mostly simple, declarative sentences.

SLI children have difficulty understanding as well as using longer and more complex sentences. For example, a TD peer would understand a kindergarten teacher's directive to "Put your papers into your folders and make sure your name is at the top of your paper before you wash your hands for lunch." An SLI child might understand that she needs to wash her hands for lunch, but forget the rest of the sentence.

> Children with SLI often use telegraphic speech, where function words are omitted.

Parents and teachers may become frustrated with SLI children because these parents and teachers do not understand that they need to simplify their language in order for SLI children to understand what they hear. In the above example, the teacher could effectively reach the SLI child by saying, "Make sure your name is at the top of your paper—name on top of the paper. [pause] Put your papers into your folders. [pause] Does everyone have their papers in their folders? Good. Please wash your hands for lunch." SLPs need to help teachers and parents understand how to simplify their language so that SLI children comprehend what they hear. Chapter 6 has specific suggestions for how to do this.

Morphology

Most SLI children have considerable difficulty with the morphological aspects of language. Difficulty with morphology is a hallmark of SLI (Eadie, Fey, Douglas, & Parsons, 2002). As Deevy and Leonard (2004) point out, all current theories of SLI attempt to account for the finding of "extraordinary difficulty" in the production of grammatical morphology (p. 802). Children with SLI will frequently omit or make errors on bound morphemes such as

- regular and irregular past tense inflections (e.g., *Yesterday he walk to the store; We drinked our lemonade at recess*)
- possessive morphemes (e.g., *That's the girl bicycle*)
- articles *a, an, the* (e.g., *Boy fell into pond*)
- third person singular forms (e.g., *She run into the classroom. He pet the kitty*)
- contractible copula forms (e.g., *Daddy not watching TV*)

There are many more bound morphemes that SLI children omit; these are just a few examples. As children with SLI grow older, their morphological problems usually become less obvious, but their difficulties with advanced sentence structures and narratives become more apparent.

When working with CLD children with potential SLI, SLPs need to consider a number of variables. For example, SLPs need to be careful not to misdiagnose CLD children who omit bound morphemes in their speech. Many children from Asian backgrounds will omit articles, plurals, and other bound morphemes because their languages do not contain these morphemes (Fletcher, Leonard, Stokes, & Wong, 2005). An Asian child who said "I have three book in car" would very probably have a language difference, not SLI, because this type of utterance is predictable for many children from Asian language backgrounds (Roseberry-McKibbin, 2008).

Children who speak African American English also demonstrate morphological patterns that differ from those of Mainstream American English (Thompson, Craig, & Washington, 2004). Coles-White (2004, p. 219) cautioned that "using morphology to identify SLI in child African American English speakers presents a problem . . ." and recommended that other more valid diagnostic measures be used instead. Chapter 4 has more specific information about these kinds of normal patterns manifested by CLD students who are learning English as a second language and by students who speak African American English.

> SLPs must be cautious in describing morphological patterns in children with SLI; these patterns differ from those of monolingual English-speaking children.

There is very little research regarding the acquisition of English morphemes by bilingual children. However, Jia (2003) conducted a study of English plural morpheme acquisition by Mandarin Chinese–speaking children. Ten native Mandarin-speaking TD children (ages five to sixteen years) who had immigrated to the United States were followed for five years. Jia found that in contrast to TD first-language learners who master the plural morpheme by approximately three years of age, only seven out of ten of her subjects did so after five years of English exposure. The younger subjects learned the English plural morpheme faster than the older subjects.

Jia suggested that if a young child second-language (L2) learner continues to make morphosyntactic errors in L2 after a long time of immersion in a rich L2 environment, that child might have SLI. However, older second language learners who still are dominant in their first language (such as Mandarin) may make morphosyntactic errors in L2 even for a long time after they have been exposed to L2; this should not be taken as a sign of SLI in these older learners. More research is needed to describe the English morphological acquisition patterns of CLD children who are learning English as a second language.

CONNECT & EXTEND

The morphological skills of CLD children from Romance and Germanic language backgrounds are described in Paradis, J., Crago, M., Genesee, F., & Rice, M. (2003). French-English bilingual children with SLI: How do they compare with their monolingual peers? *Journal of Speech, Language, and Hearing Research, 46(1),* 113–127.

Paradis, Crago, Genesee, and Rice (2003) studied morphological skills in bilingual and monolingual children with SLI. They found that both their monolingual and bilingual (French-English–speaking) SLI children had difficulty with the morphological aspects of language. They stated that cross-linguistic research on grammatical deficits in SLI in Romance and Germanic languages has shown that SLI children from various language backgrounds have difficulty with grammatical morphemes in their first languages. Bedore and Leonard (2001), in their study of SLI Spanish-speaking preschoolers, concluded that these children had substantial difficulties with grammatical morphemes in Spanish. Restrepo and Kruth (2000) also discussed the fact that Spanish-speaking children with SLI have more morphosyntactic errors than TD Spanish-speaking children have.

Thus, in sum, research has shown (for some languages) that if CLD children have genuine SLI, they will have morphological problems, even in their first language. However, Paradis (2005, pp. 183–185) cautioned that

> TD ESL (English as a second language) children's error patterns with grammatical morphology parallel what has been reported for monolingual English-speaking children with SLI at similar ages. . . . Early ESL children can be expected to make errors with grammatical morphology. . . . Difficulties in producing grammatical morphology will be evident regardless of L1 (language 1) background. . . . It becomes difficult to determine whether an early ESL child's errorful language is due to the process of L2 learning or to impaired language learning. Therefore, it is advisable to be cautious when considering the presence of errors with grammatical morphology as a sign of SLI in early ESL children.

Pragmatics

As previously stated, pragmatics refers to language use or the social rules of language. Fey (1986) described the key pragmatic characteristics of conversational assertiveness and responsiveness; SLI children frequently have a combination of difficulties with these areas. **Assertiveness** refers to the ability to initiate conversation or take a conversation turn when none has been solicited by the partner. For example, a child with appropriate assertiveness might walk up to a child at the community swimming pool and say, "Hey, wanna play with my water Frisbee?" **Responsiveness** refers to how responsive the child is to the conversational partner. In the above example, an appropriately responsive child would probably say something like "Sure, let's play in the kid pool." SLI children may be **passive**—both unresponsive and unassertive—in communicative interactions.

Other SLI children may have a different pattern of being unassertive yet responsive, or assertive yet unresponsive. In the community pool situation, the passive child would not

POINTS TO PONDER You are a new SLP in a public elementary school where the vast majority of the children have been White, monolingual speakers of Mainstream American English. In the last one to two years, there has been an influx of CLD children, especially African American and Asian children. You keep getting referrals, from classroom teachers, for Asian and African American children with "grammar problems." Upon screening these children, you find that most of them are merely demonstrating grammatical differences based on their home language/dialect, not signs of SLI. Describe what you will tell the teachers in a staff meeting to help them understand why their referrals are inappropriate.

_____

_____

_____

initiate conversation or respond to the child who asked him to play with the water Frisbee. An unassertive yet responsive child would not go up to someone else and offer to play with the water Frisbee; yet, if someone else asked him to play, he would probably say yes. The assertive yet unresponsive child might go up to another child and ask if the other child would like to play with the water Frisbee; if the other child said no or showed disinterest, the assertive yet unresponsive child would ignore these cues and try to start playing anyway.

> SLI children may have difficulty with the assertiveness and responsiveness parameters of pragmatics.

Assertiveness and responsiveness are highly influenced by culture. Sometimes teachers or even peers of TD children from CLD backgrounds will view these children as passive, when the children are acting in a way that they have been taught is polite and courteous. Brice and Montgomery (1996) evaluated the pragmatics skills of SLI and TD Spanish-speaking adolescents. They found that even the TD adolescents had difficulty regulating others through language (e.g., making classroom requests). Brice and Montgomery suggested that this may be related to a cultural trait of showing deference to authority figures.

My son just finished kindergarten, and his classroom teacher had expressed concern about several Asian children in the classroom who were "too quiet." Many Asian children are taught that in class, one must be very respectful and let the teacher be the authority figure; this often means that these children do not ask questions or volunteer to answer questions. Some teachers may view this as a sign of a pragmatics problem. The Asian children in my son's class, however, were high academic achievers who were merely showing classroom interaction patterns consistent with their cultural backgrounds.

There may be other issues impacting teachers' impressions of children from a cultural standpoint. Hwa-Froelich and Westby (2003), in their study of Southeast Asian families and Headstart staff, found that the teachers did not believe that any of the Southeast Asian children had learning problems. When asked how they knew that a child had a learning problem, the teachers said that learning problems were reflected by poor behavior. Because of the respectful and obedient way in which the Southeast Asian children conducted themselves, the teachers did not think they had learning problems. It is important for SLPs to help teachers and other school personnel to understand that CLD children come from cultures whose pragmatics rules differ from mainstream European American rules; these rules must be taken into account when attempting to decide if a student has SLI or is a TD child who is manifesting pragmatics skills consistent with those of his cultural and linguistic community.

In addition to having difficulty with the assertiveness and responsiveness aspects of conversations, SLI children may also have difficulty with **discourse skills** in general—skills such as turn-taking and maintaining the topic of discussion SLI children often interrupt, and they may use non sequiturs (utterances unrelated to the topic) in conversations. An example follows.

TD child: I saw *Shrek 2*. It was awesome, and I liked Puss 'n' Boots—

SLI child **(interrupting):**   My dad built me a new play structure; he finished it this weekend.

TD child: Shrek is cool. And what did you think of Princess Fiona? She really—

SLI child **(interrupting again):**   The monkey bars are my favorite.

CONNECT & EXTEND

Assessment and intervention for children with discourse impairments is described in detail in Bliss, L.S. (2002). *Discourse impairments: Assessment and intervention applications.* Boston, MA: Allyn & Bacon.

Pragmatics skills are heavily influenced by a student's cultural background.

Clearly, the SLI child who has these types of discourse problems is bound to have social problems, especially in interacting with peers.

Another type of social problem SLI children have is inferring or understanding other peoples' verbal and especially nonverbal cues. They may not understand, for example, that a person who crosses his arms and frowns is probably angry. SLI children's lack of ability to "read" others' cues can lead to social problems. With CLD children who are having difficulty in this area, it is important to ask if the difficulty is related to culture, SLI, or both. For example, a Mexican student who immigrated to the United States as a teenager might be very physically "touchy" with American peers and stand so close to them that they want to move away from him. He might not appear to notice their discomfort. Does this student have an SLI, or is his behavior typical of those from his cultural background?

Unfortunately, research has shown that SLI children with pragmatic and other language problems may have behavioral and social difficulties and even become targets of bullying. SLI children are less likely to initiate conversation, less liked by other children, and are more likely to play alone than their TD peers (Brinton & Fujiki, 2004). Teachers tend to rate these children as reticent, withdrawn, and less socially skilled than TD peers (Conti-Ramsden & Botting, 2004).

It is very important for SLPs to help these children learn the appropriate social rules of language so that they will fit in with their peers and succeed in school (Fujiki, Brinton,

CASES TO CONSIDER

I received a referral of an eighth-grader, Samuel, whose family had recently immigrated to the Sacramento area from Uzbekistan. Eighth grade would be over in one week, and the school wanted an assessment of Samuel's language skills so that if he had SLI, they could send him to ninth grade with an individualized special-education plan. I learned that Samuel said his first word in Uzbeki at two years of age; his mother said that in Uzbeki, "Samuel was slower to talk than all of his siblings." Samuel had struggled in school in Uzbekistan, and the English as a Second Language classroom teacher told me that Samuel was "always in trouble with the other kids; even the other Russians yell at him." What other information would be helpful to know? With just this little bit of information, do you think Samuel had a language difference or SLI? Why?

_____

_____

_____

Isaacson, & Summers, 2001). In addition, SLPs should be aware that children with SLI may have low self-esteem associated with the social and academic problems they experience at school. Research suggests that SLPs might help these children have higher self-esteem by encouraging them to persevere in difficult situations and by being generally aware of the potential self-esteem problems in children with SLI as a whole (Jerome, Fujiki, Brinton, & James, 2002). More is said about this in subsequent chapters.

Children with SLI also have difficulty with narratives, or storytelling (Greenhalgh & Strong, 2001; Swanson, Fey, Mills, & Hood, 2005). Frequently their stories lack appropriate details and the stories may not be sequenced appropriately. For example, consider the following conversation between an SLP and an SLI student, Marcos.

SLP: Hey, did you see *Shrek 2* this weekend?

Marcos: Yeah.

SLP: I have heard that it's a great movie—but I haven't had time to go. Tell me as much as you can about it.

Marcos: Well . . . there was a donkey. And Shrek and Fiona got back together in the end.

SLP: I know they got married in *Shrek 1*. Did they go away from each other in *Shrek 2*?

Marcos: Well, there was this cat named Puss 'n' Boots at the beginning. And the king turned back into a frog.

SLP: But what happened to Shrek and Princess Fiona?

Marcos: The fairy godmother didn't like Shrek. But at first, she wasn't there. Later the prince came. The queen, Fiona's mother, didn't like him. Puss 'n' Boots was supposed to kill Shrek. That's all.

For readers who have not seen *Shrek 2*, Marcos is telling the details out of sequence. He is also not giving enough detail about the movie. Frequently, children with SLI leave their listeners baffled.

When clinicians assess CLD children's narratives, they must consider the factor of which language the assessment is conducted in as well as the types of narrative tasks used. Fiestas and Peña (2004) evaluated the narrative skills of twelve TD Spanish-speaking children who were fluent in both English and Spanish. They found that for one task, the children produced narratives of equal complexity; for another task, children used more attempts and initiating events in Spanish while producing more consequences in English. Fiestas and Peña concluded that when clinicians assess the narrative skills of bilingual children, they must take into account the language and tasks used in this assessment.

Written Language

Recent research has suggested that children with SLI often have difficulty with reading and writing. It is estimated that 50 to 75 percent of children with SLI have concurrent reading disabilities (Ervin, 2001), and that these disabilities often persist over time (Catts, Fey, Tomblin, & Zhang, 2002). For example, in a follow-up study of preschoolers with SLI, Snowling, Bishop, and Stothard (2000) found that almost half of these children exhibited reading difficulties at 15 years of age. Many of these children have poor **phonological awareness**, which is the ability to think about and manipulate the sound structure of language (Goldsworthy, 2003; Reed, 2005). Phonological awareness is an important predictor of success in learning to read (Gillon, 2000; Segers & Verhoeven, 2004). Phonological awareness is described and discussed in more detail in Chapters 7 and 8.

Children with SLI often have written as well as oral language problems.

Longitudinal research has shown that children who have difficulty developing oral language in their preschool years are at increased risk for later difficulties in reading, writing, and academics in general (Flax, Realpe-Bonilla, Hirsch, Brustowicz, Bartlett, & Tallal, 2003; Goldsworthy, 2003; Windsor & Kohnert, 2004). A friend of mine who works with reading-impaired children frequently says that small children with SLI are later recategorized as "dyslexic." More is said about written language problems in Chapter 8.

SUMMARY

- Children with SLI have difficulties with semantics. This includes problems with vocabulary, abstract words, words with multiple meanings, fast mapping, and word retrieval.
- Syntax is also an area of challenge for children with SLI. They may have telegraphic speech. They may also have difficulty using and comprehending age-appropriate complex and compound sentences.
- Difficulty with morphology is a hallmark of SLI. Many children with SLI omit bound morphemes when they speak.
- Children with SLI often have difficulties with pragmatics. They may have problems with assertiveness, responsiveness, discourse skills, and narrative skills.
- SLPs must take CLD children's first language as well as culture into account when assessing semantics, syntax, morphology, and pragmatics. These parameters are often influenced by a child's first language and cultural background.
- Many children with SLI have difficulties with both oral and written language.

Add your own summary points here:

_____

_____

_____

PROCESSING CHARACTERISTICS OF CHILDREN WITH SLI

Basic Principles

As previously stated, researchers have shown that SLI children have difficulties in two primary, broad areas: linguistic skills and processing skills (e.g., Fazio, 1996; Montgomery, 2002; Roy & Chiat, 2004). Reed (2005, p. 35) states that "information processing refers to the ways in which we deal with incoming stimuli and what we do in our heads to figure them out." Children with SLI have difficulty with two specific areas of processing. One is speed of processing; children with SLI are slower than TD children at processing incoming information (Miller, Kail, Leonard, & Tomblin, 2001). Second, children with SLI have a reduced processing capacity (Montgomery, 2002). Conti-Ramsden (2003, p. 1029) stated that

> Interestingly, the search for clinical markers for SLI has traditionally been divided, conceptually and theoretically, into two main approaches: research based on processing considerations and research based on linguistic frameworks. In the processing approach, the role of memory in language performance, particularly performance on short term memory tasks such as nonword repetition, has been found to be a good indicator of SLI . . .

Marton and Schwartz (2003) argued that that children with SLI have difficulty performing tasks involving verbal working memory (processing), and that problems with verbal working memory are correlated with not only vocabulary acquisition but also language comprehension, syntactic processing, and reading comprehension. Many studies have firmly established that children with SLI have difficulty with verbal working memory, especially as it relates to nonwords (e.g., Hoffman & Gillam, 2004; Laws & Bishop, 2003; Roy & Chiat, 2004).

Specifically, children with SLI, when compared to TD children, have problems repeating back nonwords that they hear. For example, one might say to an SLI child, "This puppet is going to say three silly words. I want you to say them back just like he does: *humplah, gothu, paedish.* Now you say those." Roy and Chiat (2004) found that the use of nonword repetition tasks was effective for children as young as two years of age in predicting the presence of SLI. Dollaghan and Campbell (1998) showed that these kinds of tasks have good potential to be used successfully with bilingual children to predict SLI. However, Hwa-Froelich and Matsuo (2005) cautioned that when using invented stimuli, practitioners need to consider the level of similarity between the child's first language and English. If the stimuli are closer to English than to the child's first language—especially if the stimuli use sounds that do not exist in the child's first language—the child may have difficulty not because of an SLI but because of his lack of familiarity with English. Hwa-Froelich and Matsuo suggested that invented stimuli should use sounds that exist in the child's first language.

CONNECT & EXTEND

The use of nonword repetition tasks to assess the presence of SLI in CLD children is described fully in a study by Dolloghan, C., & Campbell, T. (1998). Nonword repetition and child language impairment. *Journal of Speech, Language, and Hearing Research, 41,* 1136–1146.

Children with SLI have difficulty recalling nonwords, digits, lists of real words, and sentences as well as facts from connected discourse (Nation et al., 2004). They have difficulty retaining the sequential order of information (Gillam, Cowan, & Day, 1995; Montgomery, 1996, 2002). For example, you might say to a child with SLI, "Tell me these words back: *horse, pencil, sky, chair.*" The child with SLI might say, "*Horse, sky, chair, pencil.*" Or you might say, "Tell these numbers back exactly the same way I say them to you: *6-9-2-4-8.*" The child with SLI might say "*6-9-4-8-2.*"

Clearly, children with SLI not only have difficulties with semantics, syntax, pragmatics, and morphology; they also have difficulty processing information that they hear. This presents a major challenge for children who are SLI and also speak English as a second language, for they have two major hurdles: an underlying SLI and a new language that they must learn with an underlying system that is inadequate for even learning one (Roseberry-McKibbin, 2003).

> The use of processing tasks such as nonword repetition is potentially a good indicator of SLI in both monolingual and bilingual children.

Conti-Ramsden (2003), in her study, examined four potential indicators of SLI in children: two linguistic indicators (ability to appropriately use past tense and plural forms) and two processing indicators (nonword repetition and digit repetition). She found that the SLI children in her study performed worse on all four indicators than a TD control group and concluded that children with SLI really do have difficulty in two broad domains: 1) language and 2) processing of information. She concluded that research is greatly needed to examine the validity of processing-dependent tasks for indicators of SLI in bilingual children. Other researchers (e.g., Dollaghan & Campbell, 1998; Kohnert, 2004; Laing & Kamhi, 2003; Meschyan & Hernandez, 2004) have stated that bilingual children with SLI indeed have difficulty with processing information, even in their first language, and that this difficulty is a reliable indicator of the presence of SLI in these children.

SUMMARY

- Children with SLI have difficulty in two broad areas: linguistic skills and processing skills.
- Children with SLI have difficulty with processing tasks such as repetition of nonwords, real words, digits, and sentences.
- Research indicates that the use of processing tasks is a valid and reliable indicator of SLI in CLD children.

Add your summary points here:

_____

_____

_____

CHAPTER HIGHLIGHTS

- The cultural and linguistic diversity in the United States is increasing, and speech-language pathologists (SLPs) are serving more children from culturally and linguistically diverse (CLD) backgrounds.

- When providing services for these children, it is important to come from a framework of evidence-based practice, which involves asking focused questions about treatment for specific clinical problems and seeking answers in high-quality evidence from the published literature.

- Linguists have traditionally described several components of language: morphology (the study of word structure), syntax (rules specifying how words may be combined to form meaningful sentences), semantics (the study of meaning), pragmatics (the study of rules that govern language use in various social situations), and phonology (the study of how sounds are put together to form words and other linguistic units such as phrases).

- Some researchers place language into three categories: 1) content (semantics), 2) form (morphology, syntax, and phonology), and 3) use (pragmatics).

- Important aspects of semantic development include vertical and horizontal expansion of vocabulary words, word and world knowledge, knowledge of synonyms and antonyms, and ability to understand and use figurative language. In addition, children must develop adequate comprehension and use of deictic words, and semantic categories, and must become proficient in fast mapping and categorization skills.

- Morphology, the study of word structure, describes bound and free morphemes and their variations, allomorphs.

- Syntax means to join or put together. Syntax involves word order and the arrangement of words to form meaningful sentences.

- Phonology is concerned with the relationships among speech sounds of a language. Children with problems in other areas of language (e.g., morphology, syntax) often have concomitant problems in phonology.

- The kernel sentence in English is subject + verb + object. Children eventually develop skill in using and understanding compound and complex sentences.

- Pragmatics involves the study of rules that govern the use of language in social contexts. Children need to develop a variety of pragmatics skills including the appropriate use of direct and indirect speech acts and turn-taking. Development of discourse and narrative skills is important as well.

- The development of skills in semantics, morphology, syntax, and pragmatics is heavily dependent on children's cultural and linguistic backgrounds.

- In discussing language disorders, researchers use two broad models: 1) the categorical-etiological model and 2) and the descriptive-developmental model.

- Some children who have difficulty with language development may be described as having specific language impairment, or SLI. These children have manifested an impairment that is specific to language, not associated with any other condition such as autism, and lifelong.

- Children with SLI have difficulties with all linguistic areas: semantics, morphology, syntax, pragmatics, and frequently phonology. Research shows that CLD children with SLI have difficulty with these linguistic areas in their first languages also. Children with SLI are a heterogeneous group, and each child's profile is different.

- Children with SLI often have difficulty with written language also. It is estimated that 50 to 75 percent of children with SLI have trouble with reading and writing. There may be a genetic basis for these difficulties.

- In addition to having difficulties in oral and written linguistic areas, children with SLI have deficient processing skills. For example, they have difficulty with repeating nonwords, real words, digits, and sentences.

- Research has shown that processing tasks such as nonword repetition are potentially a good indicator of SLI in both monolingual and bilingual children.

Add your own chapter highlights here:

_____

_____

_____

_____

STUDY AND REVIEW QUESTIONS

ESSAY

1. Describe the terms *semantics, morphology, syntax, pragmatics*, and *phonology*. What are important components of each one in a child's language development?

2. Discuss how a child's linguistic and cultural background could impact her morphological, semantic, syntactic, and semantic characteristics.

3. What do the terms *categorical-etiological model* and *descriptive-developmental model* mean in reference to children's language disorders?

4. Describe two general characteristics and two linguistic characteristics of children with SLI.

5. What have research findings shown about the processing skills of children with SLI?

FILL-IN-THE-BLANK

6. A(n) _____ is the smallest meaningful unit of a language; a(n) _____ is a variation that does not alter the original meaning of the morpheme.

7. A _____ sentence has two or more independent clauses joined by a comma and a conjunction or joined by a semicolon; a _____ sentence contains one independent clause and one or more dependent/subordinate clauses.

8. In English, the basic syntactic structure is the subject + verb + object sequence. Usually called the _____, this can also be called the _____ structure or the _____ structure.

9. The form of discourse where the speaker tells a story, telling about a logical sequence of events, is called a(n) _____.

10. Children with SLI often use _____ speech, where they talk in sentences that contain content words and omit function words.

MULTIPLE CHOICE

11. A clinician assesses a seven-year-old girl who has difficulties in the area of *discourse*. Treatment goals would most likely involve which of the following?

    a. Increasing mean length of utterance and sentence complexity
    b. Increasing accurate use of morphological structures
    c. Expanding vocabulary to be more commensurate with age level
    d. Increasing ability to converse appropriately with peers over a range of topics
    e. Increasing ability to comprehend and use metaphors and idioms

12. Pragmatics skills involve

    a. Understanding words with multiple meanings (e.g., *rock*)
    b. Use of narratives, a form of discourse where a speaker tells a story
    c. The ability to maintain coherence of sequential statements
    d. b, c
    e. a, b, c

13. A mother brings her four-year-old son Phong to you and states that his preschool teacher is concerned. Phong's family speaks Vietnamese at home, and Phong was not exposed to English until he was four years old in the preschool setting, where only English is spoken. The teacher says Phong is very quiet and does not volunteer in class. When he does speak, he "drops the endings off words; for example, he says 'play' instead of 'played.' " You find out that in Vietnamese, Phong speaks fluently; he has many friends in the Vietnamese neighborhood, and his mother says that he understands everything she says to him in Vietnamese. She states that in Vietnamese, Phong expresses himself very well. The most likely scenario in this case is that Phong

    a. Has an SLI
    b. Has a language disorder related to his use of Vietnamese in the home
    c. Is a TD child who is manifesting culturally and linguistically appropriate characteristics in the preschool setting
    d. Has processing problems that underlie both Vietnamese and English
    e. Is a child who is at risk for failure and needs to be carefully monitored

14. The father of a seven-year-old monolingual English-speaking girl brings his daughter to you for an evaluation. He states that in the state they lived in before they moved, his daughter was diagnosed with SLI. Which of the following characteristics might you see in her language?

    a. Difficulties understanding abstract meanings of words
    b. Trouble with irregular plural and past tense forms

    c. Difficulties in telling stories in sequence
    d. a, b
    e. a, b, c

15. You have been asked to assess the language of a fifteen-year-old Romanian student who immigrated to the United States with his family six months ago. He is in an English classroom for newly arrived immigrant students. The teacher says that he does not get along well with peers; however, he "catches on quickly" in class. His parents say that in Romanian, he spoke "early" and was very successful academically in Romanian schools. They share that they moved to the United States because they had undergone religious persecution in Romania, and that their children had experienced a great deal of stress. You tentatively conclude that

    a. The student is a normal language learner who may have emotional difficulties that are causing conflict with his peers.
    b. The student has a language disorder due to emotional problems.
    c. The student has an SLI that is causing him problems in his classroom.
    d. The student is bright and does not need any extra services; he just needs more time to learn English.
    e. The student needs to be placed in a classroom for students with severe emotional disturbances.

See Answers to Study and Review Questions, page 465.

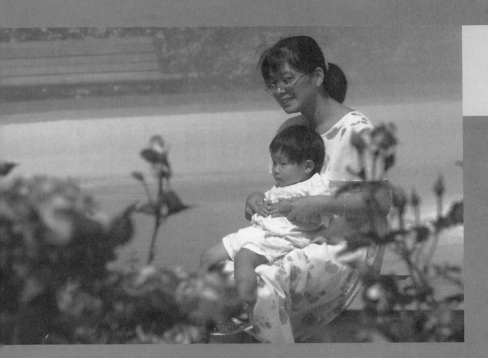

Language Development in Children: A Review

CASE STUDY

The preschool teachers were puzzled. QinQin L., a Chinese three-year-old, wasn't talking at all at the preschool. She smiled a great deal, seemed to understand basic commands in English, and was excellent with puzzles and art work. However, even after six months of an all-English preschool with warm, caring teachers, QinQin did not say even "hello" or "good-bye" in English. Despite repeated attempts by her teachers, QinQin never interacted verbally or raised her hand to speak in class. She seemed happy enough, but the teachers became concerned because of her complete lack of verbalization. They also noted that QinQin never looked them in the eye. When they spoke to her, she would always look down at the floor.

The teachers had noticed that when QinQin's mother came to pick her up, her two-year-old brother was always along—and Mrs. L., though affectionate with him, didn't speak much with him. Mrs. L. shared that they spoke only Cantonese at home and that QinQin had actually been born in Hong Kong. The family had come to the United States when QinQin was six months old. Mrs. L. worked part time for a local bank, and Mr. L. was a pharmacist for a local health maintenance organization. The teachers knew that QinQin's parents were educated and intelligent, but a home visit revealed that Mr. and Mrs. L. conversed primarily with each other and mostly gave commands to the children. Mr. and Mrs. L. did not appear to hold frequent conversations with their children and rarely asked them questions or labeled items in the environment for them. There were some children's books in the home, but Mr. and Mrs. L. said that they rarely looked at these books with QinQin or her little brother. Mr. and Mrs. L. felt that the children would engage with the books on their own when they were ready.

The teachers at the preschool were talking about a speech-language evaluation for QinQin because of her extremely sparse verbal output at school and her lack of eye contact with the teachers. They decided to first enlist the services of a local district Cantonese interpreter, Mr. Fung, who agreed to observe QinQin at school and speak with her parents. Mr. Fung observed QinQin over the period of one week at different times in the preschool day and played with her in the art corner of the classroom. He also interviewed QinQin's parents, who were very happy to speak with someone from their own cultural background.

Mr. Fung told the teachers that in her parents' opinion, QinQin was developing normally in her Cantonese language skills. Mr. and Mrs. L. said that she was able to adequately express her needs at home and that she spoke in sentences in Cantonese. Mr. and Mrs. L. were especially proud that QinQin was a "respectful, obedient child." Mr. Fung shared with the preschool teachers that in some Chinese homes, children are well loved and cared for but not necessarily encouraged to verbalize a great deal. He discussed the role of filial piety and respect in the Chinese culture, and said that in his interactions with QinQin, her relative silence and lack of verbalization were appropriate.

In Cantonese culture, Mr. Fung said, children are especially taught how to be aware of nonverbal indicators such as a slight nod or frown from their parents. Children are also taught that it is disrespectful to look an adult in the eye when he or she is talking to you. In Mr. Fung's opinion, QinQin was very aware of nonverbal cues from others, especially her teachers. In fact, he felt that "QinQin reads her teachers' body language and facial expressions better than many of her English-speaking peers." He stated that from his experience in working with other Chinese preschoolers in the district, QinQin's language skills were "just fine." In his opinion, QinQin's behavior was completely appropriate in light of her cultural and linguistic background.

INTRODUCTION

Language development begins at birth. As an infant interacts with caretakers, the exchange of communication begins. The nature of this communication is different from country to country, from culture to culture. From the hills of Cambodia to the deserts of Africa to the high-rises of New York, children and caretakers interact in unique ways that are culturally appropriate to them. Language development must always be viewed within its cultural context; to expect children all over the world to fit into US-designated expectations is to completely miss the marvelous variety that marks child language development across our globe.

> Language is a system of symbols used to represent concepts that are formed through exposure and experience.

When children develop **language**, they develop a form of social behavior shaped and maintained by a verbal community. Language can also be viewed as a system of symbols used to represent concepts that are formed through exposure and experience (Bloom & Lahey, 1978). Children from diverse cultural and linguistic backgrounds have exposure to diverse experiences, and it is this exposure that creates the concepts to which the children attach symbols, or words, as they develop language skills. This chapter reviews theories of language acquisition and normal language development milestones. There is little discussion of developmental milestones of phonology, because this topic is quite complex and deserves a more thorough coverage than is possible in this chapter. The reader is referred to other sources such as Berko Gleason (2005), Peña-Brooks and Hegde (2007), and Bernthal and Bankson (2004) for a fuller coverage of phonological development in children.

THEORIES OF LANGUAGE ACQUISITION

Practice, or "Monday morning" assessment and treatment, is built upon theory. The way that clinicians assess and treat will depend greatly on their theoretical viewpoint. Some clinicians are eclectic in their approach, blending aspects of several different theories to achieve what they view as balanced language assessment and treatment. Other clinicians depend primarily upon one theory.

In this section, five major theories of language acquisition are described: behaviorist, nativist, cognitive, social interactionist, and information processing. These theories differ in describing how language is acquired and in their implications for 1) areas that clinicians should target in assessment and intervention and 2) what procedures should be used to facilitate language teaching.

The Behaviorist Theory

The behaviorist theory, based on the work of behavioral psychologist B.F. Skinner, does not explain the learning of *language*, because language often is described by linguists and others as a mental system. Skinner (1957) did not describe language as a mental or cognitive system, because he considered that such a view would preclude an experimental study of language. Skinner's system of behavioral analysis explained the acquisition of **verbal behavior**, a form of social behavior maintained by the actions of a verbal community. Verbal behavior is typically produced under social stimulation. An audience is necessary; the audience, or person(s) interacting with the speaker, sets the stage for verbal behavior. Thus, verbal behavior is a form of social behavior shaped and maintained by the members of a verbal community.

> B.F. Skinner stated that children acquire verbal behavior, which is acquired through stimulation, response, and reinforcement.

Verbal behaviors are learned under appropriate conditions of stimulation, response, and reinforcement. Children begin with no language, and they gradually begin to imitate sounds and utterances of the persons to whom they are most frequently exposed. If the child's imitation is reinforced, he will be likely to say the sound or utterance again. If he is punished or ignored, the likelihood of the verbal behavior recurring is reduced (Kuder, 2003). Behaviorists believe that practically all forms of verbal behaviors can be increased or decreased experimentally. Social reinforcement, for example, can increase babbling, word and phrase responses, and the production of grammatic features. For instance, when my son Mark was two years old, he would say, "[I] marry Casey" (a girl friend at pre-school). Adults would always laugh at this phrase coming from a two-year-old, and Mark would say it often because of the reinforcement (laughter) that greeted his utterance.

According to behaviorist scientists, learning, not innate mechanisms, plays a key role in the acquisition of verbal behaviors. They do not believe, as nativists do, that a child has innate, inborn knowledge of the universal rules of grammar. Behaviorists focus on the *observable* and *measurable* aspects of language behavior. Unlike nativists, they emphasize performance over competence (what the child actually knows) (Bohannon & Bonvillian, 2005). Owens (2005) defines *linguistic competence* as a language user's underlying knowledge about the system of rules; it cannot be directly measured. *Linguistic performance* is linguistic knowledge in actual usage; linguistic performance is observable and measurable. Again, behaviorists emphasize linguistic performance.

> Behaviorists focus on observable and measurable of aspects of behavior, and emphasize performance over competence.

From a behaviorist perspective, the events in the child's *environment* are important (Klein & Moses, 1999; McLaughlin, 2006). Children learn only the language they are exposed to; severe social deprivation results in language deprivation as well. Thus, behaviorists question the nativist assumption that the environment offers little support to the child as she acquires language. In treatment, behaviorists teach verbal behavior to children through modeling correct responses and reinforcing children's correct productions.

Behaviorists break verbal behavior down into cause-effect (functional) units. These **functional units** include

- **Echoics.** These are imitative verbal responses whose stimuli are the speech of another person. Reinforcement for an echoic is based on a close resemblance between the stimulus and the response. Thus, a clinician will model target responses, which a child is supposed to echo or imitate. The clinician reinforces the imitations only when they at least approximate the clinician's model.

- **Mands.** Mands involve requests. The term **mand** is derived from related traditional terms such as *demand* and *command* (McLaughlin, 2006). In some cases a physiological need such as thirst or hunger stimulates speech ("Do you have something to drink?"). Needs of this sort cause various kinds of commands, demands, and requests. Skinner labeled these mands, which are reinforced by food and other biologically satisfying events and are caused by states of motivation.

- **Tacts.** Sometimes physical objects and events stimulate speaking. Verbal responses of this kind are called tacts. A **tact** is a group of verbal responses that describe and comment on the events and things around us. Tacts are reinforced socially; a nod of approval, a smile, and similar behaviors by a listener may all reinforce a tact.

> Behaviorists break language down into functional units called echoics, mands, and tacts.

Clinicians who conduct language therapy according to principles of the behavioral theory believe that one can teach language by targeting

POINTS TO PONDER If you were an SLP who subscribed to the behaviorist theory, what strategies and methods might you implement in therapy?

_____

_____

_____

any observable behavior and manipulating the elements of a stimulus, a response, and some type of reinforcement (Roseberry-McKibbin & Hegde, 2006). In treatment, the clinician selects specific target responses, creates appropriate antecedent events, and reinforces correct responses (Fey, 1986). There is a clearly established criterion for success (e.g., nine out of ten responses produced accurately). Most language development experts believe that there are inadequacies in a strict behaviorist theory of language acquisition, especially because behaviorists do not account for what the child brings to the learning task (Owens, 2005). Behaviorists focus on the external forces that shape a child's behavior into language, believing that children are passive during the language learning process (Hulit & Howard, 2002).

The Nativist Theory

CONNECT & EXTEND

Chomsky's nativist theory and later government-binding theory are described in detail by Bohannon, J.N., & Bonvillian, J.D. (2005). Theoretical approaches to language acquisition. In J. Berko Gleason, *The development of language* (6th ed.) (pp. 230–291). Boston: Allyn & Bacon.

The nativist theory, proposed by Noam Chomsky, posits the existence of a Language Acquisition Device.

The nativist theory, an influential theory of syntax proposed by Noam Chomsky in the 1950s, has had a significant impact on linguistics and on speech-language pathology. According to Chomsky, syntactic structures are the essence of language, and language is a product of the unique human mind. Chomsky stated that there are universal rules of grammar that apply to all languages. The nativist theory states that children are born with a **Language Acquisition Device (LAD)**, a specialized language processor that is a physiological part of the brain (Bohannon & Bonvillian, 2005).

The LAD knows much about languages in general, because it contains the universal rules of language. The environment provides information about the unique rules of the language the child is exposed to. The LAD then integrates the universal and the unique aspects of the language and thus helps the child learn language efficiently. Essentially, nativists believe that children are born with an innate capacity to acquire language. Because the basic knowledge necessary to acquire language is already present at birth, language is not learned through environmental stimulation, reinforcement, or teaching.

Chomsky described language **competence** and **performance**. As previously stated, competence is the underlying knowledge of the rules of universal grammar. Chomsky states that language

> Syntax is composed of both surface and deep structure; they are related through grammatic transformations.

competence is innate. Thus, the child learns language relatively independently of the environment. Language performance, the actual production of language, is imperfect because of such factors as distraction and fatigue. Chomsky also introduced the ideas of surface and deep structure. **Surface structure** is the phrase or sentence you hear; it is the actual arrangement of words in a syntactic order. Underlying this surface structure is the abstract **deep structure**, which primarily holds the rules of sentence formation. According to Chomsky, deep and surface structures are related through grammatic transformations. A **transformation** is an operation that relates the deep and surface structures and yields different forms of sentences. A transformation can further be viewed as a process by which one arranges and rearranges words to change sentences. Grammatic transformations involve adding, deleting, substituting, and rearranging words to change meaning.

Consider the following examples:

- The boy ate the Popsicle.
- Who ate the Popsicle? (a question transformation)
- Did the boy eat the Popsicle? (another question transformation)
- The boy did not eat the Popsicle. (the negative transformation)
- The Popsicle was eaten by the boy. (the passive transformation)

Each of these examples involves a transformation of either deleting, adding, substituting, or rearranging words to form a different kind of sentence. These transformations account for the creative nature of language. Because Chomsky believed that such creative transformation of sentence forms is the essence of language, his theory is often called the **transformational generative theory of grammar**. According to Chomsky, speakers can generate an endless variety of sentences through knowing the rules of grammar and transformations.

A revision of Chomsky's theory came in the early 1980s in the form of **government-binding theory** (Chomsky, 1981, 1982). Government-binding theory is a theory of how we represent language as a set of principles in our mind (Tager-Flusberg, 2005). Again, this theory attempts to describe the way that the human mind represents the autonomous system of language. As Owens states (2005; pp. 44–45):

> . . . government-binding theory attempts to describe the way in which the human mind represents the autonomous system of language. [Chomsky's] goal was to present a theory that can account for the great diversity in human languages and that can explain the development of grammars by children on the basis of limited input (Leonard & Loeb, 1988). . . . Although government-binding theory tries to incorporate many aspects of language, primary interest is still in language form. Too few child studies have been performed to make a definite statement about the contribution of government-binding theory to our understanding of language development.

> Nativists believe that in therapy with language-disordered children, it is important to focus on development of syntactic skills.

The nativist theory and its variants lead to very few specific implications for assessment and treatment of children who have language disorders. However, nativists do believe that in therapy, it is necessary to focus heavily on syntax in selecting treatment goals. Nativists also believe that reinforcement is unnecessary. Because language knowledge is innate, reinforcing a child for talking would be like reinforcing her for walking. Manipulating the child's environment is unlikely to be successful.

The Cognitive Theory

Described as a variant of the nativist theory, the cognitive theory emphasizes **cognition**, or knowledge and mental processes such as attention, memory, and auditory and visual perception. Cognitivists focus on internal aspects of behavior and on the child's regulation of learning (Klein & Moses, 1999). Cognitive theorists believe that language acquisition is made possible by cognition and general intellectual processes. Language is only one expression of a more general set of cognitive activities, and proper development of the cognitive system is a necessary precursor of linguistic expression (Bohannon & Bonvillian, 2005). Thus, the child must first acquire concepts before producing words. For example, a child who does not know about a *zoo* or a *cheetah* is not likely to say those words.

> Cognitive theorists believe that cognitive skills are foundational to language skills.

Proponents of the **strong cognition hypothesis** believe that there are cognitive abilities that are essential prerequisites to language skills. Without these prerequisite cognitive abilities, language skills will not be optimally developed. Language development is dependent on cognitive development. Jean Piaget, an advocate of the strong cognition hypothesis, described four stages of cognitive development that children must go through (see Table 2.1). Children successively acquire the necessary cognitive operations that, in turn, lead to higher levels of language development. Children must master the features of one stage in order to progress to the next stage. Children pass through each cognitive stage in the *order* given but may show variation in the *rate* at which they progress through the stages (McLaughlin, 2006; Roseberry-McKibbin & Hegde, 2006).

> Cognitive theorists generally subscribe to the strong or the weak cognition hypothesis.

The **weak cognition hypothesis** states that cognition accounts for some of a child's language abilities, but it cannot account for all of them. Some aspects of language do not develop directly as a result of underlying cognitive skills. Researchers have not proven that there is a causal relationship between cognitive and language skills; however, it has been observed that certain language skills develop at about the same time as certain cognitive skills (Owens, 2005; Reed, 2005). For example, children's use of *all gone* (a disappearance word) is associated with the emergence of object permanence.

> Belief in the cognitivist theory has major ramifications for eligibility criteria in many public school districts across the United States: deciding which children will receive intervention and which will not.

Unlike nativists, cognitive theorists believe that cognitive precursors are innate while language is not. Thus, because they believe that language is neither innate (nativist view) nor learned (behaviorist view), they view language as emerging as a result of cognitive growth. An important question with treatment implications is whether cognitive development is necessary and sufficient for language development. The answer guides eligibility criteria for speech-language therapy in

TABLE 2.1 Piaget's Stages of Cognitive Development

Sensorimotor (0–2 years)

Usually divided into six substages; children gain increased control over their environments:

- Child displays reflexive vocal and sensorimotor behavior
- Child engages in symbolic play (e.g., using a tissue for a doll's blanket; using a block to represent a car)
- Child coordinates hand-eye and hand-mouth movements
- Child begins to search for objects
- Child starts causing objects to move
- Child imitates sounds; babbling
- Object permanence occurs; child looks for an item that is out of sight
- Around 12 months, first word appears
- Child uses words for people or things that are not in present environment
- Child demonstrates means-ends behavior (e.g., pulling a string to get a toy)

Preoperational (2–7 years)

Frequently divided into two stages: preconceptual (2–4 years) and intuitive (4–7 years):

- Child is egocentric; has difficulty taking perspective of others
- Child overextends word meanings (all men are "Daddy")
- Child underextends word meanings (only the family pet, Rover, is a "dog")
- Child demonstrates concreteness of thought
- Child displays lack of conservation (e.g., lack of ability to see that a ball of clay can be rolled into a snake shape and still be the same clay)
- Child has difficulty with classification skills

Concrete Operations (7–11 years)

- Child is less egocentric, has increasing ability to see others' points of view
- Child acquires conservation skills
- Child employs logical causality
- Child uses effective classification skills

Formal Operations (more than 11 years)

- Child displays lack of egocentricity, increases in ability to see others' point of view
- Child displays ability to think and speak in the abstract
- Child can use inductive and deductive thought processes
- Child can use verbal reasoning and make "if . . . then" statements
- Child is able to use hypothetical reasoning

From Vicki A. Reed, *An Introduction to Children with Language Disorders*, 3e. Published by Allyn and Bacon, Boston, MA. Copyright © 2005 by Pearson Education. Adapted by permission of the publisher.

many school districts nationwide. There are two schools of thought on this issue (Nelson, 1998). The first holds that if cognitive development is sufficient for language development to occur, language therapy is unnecessary. As long as the student's cognitive skills continue to develop, he does not need language intervention—the cognitive growth will automatically facilitate language growth.

> **POINTS TO PONDER** Describe the nativist and cognitive theories of language acquisition. What are the clinical implications of each?
>
> _____
>
> _____
>
> _____
>
> _____

According to the second school of thought, if cognitive development is necessary for language development to occur, then children whose language skills are commensurate with their cognitive skills might be denied therapy. If the child has cognitive limitations, language therapy will not be useful. One cannot build a house (language) on a compromised foundation (cognition). On the basis of this belief, children in schools nationwide have routinely been denied language therapy. In the past, federal law has mandated that in order for a child to be eligible for certain special education services, there must be a gap between cognitive and language skills, with cognitive skills within normal range and language skills limited. It is believed that in this situation, because cognitive skills are within normal limits, there is potential for language skills to grow. However, the belief is that if cognitive skills are low, there is little or no potential for language skills to grow. The child is working to potential, thus language therapy is a waste of time and will not improve the child's language skills.

> Cognitive theorists believe that in therapy, clinicians must train cognitive precursors to language skills before language skills are directly targeted.

Another clinical implication of the cognitive theory is that clinicians must assess cognitive precursors to language and facilitate the development of these precursors before working on language itself (Van Kleeck & Richardson, 1989). Language will not improve until cognitive precursors are developed. So, for example, if a child has not said his first word and does not yet have object permanence, the clinician should establish object permanence first and only then should she work on a child's production of words.

The Social Interactionism Theory

The social interactionism theory does not focus on specific reinforcement principles (behaviorism) or innate linguistic competence (nativism). Rather, this theory states that language develops as a result of children's social interactions with the important people in their lives. Social interactionists do not emphasize language *structure*, but rather focus on language *function*. They account for the situations in which social interactions occur, believing that interactions vary depending upon the situation (Nelson, 1998).

Lev Vygotsky, a Russian psychologist, believed that language is a tool for social interaction (Vygotsky, 1962). He saw language as being intrinsically linked with the social-interactive context. Vygotsky stated that language knowledge is acquired through social interaction with more competent and experienced members of the child's culture

Eric D. was a trilingual Filipino kindergartener who wasn't talking. His teacher, Dolly C., was a Chinese American with a great deal of multicultural experience. She had been teaching for about ten years and almost never referred children for speech-language testing unless they had genuine language impairments. She was concerned about Eric and referred him to me at the end of his kindergarten year. I asked some of the other team members to test Eric so that he would have a comprehensive evaluation that would examine all his skill areas. They refused, saying that he was just a kindergartener and after all, he spoke English as his third language. They wanted to "give him time" to develop. I found out that Eric had been back and forth from the Philippines several times during his life. If you were the SLP in this situation, what questions would you have about Eric's interactions with his caretakers? What would you want to know about his background and his home life in general? What questions might you have about interaction patterns between caretakers and children in Filipino culture?

_____

_____

_____

(Van Kleeck & Richardson, 1989). He emphasized the importance of verbal guidance and adult modeling (Klein & Moses, 1999). Vygotsky held that a child's conversational partners, including the parents, are significant contributors to the language acquisition process. They contribute by *scaffolding*, or by supplying necessary communicative structure that allows the child to communicate despite limited communication skills.

> Lev Vygotsky, a proponent of social interactionism, believed that children develop language by interacting with more experienced members of their culture.

Unlike Piaget, who believed that cognitive development preceded language development, Vygotsky thought that children first learned language in interpersonal interactions and then used this language to structure thought. Vygotsky also believed that as children's language develops, they increasingly use language internally to structure their actions and direct their thoughts. For example, small children playing "house" by themselves may be observed talking to themselves as they play. Eventually, as they mature, children use language internally to mediate thought.

According to the social interactionism theory, language develops because people are motivated to interact socially with other people around them. For example, infants seek out human faces and respond to them (Bruner, 1968). Thus, the environment and its inherent social experiences are foundational to the emergence of language (Bohannon & Bonvillian, 2005). Proponents of social interactionism believe that the *child*, as well as her caretakers and the environment, plays an active role in language acquisition.

CONNECT & EXTEND

For an extended discussion of social interactionist theory and culture, see Woolfolk, A. (2004). *Educational psychology* (9th ed.). Boston, MA: Allyn & Bacon.

Vygotsky believed that cultural tools play critical roles in children's cognitive development. For example, in a culture that has only Roman numerals, certain ways of thinking mathematically are impossible. However, in a culture that has calculators and computers, many more high-level ways of mathematical thinking are possible. Children's learning is guided by the available cultural tools and child-adult interactions around these tools (Woolfolk, 2004).

Social interactionism theorists believe that oral and written language skills continue to develop across the span of a person's life. Adolescents, for example, continue to refine their skills in figurative language and pragmatics as they mature. Adults who change jobs or vocations must learn the new vocabulary relevant to their new station in life. An immigrant student from Russia who arrives in the United States at 13 years of age must develop his English written and oral skills so he can succeed in American schools.

Clinicians whose practice is driven by the social interactionism theory focus on children's *motivation* for communication. Therapy sessions are built around increasing children's motivation to communicate. To motivate children to use language, clinicians supply external situations and contexts, both verbal and nonverbal, that encourage the child to use language to meet his needs. If a clinician is working with a CLD child, she must consider his background and what needs he might have within his environmental context.

Social interactionists believe that in therapy, it is important to work on increasing the child's motivation to communicate.

For example, in the Samoan culture, children primarily interact with each other. Many Samoan mothers do not interact with their children very much until the children are old enough to communicate articulately and clearly (van Kleeck, 1994). Thus, a clinician who worked with a Samoan child might ask how motivated he would be to talk with her, an adult female. He might be more motivated to talk to peers in a group therapy situation than to talk with her in a one-on-one situation.

The Information Processing Theory

Proponents of the **information processing theory** are mostly concerned with how language is learned. They are interested in cognitive *functioning*, not cognitive structures or concepts. Information processing theorists view the human information-processing system as a mechanism that encodes stimuli from the environment, operates on interpretations of those stimuli, stores the results in memory, and permits retrieval of previously stored information. Of primary concern are the steps involved in handling or processing incoming and outgoing information. Included in these steps are organization, memory, transfer, attention, and discrimination. Long- and short-term memory are especially important (Nelson, 1998; Owens, 2005).

In recent literature, there has been a great deal of debate about the relationship between information processing and language impairments. Researchers have been interested in whether or not children with language impairments have concomitant information-processing problems (e.g., Conti-Ramsden, 2003; Hoffman & Gillam, 2004; Montgomery, 2002). In Chapter 1, we said that research has shown that language impairment and processing problems do coexist. Ellis Weismer and Evans (2002) suggested that there are two broad categories of information processing related to children's language impairments. The first category or aspect discussed is phonological processing.

Phonological processing is concerned with the processes involved in a person's ability to mentally manipulate phonological aspects of language. These include word rhyming, word segmentation, syllabication, and others. A child who has difficulty rhyming words or knowing that "c-a-t" means "cat" has phonological processing problems. The child who cannot tell you if the words *cat* and *bat* rhyme also has phonological processing problems.

The second category or aspect of information processing discussed by Ellis Weismer and Evans (2002) is **temporal auditory processing**. This deals with a person's ability to perceive the brief acoustic events that make up speech sounds and track changes in these events as they happen quickly in the speech of other people. In research on the temporal auditory processing skills of children, experts have been focused on children's 1) overall processing capacity and 2) speed of processing. In a simple example, researchers might ask if a child with a language disorder is able to listen to someone quickly say "2-5-9-3-7," remember this digit string, and repeat it back immediately and accurately. The child may have difficulty with the length of the digit string, the speed with which the string was said, or both.

Children who have difficulties in temporal auditory processing often have difficulty with other tasks. These include remembering and following long and complex directions, repeating back sentences verbatim, repeating back lists of real and nonsense words, and other tasks that tap their ability to hear, remember, and give back information that they have heard—especially if the information was given rapidly (Reed, 2005).

 # SUMMARY

- B.F. Skinner's behavioral theory explained the acquisition of verbal behavior. Behaviorists focus on aspects of language behavior that are observable and measurable. Behaviorists believe that one can teach language by targeting any observable behavior and manipulating the elements of stimulus, response, and reinforcement.
- Noam Chomsky's nativist theory stated that children are born with a Language Acquisition Device (LAD) that integrates the universal and unique as aspects of language and helps a child learn efficiently. Also called the theory of transformational generative grammar, the nativist theory categorizes children's language skills broadly into the areas of competence and performance.
- The cognitive theory, associated with Jean Piaget, emphasizes knowledge and mental processes such as attention, memory, and auditory and visual perception. Cognitive theorists believe that cognitive skills are foundational to language skills.
- The social interactionism theory, associated with Lev Vygotsky, holds that language develops because children are socially motivated to interact with those around them. In therapy, we work to increase language-impaired children's motivation to communicate.
- Information processing theorists view the human information-processing system as a mechanism that encodes stimuli from the environment, operates on interpretations of those stimuli, stores the results in memory, and permits retrieval of previously stored information.

(continued)

- Most SLPs, rather than allowing their practice to be driven by a single theory, incorporate aspects of each theory to allow an eclectic blend to serve as a foundation for optimal assessment and treatment of language-impaired children.

Add your own summary points here:

_____

_____

_____

NORMAL LANGUAGE DEVELOPMENT: DEVELOPMENTAL MILESTONES

The development of language rests upon several major variables that interact with one another. First, the individual child has innate characteristics he or she brings to the situation. Such characteristics may include a high IQ, a limited attention span, and others. Second, the child's environment plays a big role in language development. The more stimulating

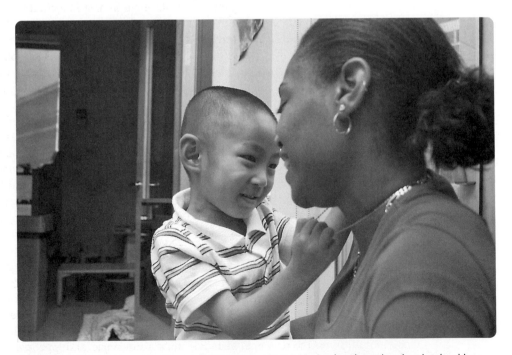

As children acquire language, they develop a form of social behavior shaped and maintained by a verbal community.

the environment, the better and more thoroughly the child will develop language skills. Language development also depends upon cultural expectations.

This section begins by briefly discussing the role of the environment in a child's developing language. Then it describes language development milestones that represent a range of expectations for times when children may develop certain language structures. This section focuses on semantic, syntactic, morphological, and pragmatic development as consistent with general mainstream American social expectations. The timeline for development of milestones in each of these areas depends very heavily upon the child's linguistic and cultural background; various cultures differ in their expectations for children's language development.

The Role of the Environment in Language Development

Children begin to interact with their environments from the day they are born. In some cultures, such as US American culture, the baby's initial interactions are with the mother. Traditional American researchers, when discussing infant interactions with others, often operate unconsciously from the paradigm of a single-family dwelling with the mother as the infant's primary caretaker.

However, in cultures where there are extended families, the baby's first interactions may take place mostly with older siblings or even grandparents who live in the home. Thus, when evaluating the role of the environment in a child's language development, clinicians must first of all ask the question: With whom does the child spend most of her time? Again, in many cultures, it cannot automatically be assumed that this is the biological mother.

> A baby's initial interactions take place mostly with the primary caretaker(s), who may or may not be the biological mother.

Numerous researchers have discussed the important role of language stimulation, or having an infant or small child talked with frequently by adults (Hulit & Howard, 2002; Kuder, 2003; Nelson, 1998; Owens, 2005). It is widely believed that the more an infant or small child is talked with by adults, the better and faster she will develop language skills. In addition, this rapid and ideal development of language skills includes the child being highly verbal; the more the child talks, the better. Children develop especially efficiently if the caretaker uses characteristics of **motherese** or **child-directed interaction**, characterized by exaggerated intonation patterns, higher pitch, shorter sentences, increased pause duration between separate utterances, repeating the child's utterances, and others (Bernstein & Levey, 2002; McLaughlin, 2006).

> Norms for interacting with infants and young children differ from culture to culture.

However, in many cultures, adult interaction with infants and young children differs from mainstream US expectations. In the dominant North American cultures (United States and Canada), parents treat children as conversational partners from the day they are born (Ochs & Schieffelin, 1984). Parents label things for children, ask them to verbally display their knowledge, and greet these displays with enthusiasm. In many mainstream homes, children are exposed to literacy activities long before they are expected to read themselves.

In contrast, adults in other cultures value different types of development and behaviors than do mainstream monolingual English-speaking White adults. For example, among many Navajo, a child's "first laugh" is very significant—much more so than the first word. Many Navajo mothers are silent with their infants (van Kleeck, 1994). Among some Western Apache Indians, children may be rebuked for "talking like a White man" if they talk too much (Harris, 1985). The Inuit people from the north of Canada live in small, remote villages where they interact with their children in a style different from that of many "mainstream" North American families (Genesee et al., 2004).

For example, Inuit mothers don't generally converse with their babies. The babies are carried around in their mothers' parkas, and the babies learn to look, listen, and observe. Mothers do not interpret their babies' early vocalizations as actual talk and do not respond verbally to these vocalizations. When the babies grow into toddlers, Inuit parents often don't address their children directly. Instead, the toddlers' needs are met silently. Children are not expected to interrupt adults' conversations or converse with adults. They play and interact primarily with their peers. Inuit adults believe that it is demeaning for an adult to sit on the floor and play with children or interact with the children as though they were adults. They consider it odd to converse with a child until the child is around five years old. Parents don't often read books with their children, and book-reading by older children may be frowned upon because the child is just sitting there instead of developing physical prowess and strength. Activities that strengthen the body and teach the child about the physical world are much more valued than literacy activities (Genesee et al., 2004).

> Some cultures have patterns of interaction with young children that differ from mainstream expectations. Children are not always treated as conversational partners.

In some other examples of home language patterns, in some African American families, "charismatic" speech and language are more valued than a child's having a large vocabulary with many labels for objects and concepts (Terrell & Hale, 1992). In Western Samoan society, if a young child appeals to her mother, the mother may not respond directly but rather direct a caregiver of lower status (such as a sibling) to respond to the child (van Kleeck, 1994). Madding (2002) describes interactions in some Hispanic homes:

CONNECT & EXTEND

To learn more about caretaker-child interactions in various cultural groups, see Lynch, E.W., & Hanson, M.J. (2004). *Developing cross-cultural competence: A guide for working with young children and their families* (3rd ed.). Baltimore: Paul H. Brookes Publishing Co.

Mother-child dyadic formations may not be an archetype in the Latino family as it is in Anglo society. The mother-child dyad may co-exist with the sibling-child dyad . . . the aunt-child dyad, or the grandparent-child dyad. . . . Multiperson socialization and care of children is more the norm than the exception. . . . Mexican-descent mothers present little teaching, rely heavily on nonverbal instruction . . . speak to their children with high percentages of adult wording. . . . Many Latinas of Mexican origin see themselves as mothers and caregivers, not as teachers.

Thus, when clinicians consider the role of the environment in a child's language development, it is extremely important to take into account the child's cultural and linguistic background. Who are the primary interactors with the child? What does that culture believe about language development? All language development milestones

CASES TO CONSIDER

Nuu F., a Samoan nineteen-month-old, was taken to a speech-language clinic by his grandmother. Nuu's mother, she explained, was unable to come for the appointment. The grandmother shared with the clinician that Nuu was the seventh child in the family and that he did not verbalize at all. She said the other six children had at least said their first word by their first birthday, but Nuu was "slow." What other questions do you need to ask the grandmother? What cultural variables might you need to consider in making recommendations for language stimulation activities in the home?

_____

_____

_____

must be viewed in this light. In Chapter 11, we will discuss the role of environmental factors in children's language acquisition in greater detail.

Traditional Language Development Milestones

As has been stated, the timeline for attaining these milestones depends heavily upon the child's linguistic and cultural background. This list of language milestones must be viewed in light of the background of each individual child. The following information regarding developmental milestones is summarized from Berko Gleason, 2005; Hulit & Howard, 2002; McLaughlin, 2006; Owens, 2005; Roseberry-McKibbin & Hegde, 2006.

Birth to One Year

The baby's first sounds are **reflexive**; they are not learned. These sounds, such as burping, coughing, and sneezing, are sometimes also called *vegetative sounds* because they are natural and made by a passive living organism. By the time the baby is two months old, he may cry less; also, the cries become more differentiated and varied. Caregivers can usually tell cries of anger from cries of fatigue and boredom. By two months of age, the baby is usually **cooing**. He is producing vowel-like sounds that are often connected to sounds that resemble "g" or "k." Cooing often occurs in response to interactions with the caregiver.

Between birth and three months of age, the baby visually tracks; he moves his eyes to the source of sound. For instance, if he hears a dog bark, he turns his head toward the dog. He also demonstrates a startle response to loud sound. Within the first three months of life, a baby will also show regard for nearby objects, including his caregiver's face. He will quiet when he is picked up. Between birth and four weeks of age, babies will smile reflexively in response to internal stimuli (e.g., gas); the first true social smile usually appears around five to six weeks of age (McLaughlin, 2006). A social smile generally occurs in response to another person.

Between four and six months of age, the child explores his vocal mechanism through vocal play such as yelling, squealing, growling, and making "raspberries" (bilabial trills). He moves or looks toward a family member when that person is named (e.g., "Where's Mommy?"). He also responds by raising his arms when mother says "come here" and reaches toward him. At around five months of age, the baby explores objects by touching and mouthing them. Most parents quickly learn that anything the baby can reach goes into his mouth!

In the **reduplicated babbling** stage, which appears at about six or seven months, the baby uses repeated CV (consonant-vowel) syllables such as "dadadada." Babies will often babble when they are alone. Many times, proud parents will think that babies are producing actual words. When my son Mark was seven months old, I was so thrilled when he said "mama." My joy quickly dissolved when he also said "mama" when he saw the dog.

> In the first six months of life, babies begin to babble and to explore objects as well as track items visually.

At around nine months of age, the baby uses a wide variety of sound combinations. The **variegated babbling** begins—e.g., "mabamabada." At nine months of age, the baby imitates the intonation and speech sounds of others. My husband swears that when our son was ten months old, he said, "Hi, Dad." I suspect that the proud father was hearing variegated babbling which contained the syllables "Idada."

Between ten and twelve months of age, the baby jabbers loudly, using a wide variety of sounds and pitch variations when vocalizing. He will not produce his first true word until about twelve months of age but will produce **protowords**. Protowords, though not recognizable as adult words, are consistent productions the child uses in response to various situations. For example, when our dog walked into the room, Mark would say "ah" each time.

As babies approach one year of age, they will use all consonant and vowel sounds in vocal play. They may understand between ten and fifty words such as "bye-bye, pat-a-cake, hot, no." They will usually understand one simple direction like "sit down," especially when commands are accompanied by gestures. At twelve months of age, babies begin to relate symbols and objects; the first true word is spoken. They will look in the correct place for toys or objects that are out of sight (**object permanence**). For example, if a mother shows a twelve-month-old child a puppet and then puts it behind her back, the child will come and look for it. He knows that even though he can't see the puppet, it still exists.

In terms of pragmatics or social language skills, babies between birth and six months of age use **perlocutionary behaviors**—signals issued by the child that have an effect on the listener but lack communicative intent. For example, if a mother puts her baby into the bath and he begins to cry, she might say, "Uh-oh, that water is too cold and you don't like it. I'd better warm it up." But the baby could be crying for any number of reasons; his mother has interpreted his cry as indicating that he doesn't like the temperature of the bathwater, and she is now adding warm water in hopes that he will like the bath better.

> By one year of age, most children will speak their first word and demonstrate object permanence as well as joint reference.

At nine to ten months of age, the baby uses **illocutionary behavior**—a signal to carry out some socially organized action. This is intentional communication (e.g., pointing to a desired object). For example, a baby may point to a balloon; his intent is to obtain the balloon. At approximately twelve months of age, the baby enters the **locutionary** stage as he begins to use true words. Babies also learn to establish **joint reference**, or the focusing of joint attention on an object or event. Caretakers begin to establish joint reference by establishing eye contact with the baby in the early months. Then, later, caretakers point to or name objects that both the caretaker and child focus upon. In Chapter 11, we will discuss how parents of blind children can help their children develop language without the use of joint reference.

One to Two Years (12–24 months)

Semantics The period between twelve and twenty-four months of age is one of great growth. With regard to semantics, at around eighteen months, the child produces about fifty words expressively. At approximately eighteen months of age, she understands about two hundred words. By twenty-four months of age, the child should produce (expressively) between 150 and 300 words. The child between twelve and twenty-four months of age verbalizes immediate experiences. Her most frequent lexical categories are verbs (e.g., *run, eat*) and nominals (e.g. *doggy, Grandma.*) Young children may use **overextensions** (e.g., all round items are balls) or **underextensions** (only an Oreo is a cookie). When my son was between one and two years old, he gave me an excellent example of an overexten-

> Between one and two years of age, children's receptive and expressive vocabulary expands dramatically.

sion. We were in a store where there was a magazine with Sharon Stone on the front cover. He pointed to her excitedly and said, "Mommy!" Naturally, after that overextension, we had to visit the toy store immediately.

The child also begins to use some adjectives (e.g., *hot, yucky*). She starts to use **semantic relations**, or utterances that reflect meaning based on relationships between different words (e.g., cause-effect relationships). She begins with one-word utterances and gradually progresses to two-word utterances (see Table 2.2 and Table 2.3).

Syntax Between twelve and eighteen months of age, the child's average MLU (mean length of utterance in morphemes) is 1.0 to 2.0. The sentencelike word exists in the single word or **holophrastic phase**; children communicate relationships by using one word plus vocal and bodily cues. The sentencelike word can have several basic functions:

- The question: e.g., "Car?" (child asking if that's a car)
- The emphatic or imperative statement: e.g., "Car!" (child telling you to look at a car)
- The declarative statement: e.g., "Car." Child saying it's a car and not something else.

At approximately eighteen months of age, the child begins to put two words together (she must have an expressive vocabulary of fifty words first). Most words in a child's first

> Most children begin putting two words together at eighteen months of age.

fifty spoken words refer to things that she can act upon (e.g., toys, objects). At two years of age, the child may use three- or four-word responses.

Pragmatics Between one and two years of age, the child begins to understand some rules of dialogue, e.g., "when someone talks, you

TABLE 2.2   Relations Expressed by Single-Word Utterances

Before children reach the two-word-utterance stage, they typically use single words to express themselves. The relations expressed by single words are as follows:

Relation	Definition	Example
Attribution	An adjective; a property or characteristic of an event, person, or object	*Big* doggy *Clean* dolly Face *dirty*
Action	Child requests or labels an action; indicates movement relationships between objects and people	*Open* box Kitty *run* *Close* door
Locative action	Child refers to a change in an object's location	*There* doggy Ball *up*
Existence	Child is attending to item or object present in the immediate environment, especially a novel one	What's *that?* *This* kitty
Nonexistence or disappearance	An action or object is expected to be present but is not; something was present but disappeared	*All gone* juice *Bye bye* Mom *No* doggy
Denial	Child denies a statement or previous utterance (e.g., in response to a parent saying, "Is this a kitty?")	*No* kitty
Rejection	Child does not want something to happen; child refuses an object or action	*No* bath *No* beans
Recurrence	An event happens again; an object reappears or replaces another	*More* cookie *Another* doggie
Possession	Child identifies something as belonging to him or her, or to another person	*His* block Doll *mine*

From Vicki A. Reed, *An Introduction to Children with Language Disorders*, 3e. Published by Allyn and Bacon, Boston, MA. Copyright © 2005 by Pearson Education. Adapted by permission of the publisher.

need to listen." She starts to be able to take the role of both speaker and listener. **Presuppositions** emerge—the child uses expressions that have shared meaning to listener and speaker. The child also uses both verbal and nonverbal communication to signal intent. Halliday considered *listener's responses* in describing the following seven functions of communicative intent that develop between nine and eighteen months of age (adapted from Halliday, 1975):

- **Regulatory**—children attempt to control behavior of others ("do as I tell you to do")
- **Personal**—self-awareness; children express own feelings and attitudes (Child says "yummy" as he eats an ice cream cone)

TABLE 2.3   Semantic Relations Expressed by Two-Word Utterances

Semantic Relation	Structure	Example
Notice	Hi + noun	Hi doggy
Nomination	Demonstrative + noun	That chair
Instrumental	Verb + noun	Cut [with scissors]
Conjunction	Noun + noun	Knife spoon
Recurrence	More + noun	More juice
Action-object	Verb + noun	Pet kitty
Action-indirect object	Verb + noun	Give [to] Mommy
Agent-action	Noun (agent) + verb	Doggy bark
Agent-object	Noun (agent) + noun	Baby [drink] juice
Possessor-possession	Noun (possessor) + noun	Mommy sock
Attribute-entity	Adjective/attributive + noun	Red ball
Entity + locative	Non + locative	Juice [in] glass
Action + locative	Verb + noun	Jump [on] bed

From Vicki A. Reed, *An Introduction to Children with Language Disorders*, 3e. Published by Allyn and Bacon, Boston, MA. Copyright © 2005 by Pearson Education. Adapted by permission of the publisher.

- **Imaginative**—children do pretend or play-acting; they use language to create an environment; there is communicative function ("Let's pretend"; child may vocalize to herself while playing with dolls)

> Halliday described seven functions of communicative intent that develop between nine and eighteen months of age; these functions consider the listener's responses.

- **Instrumental**—children attempt to get assistance, material things from others ("I want cereal")
- **Heuristic**—children attempt to have their environment, events in the environment explained to them; they organize and investigate the environment ("Tell me why?" "What that?" [pointing to a horse])
- **Informative**—children tell someone something, communicate experiences ("I have something to tell you")
- **Interactional**—children initiate interactions with others ("Hi Daddy")

Dore (1975) focused on the twelve- to twenty-four-month period where children used early words to signal communicative intent. Rather than focusing on listeners' reactions, Dore focused more on children's intentions:

> Dore described children's communication intentions that develop from twelve to twenty-four months of age.

- **Requesting an answer** (child: "Sheep?" adult: "Yes, it's a sheep.")
- **Labeling** (child is playing with a doll and labels "mouth," "nose," etc.)
- **Protesting** ("no" and resisting)
- **Greeting** ("Hi Mama" as mother comes in door)
- **Practicing** (language)

POINTS TO PONDER Describe one important milestone in each area (semantics, syntax, morphology, pragmatics) that occurs in the first two years of life.

_____

_____

_____

- **Answering** (adult: "What's this?" child: "elephant")
- **Calling/addressing** ("Daddy!")
- **Requesting action** (child says "cookie" when wants to be given a cookie)
- **Repeating/imitating** (child overhears and repeats the word "car")

Two to Three Years

Semantics At thirty months of age, the child comprehends up to 2,400 words. At thirty-six months of age, he comprehends up to 3,600 words. The child's expressive vocabulary ranges between 200 and 600 words; the average is 425 words at thirty months of age. By three years of age, the child has an expressive vocabulary of 900 to 1,000 words. Meanings seem to be learned in sequence: 1) objects, 2) events, 3) actions, 4) adjectives, 5) adverbs, 6) spatial concepts, and 7) temporal (time) concepts. The first pronouns used are self-referents like "I, me." The child can answer simple "wh-" questions—e.g., "What walks?" At thirty months of age, he begins asking wh- questions of adults.

> Between two and three years of age, children develop several hundred additional words expressively and communicate in two- to four-word sentences.

He can comprehend and carry out one- and two-part commands such as "Pick up the truck and give it to Grandma." He understands plurals and can identify simple body parts (e.g., "show me your tummy"). By thirty-six months of age, the child can give a simple account of experiences and tell understandable stories.

Syntax Between two and three years of age, word combinations are primarily used. The child has beginning phrase and sentence structure. Her average MLU (mean length of utterance in morphemes) is 2.0 to 4.0. At thirty-six months, sentences often average three or four words per sentence (see Table 2.4). The child combines three or four words in subject + verb + object format; e.g., "*Mommy wash clothes*." Telegraphic speech is frequently used—word order is often object-verb (e.g. "*kitty eat*"), verb-object (e.g., "*comb hair*"), or subject-verb. Most sentences are incomplete.The child expresses negation by adding "no" or "not" in front of the verb—e.g., "*she not do that*," or "*he no push*." The child frequently asks yes-no questions and wh- questions. As the weary parent of a child this age will tell you, "Why?" is a favorite wh- question.

TABLE 2.4   Sequence of Acquisition for Fourteen Grammatical Morphemes

Morpheme	MLU	Maximum Length in Morphemes	Stage
1. Present progressive ending (-ing)			
2. 3. *In* and *on*	2.25	7	II
4. Noun plurals			
5. Past-tense irregular verbs			
6. Possessive nouns	2.75	9	III
7. Uncontractible copula ("Here I <u>am</u>")			
8. Articles			
9. Past-tense regular verbs	3.50	11	IV
10. Regular third-person singular present-tense verbs			
11. Irregular third-person singular present-tense verbs			
12. Uncontractible auxiliary ("He <u>was</u> running")	4.00	13	V
13. Contractible copula ("She<u>'s</u> big")			
14. Contractible auxiliary ("The boy<u>'s</u> eating")			

From Vicki A. Reed, *An Introduction to Children with Language Disorders*, 3e. Published by Allyn and Bacon, Boston, MA. Copyright © 2005 by Pearson Education. Adapted by permission of the publisher.

CASES TO CONSIDER

A few weeks ago, I took my son to a nearby community pool to help him cool off on a 102-degree day. I ran into Richard, the father of one of Mark's classmates (Robby) at school. Robby's two-year-old sister was there too. As Richard and I began to chat while we watched our children in the kiddie pool, he told me that the sister only spoke about ten to twelve words. He said that she appeared to understand everything, but shared that "she just doesn't like to talk." He asked my advice and wondered if he and his wife should take her for a formal speech-language evaluation. What would you tell Richard? What language milestones should a child have achieved by thirty months of age?

_____

_____

_____

Morphology Between two and three years of age, the child develops consistent use of regular past tense verbs (e.g., walk*ed*, look*ed*). He demonstrates overregularization of past tense inflections—for example, he will say things like "*goed, throwed, falled.*" However, he may correctly produce simple, irregular past tense verbs such as "went." Overgeneralization of plural morphemes occurs also (e.g., "*mans, foots*"). The child develops inflections such as *-ing*, spatial prepositions "in" and "on," plural, possessive *'s*, articles, pronouns (see Table 2.4). There is general emergence of bound morphemes, and the child may use some memorized contractions like "*don't, can't, it's, that's.*"

> Between two and three years of age, children develop use of some basic morphemes and communicate, on average, in three- to four-word sentences.

Pragmatics In terms of pragmatics skills, the child's communication expands; she learns to adopt a role to express her own opinions and personality. Her utterances generally have a communicative intent, although some utterances are still egocentric. There are rapid topic shifts; a three-year-old can only sustain the topic of conversation about 20 percent of the time. Communication includes questions, answers, criticism, commands, requests, and threats.

Three to Four Years

Semantics At thirty-six months of age, the child will have an expressive vocabulary of approximately 900 to 1,000 words. She will use approximately 12,000 individual words per day. At forty-two months of age, she comprehends up to 4,200 words; at forty-eight months, she comprehends up to 5,600 words. The child may understand some common opposites—for example, day/night, little/big, fast/slow. She will be able to state her full name, the name of the street she lives on, and several nursery rhymes (if her environment has included teaching of these concepts). It is important to note that in some cultures, caregivers do not believe that it is important for children to be able to state their name and address. Thus, SLPs must be very careful to not label these children as deficient in their language skills if they do not demonstrate these "normal" milestones.

Between three and four years of age, the child can relate experiences and tell about activities in sequential order. She learns to answer questions appropriately (e.g., "What color is this?", "Where is the doggy?", "What is your favorite toy?") She can also appropriately answer simple cause-and-effect or "what-if" questions such as "What would you do if you fell down?" Most children also understand preschool children's stories and comprehend concepts such as more-less, around, next to, big-little, in front of-in back of, heavy-light, empty-full, hard-soft, rough-smooth. They should understand agent-action relationships (e.g., "Tell me what swims, bites, flies," etc.).

> From three to four years of age, children begin to tell stories, ask questions, and comprehend a variety of basic concepts.

Syntax The child between three and four years of age uses mostly complete sentences, and her MLU is approximately 3.0 to 5.0. The child's expressive syntactic skills are heavily dependent upon the amount and type of language stimulation in the environment. I'll never forget the story I heard about a precocious three-year-old farm girl who told her mother, "Mommy, we can't milk Flicker because her orifices are too small." Again, the amount and type of language stimulation in a child's environment greatly influence her syntactic skills.

The average three- to four-year-old child begins using complex verb phrases (e.g., "I should have been able to do it"). She also begins using modal verbs (*could, should,* etc.; modals are *can, may, will, shall, must*). The child learns clause-connecting devices: coordination (e.g., "and"), and subordination (e.g., "because"). So, for example, she can say, "I played with Billy *and* I ate with Kathy at preschool today." She can also say, "I didn't finish my coloring *because* it was time for snacks." The conjunction *because* typically emerges between forty-three and forty-eight months of age.

> Three- to four-year-old children begin using complex and compound sentences as well as regular past tense and plural forms.

The three- to four-year-old child begins using **embedded** forms, or forms that rearrange or add elements within sentences. For example, the child might say, "The woman *who was using crutches* fell down." The child also begins using the passive voice, e.g., "My dad was hit by a baseball" or "The piano was played by my big brother." Do-insertions are acquired and transformation occurs–e.g., "Does the bus stop by our house?" The child also begins using complex and compound sentences—7 percent of sentences are compound or complex. You will recall that we discussed these sentence types in Chapter 1.

Morphology The child who is between three and four years of age uses simple (regular) plural forms correctly; for example, she accurately says *boys, houses, lights*. Irregular plural forms emerge; for example, she will say the words "feet" and "mice" instead of *foots* and *mouses*. She is beginning to use "is" at the beginning of questions and consistently uses "is, are, am" in sentences. The child uses contracted forms of modals (e.g., "can't, won't"). The possessive marker *'s* is consistently used (e.g., the *man's* motorcycle; the *dog's* dish). The reflexive pronoun "myself" emerges between forty-three and forty-eight months of age.

Pragmatics

The three- to four-year-old is beginning to modify her speech to the age of the listener (e.g., using simplified language with a younger child). He is also beginning to produce indirectives (e.g., "Do I smell pie?" meaning "I want some pie."). My son Mark loves Icees. When he was three years old, we drove past a gas station that had a large, plastic replica of an Icee on the roof. Mark said, "Does anyone need some gas?"

The three- to four-year-old can maintain a short conversation without losing track of the topic; he can produce short narratives. His responses contain structures such as "*yes/no,*

POINTS TO PONDER Summarize the overall language development milestones that a three-and-a-half-year-old child should have achieved by traditional, mainstream timelines.

_____

_____

_____

because," agreement or denial, such as "*I didn't really spill that juice,*" compliance or refusal (e.g., "*I won't take a bath!*"). Conversational devices used by the three- to four-year-
old child include

- *calls*–"hey Grandpa!"
- *politeness markers*–"please, thank you" (if caretakers have taught this)
- *boundary markers* like "hi, bye"–indicate beginning, end of communication

Four to Five Years

As we have repeatedly said, a child's environment is a major variable in determining his
language skills. You will recall that many children between four and five years of age attend preschool. However, as we discuss elsewhere in this book, not all cultures believe that
young children should spend time away from their immediate families. Thus, the "typical"
milestones described at this age level will probably be most applicable to children who
have had some formal preschool experience.

Semantics At forty-eight months of age, the child uses 1,500 to 1,600 words expressively.
She comprehends about 2,500 to 2,800 words. By fifty-four months of age, the child comprehends approximately 6,500 words; by 60 months (5 years), she can comprehend up to
9,600 words. She can name items in a category (e.g., food, animals). For example, if you say,
"Tell me all the animals you can think of," the child is able to name some. She can point to
categorical items (e.g., "show me furniture" or "show me some fruits").

By four to five years of age, most children can name primary colors and label some
coins. Most children use pronouns, including possessives (e.g., "mine, his, her"). The child
uses "how" and "why" questions (such as when Mark, after eating candy, said, "Why can't
we just rinse our teeth with root beer?"). If the child comes from a home and/or preschool
environment where time is referenced, he will understand time concepts such as "early in
the morning, tomorrow, after." As we shall discuss in Chapter 10, children who come from
low-income homes may have difficulty with this because many low-income homes are
fairly unstructured. This is yet another example of how a child's environment impacts his
acquisition of "typical" language milestones.

> Between four and five years of age, children be-gin to categorize items as well as understand the concepts of right and left.

By four-and-a-half years of age, the child can define common
words (e.g., "What is a ball?"). He begins to understand right and left
on himself but has difficulty telling right and left on others. Thus,
even if a child can correctly identify his left and right foot, he might
have difficulty with the command "Point to Mommy's left shoe." Between four and five years of age, the child can identify objects by use
and function (e.g., "show me what you use to cook with"; "show me
which one gives us milk"). He can also identify past and future verbs
("show me the girl who threw the ball"; "who will throw the ball?").

Syntax The four- to five-year-old child generally speaks in complete sentences. She uses
complex sentences expressively and comprehends complex sentences correctly. By four-
and-a-half years of age, only about 8 percent of the child's sentences are incomplete. Her
average MLU is 4.5 to 7.0; by five years of age, her sentences average six or six-and-a-half

Four- to five-year-olds generally speak in complete sentences and use irregular plurals fairly consistently.

words. She consistently uses future tense correctly (e.g., "He will take me to the store").

Morphology The four- to five-year-old child consistently uses "could, would" in sentences. Irregular plurals (e.g., *feet, women*) should be used fairly consistently. The child also usually uses comparatives correctly (e.g., "shorter, skinnier, faster").

Pragmatics The four- to five-year-old child is able to maintain a topic over successive utterances. Her narrative skills improve; she is able to tell long stories. She uses egocentric monologue about one-third of the time; this monologue does not communicate information to the listener. Generally, the four- to five-year-old plays well in a group and cooperates with others. At five years, she begins to tell jokes and riddles.

CONNECT & EXTEND

To learn more about patterns of narrative development in various cultural groups, see McCabe, A., & Bliss, L. (2003). *Patterns of narrative discourse: A multicultural, life-span approach.* Boston, MA: Allyn & Bacon.

Five to Six Years

Semantics The typically developing (TD) five- to six-year-old has an expressive vocabulary of approximately 2,000 words. By age six, he comprehends 13,000 to 15,000 words. He knows spatial relations/prepositions such as "on top, behind, far, near," and can distinguish "alike, same-different" and understands "opposite of." For example, he will be able to correctly answer the question, "what's the opposite of cold?" The five- to six-year-old knows concepts such as yesterday/tomorrow, more/less, some/many, several/few, most/least, before/after, now/later. He can state his complete address and phone number.

The five- to six-year-old can usually name the days of the week in order. He may also know months of the year. He can define objects by composition and use (e.g., "napkins are made of paper; you wipe your mouth with them"). He is able to tell a long story; he retells tales of past and present events, and creates imaginary stories. The child can state similarities and differences between objects and name their position (e.g., first, second, third).

Between five and six years of age, children begin to understand spatial relationships and opposites.

Syntax The average MLU for a five- to six-year-old is 6.0 to 8.0. He is very consistent in using conjunctions to string words together (e.g., "a bear and a wolf and a fox"). "If" sentences occur—for example, my 5-year-old Mark said, "Mommy, I would make you into a tomato if you did that." The child uses present, past, and future tense consistently. His understanding and use of complex sentences improves; grammatical errors continue to decrease as sentences and vocabulary become more sophisticated. The child comprehends verb tenses in the passive voice (e.g., "Robin Hood was hit by the mean sheriff of Ham"; "The dog was fed by the boy"). Language often sounds very adult like (e.g., when Mark said, "Mercury has no atmosphere. It's just a rocky ball.").

Morphology The five- to six-year-old uses irregular plurals, possessives, and negatives with general consistency. All pronouns are used consistently. The child knows the passive

CASES TO CONSIDER

John and Carol Brown, friends of yours, have just adopted a little boy (Viktor) from a Russian orphanage. Viktor has some basic English skills and is almost ready to go to a U.S. kindergarten. John and Carol ask you to work with Viktor to help him become ready for kindergarten in his local neighborhood. What goals might you have for Viktor's language development?

_____

_____

_____

> Five- to six-year-olds use conjunctions and indefinite pronouns accurately.

forms of main verbs and knows indefinite pronouns—*every, both, few, many, anything, anybody,* etc. Superlative *-est* is used consistently (e.g., "tight*est*"). Adverbial word endings are emerging (e.g., nice*ly*).

Pragmatics The five- to six-year-old rewords socially offensive messages in polite form. For example, if the child says to his mother, "Gimme some toys," his mother will probably say, "I need to hear you say that more politely." The child will be able to then say something like, "I'd like some toys, please." The child consistently uses expressions such as "thank you; I'm sorry; may I please." The child demonstrates basic understanding of humor and surprise and likes to tease. He can correct potential errors by modifying the message.

The five- to six-year-old child continues to gain greater facility with indirect requests, and formal levels of address become significant (e.g., Mr., Mrs.). He often asks permission to use objects belonging to others and contributes to adult conversation.

Six to Seven Years

Semantics The six- to seven-year-old child generally has an expressive vocabulary of 2,600 words. Her receptive vocabulary is about 20,000 words (McLaughlin, 2006). She counts to 100 by rote and tells time related to a specific daily schedule. In terms of writing, she forms her letters from left to right; reversals are common (e.g., "b" instead of "d"). She can print the alphabet and numerals from previously printed model. She is able to recite the alphabet sequentially. She can name capital letters and match lower to uppercase letters.

> Six- to seven-year-olds begin to recite the alphabet and to print.

Syntax The six- to seven-year-old child uses many complex, well-formed sentences. She is well-developed in her use of reflexive pronouns (e.g., "himself, myself"). Use of the passive voice is fully developed in most children, and their average MLU is 7.3 words. Embedding is used more frequently (e.g., "The lady *who bought a hat* went to the party.").

Six- to seven-year-olds have generally developed use of the passive voice as well as embedded structures in sentences.

Morphology The six- to seven-year-old child shows consistent use of most morphological markers. She is beginning to produce **gerunds** (verbs to which -ing is added to produce a form that fulfills a noun function; e.g., *fish—fishing*). She is also using **derivational morphemes**, where verbs are changed into nouns (e.g., "teach" becomes "teacher"). Most of the time, the child uses irregular comparatives (*good, better, best*) correctly. There is continued improvement in correct usage of irregular past and plural forms.

Pragmatic As any parent can tell you, the six- to seven-year-old tends to use slang and mild profanity (as modeled by members of her peer group). She is aware of mistakes in other people's speech. She can fairly consistently match her conversational style to the demands of the situation.

Seven to Nine Years

Semantics The seven- to nine-year-old enjoys telling stories and anecdotes. She can retell a story, keeping the main ideas in correct sequence. She anticipates story endings; for example, she is able to predict what will happen at the end of a story she hears. She uses some figurative language and describes things in detail. She readily verbalizes problems and ideas.

Seven- to nine-year-olds verbalize readily, use predominantly complex sentence forms, and use appropriate discourse styles with their interlocutors.

Syntax and Morphology The seven- to nine-year-old uses predominantly complex sentence forms. She uses most irregular verb forms correctly, although may make mistakes on irregular past tense verbs. She correctly uses adverbs on a regular basis.

Pragmatics The seven- to nine-year-old determines and uses appropriate discourse codes and styles; for example, she is informal with friends and formal with adults. More care is taken in communicating with unfamiliar people; topic shifts are announced. Generally, there is appropriate use of nonlinguistic/nonverbal behaviors—posture and gestures are appropriate to the situation. The seven- to nine-year-old initiates and maintains conversation in small groups. She is able to consistently take the listener's point of view.

An eight-year-old can sustain a topic through a number of conversational turns, but her topics tend to be concrete. Nine-year-olds will usually appear to be capable of repairing communication breakdowns; they can define terms, provide background context, and monitor their own communication. After age eleven, discussions involving abstract topics can be sustained.

CONNECT & EXTEND

Information regarding language development in school-age children and adolescents is detailed in Nippold, M.A. (1998), *Later language development: The school-age and adolescent years*. Austin, TX: Pro-Ed.

Education, Language, and Literacy Development in the School-Age Years

It is very important for SLPs who work with school-age children to not only be familiar with oral language milestones in the early years, but to also be familiar with language development expectations in the school-age years. When children enter school, they grow and change in a number of areas. Some of the major changes children undergo are as follows (McLaughlin, 2006; Morrison, 2003; Owens, 2001; Reed, 2005; Roseberry-McKibbin & Hegde, 2006; Woolfolk, 2004).

First, when a TD child enters kindergarten, she should have solid speaking and listening (**auditory-oral**) skills. Good auditory-oral skills are strongly related to learning to read and write. Research shows that children who have poor auditory-oral skills often have more difficulty learning to read and write. In Chapter 12 we will discuss the fact that in school, children receive little or no formal instruction in speaking and listening—schools expect that those skills have been mastered. But some students have not mastered those skills, especially listening skills. In Chapters 6 and 12, we will discuss some specific strategies that professionals can use to help these children develop their listening skills.

Hopefully, during the preschool years, children have had good exposure to prereading and prewriting skills and activities (e.g., coloring, being read to, etc.). This exposure impacts a child's development of *emergent literacy* or *preliteracy skills* that are foundational to later reading and writing in school. In the last decade in the United States, there has been a much greater emphasis on literacy skills at the preschool level. Some preschools now actively teach the alphabet, for example. The child who has not attended preschool may be at a distinct disadvantage in kindergarten. When my son started kindergarten in a California public school, children in his class were expected to walk in the door on the first day knowing their colors, shapes, numbers, and letters. All these basic concepts were reviewed only very briefly the first few weeks of school.

In kindergarten, teachers work on strengthening children's oral language skills. They also address basic reading and writing. In some states, such as California, children are expected to be able to write short paragraphs by the end of kindergarten and read simple books. In other states, reading and writing are postponed till first grade. In many states, kindergarteners are asked to learn basic computer skills.

In first grade, teachers focus more heavily on reading and writing although there is still work on oral language skills as well. Children are expected to do math problems involving addition and subtraction, and some teachers also introduce two-digit numbers at this time. Research shows that first grade is a very important time for children; children who have difficulty in first grade usually have difficulty in the later grades also. Early intervention is critical for children who are struggling in first grade (Woolfolk, 2004).

Second-grade teachers emphasize increased skill in reading and writing. Independent reading is encouraged, and children also learn to spell. They are expected to develop independent word-recognition skills and to comprehend more abstract language. Third grade is a transition grade where children are expected to read longer, more complex stories and write longer, more complex paragraphs. They are asked to proofread and correct their written work as well as spell more complicated words. Most children learn cursive writing in third grade.

In grades four through six, children go from "learning to read and write" to "reading and writing to learn." The emphasis shifts from a focus on *how to* read and write to using reading and writing as tools for learning more about content areas such as social studies and science. Students often have to write reports. By sixth grade, a child should understand about 50,000 words. It is in grades four through six that children with language impairments are often identified. This is because their weak auditory-oral and written language skills do not serve as a strong enough foundation to help them learn information in content areas such as social studies. For example, if a child is struggling with the skills of listening, speaking, reading, and writing, she will have difficulty reading about the continent of Australia, writing a report on it, and presenting her report to the class.

In junior high and high school, teachers generally lecture and students must take notes on what they hear. There may be a different teacher for each subject. Students are tested frequently. Written language becomes extremely important. A high school student should understand about 80,000 words.

 SUMMARY

- Children develop language based upon their innate characteristics, the environment they are exposed to, and expectations of their particular cultures.
- Caretaker-child interactions vary between cultures, and these interactions play a major role in shaping a child's developing language. Mainstream US clinicians expect that a high level of verbosity is the ideal goal for a child; not all cultures agree with this, and caretakers interact with children accordingly.
- The development of semantic, syntactics, morphological, and pragmatics skills depends in large part upon the above factors. Each child develops at his individual rate, and variation among children is to be expected.
- When a child enters school, she ideally has well-developed auditory-oral skills and preliteracy skills. These are critical to later success in reading and writing. In fourth grade, children stop learning to read and write and begin writing and reading to learn. Children with language disorders are often identified between fourth and sixth grade.

Add your own summary points here:

_____

_____

_____

CHAPTER HIGHLIGHTS

- Language is a system of symbols used to represent concepts that are formed through exposure and experience. Children from CLD backgrounds have diverse experiences that impact their language acquisition.
- Various theories of language development provide the foundational underpinnings for assessment and treatment of children with language problems. Key theories that have influenced clinical practice include the behaviorist theory (B.F. Skinner), the nativist theory (Noam Chomsky), the cognitive theory (Jean Piaget), the social interactionism theory (Lev Vygotsky), and the information processing theory.
- The behaviorist theory, proposed by Skinner, explained language acquisition as the development of verbal behavior. He suggested that learning, not an innate unobservable

mechanism such as the Language Acquisition Device, played a major role in children's acquisition of language. He emphasized the importance of the environment.

- According to Chomsky's nativist theory, children are born with a Language Acquisition Device that contains the universal rules of language. Chomsky described concepts of language competence and language performance as well as the concepts of deep and surface structure.

- Advocates of the cognitive theory (Piaget) state that cognition and intellectual processes make language acquisition possible. Piaget, a supporter of the strong cognition hypothesis, said that children pass through four overlapping developmental cognitive stages: the sensorimotor, preoperational, concrete operations, and formal operations stages.

- Vygotsky's social interactionism theory emphasized language function over language structure. Vygotsky believed that language develops as a function of social interaction between a child and his environment (including significant others in that environment). He stressed the role of the child's motivation in language acquisition.

- Information-processing theorists view the human information-processing system as a mechanism that encodes stimuli from the environment, operates on interpretations of those stimuli, stores the results in memory, and permits retrieval of previously stored information.

- A child's language development depends upon several major interacting variables: the child's innate characteristics, her environment, the expectations of her cultural milieu, and cultural expectations for a child's developing language.

- There are language developmental milestones that clinicians can use to guide their expectations about language characteristics of children at certain chronological ages. However, there is a great deal of individual variability among children, and developmental milestones can only serve as a *general* frame of reference. Children's time of arrival at various language milestones depends heavily on their cultural and linguistic background.

Add your own chapter highlights here:

_____

_____

_____

_____

STUDY AND REVIEW QUESTIONS

ESSAY

1. When evaluating the role of the environment in a child's development of language, what must we remember about how other cultures may differ from mainstream US culture with regard to a baby's primary caregivers?

2. In the United States we believe it is important for children to be verbose, to have a large vocabulary, etc. What child language characteristics might other cultures value? Give several examples.

3. Contrast the nativist theory with the behaviorist theory of language development. How do these two theories differ?

4. Discuss how a clinician whose therapy is based on social interactionism might motivate a child from the Samoan culture to talk more in therapy sessions.

5. Briefly describe the syntactic skills of a TD child between two and three years of age.

FILL-IN-THE-BLANK

6. _____ is a system of symbols used to represent concepts that are formed through exposure and experience.

7. _____ proposed the nativist theory, which stated that children are born with a(n) _____, a specialized language processor that is a physiological part of the brain.

8. _____ are imitative verbal responses whose stimuli are the speech of another person.

9. Psychologist B.F. Skinner proposed the _____ theory of language acquisition and said that verbal behaviors are acquired under appropriate conditions of _____, _____, and _____.

10. Social interactionism theory, associated with Russian psychologist _____, focuses on language _____ rather than language _____.

MULTIPLE CHOICE

11. You are evaluating the language of a five-year-old who says, "Him can't eat cookies." This is an example of
    a. Four words, five morphemes, personal prounoun + negative + verb + plural noun
    b. Four words, six morphemes, modal + negative + verb + auxiliary
    c. Four words, four morphemes, personal pronoun + copula + negative + noun
    d. Four words, five morphemes, negative + personal pronoun + copula
    e. Four words, five morphemes, personal pronoun + auxiliary + negative + plural noun

12. Halliday described seven functions of communicative intent that develop between nine and eighteen months of age. Which of the following is an example of a child using the *heuristic* function?
    a. Yummy cookie!
    b. I want juice.
    c. Why airplane fly?
    d. Hi Mommy.
    e. I go store.

13. A child says "red crayon." This is an example of which type of semantic relations?
    a. Action + locative
    b. Agent + action
    c. Possession + attribute
    d. Attribute + entity
    e. Attribute + action

14. An example of a sentence using an embedded form would be
    a. I saw the squirrel climbing the tree.
    b. The girl ate a cookie, three crackers, and some fruit.
    c. Mom and Dad are going to the store to buy some groceries.
    d. Because he was on time, they were happy with him.
    e. The boy who got a haircut looks nice.

15. Which one of the following does NOT occur between eight and ten months of age in the TD child?
    a. Comprehension of "no"
    b. Using the phrase "all gone" to express emerging negation
    c. Using variegated babbling (e.g., "madamada")
    d. Uncovering a hidden toy (beginning of object permanence)
    e. Use of gestural language such as shaking head "no," playing peek-a-boo

See Answers to Study and Review Questions, page 465.

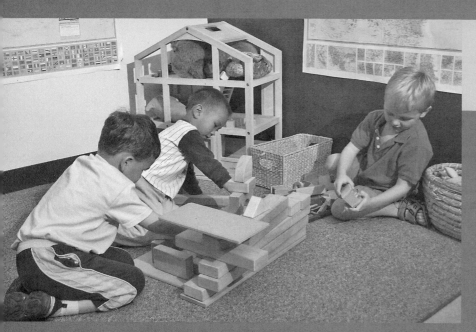

The Impact of Second Language Acquisition and Bilingualism on Children's Developing Language

CASE STUDY

Mr. F., the fifth-grade teacher, thought Mona had a problem. He told me that she did not contribute much to class discussions and couldn't keep up with the class assignments. He said she especially struggled with science and social studies. Retention was being considered.

Upon doing some research, I found that Mona and her family had come to the Sacramento area from the Philippines a year and a half ago. Mona had immediately been put into an all-English-speaking fourth-grade classroom, with little outside support. Thankfully, she did work with Jocelyn R., a district Filipino Bilingual As-

sociate, once or twice a week. Ms. R., an experienced employee, helped Mona with her classwork and taught her in both Ilocano and English.

When I spoke with Ms. R., she said Mona did an "excellent" job in Ilocano—spoke with age-appropriate complexity and fluency, and understood directions and instructions. I asked Ms. R. this question: in the five to ten years you have been in this school district, how does Mona compare to the other several hundred Filipino children you have worked with? Does she learn readily like they do, or does she seem 'slow' to you?" Ms. R. said that in comparison to Filipino peers, Mona "keeps up and does well." She said that in her opinion, Mona just needed more time to learn English. She said that Mona had both Filipino and American friends and had excellent interpersonal skills; it was academic English that gave her difficulty.

When I spoke with Mona's mother on the phone, she said that Mona "did a very good job in the Philippines" (in school). She said that Mona had good language comprehension and expression in Ilocano and also in Tagalog (the other language spoken in the home). According to Ms. T., Mona met her language development milestones in Tagalog and Ilocano in a timely manner. She said Mona's main problem was understanding the fifth-grade English assignments she brought home.

When I fetched Mona from her classroom to assess her, she was friendly and courteous. During the assessment (Ms. R. did the Ilocano portion and I did the English portion) I noticed that Mona did an excellent job communicating meaning in English. She sequenced stories appropriately and described things to me in adequate detail. Her pragmatics skills were quite good. I did notice a number of grammatical "errors" in English that I knew (from growing up in the Philippines myself) were directly traceable to the influence of Ilocano and Tagalog (I was exposed to both those languages myself).

Extensive assessment in English and Ilocano revealed that Mona was developing well and progressing along typical timelines for a learner of English as a third language. She was not placed into speech-language therapy; however, she was placed in an additional non–special education support service to help her gain more facility in her English vocabulary and academic skills. I also recommended that the services of Ms. R. continue so that Mona's Ilocano skills could be supported and so that she would not experience too much language loss in Ilocano.

INTRODUCTION

When assessing a child for a possible specific language impairment (SLI), it is necessary to understand typical language behavior as a frame of reference (Roseberry-McKibbin, 2008). A major challenge confronting professionals is that typical language behavior varies widely even among monolingual children. When working with culturally and linguistically diverse (CLD) students who are learning English as a second language, the picture becomes far more complex. In order to avoid an inappropriate diagnosis of SLI, it is important to recognize typical second-language acquisition and bilingualism phenomena (Restrepo & Kruth, 2000).

When a child's language is characterized or impacted by one or more of these phenomena, she can erroneously be labeled SLI when in fact she is a typically developing (TD) bilingual learner who displays a **language difference**, not an SLI. Windsor and Kohnert (2004) describe children with SLI as having " . . . some breach in their internal language processing system . . . the poorer language skills cannot be attributed to observable differences in language input" (p. 878).

Many errors in assessment and diagnosis can be avoided if speech-language pathologists (SLPs) are aware of normal second-language acquisition and bilingualism phenomena. In this chapter, relevant information is discussed to help the SLP learn to understand the experience of a TD CLD child. This information is divided into four major sections: language proficiency in the CLD child, normal processes in second language acquisition, cognitive-linguistic variables impacting second language acquisition, and affective variables impacting second language acquisition.

LANGUAGE PROFICIENCY IN CLD CHILDREN

Most CLD students are bilingual. A bilingual child has the ability to speak, listen, read, and/or write in more than one language with varying degrees of proficiency (Brice, 2002). Bilingual learners are quite heterogeneous, and each learner must be viewed individually according to his language history, measures of spontaneous language, and other parameters (DeGroot & Kroll, 1997; Gutierrez-Clellen, Calderon, & Ellis Weismer, 2004). Kohnert (2004) points out that not only is there significant variability *between* children learning two languages; there is also substantial variability *within* each child.

As Goldstein (2004, p. 7) puts it, " . . . acquiring one language is a life-long, complex task with great individual variation and a developmental trajectory that is not uniform; skills ebb and flow over time." Language proficiency is a complex phenomenon that has been defined in a variety of ways. In this section, several models of language proficiency are described. When differentiating between a language difference and an SLI, knowledge of what constitutes proficiency in the two languages is critical.

Separate Underlying Proficiency versus Common Underlying Proficiency

Cummins (1992, 2000) described the ***Separate Underlying Proficiency*** (SUP) and the **Common Underlying Proficiency** (CUP) models. In the SUP model, proficiency in the first language is viewed as entirely separate from proficiency in the second language. Thus, skills learned in the first language will not transfer to the second language. One implication of this model is that language development activities in the first language will not enhance learning of a second language and vice versa.

Supporters of the CUP model have often tried to eradicate languages other than English by encouraging students and their families to speak English only. Children who learn English from models who lack proficiency in the language will speak the language as they hear it used in their environment. Supporters of the SUP model believe that exposure to poor language models in English will be more beneficial to the child in developing English language skills than a language environment in which only the first language is used.

> Some professionals believe in Separate Underlying Proficiency, a belief that holds that supporting one of the child's languages does not help the other.

Sadly, many professionals tell CLD parents to discontinue use of the primary language in the home and "just speak English." This may happen in other parts of the world, too—for example, in Flanders, speech pathologists may tell CLD parents to stop speaking their first language of English in the home and speak only Dutch (Houwer, 1999). Cummins (2000) talked about conducting a workshop in a large school district near Los Angeles. Several workshop participants shared that in their school districts, teachers were being instructed to not send Spanish books home for parents and children to read together. Teachers were also being told to discourage parents from reading to their children in Spanish and even refrain from speaking to their children in Spanish.

This advice is extremely deleterious on many levels. In terms of cognitive-linguistic skills, children benefit far more from a linguistically rich, proficient language model (usually the primary language) than from an impoverished, hesitant, perhaps even grammatically incorrect model of the second language.

Also, if a child's parents abruptly stop using the home language in favor of the second language, there can be profound emotional and psychological difficulties for both the child and the parents (Houwer, 1999). This is especially true if the child has an SLI (Restrepo & Gutierrez-Clellen, 2004). Despite this, supporters of the SUP model tell CLD parents to speak only the second language at home. And school districts nationwide overtly or covertly do not support the child's first language, believing that "the more English the better."

> Professionals who believe in the SUP model usually tell parents to stop speaking their first language in the home and speak only English.

There is no evidence at all to support the SUP model (Cummins, 1992, 2000). As children learn their first language, they acquire concepts and strategies that will facilitate the learning of a second language. Concepts are acquired through interaction with the environment, and the nature of this interaction may vary from culture to culture. High-quality exposure enhances the learning of concepts that are important for cognitive and linguistic development. As children hear and use their native language in a variety of contexts, they develop the conceptual knowledge and cognitive strategies necessary for success in acquiring new information and linguistic skills (Baker, 2000; Coltrane, 2003; Gibbons, 2002; Owens, 2004).

CONNECT & EXTEND

Second language acquisition and bilingual development are explained in detail in Cummins, J. (2000). *Language, power, and pedagogy: Bilingual children in the crossfire.* Clevedon, England: Multilingual Matters.

Cummins (1992) described the CUP model as an alternative to the SUP model (see Figure 3.1). In describing the CUP model, Cummins stated that " . . . the literacy-related aspects of a bilingual's proficiency in L1 and L2 are seen as common or interdependent across languages . . . experience with either language can promote development of the proficiency underlying both languages, given adequate motivation and exposure to both either in school or in the wider environment" (1992, p. 23–25).

POINTS TO PONDER Discuss the negative ramifications of the Separate Underlying Proficiency (SUP) model for CLD students. If professionals subscribe to the SUP model, what kinds of mistakes might they make when working with CLD students?

_____

_____

_____

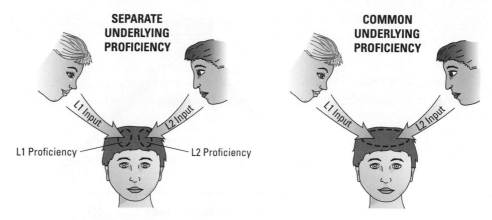

FIGURE 3.1   Two Models of Language Proficiency

Adapted from Cummins, J. (1992). The role of primary language development in promoting educational success of language minority students. In *California State Department of Education Schooling and language minority students: A theoretical framework.*

This underlying proficiency is that which is involved in cognitively demanding communicative tasks, and it is interdependent across languages.

> According to the Common Underlying Proficiency model, underlying proficiency for demanding communicative tasks is interdependent across languages.

For example, ample research supports a strong correlation between reading skills in the first and second language; the better the reading skills in the first language, the better will be the reading skills in the second language (Cummins, 2000; Kayser, 2004; Walqui, 2000; Zecker, 2004). Also, the student who does not read in the first language at all is likely to have a more difficult time reading in English than the student who reads fluently in the first language (Kayser, 2004; Ramirez, Yuen, & Ramey, 1991).

The CUP model has major implications for SLPs working with CLD students. If a student has had limited exposure and experience in the first language, the conceptual foundation necessary for success in the classroom will be underdeveloped. Many experts (e.g., Baker, 2000; Coltrane, 2003; Cummins, 2002; Gibbons, 2002) recommend strengthening the foundation in the first language before instruction is attempted in the second language. Negative cognitive consequences may result if efforts are made to switch the child to English before the first language is fully developed (see Figure 3.2).

> Ideally, CLD students will be exposed to English when they have a strong foundation in their first language.

Using the second language for instruction when the first language has not yet been fully developed is like building a house on an unstable foundation. By building a solid foundation in the first language, the child acquires concepts and strategies that will facilitate learning another language. Research has shown that children who possess first-language literacy skills perform much better academically in American schools than children who do not have literacy skills in

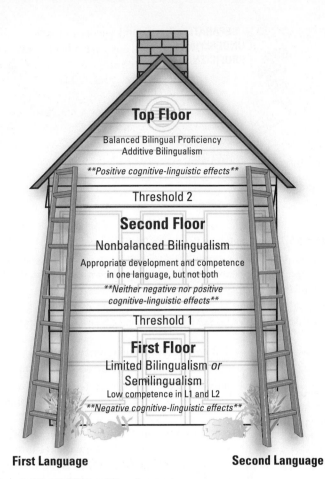

Top Floor

Balanced Bilingual Proficiency
Additive Bilingualism

Positive cognitive-linguistic effects

Threshold 2

Second Floor

Nonbalanced Bilingualism

Appropriate development and competence
in one language, but not both

***Neither negative nor positive
cognitive-linguistic effects***

Threshold 1

First Floor

Limited Bilingualism *or*
Semilingualism

Low competence in L1 and L2

Negative cognitive-linguistic effects

First Language   **Second Language**

FIGURE 3.2   Thresholds of Bilingual Development

Used with permission. From Roseberry-McKibbin, C. (2008) *Multicultural students with special language needs: Practical strategies for assessment and intervention* (3rd edition), Oceanside, CA: Academic Communication Associates, Inc.

> Professionals should support the child's continued development of the first language, ensuring a strong foundation upon which to build second language competence.

their first languages (Garcia, 1999; Ramirez et al.,1991; Zecker, 2004). By suddenly switching the child to a new language, school professionals deprive students of opportunities to make use of their previously acquired knowledge when confronted with learning situations in the classroom. When children have difficulty relating new experiences to what they already know, learning is a slow process.

Rather than eradicate the first language, professionals should encourage students to become fluent bilingual speakers. If they develop high levels of proficiency in the first and second languages, students may experience growth in various cognitive skills that have

CONNECT & EXTEND

Biliteracy in young children is described in the research of Zecker, L.B. (2004). Learning to read and write in two languages: The development of early biliteracy abilities. In C.A. Stone, E.R. Silliman, B.J. Ehren, & K. Apel (Eds.), *Handbook of language and literacy: Development and disorders* (pp. 248–265). New York: The Guilford Press.

been associated with success in school. Children who speak two or more languages fluently have been found to outperform monolingual children in some cognitive and linguistic tasks (Baker, 2000; Thomas & Collier, 1998; Woolfolk, 2004).

Research shows that bilingual children younger than six years of age tend to outperform monolingual children on isolated tasks of metalinguistic awareness related to reading (Garcia, 1999; Garcia, Jimenez, & Pearson, 1998). Bialystok (1997) found that four- and five-year-old bilingual preschoolers in Canada (French-English and Mandarin-English speakers) outperformed monolingual English-speaking preschoolers on a metalinguistic task related to beginning reading. Bialystok (2001) showed that bilingual children had an advantage in performing a variety of cognitive tasks when selective attention was required during information processing so that misleading information was inhibited in favor of relevant information.

The ramifications for CLD students in the schools are clear. If a student is struggling academically or not learning English as rapidly as would be expected, the SLP might suspect that the student has an SLI. However, it can be seen from the above discussion that limited progress in school is often due, at least in part, to incompletely developed skills in the first language and lack of opportunities for continued development of skills in that language. Thomas and Collier (1998) found that one of the three key predictors of academic success for CLD students is English language support through subject areas in conjunction with support in the first language. Most CLD students in the United States do not receive this type of support.

To experience optimal success in school, CLD students need continuous support in their first language as well as in English.

Thomas and Collier (1998) stated that the average English speaker generally gains ten months of academic growth in a ten-month school year. Second-language learners must outgain native speakers by making one and one-half years' progress on academic tests in English for six successive school years. Thus, in order to perform at a level commensurate with that of native speakers, CLD students must make

POINTS TO PONDER Discuss the advantages of being bilingual. What happens to CLD students when their first language is not supported and developed along with English?

_____

_____

_____

nine years' progress in six years. It is no wonder that US schools create deficits in students that are not caused by SLI, but rather by an educational system that does not even begin to adequately meet the needs of CLD students. This is an especially important consideration in cases where the student is a sequential bilingual learner.

Simultaneous Language Acquisition versus Sequential Language Acquisition

Bhatia and Ritchie (1999) remind us that we have to understand the *pattern* of exposure to both languages that a child has received in order to truly understand her bilingual development. Broadly, patterns of exposure to two languages can be characterized as involving simultaneous or sequential language acquisition.

Patterson and Pearson (2004) describe a simultaneous bilingual learner as one who has had significant input in two languages before she is three years old. A student who has experienced **simultaneous acquisition** of two languages from infancy and has learned these two languages in naturalistic situations seems to experience minimal interference between the languages. These children commonly manifest generally equivalent levels of proficiency in both the first and second language.

> Simultaneous learners acquire two languages from birth, while sequential learners are exposed to one language at birth and learn the second language later in childhood.

Children who experience **sequential acquisition** are introduced to the first language as infants and learn the second language later in childhood (Kayser, 2002). Patterson and Pearson define a sequential learner as a child whose major exposure to a second language occurs after three years of age, after a great deal of learning of the first language has taken place.

Sequential bilingual learners experience some variation in the quality and quantity of acquisition of the two languages (Kohnert, 2002; Kan & Kohnert, 2005) and show greater diversity in rates and stages of language acquisition (Kayser, 2002; Owens, 2004). Regarding learning two languages, Gutierrez-Clellen, Restrepo, Bedore, Peña, & Anderson (2000, p. 89) state that

CONNECT & EXTEND

A research study examining sequential learning in CLD children was conducted by Kan, P.F., & Kohnert, K. (2005). Preschoolers learning Hmong and English: Lexical-semantic skills in L1 and L2. *Journal of Speech, Language, and Hearing Research, 48,* 372–383.

> The timing and process of acquisition of the language(s) has important implications for the assessment of a child's language development. Children with limited exposure to a second language (L2) or whose native language exposure was interrupted when an L2 was introduced may not perform the same as children who were raised learning two languages from birth.

Some students acquire the second language with minimal difficulty, while others experience problems. Students tend to experience more difficulty when the second language is introduced before there is a solid foundation in the first language. If the second language is introduced while the child is still developing the first language, the development of the first language may be arrested or even regress while the child is focused on learning the second language (Schiff-Myers, 1992; Owens, 2004). Sequential learners may also have challenges with traditional assessment measures (Windsor & Kohnert, 2004). This is explained further in Chapter 5.

Children who are not competent in either their first or second language have been described as being in a state of **semilingualism** or **limited bilingualism** (Portes & Rumbaut, 2001; Skutnabb-Kangas & Toukomaa, 1976). These terms are not as widely used today. Genesee et al. (2004, pp. 142–143) describe why these terms should be avoided:

> Many researchers and practitioners working with L2 [language 2] children have noticed that some of these children can go through a transitional period when their L1 [language 1] ability has declined considerably and rapidly, but their L2 ability is nowhere near complete or native-like. This transitional period has often been labeled semilingualism. . . . . [This term is] very controversial because it implies that the child is in a kind of a linguistic vacuum from which there may be no escape. . . . The concept of semilingualism is misleading because it is often taken as a description of a state that all early bilinguals are in, possibly forever. This is usually not the case. . . . [Children's] L1 abilities do not decline so precipitously that they could validly be deemed to lack functional competence in that language, and their L2 abilities usually increase sufficiently during the transition period that they are proficient enough in the L2 to satisfy their interpersonal communication needs.

If a CLD student is in the transitional phase as described by Genesee et al. (2004), where the second language has been introduced in a sequential situation where the first language is not well developed, the student will probably obtain low test scores in both English and her first language, thus appearing to have an SLI (Gopaul-McNichol & Armour-Thomas, 2002). This is especially common when a second language is introduced when the child is in preschool. I have received many e-mails and phone calls from concerned SLPs who worked with preschool children who appeared to be weak in both their first language and English. It is important not to misdiagnose these sequential bilingual learners as having SLI when they are probably merely displaying normal characteristics of sequential bilingual learning.

> Sequential bilingual learners may have more challenges than simultaneous bilingual learners.

Generally, it is considered ideal for a child to be exposed to two languages from birth onward. If the child is exposed to only one language at birth, some researchers believe it is best to wait until the child is between five and six years of age before introducing a second language. Coltrane (2003, pp. 1–2) states that

> For children younger than 5, many aspects of their first language have not yet fully developed. So while older learners have the foundation of a fully developed first language when they begin acquiring a new language, younger English language learners are working toward two milestones at the same time: the full development of their native language and the acquisition of English. . . . . Educators must keep in mind that young children do not have a fully developed native language on which to base the learning of a second.

Ideally, eventually the child will be proficient in both the first and second language. In these cases, the child is said to experience additive bilingualism.

Additive and Subtractive Bilingualism

Additive bilingualism is defined as achievement of high levels of proficiency in the first and second languages. The student's first language is not eradicated; rather, it is nurtured and encouraged, and continues to grow throughout the school experience. The student also achieves a high level of second language proficiency, thus becoming a fluent and balanced bilingual. This is the ideal for all students. By becoming fully bilingual, individuals develop high-level metalinguistic skills as we described earlier in this chapter. Bilingual individuals enhance their employability and increase their potential for making valuable contributions to society (Coltrane, 2003; Genesee et al., 2004). In today's global economy, bilingualism is a great asset. In many parts of the world, multilingual individuals are considered educated and cosmopolitan (Roseberry-McKibbin, 2008). Being a fluent bilingual individual has many advantages (Zentella, 2002).

> Additive bilingualism is an ideal situation where the student is a balanced and proficient speaker of more than one language.

What occurs much more frequently is **subtractive bilingualism**, a situation in which a student's first language is replaced by the second language. Acquisition of the majority language comes at the cost of the minority language (Genesee et al., 2004). In this situation, language loss in the first language occurs, and the student gradually becomes a monolingual speaker of English or the majority language. However, if English skills continue to be limited, the student's cognitive and linguistic growth is likely to be negatively affected. One can see how students who struggle academically and linguistically, then, may not actually have an SLI; rather, they may be normal learners who have simply experienced subtractive bilingualism, consequent negative cognitive effects, and reduced conceptual foundation on which to build academic and linguistic skills (Owens, 2004; Roseberry-McKibbin, 2003).

Children who are sequential language learners and belong to a minority ethnolinguistic community may be especially vulnerable to experiencing subtractive bilingualism. Genesee et al. (2004) explain that bilingual children can differ from one another on a very important parameter: whether they belong to a majority or minority ethnolinguistic community. A **majority ethnolinguistic community** is one where the language has high social status and is widely used. Typically the language has institutional support from the government. It is the language of business. Speakers of Mainstream American English in the United States are members of a majority ethnolinguistic community.

In the Philippines, Tagalog is the national language. A person from the Visayan Islands who learns Hiligaynon will be taught Tagalog in school so he can be a member of the majority ethnolinguistic community. In the little town of Odiongan where my family lived for a while, we spoke the local dialect of Odionganon. Church services were conducted in Hiligaynon, and in school we were taught Tagalog as part of the curriculum. In Germany, Hoch Deutsch is the language of business and government. Children who come to school speaking Schweitzer Deutsch (a dialect of German) must learn Hoch Deutsch to become members of the majority ethnolinguistic community.

A **minority ethnolinguistic community** is one in which the language has lower social status, is less widely spoken and valued, may be associated with little socioeconomic power, and may receive little or no institutional support. Genesee et al. give the examples

> Students who experience subtractive bilingualism often struggle in school because they are not strong in either the first or the second language.

of speakers of Cantonese in Canada, Spanish-speaking children in the United States, and Turkish-speaking children in Germany as members of minority ethnolinguistic communities. Hammer, Miccio, and Rodriguez (2004) make the point that for Spanish-speaking children in the United States, it can be a struggle for the parents to maintain the children's Spanish skills because the schools provide little or no support for maintenance of Spanish.

When working with CLD students, SLPs must take these language proficiency factors into account. TD language learners who have experienced subtractive bilingualism and consequent reduced proficiency in both languages do not need special education; they need assistance in the first language to enhance conceptual development (Coltrane, 2003). They also need comprehensible second-language input and interactive experiences that will promote communicative competence. Table 3.1 on page 78 is an example of a checklist that SLPs can use to evaluate a CLD student's conceptual development.

Comprehensible Input

It is important to provide CLD students with **comprehensible input** in English (Coltrane, 2003; Krashen, 1992). CLD students are often placed in "sink or swim" situations where they speak only their primary language, and classes are all conducted in English. The students do not understand what they hear, and thus fall behind academically. The reader can imagine traveling to the Philippines and going into a classroom

> Students must receive comprehensible input in the classroom in order to succeed academically.

where history is taught in the language of Hiligaynon. The class would be incomprehensible, and the reader would learn nothing but would be responsible for the material. As ludicrous as this sounds, this type of situation occurs routinely, daily, in US schools. School personnel expect CLD children to understand what they hear, make sense of it, and succeed academically.

Krashen's input hypothesis proposes that people acquire language by understanding messages (Krashen, 1992). The learner's focus is on the meaning of what is heard rather than on the grammatical form. According to Krashen, optimal comprehensible input in the second language includes the following characteristics:

1. It occurs naturally; the learner has practice opportunities in natural, conversational, everyday situations that are communicatively meaningful.
2. There are available, concrete referents such as visuals and hands-on materials.
3. The input is interesting, meaningful, and relevant to the learner.
4. The input is not grammatically sequenced, but rather occurs naturally.
5. There are sufficient quantities of this input to ensure optimal learning.

Experts believe that comprehensible input alone is not enough to help the CLD student succeed; the student must also be an active agent in his environment in terms of language output and interaction with others (Baker, 2000; Coltrane, 2003; Garcia, 1999; Walqui, 2000).

TABLE 3.1   Linguistic and Conceptual Development Checklist

Student's Name:_____ Date of Birth: _____ Chronological Age: _____
Language Spoken: _____

Questions	Yes	No	Don't Know
• Has the child been regularly exposed to L1 literacy-related materials?	____	____	____
• Is the child's vocabulary in the first language well-developed?	____	____	____
• Was the child's L1 fluent and well-developed when s/he began learning English?	____	____	____
• Have the child's parents been encouraged to speak and/or read in L1 at home?	____	____	____
• Has the child's L1 been maintained in school through bilingual education, L1 tutoring, and/or other L1 maintenance activities?	____	____	____
• Does the child show interest in L1 maintenance and interaction?	____	____	____
• Is the English classroom input comprehensible to the child?	____	____	____
• Does the child have frequent opportunities for negotiating meaning and practicing comprehensible output in English?	____	____	____
• Has the child had frequent exposure to enriching experiences such as going to museums, libraries, etc.?	____	____	____
• Has the child's school attendance been regular?	____	____	____
• Has the child had long-term exposure to standard English models?	____	____	____

The more "yes" answers that are checked, the more likely it is that the child has a good conceptual foundation for language and academic learning. The more "no" answers that are checked, the more likely it is that the child has underdeveloped conceptual and linguistic abilities due to limitations within the school and/or home environment, language loss, limited English practice opportunities, inadequate bilingual services, or a combination of these factors.

Used with permission. From Roseberry-McKibbin, C. (2008) *Multicultural students with special language needs: Practical strategies for assessment and intervention* (3rd edition), Oceanside, CA: Academic Communication Associates, Inc.

CASES TO CONSIDER

Falda was referred to me for speech-language testing by her sixth-grade teacher, who was afraid that "Falda just won't cut it academically in junior high school. I think she needs special education." I examined the contents of Falda's school file, which indicated that the family had come from Saudi Arabia two years ago and spoke primarily Arabic, although there was some mention of English. What questions would you want to ask about Falda's exposure to Arabic and English? What do you need to find out about her school situation in Saudi Arabia and the United States?

_____

_____

_____

The main point is that the CLD student must understand what he is hearing in the classroom and be able to make sense of it so he can be an active interactor in the classroom environment. If CLD students are not understanding the English that they hear, they will not develop optimal English proficiency and they may even appear SLI.

Thus, when a CLD student is referred for SLI assessment because she is struggling academically, SLPs can ask if the classroom language is comprehensible to the student. If it isn't, the student's difficulties may stem directly from a lack of comprehension and consequent reduced success in the classroom setting. This is illustrated by the case of Falda (above).

Developing Bilingual Language Proficiency

Monolingual Norm Assumption

Some US citizens have a negative attitude toward bilingualism and believe that being bilingual has negative cognitive and social effects on children (Houwer, 1999). Malakoff & Hakuta (1991, p. 141) described the **monolingual norm assumption**: the belief that monolingualism is the cognitive-linguistic norm and that the child's cognitive system is fragile and only designed to cope with one language.

Genesee et al. (2004) call this belief the **limited capacity hypothesis**: the belief that the language faculty has a limited capacity, so acquiring two languages is problematic. They describe this further as the belief that a child's underlying mental capacity for learning language is like a balloon that can only contain so much air; when the balloon gets bigger as a result of acquiring one language, there is limited space to acquire another language.

> Many Americans believe that bilingualism is damaging to children and that monolingualism is the norm.

The monolingual norm assumption/limited capacity hypothesis has given rise to the negative myths surrounding bilingualism: bilingualism has been blamed for cognitive, social, and emotional damage to children (Houwer, 1999). For example, when I was pregnant, I told an SLP friend of mine that I hoped to find a Spanish-speaking part-time sitter so my son could be exposed to two languages from infancy. My friend exclaimed in horror: "What are you thinking? Won't that delay the baby's language skills?" The fact is that the United States is one of the only monolingual countries in the entire world. Citizens of most countries speak at least two languages. In many European countries, students cannot graduate from high school unless they speak three languages fluently.

Bilingual Education

In order to maintain students' first languages and also help them become proficient in the second language (English in the United States), ideally these students should participate in bilingual education throughout the elementary years and beyond if possible (Baker, 2000; Gibbons, 2002; Woolfolk, 2004). Such **maintenance bilingual education** provides students with culturally appropriate learning experiences, opportunities for continued use of the first language, and experiences designed to promote the learning and effective use of a second language.

Programs of bilingual education appear to promote the greatest linguistic, cultural, and cognitive benefits when there is active parent and community involvement (Coltrane, 2003). Cummins (2000) states that in his opinion, ideal bilingual programs take steps to develop both oral and written skills in both languages at early ages. He recommends having children read and write in both languages by at least second grade.

Cummins (2000) points out the irony that some bilingual education programs are considered prestigious, while others are not. For example, in California's Silicon Valley, there is a private school called the French-American School of Silicon Valley. Parents are urged to give their children the benefit and gift of bilingual education. However, as we have stated, some teachers of Spanish-speaking Mexican children near Los Angeles have been encouraged to tell parents not to speak Spanish or read in Spanish with their children in the home. As Cummins (2000, p. 16) states, "Bilingualism is good for the rich but bad for the poor."

It is indeed thought-provoking to realize that at least in some places, children from majority ethnolinguistic communities are encouraged to participate in bilingual education programs such as in the example above. Children in minority ethnolinguistic communities and their parents are told—implicitly or explicitly—that being bilingual is "bad" and that they should forsake their language and culture in exchange for those of the majority (Cummins, 2000; Genesee et al., 2004). Cummins (2000, p. 23) states that

> The very positive media picture of bilingual education for affluent children in countries around the world is similar to the way French immersion programs have typically been depicted in the Canadian context. These programs serve the interest of dominant middle-class majority language children. By contrast, when bilingual education aims to serve the interests of marginalized students from minority groups, the media appear to have extreme difficulty understanding the rationale for these programs.

Ideally, CLD students would experience maintenance bilingual education.

Most professionals are aware that the optimal situation of maintenance bilingual education rarely exists in school in the United States. Bilingual programs in US schools, when they do exist, are often transitional programs wherein the first language is used to teach academic subjects but an emphasis is placed on transitioning the student into English as quickly as possible.

Some schools have Sheltered English classrooms, where subject matter is taught in English that is comprehensible to students who are learning English. Some school programs do not have any support services at all. Thus, the question becomes one of helping CLD students to achieve language proficiency and academic success with resources that are often quite limited and perhaps even nonexistent. These students may develop conversational English skills, but struggle with more advanced, complex, academic English.

Basic Interpersonal Communication Skills (BICS) and Cognitive Academic Language Proficiency (CALP)

One useful model of language proficiency distinguishes **Basic Interpersonal Communication Skills** (BICS) from **Cognitive Academic Language Proficiency** (CALP). Some experts describe these skills as being on a continuum instead of being discrete and separate entities (Cummins, 2000; Genesee et al., 2004). This is the most accurate description of BICS and CALP; however, for ease of discussion here, I have used the terms BICS and CALP.

BICS take approximately two years (in an ideal situation) to develop to a level commensurate with that of native speakers of the language (Cummins 1992, 2002; Gibbons, 2002); CALP takes between five and seven years to develop to a nativelike level (Cummins, 2002; see Figure 3.3). This five-to seven-year time frame is common for students from enriched backgrounds. Some researchers are even positing that it can take up to seven to ten years for CALP to develop to a nativelike level under less than optimal conditions (Peregoy & Boyle, 1997). Cummins (2000, p. 13) described a conference where an Israeli speaker reported that in the Israeli context, a period of seven to nine years is typically required for immigrant students to catch up academically with native students.

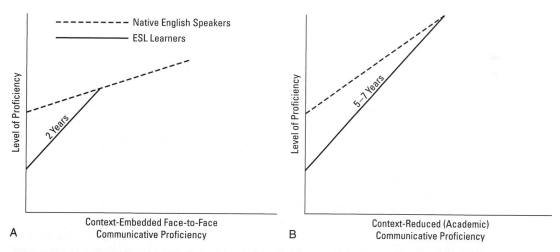

FIGURE 3.3   Length of Time Required to Achieve Age-Appropriate Levels of Context Embelled and Context Reduced Communicative Proficiency

Adapted from Cummins, J. (1992). The role of primary language development in promoty educational success of language minority students. In *California State Department of Education, Schooling and language minority students: A theoretical framework*. Reprinted with permission.

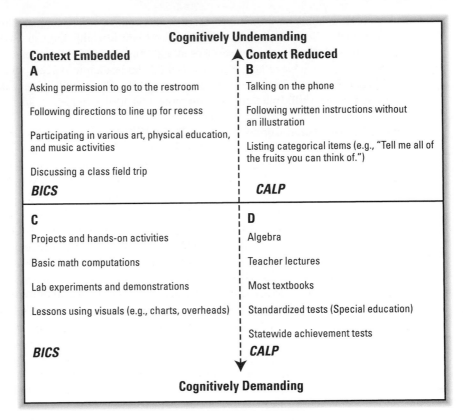

FIGURE 3.4   Illustration of Cummins' Grid of Cognitive Demands

Used with permission. From Roseberry-McKibbin, C. (2008) *Multicultural students with special language needs: Practical strategies for assessment and intervention* (3rd edition), Oceanside, CA: Academic Communication Associates, Inc.

Basic Interpersonal Communication Skills are cognitively undemanding, context-embedded forms of communication. Cognitive Academic Language Proficiency refers to the cognitively demanding, context-reduced forms of communication (see Figure 3.4). In **context-embedded communication**, participants can actively negotiate meaning and they have a shared reality.

> Basic Interpersonal Skills, or BICS, take two or three years to develop to a nativelike level. Cognitive Academic Language Proficiency, or CALP, takes at least five to seven years to develop to a nativelike level.

Context-embedded communication is typical of that found in the everyday world outside the classroom, where language is supported by a wide range of meaningful situational cues and paralinguistic gestures. Gestures and facial expressions facilitate the communication of meaning in context-embedded situations. For example, on the playground, some students may want to play tetherball and others may want to play tag instead. In the discussion, there is a shared reality, a concrete and visible situation, and facial expressions and gestures to accompany words (Roseberry-McKibbin, 2003).

Context-reduced communication, on the other hand, does not assume a shared reality. It may rely exclusively on linguistic cues for meaning (Cummins, 2002). For example, a teacher might discuss a field trip to the aquarium that will take place next week. For the CLD student, there is nothing to look at; there are no visible cues to support the teacher's words. The teacher's explanation is very hard to understand in this case.

Proficiency in context-reduced communication involves the ability to make complex meanings clear by means of language itself rather than by use of paralinguistic cues or contextual support (Cummins, 2000). Long-term academic success ultimately depends upon the ability to read about or express (verbally or in writing) complex, abstract ideas in the absence of past experience or contextual support (Genesee et al., 2004).

> Communication can be context embedded or context reduced.

Cognitive demands, in a communication situation, are related to the amount of information that a student needs to process simultaneously or in close succession in order to do an activity. **Cognitively undemanding** tasks are those that are generally automatized and require little active cognitive involvement for adequate performance.

For instance, a cognitively undemanding task for most people is to state their name and Social Security number when asked for this information. Cognitively demanding tasks, however, do not involve automatized where knowledge; the person must make use of various cognitive strategies to perform them. For example, writing an essay in a foreign language is cognitively demanding for a student who has not yet mastered that language. For the average reader of this book (if you are anything like me), advanced algebra and calculus are cognitively demanding.

> SLPs must ascertain whether the CLD student is exposed to communication that is cognitively undemanding or cognitively demanding.

Thus, when SLPs are assessing a student because of a suspected SLI, it is important to examine the school environment. Is the student in a classroom situation where cognitively demanding tasks are routinely presented? How much contextual information is available to facilitate comprehension? If the student has not yet acquired the cognitive academic skills necessary to complete classroom assignments, she will struggle in school and the teacher may erroneously suspect an SLI.

POINTS TO PONDER Describe BICS and CALP. How are these types of language proficiency different? Why is it so important to be aware of them when a CLD student is referred for assessment for a possible SLI?

_____

_____

_____

As was previously mentioned, students are often placed into submersion or sink-or-swim classrooms where only English is spoken and no special provisions are made to help them learn the English they need for school. Students who speak no English are often expected to learn English in the classroom setting where the linguistic input is often context reduced and cognitively demanding.

> Many CLD students struggle academically because their initial exposure to English is cognitively demanding and context reduced; these students may appear to be SLI when they are not.

Because a student's initial exposure to English is often of this nature, many students fail to acquire a solid conceptual foundation, and thus they struggle academically. The acquisition of CALP is difficult if the student's primary exposure to the language occurs within situations where contextual cues are limited. Helping students to develop a basic conceptual foundation is critical if they are to acquire the strategies necessary for academic success (Coltrane, 2003; Gibbons, 2002)

When SLPs make judgments about overall proficiency in English based on a student's performance in face-to-face communication situations (BICS), they risk creating academic

CASES TO CONSIDER

Phaiwanh L., a somewhat shy speaker of Khmer, was referred for assessment by her second-grade teacher, who said that Phaiwanh "just isn't keeping up with her classmates. I worry that she is slow." The SLP knew that Phaiwanh's strongest language was Khmer, but he did not request the services of an interpreter. Instead, he went to the classroom and spoke with Phaiwanh for fifteen minutes, using attractive picture books and a game to help Phaiwanh talk comfortably. Phaiwanh was flattered by the attention and spoke at length during the conversation. Although she made some grammatical errors, she communicated meaning very well, and the SLP was impressed by Phaiwanh's conversational skills. But because Phaiwanh was not progressing along with the rest of her monolingual English-speaking peers in math and science, the SLP decided to evaluate her for the presence of an SLI. He gave Phaiwanh several standardized tests in English. These tests presented Phaiwanh with such tasks as "Listen: **circus**. Tell me what that word means" and "Give me a word that means the same thing as "**large**." The SLP read Phaiwanh a ten-sentence paragraph about ice skating and then asked her to retell the story. Because the tasks were given in English and were cognitively demanding and context reduced, Phaiwanh achieved very low scores on each test. The special education team concluded that Phaiwanh had an SLI and placed her into special education.

What second-language and bilingualism phenomena influenced Phaiwanh's acquisition of English? How was her performance in the classroom and on the SLP's tests influenced by BICS and CALP? What mistakes did the teacher and SLP make?

_____

_____

_____

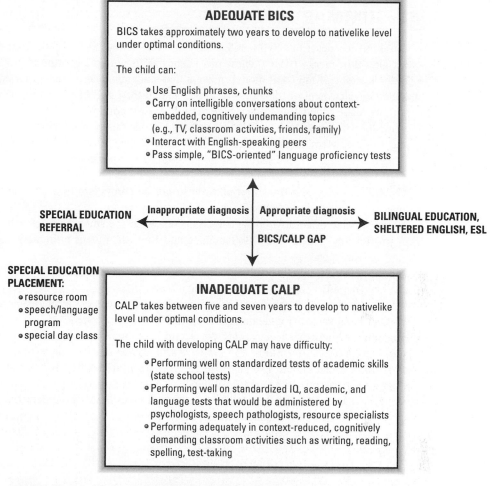

ADEQUATE BICS

BICS takes approximately two years to develop to nativelike level under optimal conditions.

The child can:

- Use English phrases, chunks
- Carry on intelligible conversations about context-embedded, cognitively undemanding topics (e.g., TV, classroom activities, friends, family)
- Interact with English-speaking peers
- Pass simple, "BICS-oriented" language proficiency tests

SPECIAL EDUCATION REFERRAL ← Inappropriate diagnosis | Appropriate diagnosis → **BILINGUAL EDUCATION, SHELTERED ENGLISH, ESL**

BICS/CALP GAP

SPECIAL EDUCATION PLACEMENT:
- resource room
- speech/language program
- special day class

INADEQUATE CALP

CALP takes between five and seven years to develop to nativelike level under optimal conditions.

The child with developing CALP may have difficulty:

- Performing well on standardized tests of academic skills (state school tests)
- Performing well on standardized IQ, academic, and language tests that would be administered by psychologists, speech pathologists, resource specialists
- Performing adequately in context-reduced, cognitively demanding classroom activities such as writing, reading, spelling, test-taking

FIGURE 3.5   Language Proficiency Misdiagnos is Model

Used with permission. From Roseberry-McKibbin, C. (2008) *Multicultural students with special language needs: Practical strategies for assessment and intervention* (3rd edition), Oceanside, CA: Academic Communication Associates, Inc.

deficits in these students. It is important to keep in mind that skill in BICS is acquired in about two years, but CALP takes much longer. Thus, a student may have good English conversational skill, and perform well in context-embedded and cognitively undemanding situations, but continue to face challenges in subjects such as social studies and science (see Figure 3.5).

It is important to not make the error of assessing a student for an SLI using tests that are context reduced and cognitively demanding when the student has only been exposed to English for one to two years. The student's adequate conversational skills do not mean that she can succeed with tasks such as answering questions after hearing a complicated story only one time with no accompanying visual cues. The example of Phaiwanh L. (see page 84) illustrates this type of mistake that SLPs commonly make.

SUMMARY

- Cummins has described Separate Underlying Proficiency (SUP) versus Common Underlying Proficiency (CUP). These proficiency skills are on a continuum.
- Ramifications of the CUP model indicate that students need to be supported in continued development of their first language so that they will have a strong conceptual and linguistic foundation upon which to build their second language of English.
- Students who experience simultaneous language acquisition of their first language and English seem to experience minimal interference between the two languages. Students who experience sequential acquisition may experience more variation in the quality and quantity of acquisition in the two languages.
- The child who is in a transition phase may not be competent in either the first language or English; she may experience difficulty in school.
- The ideal state of additive bilingualism occurs when the student achieves high levels of proficiency in both the first language and English. Fluent bilinguals experience many advantages.
- In subtractive bilingualism, the student's first language is replaced by English. This can have negative cognitive and linguistic effects.
- Ideally, students who are developing English should hear comprehensible input, or English input specially designed for English Language Learners.
- Students develop two basic kinds of second-language proficiency. Basic Interpersonal Communication Skills (BICS) represent day-to-day language that is context embedded; it takes about two years for a CLD student to develop appropriate BICS.
- Cognitive Academic Language Proficiency (CALP) refers to language that is context reduced, academic, and cognitively demanding. It takes the CLD student five to seven (or even 10) years to become proficient in CALP.

Add your own summary points here:

_____

_____

_____

NORMAL PROCESSES OF SECOND LANGUAGE ACQUISITION

Normal processes involved in acquiring a second language must be understood if one is to differentiate between a language difference and an SLI (Brice, 2002; Genesee et al., 2004; Saenz, 1996). Normal second-language acquisition processes often result in differences that can mask as symptoms of a communication disorder. These differences need to be recognized as normal behaviors for students who are not yet proficient in English. Some

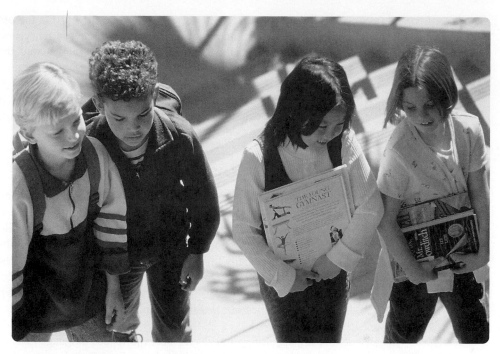

Acquisition of a second language is affected by many variables, including opportunities for interaction with native speakers of the second language.

of the most commonly observed processes are the silent period, language loss, language transfer, interlanguage, and codeswitching.

Silent Period

Some students, during the initial stages of learning a second language, go through a *silent period* in which there is much listening/comprehension and little output (Brice, 2002; Genesee et al., 2004; Krashen, 1992). It is believed that during this time, students are learning the rules of the language and focusing on comprehension. The silent period can last anywhere from three to six months, although this depends on the individual student.

The younger the child when she is exposed to the second language, the longer the silent period generally lasts (Tabors, 1997). SLPs might believe that a student has an expressive language delay, when in reality the student is focusing her attention on understanding the language.

Tabors (1997) gives the example of a child who came to the United States from Greece when he was two years old. His silent period lasted almost one and a half years as compared to six to eight weeks for several elementary-age children who began learning a second

> Many second-language learners go through an initial silent period, where they focus on comprehension of the second language.

CONNECT & EXTEND

An excellent, detailed description of the phenomena of bilingualism, second language acquisition, and language disorders can be found in Genesee, F., Paradis, J., & Crago, M.B. (2004). *Dual language development and disorders: A handbook on bilingualism and second language learners.* Baltimore, MD: Brookes Publishing Co.

language at five and six years old respectively. On the other hand, I know a Ukrainian family whose daughter was ten years old when they came to the United States. The mother shared that the girl spoke little in either language for a whole year but is now performing successfully in school. If a teacher refers a student who is "not talking like she should," the SLP should ask how long the student has been exposed to English and ascertain whether or not she is in the silent period.

Language Loss

If a student begins to use the first language less frequently, she will lose skills in that language as she is acquiring skills in the second language (Anderson, 1999; Coltrane, 2003). Many CLD children, when they come to school, are surrounded only by English; bilingual education is often nonexistent, especially for the less common languages. Since English is the dominant language of society in the United States, children often experience **language loss** in their first language; that language is gradually replaced by English. This is particularly true for children whose families are members of minority ethnolinguistic communities (Anderson, 1999).

If a student is still acquiring English and has experienced language loss, then the student may appear to be low functioning in both languages. Based on low language test scores, the SLP may conclude that the student has an SLI.

For example, Gutierrez-Clellen et al. (2000) discuss Spanish-speaking children and state that a child may show adequate use of a language target form at an earlier time, while failing to show productive use of this same form at a later time. They state that this can mean that older children can demonstrate lower language skills in L1 than younger children. As a clinician, I have seen this often in my work. For example, if I use a Spanish language test with a kindergartener who comes to school speaking only Spanish, she will often do better than the Spanish-speaking fourth grader who has had greater English exposure and decreased Spanish exposure because she is not at home as much.

> Many students undergo loss of skills in their first languages, because these languages are not supported in school.

Differentiating between language differences and language learning disabilities in a situation where language loss has occurred is challenging. CLD students are at risk of being diagnosed with SLI when they are in the process of losing the first language and still developing proficiency in the second language or English (see Figure 3.6).

Language Transfer

Language transfer or **interference** refers to a process in which a communicative behavior from the first language is carried over into the second language. Language transfer involves the cross-linguistic influence that two or more languages may have on each other.

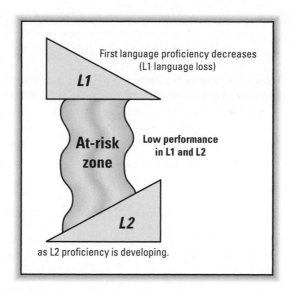

First language proficiency decreases
(L1 language loss)

L1

At-risk zone

Low performance in L1 and L2

L2

as L2 proficiency is developing.

FIGURE 3.6   English Language Learners at Risk

Used with permission. From Roseberry-McKibbin, C. (2008) *Multicultural students with special language needs: Practical strategies for assessment and intervention* (3rd edition), Oceanside, CA: Academic Communication Associates, Inc.

CONNECT & EXTEND

Many examples of language transfer from Spanish to English are given in Brice, A. E. (2002). *The Hispanic child: Speech, language, culture, and education.* Boston, MA: Allyn & Bacon.

Sometimes a student's English errors are the result of transfer from her first language.

Transfer can occur in all areas: syntax, morphology, phonology, pragmatics, and semantics. Language patterns from the first language may influence how a student formulates a particular message in the second language.

In German, for example, *Ich habe Hunger* means *I'm hungry*. A literal translation of the German, however, would be *I have hunger*. Thus, a German-speaking student who says, "I have hunger—let's eat!" would be manifesting transfer from German into English. Brice (2002) gives the example of how Spanish syntax can be superimposed onto English when a Spanish-speaking child says, "The ball red is mine." (see Table 3.2 for more examples of language interference between Spanish and English).

When second language learners produce errors in English, it is important to consider the possibility that these errors result from transfer from the first language. Information about the student's first language can sometimes be obtained from a local library or possibly from a local university with a foreign language program. Bilingual paraprofessionals who speak the same dialect as the student can be of great assistance in helping the SLP determine the possibility of first language transfer.

TABLE 3.2   Examples of Language Interference (Bricc & Montgomery, 1998; Dulay & Burt, 1974)

Type of Error	*Construction*	*Examples*
Interference	Possessive pronoun + agreement. Not allowed in English; obligatory in Spanish.	Now she's putting hers clothes on. (*Ahora ella se esta poniendo su ropa.*)
	Omission of obligatory "how" in English; obligatory in Spanish	I know to do all that. (*Yo sé qué hacer todo eso.*)
	Use of infinitive for gerund. Not allowed in English; obligatory in Spanish.	I finish to watch tv when it's four o'clock. (*Yo termino de ver la tv cuando es la cuatro.*)
	Do–subject agreement missing.	Where the spiders go.
	Object pronoun missing.	My mother can fix.
	Trouble with irregular past tense and prepositions.	Yesterday, we go see my grandma. (*Ayer, nosotros fuimos a ver mi abuela.*)
		We went to. I calling to you later. Last week we seeing some good movie.
	Trouble with future tense marker.	I will called you.
	Copula "be" and possessive "s" marker.	This is the car of my mother. (*Ésto es el carro de mi madre.*)
	Trouble conjugating the "to be" verb.	When we beauty the room it pretty. (*Cuando arreglamos el cuarto está bonito.*)
	Trouble with negation forms.	In my country not we eat pork. (*En mi país no comemos puerco.*)
	Trouble with negation and singular possession.	This house no is my. (*Esta casa no es mía.*)
	Trouble with "s" markers and articles.	This three boy is playing on basketball team.
	Trouble with verb-subject forms; past tense inversion; wh-questions.	For why you asking me this question before? (*Por qué me estás preguntando esta pregunta antes?*)
	Wrong "no" placement; "no-not" distinction; "do" missing.	It no cause too trouble. (*Éso no me causa mucha problema.*)
	Use of noun for possessive pronoun.	She name is Maria. (*Su nombre es María.*)
	Overuse of "do."	We do got no more book. (*Nosotros no tenemos mas libros.*)
	"-ing" with modal.	Now we will talking about. (*Ahora nosotros estamos hablamos de éso.*)

TABLE 3.2   Examples of Language Interference (Bricc & Montgomery, 1998; Dulay & Burt, 1974) (*continued*)

Type of Error	Construction	Examples
Developmental Errors	Irregular treated as regular form.	She took her teeths off.
	Two verbal words tensed where only one is required.	I didn't weared my any hat.
	Accusative pronoun with nominative.	Me needs crayons now.

From Alejandro E. Brice, The Hispanic Child: Speech, Language, Culture and Education. Published by Allyn & Bacon, Boston, MA. Copyright © 2002 by Pearson Education. Reprinted by permission of publisher.

Interlanguage

Interlanguage is defined as the period in second language development when the learner starts to use language productively until she achieves competence similar to that of a native speaker (Genesee et al., 2004). Interlanguage involves the approximation of the target language while it is still being learned (Brice, 2002). Interlanguage is constantly changing and is developmentally idiosyncratic (Gorbet, 1979). When learning a second language, the learner tests hypotheses about how language works and forms her own set of rules for using language. The individual's production changes over time as language is experienced in different contexts. Inconsistent errors reflect the progress that the student is making in learning a new language and should not be viewed as evidence of an abnormality.

> A student in the interlanguage phase may make inconsistent errors in the second language; these errors reflect the language learning process.

CASES TO CONSIDER

A kindergarten teacher has referred Mmaete to you. Mmaete is five years old and has been in the all-English-speaking kindergarten for four months. Her family speaks Ibo, and they are from Nigeria. Mmaete has never been exposed to English before kindergarten. The teacher is concerned because "Mmaete is quiet and when she does talk, I hear mistakes in pronunciation and grammar. I'm afraid she has a speech impediment." How will you deal with this situation?

_____

_____

_____

Codeswitching

The use of two languages alternately in discourse can be divided into two major categories. **Codeswitching** is the alternation of two languages within a single constituent, sentence, or discourse. Language alternation within a sentence is also called **code mixing** (Brice & Anderson, 1999). The term codeswitching is used here. During the early stages of second language learning, the learner may substitute structures, forms, or lexical items from the first language for forms in the second language that have not yet been learned. Bilingual children commonly use codeswitching as a strategy, and the use of code mixing seems to help bridge the two languages that a child is learning (Brice & Anderson, 1999).

In the later stages of second language learning, when the child has gained proficiency in the second language (e.g., English), she may still codeswitch—not as a strategy of substituting lexical forms in her first language for unknown items in English, but as a pattern found in most bilingual speakers. Genesee et al. (2004) state that codeswitching is common in bilingual communities across the globe. In general, codeswitching behavior is used by normal bilingual speakers throughout the world (Goldstein, 2000; Wyatt, 2002). Switching between two languages is commonly observed among fluent bilingual speakers and, therefore, is not necessarily an indicator of a problem (Houwer, 1999). In fact, codeswitching in fluent bilinguals is often thought to be a sign of linguistic sophistication.

> **CONNECT & EXTEND**
>
> Codeswitching is explained in an article by Brice, A., & Anderson, R. (1999). Code mixing in a young bilingual child. *Communication Disorders Quarterly, 21*(1), 17–22.

> Codeswitching, or alternating between languages during a conversation, is a normal phenomenon observed in bilingual speakers worldwide.

 SUMMARY

- During the initial stages of learning a new language, some students go through the silent period, where they focus on comprehension and talk very little.
- In the situation of language loss, the student's first language is replaced by English.
- Language transfer or interference is a process where a communicative behavior or structure is carried over from the first language to the second language.
- Interlanguage involves the approximation of the target language while it is still being learned. Second language learners may have variable second language errors during this time.
- Codeswitching, a behavior used by sophisticated bilinguals worldwide, involves changing languages within a single constituent, sentence, or discourse.

Write your own summary points here:

_____

_____

_____

COGNITIVE-LINGUISTIC VARIABLES IN SECOND LANGUAGE ACQUISITION

Students bring a variety of language learning styles and strategies to the second language learning situation (Walqui, 2000). This section delineates learning styles and strategies that might influence the CLD student's communication. SLPs need to be sure that they are not identifying these normal styles and strategies as signs of SLI. These styles and strategies include use of routines, performance as a high- or low-input generator, use of practice opportunities, avoidance of speaking English, and imitation of environmental models.

Use of Routines

Routines are phrases such as "Have a good day!" that are learned as a whole. My son Mark, when he was two years old, would say to store clerks, "Thanks, and have a nice day!" (They just about got whiplash from hearing this sentence from a toddler.) Clearly, Mark was able to use a phrase appropriately even though he did not understand the individual words.

> Some children use routines, or memorized phrases in English, to communicate in social situations.

In the same way, second language learners may use whole phrases appropriately, although they may not know the meaning or grammatical function of individual words within the phrase (Ventriglia, 1982). Students who use these memorized phrases are often able to initiate and sustain simple conversation and, therefore, give the false impression that they are fluent speakers of the language. I was working with little Joanna, a first-grade Vietnamese student with extremely minimal English skills. Out of the blue one day, she said, "Your hair is just lovely." I was shocked to hear this memorized sentence out of a child who was still in the very early stages of English development.

High- versus Low-Input Generators

CLD students who are **high-input generators** use the learning strategy of creating many opportunities for practicing language. Often, these students are extroverted and initiate conversations with speakers of the second language. This initiation, in turn, generates an interchange that gives the CLD students increased opportunities to practice communication. On the other hand, **low-input generators** are usually not assertive, generate few opportunities to practice using language, and acquire language skills more slowly than high-input generators.

> A high-input generator avails herself of many opportunities to practice speaking English. She tends to learn English faster than a low-input generator.

I have worked with a number of CLD students who were introverted and initiated few if any conversations with native English speakers. These students can appear to have SLI because their acquisition of English is slower than that of students who are outgoing and create many conversational exchanges and interactions with native English-speaking students.

POINTS TO PONDER Discuss how a child who was a low-input generator with few language-practice opportunities might appear to have an SLI. What mistake might professionals make in assessing this child?

_____

_____

_____

Practice Opportunities

Much of a student's progress in second language acquisition depends on the availability of functional opportunities for second language practice (Baker, 2000; Gibbons, 2002). Some students speak English in the classroom but not in any other contexts. Even then, they may speak very little. The learning of English is likely to be slow if the student speaks very little English in the classroom and little or no English outside the classroom.

Avoidance

A student may avoid communicating in the second language so she will not be made fun of by others. Students don't want to be laughed at when they speak. This may be particularly

> Some students may comprehend English well but avoid speaking for fear of being ridiculed because of how they sound.

true of older students who speak English with a pronounced accent. Students who use the strategy of **avoidance** of speaking in English may appear to have expressive language problems, but their comprehension of English may be intact. Speech-language pathologists should ascertain whether or not students who appear to be slow to speak English actually have an SLI or are just avoiding speaking for fear of being ridiculed.

Modeling

When assessing CLD students for the possible presence of SLI, it is important for SLPs to familiarize themselves with the students' daily speech and language models. Many professionals have assessed a student and subsequently talked with a caretaker about the child's performance–the caretaker's speech and language patterns often sound very similar to those

> A child's daily language models have a great impact on her own language.

of the child. It is very important to consider not only the impact of parents' modeling, but also that of siblings, neighborhood friends, school peers, grandparents, and babysitters.

Students may come from extended families where they spend much time with grandparents or babysitters who are not native speakers of English. I recently assessed Nolan H., who spent most of the first

CASES TO CONSIDER

At the high school, the English teacher refers Tran to you because of "slow academic progress." Tran is being considered for placement in a self-contained, special education classroom. As you review Tran's history and interact with him, you discover the following. Tran is very shy, speaks only Vietnamese in the home, and associates primarily with Vietnamese peers at the high school. He has no native English-speaking friends and tells you that he doesn't speak in English much because "I am afraid I will pronounce words wrong." You discover that Tran's skills in Vietnamese are excellent and that he does not have an SLI. What will you recommend for Tran?

_____

_____

_____

five years of his life at home with his Cantonese-speaking grandparents while his parents worked. The interpreter, who knew the family well, shared that the grandparents' Cantonese oral skills were "limited." Thus, Nolan's first language foundation had been heavily influenced by these home models, and this had to be considered in the assessment.

 SUMMARY

- Students bring a variety of strategies to the language learning process. One of these is the use of routines, or whole memorized phrases or sentences that help them communicate with speakers of the second language.
- Students who are high-input generators create many opportunities to practice the second language. Low-input generators generate few opportunities for practicing the second language and tend to develop the second language more slowly than high-input generators.
- Low-input generators usually have fewer practice opportunities to use and develop their second language skills.
- Some students will avoid speaking in the second language for fear of being laughed at. This also may slow down their second language acquisition.
- Students speak like their models do. It is critical that SLPs find out what kind of language models students are exposed to.

Add your own summary points here:

_____

_____

_____

AFFECTIVE VARIABLES IN SECOND LANGUAGE ACQUISITION

The influence of affective variables in second language acquisition has been documented by many researchers (Brice, 2002; Coltrane, 2003; Cummins, 2002; Hearne, 2000; Langdon, 2000; Roseberry-McKibbin, 2008). In this section, these variables are described in terms of their effect on the academic and linguistic performance of CLD students.

Personality

A student's personality impacts her learning of a second language. The following personality variables will influence how quickly and well a second language is learned.

a. *Self-Esteem.* To maximize learning, students need to have a positive attitude and a positive self-concept. The more positive that students feel about themselves, the more rapidly and completely second language acquisition is likely to take place. Students whose first language and culture are rejected may have low self-esteem and consequently learn English more slowly than children whose backgrounds are accepted.

> Self-esteem, extroversion, and assertiveness impact second language learning.

b. *Extroversion.* There is some evidence that extroverted students learn English conversational skills faster than introverted students (Wong Fillmore, 1976; Ventriglia, 1982). Shy students may take longer to develop conversational competence than outgoing students.

c. *Assertiveness.* Being assertive can be very helpful in facilitating second language learning, as assertive learners avail themselves of increased opportunities for second language practice. If a student is not assertive, there may be fewer opportunities to practice English skills with native speakers.

Anxiety Level

Motivated students with a low anxiety level are able to learn a second language with more ease and speed than anxious students, even if these students are motivated to learn. Krashen (1992) described such students as having a low affective filter. These students learn better because they are in an environment that is accepting and appropriately geared toward their needs.

> Anxiety can inhibit the learning of a second language, as can lack of motivation.

If a student is not learning English quickly or well enough in the professional's judgment, this may be due in part to anxiety. Students may be anxious if they are in an all-English-speaking classroom where they understand very little and the academic demands are high. Monolingual English-speaking readers may imagine going to China, learning conversational Mandarin, and then being expected to take and pass a geometry or chemistry class taught in Mandarin. This would be quite anxiety provoking.

Motivation

Children's motivation to communicate and fit in with peers who speak the second language has a powerful influence on their acquisition of that second language. Students who are intrinsically motivated to learn English will fare best because they learn English due to its challenge, interest, and value (Walqui, 2000). Students who are only extrinsically motivated to learn English (e.g., because the school demands it) may learn more slowly.

Genesee et al. (2004) point out that refugee and immigrant children who have been traumatized in their home countries may have some challenges with adapting to a new culture and being motivated to learn the second language. When attempting to determine a student's level of motivation for learning English, the following questions can be asked:

a. *Is the student becoming acculturated into the English cultural and linguistic environment?*

> **CONNECT & EXTEND**
>
> Affective variables in second language acquisition are explained in further detail in Roseberry-McKibbin, C. (2008). *Multicultural students with special language needs: Practical strategies for assessment and intervention* (3rd ed.). Oceanside, CA: Academic Communication Associates.

Acculturation (described in more detail in Chapter 4) refers to psychological integration with speakers of the second language (Schumann, 1986). According to Schumann, second language learners acquire the second language to the degree that they acculturate. Thus, if a student is not integrated into situations with English-speaking peers, she may be somewhat unmotivated to learn English. Some parents of CLD students may discourage them from playing and interacting with native English-speaking students. In these cases, motivation to learn English may be quite low and the student's progress will be slowed down.

b. *Does the student feel that learning a second language will threaten her identity?*

If a student is rejected by family and/or peers for speaking English, motivation will be affected. For example, teenagers are heavily influenced by their peer groups; if a teenager begins to speak English like a native speaker, she may no longer be regarded as belonging to the native-language peer group because speaking fluent English threatens the group's identity (Walqui, 2000).

c. *Is there congruence between the student's cultural group and the dominant group?*

The more **congruent** or similar two cultures are, the more likely that social contact will occur and second language learning will be facilitated. Likewise, the more dissimilar the cultures, the less social contact there will be and the less English learning will take place. For example, many Filipinos who come to the United States have learned English in the Philippines, watched American movies and television, and worn clothing that is similar in style to that of Americans.

As a group, Filipinos tend to acculturate and speak English quite well because their culture is fairly congruent with that of the United States. On the other hand,

CASES TO CONSIDER

A teacher has referred a ten-year-old boy to you for assessment. She says he is "slow" to catch on in class. You learn that the boy, whose family is from Laos, speaks primarily Hmong at home. He tells you that his parents and friends don't think English is "cool." What other information will you try to find out? How might you deal constructively with this situation?

_____

_____

_____

> The more congruence there is between the student's culture and US culture, the greater will be the student's motivation to learn English.

a student may be from a country where English is rarely spoken and not taught in school, Americans are hated, and clothing is dramatically different in style and fashion. This student may have a longer and more difficult English learning experience than the Filipino student.

d. *How long does the student's family intend to stay in the United States?*

Will the family be going back to the home country? If the family plans to remain in the United States, motivation to learn English is often higher than in families that plan to return to their homeland.

 SUMMARY

- Extroverted, assertive students with good self-esteem tend to acquire second language skills faster than introverted, passive students with low self-esteem.
- Students who are anxious in second-language learning situations often learn more slowly than those who are relaxed.
- A student's motivation to learn the second language impacts quality and quantity of acquisition. Motivation may be impacted by the student's acculturation and the congruency of her culture and mainstream US culture.

Add your own summary points here:

_____

_____

_____

CHAPTER HIGHLIGHTS

- Many errors in assessment of CLD students can be avoided if SLPs take into account normal second-language learning phenomena as well as characteristics of bilingualism.
- Language proficiency in children can be viewed through several different models. One of these models is Separate Underlying Proficiency vs. Common Underlying Proficiency.
- It is important to consider the model that differentiates Basic Interpersonal Communication Skills (BICS) from Cognitive Academic Language Proficiency (CALP). Under ideal conditions, BICS takes two to three years to develop to a nativelike level while CALP takes five to seven or even up to ten years.
- It is important to ascertain how a child has learned two languages. Children acquire two languages either sequentially or simultaneously. Sequential learners experience more variation in the quality and quantity of their language acquisition than simultaneous learners.
- Ideally, CLD students experience additive bilingualism, where they develop high-levels of proficiency in their first language as well as English through maintenance bilingual education.
- Subtractive bilingualism, where the second language eventually replaces the first language, is more the norm in US schools, and this often leads to negative academic consequences. This is due to a number of factors such as the erroneous assumption that bilingualism is damaging to children and that monolingualism is the norm.
- Normal processes of second language acquisition that need to be considered in evaluating CLD students are the silent period, language loss, language transfer or interference from the first language, interlanguage, and codeswitching.
- Cognitive-linguistic variables that need to be considered in evaluating CLD students are the use of routines, the child's status as a high- or low-input generator, practice opportunities, avoidance, and the child's language models.
- Affective variables that impact a child's acquisition of a second language are personality, anxiety level, motivation, and acculturation.

Add your own chapter highlights here:

_____

_____

_____

_____

STUDY AND REVIEW QUESTIONS

ESSAY

1. Define the terms *simultaneous* and *sequential bilingualism*. Which type of child may have more difficulty, the child who is a simultaneous language learner or the child who is a sequential language learner?

2. Discuss the negative myths about bilingualism in the United States. How have these negative myths impacted actual practice in US school systems?

3. Describe the terms Separate Underlying Proficiency and Common Underlying Proficiency. Which one is accurate? Why?

4. What are the advantages of being a proficient bilingual? Discuss the ideal school situation for a student who comes to school speaking a language other than English.

5. Describe Basic Interpersonal Communication Skills and Cognitive Academic Language Proficiency. How do they differ? Why are these types of language proficiency so important to consider when working with students who are acquiring English as a second language?

FILL-IN-THE-BLANK

6. _____ refers to psychological integration with speakers of a second language.

7. _____ refers to a process in which a communicative behavior from the first language is carried over into the second language.

8. The alternation of two languages within a single constituent, sentence, or discourse is called _____.

9. When a student's first language is replaced by the second language, this is called _____.

10. The _____ includes the belief that the child's cognitive system is fragile and only designed to cope with one language.

MULTIPLE CHOICE

11. A teacher refers a student to you. She is from Somalia, and she and her family have been in the United States for five months. She is in third grade here in the United States, and the teacher suspects that she has SLI because she is very quiet in class, makes some grammatical errors in English, and sometimes "mixes Somalian and English when she talks" (according to the teacher). The student's parents report that she was a high achiever in Somalian schools. The Somalian interpreter tells you that the student is "high level" in Somalian. Which of the following are TRUE? The student is probably

    I. In the silent period
    II. Experiencing interference or transfer from Somalian to English
    III. Codeswitching between Somalian and English
    IV. A student with an SLI who needs speech-language services
    V. A normal second language learner who needs more time to learn English

    a. I, II, III, IV
    b. II, III, V
    c. I, III, IV
    d. I, II, III, V
    e. II, III, IV

12. You have a student from the Mexico who runs into class one day, very excited about something. You overhear her talking to her friends. She says, "It was wonderful! Esta casa es más grande! I want to go back soon! Es muy bonita!" This student

   a. Has an SLI as evidenced by her language confusion

   b. Clearly has deficient skills in English

   c. Is demonstrating codeswitching, a normal behavior among bilingual speakers

   d. Should be watched for signs of a developmental delay

   e. None of the above

13. Which one of the following is FALSE?

   a. If a child comes to school speaking a language other than English, school personnel should discourage use of that language because it will interfere with his English acquisition.

   b. Students who experience simultaneous acquisition of two languages seem to do so with minimal interference between the languages.

   c. A child who is semilingual is not competent in either her first language or English and may be at risk in school.

   d. Input that is comprehensible is not grammatically sequenced, but rather occurs naturally.

   e. Maintenance bilingual education programs provide students with opportunities to continue to use the first language as well as experiences designed to promote effective use of the second language.

14. Basic Interpersonal Communication Skills (BICS) are characterized by

   a. Context-embedded communication

   b. Cognitively undemanding communication

   c. Situations where the student is called upon to use various cognitive strategies to perform tasks where knowledge is not automatized

   d. a, b

   e. a, b, c

15. Which is FALSE regarding affective variables that play a role in second language acquisition?

   a. Extroverted students will probably acquire second language conversational skills faster than introverted students.

   b. Second language learners who are anxious generally learn the second language faster than relaxed students because their anxiety motivates them to work harder.

   c. The more congruent the student's culture is with US culture, the more likely she is to learn English faster.

   d. Students who are extrinsically motivated to learn English may learn more slowly than intrinsically motivated learners.

   e. Being assertive is helpful in learning a second language.

See Answers to Study and Review Questions, page 465.

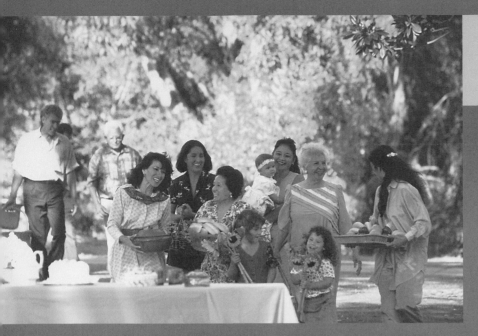

Factors Impacting Language Development in Culturally and Linguistically Diverse Children

CASE STUDY

Tran was struggling in his fourth-grade class. His teacher, Ms. West, was sympathetic but under pressure herself. With the rising academic standards and pressures on teachers to have students achieve high test scores, she felt both sympathy and frustration with Tran's slow progress. The school did have a special day class for students with "communication handicaps," and Ms. West was seriously considering referring Tran for placement in this class. After all, she did not have time to give him any one-on-one attention; plus, the school did not have many resources for English Language Learner students. Ms. West had also noticed that Tran "confuses /r/ and /l/ and leaves endings off of some of his words."

That day at lunch, Ms. West shared her frustrations with Shelley, the speech-language pathologist (SLP) at the school. Shelley, a recent graduate, had had a course in multicultural issues in speech-language pathology. She remembered the professor saying that many culturally and linguistically diverse (CLD) students are incorrectly placed into special education settings, but she also understood Ms. West's frustration with the situation. Shelley assured Ms. West that she would bring Tran in for screening and also conduct a classroom observation.

When Shelley went into the classroom to observe, she found that Tran was sitting in the back of the class. He never raised his hand to share, and was extremely quiet. At recess, Tran played well with his friends and was clearly well liked by his peers. Though he was fairly quiet, it was obvious that socially he was successful and popular. Knowing that students with true SLI are often rejected by their peers, Shelley decided to do some additional research.

She went to Tran's school records and also arranged a meeting with Tran's father and the Khmer interpreter. The interpreter told Shelley that according to Tran's father, the family come to the United States from Cambodia seven years ago as refugees. When Tran was five years old, he had kidney failure and the doctors recommended a kidney transplant for him. But the Buddhist family, who believed in reincarnation, did not want Tran to undergo this procedure. They felt that if Tran died, he would be reincarnated into a better body; they were also reluctant to have him "cut into."

Eventually the American doctors prevailed, and Tran had the kidney transplant. However, he became electively mute and did not speak in Khmer or English for almost one year. When he did begin to speak again, his Khmer was normal but his English was understandably quite rudimentary. According to Tran's father, in Khmer Tran spoke "just fine; he's a bright boy who expresses himself well." However, the father shared that Tran's English lagged considerably behind that of his siblings due to his medical problems and subsequent period of elective mutism.

The Khmer interpreter spoke with Tran, who came from his classroom for a brief screening in Shelley's room. The interpreter and Tran played a game, looked at several books, and conversed about familiar topics. Though Shelley did not understand what she was hearing, she observed Tran talking animatedly with no hesitation. After Tran left the room to go back to class, the interpreter told Shelley that in his opinion, Tran was "above average" in his Khmer speaking skills and that Tran had excellent ability to follow directions that were given in Khmer. The interpreter, who had been in the school district for five years and had worked with approximately two hundred to three hundred Khmer students during that time, shared with Shelley that Tran was very

much within normal limits in his experience with other Khmer-speaking students in the district. The interpreter said, "I think he just needs more time to learn English; his Khmer language skills are good." When Shelley spoke with Tran in English, she noted that he did omit some of the final consonants from words and that he sometimes substituted /r/ for /l/ and vice versa. But Shelley knew that many speakers of Asian languages do this, as many Asian languages end in vowels and do not contain the /r/ and /l/ sounds.

Shelley shared this information with Ms. West, who was relieved to hear that Tran had typically developing skills in his primary language. Ms. West also understood that Tran's articulation differences in English were due to the influence of his primary language of Khmer, not to an articulation disorder. Shelley and Ms. West worked together to create additional opportunities for Tran to improve his English skills so that he could experience greater success in the classroom. They agreed that Tran did not need special education. They wanted to involve Tran's parents in assisting him in the home, but the interpreter cautioned them that the parents viewed school personnel as "the experts" and that the parents might resist efforts to become involved.

Thus, it was decided that Tran would begin receiving extra support from the Khmer interpreter several times a week so that he could use his Khmer language skills to facilitate learning of academic information. In addition, Tran was placed into the school's Reading Clinic, a non–special education support laboratory for students to receive additional small-group support in reading comprehension. Tran attended the school's Discovery Club, an after-care program for students whose parents worked full time. At Discovery Club, the teachers who worked with the students after school made a special point of encouraging Tran to speak in English as much as possible in peer-group activities. Six months later, Tran had made noticeable progress in the classroom. Though he needed continued extra support, Ms. West felt that he would be ready for fifth grade the next fall.

INTRODUCTION

Many times when SLPs work with CLD students, it is easy to overlook variables that contribute to these students' academic and linguistic performance. Teachers in public schools nationwide experience a great deal of pressure to have students achieve high scores on statewide standardized tests that are administered in English. When a student does not perform well on these tests, many teachers automatically consider special education as an option.

The teachers may believe that a particular student has an SLI or other special need that prevents her from performing adequately in the classroom. Often, the SLP is the first person the teacher turns to for assistance. Part of differentiating a normal language difference from SLI involves viewing the student holistically in terms of cultural, religious, environmental, and linguistic background factors. Thus, this chapter is devoted to the topics of 1) culture and cultural diversity among students, 2) developing cultural competence, 3) the impact of family refugee/immigrant status, 4) the impact of religion, and 5) influences of other languages on English production.

CULTURE AND CULTURAL DIVERSITY

Variables Impacting Behavior of Members of Various Cultural Groups

Experts have defined culture in many different ways. Simply, **culture** is a dynamic set of values and belief systems that shape the behavior of individuals from various groups and communities. In the United States, the concept of **cultural pluralism** means that instead of being a "melting pot," where individuals forsake their primary culture to blend into the mainstream, the United States is more of a "salad bowl" where we all live together, but the distinguishing characteristics of each group are preserved and valued.

> Culture is a dynamic set of values and belief systems that shape the behavior of individuals from various groups and communities.

A number of variables influence the behavior of individuals within the cultural groups (Lynch, 2004; Parkay & Stanford, 2004; Roseberry-McKibbin, 2008; Woolfolk, 2004). When SLPs provide services to CLD students, they must consider the following for each individual student and family:

- Languages spoken in the home
- Parents' educational level
- Country of birth of the student and parents
- Length of residence in the United States
- Socioeconomic status
- Student's age and gender
- Generational membership (first, second, third generation in the United States)
- Neighborhood and peer group
- Degree of acculturation into American life

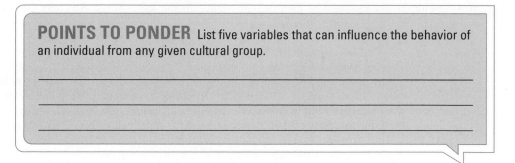

POINTS TO PONDER List five variables that can influence the behavior of an individual from any given cultural group.

_____

_____

_____

Some students come from homes like Tran's, where only the primary language is spoken. The parents might not have received a formal education and might have come from a rural background in their home country. Perhaps they have not acculturated and become integrated into mainstream American life; this will impact their children's linguistic and academic development. If the family is also experiencing poverty, the student's education may be impacted by this factor as well.

Other students come from homes where the parents are literate, educated professionals who were of middle–upper class financial status in their home country. These parents may or may not have middle–upper class socioeconomic status (SES) in the United States; a family's SES in the United States depends very heavily on whether the parents can obtain jobs in the United States that are commensurate with the jobs they had in their home countries.

I once had a good wake-up call that forced me to reexamine my stereotype about most immigrants/refugees being low SES. A former student called me to ask about a Southeast Asian refugee girl; there had been a visit with the girl's mother, and it was apparent that the girl needed medical services. I assumed that the family was low SES and had no health insurance. My former student quickly assured me that this was not the case; in fact, the mother had worn diamonds and a fur coat (yes, here in California) to the meeting. We as SLPs can never make assumptions; each student and family is unique, and part of being a culturally competent SLP is continuously remembering this fact.

> Part of being a culturally competent professional is recognizing individual variation within a culture as well as variables that impact a student's performance.

Increasing Cultural Competence

It is important for all professionals to be culturally competent as they work with students from diverse cultural backgrounds (Madding, 2002). For example, in the school district where I work part time, students represent more than 80 different linguistic and cultural groups. As previously stated, part of being a culturally competent professional is recognizing that each person in each culture is an individual, and that great heterogeneity exists within each cultural group. Hanson (2004) reminds us that although people of the same cultural background may share tendencies, not all members of a group who share a common cultural background or history will behave in the same ways. Sue and Sue (2003, pp. 16–17) discuss **cultural competence:**

> . . . a culturally competent helping professional is one who is actively in the process of becoming aware of his or her own assumptions. . . . Second, a culturally competent helping professional is one who actively attempts to understand the worldview of his or her culturally different client. . . . Third, a culturally competent helping professional is one who is in the process of actively developing and practicing appropriate, relevant, and sensitive intervention strategies and skills in working with his or her culturally different client.

Clearly, being a culturally competent SLP is an ongoing process. As stated in Chapter 1, a professional should never stop growing and learning. I remember a student from several years ago who said to me in frustration, "How can I keep from messing up? There's no way to remember all this information about every cultural group!" Probably we will all "mess up" at one time or another. But there are ways to increase one's cultural competence, and these practical suggestions are as follows (Brice, 2002; Huer & Saenz, 2003; Roseberry-McKibbin, 2008):

1. **Evaluate your own values and assumptions.** Consider how these affect the way you interact with students and their families. For example, many Americans consider early independence in children to be highly desirable. As an illustration, I read in one child-raising book that parents should encourage their two-year-old children to learn how to scramble eggs. American babies are often transitioned to solid foods as quickly as possible. But you may work with a Middle Eastern family where a four-year-old child still drinks from a bottle because this type of behavior would be considered appropriate in some areas of the Middle East (Sharifzadeh, 2004). Will you communicate that the family's ways are inferior to yours, or will you allow for cultural differences in child rearing? In one school where I

CONNECT & EXTEND

A source that has detailed information about the cultural and linguistic characteristics of various groups such as Middle Easterners, Asians, Pacific Islanders, and others is Lynch, E.W., & Hanson, M.J. (2004). *Developing cross-cultural competence: A guide to working with young children and their families* (3rd ed.). Baltimore, MD: Paul H. Brookes Publishing Co.

worked, on the first day of school, a boy from a certain cultural group was literally carried into kindergarten on a pillow. We might want to have a chat with that family; however, we should be aware that in that culture, boys are routinely catered to and encouraged to be dependent on their caregivers.

2. **Read as much as you can about the family's linguistic and cultural background.** There are many books, articles, and Web sites that can help SLPs increase their understanding of various cultural groups and languages.

3. **Team up with persons from the local cultural community who can act as interpreters and informants.** I have found that this is an invaluable way to gain insight into a family's or student's situation. For example, I worked with a kindergarten Hmong-speaking boy who was quite hoarse. In accordance with my wishes, the Hmong interpreter called the home and asked the family if the boy had seen an ear, nose, and throat doctor (ENT). The family told him yes, and that their son was "fine." After he hung up, the interpreter told me that in this cultural group, a problem does not exist unless it is directly visible. Therefore, the family

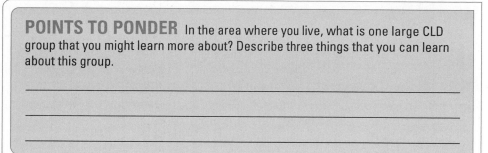

POINTS TO PONDER In the area where you live, what is one large CLD group that you might learn more about? Describe three things that you can learn about this group.

_____

_____

_____

An excellent way for SLPs to increase their cultural competence is to team up with persons from local cultural communities to act as interpreters and informants.

was probably just being polite but had never taken their son to an ENT and had no intention of ever doing so.

4. Consider the value system of the family and larger community when setting intervention goals. For example, a Filipino SLP shared with me that for many Filipino families, early intervention with toddlers and preschoolers is not a priority because in the Philippines, many children do not begin attending school until age seven. Thus, if you are working with a three-year-old Filipino child who does not speak in complete sentences in any language, language intervention might be much more important to you than to the family, who believes in "letting children be children."

There are many practical ways for SLPs to increase their cultural competence.

5. Ask students, family members, and interpreters to share important aspects of their culture with you. I have found that they often love to share; rarely does anyone in the United States ask them about themselves and their culture. They are especially appreciative when I attempt to learn a few words in their language. It is my experience that Mandarin and Russian are very challenging indeed! I always feel a newfound respect for immigrants who have to learn English.

 ## SUMMARY

- Culture is a dynamic set of values and belief systems that shape the behavior of individuals from various groups and communities.
- A number of variables influence the behavior of individuals within the cultural groups. These include things like length of residence in the United States, generational membership, gender, educational level, and others.

(continued)

- It is important for SLPs to develop cultural competence. This includes actively developing and practicing appropriate, relevant, and sensitive intervention strategies and skills in working with CLD students and their families.
- Practical ways to increase cultural competence include reading, teaming up with persons in various cultural communities, and asking families and students to share aspects of their culture with you.

Add your own summary points here:

_____

_____

_____

CONSIDERATIONS IN WORKING WITH IMMIGRANTS AND REFUGEES

General Issues

As we consider the unique and individual backgrounds of our CLD students, we must remember that many of them will be from immigrant and refugee families. The number of immigrants and refugees in the United States is increasing. In the year 2000, 28.4 million immigrants came to the United States. Between 2000 and 2003, a total of 4.5 million new immigrants arrived in the United States. Unemployment is rising among immigrants. In terms of being in poverty, 11.5 percent of US-born natives are in poverty while the rate among immigrants is 16.6 percent. In native-born households, welfare use is 16.7 percent; in immigrant households, welfare use is 25.5 percent. Health insurance is also an issue. In 2003, 12.8 percent of native-born Americans were uninsured as compared to 33.4 percent of immigrants (Camarota, 2003). Clearly, poverty and lack of health insurance are major issues for many families who immigrate to the United States.

Immigrant families come to the United States with the intention of becoming permanent residents. Refugees are individuals who flee from a country because of persecution (religious, political). In this section, the term immigrants/refugees is used for the purposes of brevity, but it is important to keep in mind the distinction between the two groups.

When a student from an immigrant/refugee family is being evaluated for speech-language services, it is important to consider the impact of the immigrant/refugee status on the student's whole family. First, it is important to be aware of the family's socioeconomic status, which is dependent upon whether the parents have jobs that pay adequately (Portes & Rumbaut, 2001).

The number of immigrants to the United States is increasing. If a student is from an immigrant family, the SLP needs to be aware of certain issues such as poverty that may impact the student's language development.

It is important to note that there are two basic kinds of poverty: situational and generational. **Generational poverty** refers to the situation where at least two generations of a family have been in poverty and have probably received welfare. Poverty is a way of life, and there may be few efforts to change this. **Situational poverty**, on the other hand, occurs for a shorter time and is caused by circumstances such as moving to a country where one's professional credentials are not accepted (Payne, 2003). Many immigrants/refugees live in situational poverty. They work extremely hard to get out of poverty.

At the church my parents attend, there is a woman named Celeste P. who is from a country in Africa. Her husband is still in Africa, and she is here in California trying to support herself and four boys on the salary she earns from her paper route. She would like to return to Africa; however, if she and her boys go back to their country, her son who is going into fifth grade will be drafted into the army. So Celeste stays in California, working at her paper route and doing the best she can to feed and clothe herself and her four sons. Most Americans have little or no understanding of this type of pressure and hardship, which is so commonplace among immigrants/refugees.

> Immigrant and refugee families often experience many stressors, including poverty and lack of familiarity with US culture as well as with English.

I have known of immigrants/refugees who were dentists and architects in their home countries but worked as custodians and taxi drivers in the United States because their credentials were not considered adequate for practice in the United States. Many of these immigrants/refugees who work low-paying jobs must hold down several jobs to support themselves and their children. These families experience a great deal of financial and emotional stress, and I have frequently found that the parents are very tired and have little or no time to spend with their children beyond "the basics."

One girl I worked with was from a Nigerian family. Her father, an architect in Nigeria, was a truck driver in Sacramento. The girl's mother had major medical problems. The father drove trucks all night and had to take care of his daughter during the day. I remember him practically falling asleep when he had been sitting down for more than two minutes. It is important to be sensitive to these issues when recommending such things as homework programs for students with speech-language disorders.

Another issue to consider is that many immigrant/refugee families come from countries where school personnel are considered the "experts," and thus parents feel uncomfortable

POINTS TO PONDER Describe the differences between situational and generational poverty. Why do so many immigrant and refugee families live in situational poverty?

_____

_____

_____

with working with their children at home. In terms of viewing this issue from the perspective of the families, Lynch (2004, p. 29) states:

> Everyone keeps suggesting programs and services for this "baby," but she is only 4 years old. Why should a 4-year-old child go to school? And why do all of these well-educated people [professionals] keep asking the family's opinion, wanting them to participate, to set goals? That is a job for them, not a job for the family. How presumptuous it would be to tell those professionals what they should do to help! The professionals are the experts.

Immigrant families often experience situational poverty, which is caused by circumstances such as moving to a country (the United States) where one's professional credentials are not accepted.

One of the best ways that SLPs can assist students and their families in these and other situations is to provide connections with local support groups or networks consisting of persons from their own culture who can provide necessary resources and information.

CASES TO CONSIDER

Cresandro P., a Filipino boy, was referred to me by his kindergarten teacher because he "isn't talking" and "doesn't understand what's going on." Upon talking with Cresandro's mother, I found out that his parents were well-educated professionals who held full-time jobs in the community. Cresandro spent the first years of his life being cared for primarily by his Ilocano-speaking grandparents, and he did not attend preschool. Cresandro's mother said that she spoke Tagalog, and her husband spoke Pampango. Thus, Cresandro entered kindergarten at age 4:10 years from a trilingual environment where he was not exposed to English and did not master any of the Filipino languages in his environment. The Filipino interpreter told me that Cresandro did not speak any of his Filipino languages adequately enough for her to assess him in any of them. Cresandro showed excellent fine-motor skills and was able to name many common objects in English and also count to fifty in English. He recited the alphabet perfectly and followed basic directions in English. His nonverbal intelligence testing revealed an above-average IQ. Cresandro's mother ruefully shared with me that when his older sister was born, she had much more time to spend with her than with Cresandro. When she came home from work after the graveyard shift, she was too tired to spend much time with Cresandro. His father was also tired from working. What recommendations would you make for Cresandro? Do you think he might need speech-language therapy? Why or why not?

_____

_____

_____

Acculturation

When we work with students and families who have immigrant/refugee status, we want to consider their level of acculturation. We did introduce this concept in Chapter 3, and I want to extend it here. Locke (1998) proposed a model of acculturation that is based on attitudes and involvement with one's culture of origin and also with the larger society in which one is currently living. Locke delineated four levels of acculturation within these parameters:

- **Traditional;** individuals do not adapt to a new culture and continue to adhere to the values and practices of their culture of origin
- **Acculturated;** individuals adapt to the new culture but lose some parameters of their culture of origin
  - **Marginal;** the individual adapts minimally to either the new culture or the culture of origin
  - **Bicultural;** individuals retain strong ties with the culture of origin and successfully adapt to the new culture as well

> There are four levels of acculturation: traditional, acculturated, marginal, and bicultural.

I have found that a family's level of acculturation impacts their willingness for a child to receive speech-language services. Level of acculturation also impacts the family's willingness to partner with the SLP in the intervention process for those students with language impairments. I have worked with families who were truly bicultural; they were vocal about their beliefs and values but also willing to listen to my recommendations for their children.

CONNECT & EXTEND

The conflict between traditional families and US values is described in Fadiman, A. (1997). *The spirit catches you and you fall down: A Hmong child, her American doctors, and the collision of two cultures.* New York: Farrar, Straus, and Giroux.

In contrast, I worked with one family with "traditional" acculturation whose daughter underwent a period of not speaking at all during a time when she was experiencing life-threatening medical problems. Meuy needed a kidney transplant, but her parents did not want her to have the transplant even though her life depended on it. According to their religious belief system, if she died, she would be reincarnated into a more whole form and death was preferable to major surgery. Fadiman (1997) discusses these kinds of conflicts in a beautiful, sensitively written story about a Hmong child with epilepsy. This story embodies the conflict that traditionally acculturated families may feel when confronted with new practices in the United States.

Considerations in Working with Internationally Adopted Children

A trend that has become more pronounced in the United States is international adoptions. Many Americans, unable to have their own biological children, have increasingly turned to international adoption as an alternative. Each year, approximately 12,500 overseas children are considered for adoption by prospective American parents (Pearson, 2001). These children are not technically immigrants or refugees; however, they do experience some issues of acculturation that are similar to those experienced by children from immigrant and refugee families.

Frequently, within twenty-four to twenty-eight hours, internationally adopted children (IAC) have been completely and abruptly taken out of familiar surroundings and placed in a totally new environment. This type of adjustment is especially hard on older IAC, who may miss the familiarity of the surroundings they have known all of their lives. It is important to consider the impact of acculturation on language development. Other factors impact language development also.

> Many internationally adopted children, especially older ones, experience acculturation issues when they arrive in the United States.

Many IAC come from institutionalized settings such as orphanages. The children may be in orphanages because their parents are dead. However, many are there because they were not planned and their families cannot afford to feed them. Research regarding the language skills of these children is very sparse; however, the few available sources in the speech-language pathology literature do point to certain general characteristics of this population.

First, it must be remembered that language characteristics of IAC depend very heavily on their prior experience in their home country. Friends of mine adopted a beautiful baby girl from a Taiwanese orphanage. The result of an unplanned pregnancy, she was very well cared for in the Taiwanese orphanage and is developing normally at this time. Other friends of mine adopted a four-year-old boy from a Russian orphanage; his mother, a widow, could not afford to keep him. This boy has shown excellent development and is doing well in school.

These "success stories" are very encouraging, for the little existing information about IAC indicates that they may often have profound and all-encompassing problems. Many exhibit severe developmental delays; for example, some young children have such low oral muscle tone that they refuse to even chew, let alone speak. Some have severe cognitive-linguistic delays. By some estimates, upon arrival in their adoptive homes, IAC with prior challenges show varied improvement. Twenty percent thrive upon placement in their adoptive homes; 60 percent experience continuing delays with only partial improvement, and the other 20 percent show little or no improvement (Pearson, 2001).

CONNECT & EXTEND

Information about IAC is available in Glennen, S. (2002). Language development and delay in internationally adopted infants and toddlers: A review. *American Journal of Speech-Language Pathology, 11*(4), 333–339, and Glennen, S., & Masters, M.G. (2002). Typical and atypical language development in infants and toddlers adopted from Eastern Europe. *American Journal of Speech-Language Pathology, 11*(4), 417–433. A highly informative Web site is www.familyhelper.net.

In one of the few existing pieces of research in the field of speech-language pathology about language development in IAC, Glennen and Masters (2002) conducted a longitudinal study of 130 infants and toddlers adopted from Eastern Europe. The children were followed up through the age of thirty to forty months. The findings of the study indicated that age of adoption was a critical factor in language development. By thirty-six to forty months of age, the children who were adopted younger were fully caught up to English language norms. The children who were adopted older lagged behind, with the length of their delay related to the age of adoption.

Roberts, Pollock, Krakow, Price, Fulmer, and Wang (2005) studied the language development of fifty-five preschool-age children adopted from China by American parents. All children had lived in their permanent homes for two or more years. The results of Robert et al.'s research showed that most (94.5 percent) of the children were within or above the normal range for native-born monolingual speakers after approximately two or more years of exposure to English. Slightly over one-fourth of the subjects performed significantly above average on at least two standardized language tests. Roberts and her colleagues hypothesized that perhaps one important factor that might have contributed to the language outcomes was the age at which the children were adopted (between six and twenty-five months of age). On all three language measures in this study, age of adoption was a significant predictor variable. Thus, early adoption was found to be advantageous with regard to learning English.

CASES TO CONSIDER

Recently at an outpatient rehabilitation center, I met Susan, who brings her eight-year-old son Alexi for weekly physical therapy. A few weeks ago, Susan and Alexi both arrived in tears and had clearly had a rough day. After Alexi went into the physical therapy room, I asked Susan if she would like to talk—she said she would. I was glad to be there so I could hear her story and perhaps help her feel better just by listening.

Susan shared that she and her husband had adopted Alexi from a Bulgarian orphanage when he was a preschooler. When they went to Bulgaria to bring him to the United States, they found him living in conditions of squalor, filth, and abuse. When Alexi arrived in the United States, he would not let Susan out of his sight. She could not let him hear the sound of a door shutting or he would scream and cry inconsolably. Alexi had many attachment issues and behavior problems. Even at four years of age, Alexi could hardly walk and he didn't speak at all.

Susan found out that in the Bulgarian orphanage, Alexi had been kicked in the head, beaten, and sexually abused. To this day, Alexi has scars on his head from the beatings. In the orphanage, he was regularly locked in small, dark closets. Currently, Alexi has profound delays in all areas: gross and fine-motor, cognitive, and language skills. Susan told me that "he still won't let me out of his sight," adding that she cannot even take a few minutes by herself or Alexi will scream and cry. Susan shared that the day before we spoke, she had taken Alexi to a psychiatrist who diagnosed him with significant post-traumatic stress syndrome and mental retardation. Susan wonders if she can ever reach Alexi; if he will ever be "normal."

In terms of speech and language, Alexi's delays are profound. I have spoken to him and have noticed his lack of intelligibility and sparse verbal output. At eight years of age, he speaks in three- or four-word utterances. I would like to recommend speech-language therapy, but Susan is exhausted, depressed, and depleted. Her financial

(continued)

resources are stretched to the breaking point because Alexi has such profound needs in so many areas. She spends most of her time taking him to various professionals for help. Would you advise Susan to seek formal speech-language therapy in addition to the physical therapy, occupational therapy, and psychological counseling that she is already obtaining for Alexi? If not, what suggestions might you give her to help her provide additional language stimulation for her child?

_____

_____

_____

A major challenge for SLPs is service delivery to older IAC. They are often delayed in their first language and thus do not have a strong foundation upon which to build English skills. For many, the linguistic input they have received in their orphanages is impoverished (Glennen, 2002). You will recall that we stressed in Chapter 3 that such children often experience difficulties because the first language foundation is weak, and thus the second language is weak also. This has negative cognitive and linguistic effects. For IAC it is often compounded by malnutrition, physical abuse, neglect, and very few emotional bonding opportunities. Anecdotally, I have heard of older children like this whose needs are so profound and extensive that they severely strain family relations. SLPs usually need to work as part of a multidisciplinary team to meet the needs of these children.

SUMMARY

- The number of immigrants to the United States is increasing. Poverty is a challenge that many of them face.
- When working with students from immigrant families, it is extremely helpful to partner with an interpreter or other person from the family's own cultural background.
- There are four different levels of acculturation: traditional, acculturated, marginal, and bicultural.
- Internationally adopted children can experiences issues in acculturation when they arrive in the United States. Many of them, especially older ones, also face challenges such as language delays as well as medical and emotional problems.

Add your own summary points here:

_____

_____

_____

IMPACT OF RELIGIOUS AND CULTURAL BELIEFS ON SERVICE DELIVERY

In the United States, two taboo subjects for most people are religion and politics. Most SLPs do not consider a family's religious or even cultural beliefs when making decisions about assessment and intervention for children. However, for some students and their families, religious and cultural beliefs can impact decisions about service delivery for students who need language intervention. Sometimes the family's belief about causes of disabilities can have an effect on whether or not language assessment and intervention can be carried out.

Beliefs about Causes of Disabilities

Salas-Provance, Erickson, and Reed (2002) state that SLPs must be careful not to stereotype families' beliefs about causes of disabilities based upon cultural, religious, or linguistic background. Salas-Provance et al., who studied forty people from four generations of one Hispanic family, found that beliefs in folk causes and cures of disabilities varied according to gender, age, income, and education. For example, the older, less-educated Hispanics in this study tended to believe strongly in folk remedies for ear problems. In contrast, younger and better-educated family members used traditional medical care more frequently for curing disabilities, including middle ear problems.

The older family members placed a great deal of emphasis on religion and religious rites as related to health and illness; in contrast, more than half of the younger family members were unfamiliar with the important cultural ritual of praying a *novena*. This study illustrates the importance of not stereotyping persons from various CLD backgrounds according to language and ethnicity; again, gender, age, income, and education are important variables that also influence people's beliefs.

With this in mind, SLPs should remember that individuals from some religious backgrounds may believe that a child's disability is the will of God or fate. Kayser (1998) tells the story of a Hispanic mother who prayed for another baby. Her four-year-old son ingested peroxide and, due to massive brain damage, regressed to a four-month-old level in all areas. The mother did not want treatment for him because she believed that this was the answer to her prayer—her son had become a baby again, and would always be a baby.

Families who believe that God (or Allah) or fate has caused or allowed a child's disability may not be open to intervention of any kind. This depends on the exact nature of the family's religious beliefs. For these families, attempting to exercise control or change a situation might seem irreverent or even blasphemous (Roseberry-McKibbin, 2008; Lynch, 2004). Thus, for religious reasons, some families may decline services offered by SLPs.

> Some families may believe that a disability is caused by fate or the actions of a higher power. This may discourage them from seeking treatment.

Sharifzadeh (2004) reported that many "Middle Eastern" families might not be open to intervention for various reasons. However, a recent study (Khan, Roseberry-McKibbin, O'Hanlon, Roy, & Roberts, 2005) found that Sunni Muslim immigrants from Afghanistan and Pakistan in two California cities strongly supported rehabilitation/intervention for children with disabilities. SLPs must consider the needs and beliefs of individual families; if a family does not believe in the necessity of intervention, the SLP must not pressure the family to accept it.

Parents from certain religious backgrounds may feel personally responsible for a child's disabling condition. I had an Asian university student tell me that her sister was born with a cleft palate because of something the mother did wrong during the pregnancy. Vining (1999) discussed some of the beliefs of Navajo Indians; for example, a child is born with a disability because of curses placed on the child or taboos violated by parents. If parents feel shame, that they have somehow caused the child's disability through their own wrongdoing or the sins of ancestors, then they may be embarrassed to seek intervention. Children with disabilities may be hidden for quite some time until the family is forced by law to send them to school, where the disability is finally discovered.

CONNECT & EXTEND

Research comparing the beliefs of Mexican American and Anglo-American mothers can be found in Rodriguez, B.L., & Olswang, L.B. (2003). Mexican-American and Anglo-American mothers' beliefs and values about child rearing, education, and language impairment. *American Journal of Speech-Language Pathology, 12*(4), 452–462.

Rodriguez and Olswang (2003) investigated the cross-cultural and intracultural diversity of mothers' values and beliefs regarding education, child rearing, and the causes of language impairment. Two groups of mothers were compared: Anglo-American and Mexican American. One major finding from this study was that 80 percent of the Mexican American mothers attributed their child's language problems to extrinsic factors. These included God's will or spirituality, mismatches between the home and the school, and the lack of a stimulating home environment. In contrast, only 40 percent of the Anglo-American mothers attributed their children's language problems to extrinsic factors.

Beliefs about Treatment for Children with Disabilities

Most SLPs approach treatment for children with any type of disability—including an SLI—with the attitude that the goal is to help the child function as independently as possible. But we have to remember that in some cultures, as we have said, independence for children is not a high priority. For example, in other cultures, less emphasis is placed on toilet training. Young children do not wear diapers—they relieve themselves freely wherever they are and are washed as needed. Breastfeeding may occur for an extended period of time—in some cultures, it is not unusual for three- and four-year old children to still be nursing. In many cultures, children are not cared for by anyone except family members until they are six or seven years old, at which time they begin attending elementary school. Because cultures such as these value *interdependence* more than *independence,* families may hold the view that caring for a child with a disability is not a burden (Lynch, 2004). Thus, these families might be less likely to bring a child to an SLP for intervention, especially if the child is young.

Along these lines, Salas-Provance et al. (2002, p. 152) describe the attitude toward disabilities among some Hispanic families:

Because some members of the Hispanic culture often distinguish between the disability and what they describe as the normal child within, children with disabilities may be considered healthy and normal. Being healthy could simply refer to a lack of physical illness or disease, and being normal may be culturally defined as being able to attend to daily living at their present level of functioning. . . . In addition, a close relationship exists between religion and illness. Therefore, a disability may be viewed as a divine punishment for sin, and the family may believe they should not interfere with God's will.

Other families may believe in varying forms of treatment that differ from Western intervention methods (Hanson, 2004). A nurse friend of mine worked in a central California hospital. One day he smelled smoke coming from the room of a Southeast Asian child. He rushed in to find that the family had literally lit a fire under the child's bed, hoping to drive away the evil spirits that caused the illness. Other families may believe that herbal remedies, religious ceremonies, and other forms of treatment are more effective than speech-language services, and act accordingly. In these situations, SLPs must try hard to work sensitively with the family, recommending speech-language intervention in conjunction with the family's preferred method of intervention. A friend of mine says that when the family says to her, "God can heal my child," she says, "Yes, God can—and He can use speech-language therapy as His tool to do so."

> Some CLD families may believe in forms of healing and intervention that differ from traditional Western methods.

Gender issues are always important to consider in working with families from some religious backgrounds (Lynch, 2004; Nellum-Davis, Gentry, & Hubbard-Wiley, 2002; Shipley & Roseberry-McKibbin, 2006). Some children from conservative religious families have parents who believe that female clinicians should not work with male children and vice versa. In other families, fathers may want their children to receive intervention from a male, not female, SLP. Lynch (2004) points out that in the United States, most service providers are women. They are accustomed to speaking their minds freely, earning money, and making their own choices.

However, in some cultures, wives defer to their husbands, who are considered the heads of the house. The wives have little or no role in decision making, even if they are the ones to carry out whatever is decided upon. These situations can be difficult for mainstream US female service providers, who naturally want to provide services themselves and also advocate for the mothers in the families they serve. However, this desire for personal service provision and advocacy may cause the female SLP to offend the family's cultural values and upset the mother, who is accustomed to a particular role and place. Female SLPs in the

CONNECT & EXTEND

Specific issues of how cultural and religious values of various groups may impact service delivery are described in Nellum Davis, P., Gentry, B., & Hubbard-Wiley, P. (2002). Clinical practice issues. In D.E. Battle (Ed.), *Communication disorders in multicultural populations* (3rd ed.) (pp. 461–486). Woburn, MA: Butterworth-Heinemann.

POINTS TO PONDER Describe two beliefs that might cause families not to seek intervention for a child with a disability.

_____

_____

_____

> In some families from certain religious backgrounds, it may be considered unacceptable for SLPs to work with a child or adult of the opposite gender.

United States must keep in mind that even if they disagree with the family's values, it is still important to be supportive and sensitive.

Some students may come from religious backgrounds where traditional American holidays such as Christmas and Easter are not celebrated. One sixth-grader told me that he could not complete an Easter crossword-puzzle activity because his family did not celebrate Easter. Speech-language assessment and intervention activities that involve holiday materials must be carefully considered when working with children from some religious backgrounds. Also, SLPs should remember that some children may be pulled out of school for one or more days while religious holidays are celebrated or religious ceremonies are held.

SUMMARY

- A family's cultural or religious beliefs can impact their receptivity toward intervention for a child with a disabling condition such as an SLI. A family may believe that God or fate caused a disability, and nothing should be done to intervene.
- A family may also believe in nontraditional forms of intervention that do not include speech-language services. In all these cases, SLPs must attempt to incorporate the family's belief system into optimal intervention services for the child involved.
- Families from some conservative backgrounds may not think it is acceptable for an SLP to work with a child of the opposite sex.
- Some families, due to their religious and cultural backgrounds, may also not celebrate certain holidays that mainstream Americans consider "standard."

Add your own summary points here:

_____

_____

_____

WORKING WITH STUDENTS WHO SPEAK AFRICAN AMERICAN ENGLISH

General Characteristics

Some children speak African American English (AAE). AAE is a rule-governed form of English that has been influenced by a number of languages of West Africa. Some African American children speak AAE; others do not. Some African American children codeswitch back and forth between AAE and mainstream English depending on the context (van Keulen et al., 1998). Many experts consider AAE to be a dialect of Mainstream American English. Battle (2002, pp. 360–361), states that

A dialect is a rule-governed variation in a language used by a racial, ethnic, geographic, or socioeconomic group. Although dialects of a language are generally intelligible to individuals outside the speech community, they reflect variations in almost every aspect of language. . . . Dialects of the same language may differ in form, pronunciation, vocabulary, and/or grammar from each other; however, they are enough alike to be mutually understood by speakers of different dialects of the same language.

Use of AAE is influenced by such factors as gender, age, socioeconomic status, and geographic region. Craig, Washington, and Thompson-Porter (1998) found in their study that African American children from low-income homes used more "dialectal forms" than their peers from middle class homes. Boys' discourse showed more evidence of these forms than girls' discourse. Craig, Thompson, Washington, and Potter (2003) stated that preschool and kindergarten African American students produce up to sixteen different morphosyntactic types of AAE. The research of Isaacs (1996) indicates that children who speak AAE use it most frequently between the ages of three and eight; after age eight, children may use AAE less as they are increasingly exposed to Mainstream American English in school.

> Children's use of African American English is influenced by a number of factors, including socioeconomic status and gender.

Jackson and Roberts (2001) examined changes in the complex syntax production of eighty-five three- and four-year-old African American children and the role of family and child factors in the children's production of complex syntax. Child factors included age, gender, and use of AAE. Family factors included home environment factors such as the stimulation and responsiveness available in children's homes (e.g., acceptance of the child's behavior, emotional/verbal responsiveness of the parent, provision of appropriate play materials, variety in daily experience).

Jackson and Roberts found that children from more responsive homes used more complex syntax forms; the amount of complex syntax a child used was not related to the use of AAE. Girls produced more complex sentences than boys did. Jackson and Roberts concluded that gender and home environment affected the complex syntax development of the children they studied and suggested that "the finding that complex syntax use was not affected by dialect use suggests the usefulness of examining this area of language development across different cultural groups" (p. 1094).

> Ideally, children who speak African American English (AAE) learn to be proficient in both AAE and mainstream English. In this way, they retain optimal linguistic flexibility and cultural identity.

Ideally, children who speak AAE are able to become "bidialectal"; that is, they learn and use mainstream English and retain AAE also. In this way, they have maximum linguistic flexibility and cultural identity. Campbell (1993) stated that children who speak AAE can be taught the difference between "home language" and "school language," a nonpejorative way of helping children be confidently bidialectal.

Many standardized articulation and language tests are biased against children who speak AAE (Craig & Washington, 2002; Thompson, Craig, & Washington, 2002; Thomas-Tate, Washington, & Edwards, 2004; Stockman, 2006; Wyatt, 2002). Most of these tests are based on the characteristics of Anglo children who speak Mainstream American English. When SLPs assess AAE speakers, it is critical to know which speech and language characteristics reflect the influence of AAE, and which characteristics reflect signs of SLI (Johnson, 2005). Table 4.1 describes characteristics of AAE morphology

TABLE 4.1   Characteristics of African American English (AAE) Morphology and Syntax

AAE Feature/Characteristic	Mainstream American English	Sample AAE Utterance
Omission of noun possessive	That's the woman's car. It's John's pencil.	That **the woman** car. It **John** pencil.
Omission of noun plural	He has two boxes of apples. She gives me five cents.	He got two **box** of **apple**. She give me five **cent**.
Omission of third-person singular present-tense marker	She walks to school. The man works in his yard.	She **walk** to school. The man **work** in his yard.
Omission of "to be" forms such as "is, are"	She is a nice lady. They are going to a movie.	**She a** nice lady. **They going** to a movie.
Present tense "is" may be used regardless of person/number.	They are having fun. You are a smart man.	**They is** having fun. **You is** a smart man.
Utterances with "to be" may not show person-number agreement with past and present forms.	You are playing ball. They are having a picnic.	**You is** playing ball. They **is** having a picnic.
Present-tense forms of auxiliary "have" are omitted.	I have been here for two hours. He has done it again.	I been here for two hours. He done it again.
Past-tense endings may be omitted.	He lived in California. She cracked the nut.	He **live** in California. She **crack** the nut.
Past "was" may be used regardless of number and person.	They were shopping. You were helping me.	They **was** shopping. You **was** helping me.
Multiple negatives (each additional negative form adds emphasis to the negative meaning).	We don't have any more. I don't want any cake. I don't like broccoli.	We **don't** have **no** more. I **don't never** want **no** cake. I **don't never** like broccoli.
"None" may be substituted for "any."	She doesn't want any.	She don't want **none**.
Perfective construction; "been" may be used to indicate that an action took place in the distant past.	I had the mumps last year. I have known her for years.	I **been had** the mumps last year. I **been known** her.
"Done" may be combined with a past-tense form to indicate that an action was started and completed.	He fixed the stove. She tried to paint it.	He **done fixed** the stove. She **done tried** to paint it.
The form "be" may be used as the main verb.	Today she is working. We are singing.	Today **she be** working. **We be** singing.
Distributive "be" may be used to indicate actions and events over time.	He is often cheerful. She's kind sometimes.	**He be** cheerful. **She be** kind.
A pronoun may be used to restate the subject.	My brother surprised me. My dog has fleas.	My brother, **he** surprise me. My dog, **he** got fleas.
"Them" may be substituted for "those."	Those cars are antiques. Where'd you get those books?	**Them cars**, they be antique. Where you get **them books**?
Future tense "is, are" may be replaced by "gonna."	She is going to help us. They are going to be there.	She **gonna** help us. They **gonna** be there.

TABLE 4.1   Characteristics of African American English (AAE) Morphology and Syntax (*continued*)

AAE Feature/Characteristic	Mainstream American English	Sample AAE Utterance
"At" is use at the end of "where" questions.	Where is the house? Where is the store?	Where is the house **at**? Where is the store **at**?
Additional auxiliaries are often used.	I might have done it.	I **might could have** done it.
"Does" is replaced by "do."	She does funny things. It does make sense.	**She do** funny things. **It do** make sense.

Used with permission. From Roseberry-McKibbin, C. (2008) *Multicultural students with special language needs: Practical strategies for assessment and intervention* (3rd edition), Oceanside, CA: Academic Communication Associates, Inc.

CONNECT & EXTEND

The phonological characteristics of children who speak AAE are described in depth in a study by Craig, H.K., Thompson, C.A., Washington, J.A., & Potter, S.L. (2003). Phonological features of child African American English. *Journal of Speech, Language, and Hearing Research, 46*(3), 623–635.

and syntax. Table 4.2 shows examples of utterances that would be considered acceptable in children who speak AAE. Speakers of AAE who manifest these characteristics show signs of linguistic difference, not SLI.

Characteristics of Communication

As we discussed in Chapter 1, communication style is influenced by pragmatics, or the social rules governing language use in context. Communication style may differ between speakers of AAE and Mainstream American English. For example, in a conversation involving AAE-speaking participants, traditional turn-taking may not be observed and interruptions may be very frequent. Conversational partners are expected to participate verbally in conversations, and verbal competition may prevail as the most assertive participants do most of the talking (van Keulen et al., 1998). SLPs must be careful not to judge this behavior as "rude" or as a sign of a "pragmatics disorder."

POINTS TO PONDER Describe four grammatical characteristics of African American English that an SLP might mistake for signs of SLI.

_____

_____

_____

TABLE 4.2   Examples of Acceptable Utterances by Speakers of African American English

Mainstream American English	African American English
That boy looks like me.	That boy, he look like me.
If he kicks it, he'll be in trouble.	If he kick it, he be in trouble.
When the lights are off, it's dark.	When the lights be off, it dark.
It could be somebody's pet.	It could be somebody pet.
Her feet are too big.	Her feet is too big.
I'll get something to eat.	I will get me something to eat.
She is dancing and the music's on.	She be dancin' an' the music on.
What kind of cheese do you want?	What kind of cheese you want?
My brother's name is Joe.	My brother name is Joe.
I raked the leaves outside.	I rakted the leaves outside.
After the recital, they shook my hand.	After the recital, they shaketed my hand.
They are standing around.	They is just standing around.
He is a basketball star.	He a basketball star.
They are in cages.	They be in cages.
It's not like a tree or anything.	It not like a tree or nothin'.
He does like to fish.	He do like to fish.
They are going to swim.	They gonna swim.
Mom already repaired the car.	Mom done repair the car.

Used with permission. From Roseberry-McKibbin, C. (2008) *Multicultural students with special language needs: Practical strategies for assessment and intervention* (3rd edition), Oceanside, CA: Academic Communication Associates, Inc.

> Speakers of African American English have communication styles that differ from mainstream English. These include nontraditional turn-taking and narrative differences.

African American culture contains communication rituals and distinctive styles that affirm cultural identity and allegiance to the group. For example, in many African American churches, the congregation engages in **call-and-response** where they echo part of the preacher's previous utterance. If the preacher says, "Jesus rose from the dead on Easter morning," the congregation might say, "on Easter morning" (van Keulen et al., 1998). An African American child, in class, might echo part of what a teacher says. This is part of his culture. It is not echolalia or a sign of an SLI.

Some AAE-speaking students are quiet in front of unfamiliar adults and may make little eye contact. SLPs must not misjudge these students as having expressive language or pragmatics problems. AAE-speaking students also have narrative styles that differ from those of mainstream English-speaking students. SLPs must be aware of these stylistic

CONNECT & EXTEND

Thorough explanations of characteristics of communication styles of African American English speakers are found in van Keulen, J.E., Weddington, G.T., & DeBose, C.E. (1998). *Speech, language, learning, and the African American child.* Boston: Allyn & Bacon.

Children who speak African American English may differ from Mainstream American English speakers along many parameters, including narrative style, discourse style, and areas of pragmatics.

differences so that AAE-speaking students are not misdiagnosed as having clinically significant narrative problems (Gutierrez-Clellen & Quinn, 1993; Kamhi, Pollock, & Harris, 1996; Terrell & Jackson, 2002; van Keulen et al., 1998):

- AAE-speaking students may include personal judgments in their stories as well as personal evaluations of the characters.
- These students often rely on gestures to accompany and augment narratives.
- AAE-speaking students may also tell stories with a topic-associating style, characterized by lack of consideration for detail, presupposition of shared knowledge between listeners and speakers, and structured discourse on several linked topics. This contrasts with the mainstream narrative style, which is characterized by topic elaboration, lack of presupposition of shared knowledge between speakers and listeners, and structured discourse on a single topic. SLPs must be aware of these differences in narrative communication styles of AAE- and mainstream English-speaking students so misdiagnoses will not be made.

It is also important to think about the effect of AAE on children's interaction with print. Children who speak Mainstream American English at home have congruence in the language they speak at home and the language of books in school. AAE-speaking children who come from print-rich environments where parents model and reinforce emergent literacy skills will likely enter first grade equal to their counterparts who have had the same or similar experiences. However, for children who speak AAE and have not been taught emergent literacy skills, their spoken home language is not represented in conventional textbooks or storybooks. This lack of congruence for AAE-speaking children can cause teachers to misjudge them as having SLI or learning disabilities. Teachers need

CASES TO CONSIDER

I remember a five-year-old AAE-speaking boy in one of my therapy sessions. Isaiah, a kindergartener with a wide grin and charming personality, was constantly interrupting me when I was talking to his small group. What would you do in my place? Would you tell Isaiah that he was rude? Would you let him continue to interrupt the therapy session frequently? How might you handle the situation?

_____

_____

_____

to understand cultural differences to prevent misconceptions about AAE-speaking students and their ability to learn (van Keulen et al., 1998).

SLPs must also keep the factor of SES in mind when assessing the language abilities of children who speak AAE. Hammer and Weiss (1999) studied low- and mid-SES African American mothers and their interactions with their children. Hammer and Weiss showed that mid-SES mothers tended to include significantly more language goals (for example, labeling objects) in their interactions with their children than low-SES mothers. Hammer and Weiss speculated that as the children in the low-SES group grew older, they might be at risk for lower gains in language skills as measured by standardized tests. When interaction styles at home differ from those expected at school, children may not develop language skills that will help them to perform well on standardized tests in the school setting.

 SUMMARY

- African American English (AAE) is a rule-governed form of English that has been influenced by a number of languages of West Africa.
- Some African American children speak AAE; others do not. Some African American children codeswitch back and forth between AAE and mainstream English.
- Use of AAE is influenced by such factors as gender, age, socioeconomic status, and geographic region.
- Speakers of AAE have many language characteristics that differ from Mainstream American English. For example, speakers of AAE may delete plural and possessive -*s*.
- Many standardized language tests are biased against students who speak AAE.
- Parameters of language use such as turn-taking and narrative style are distinctive to students who speak AAE. It is important to not interpret these as signs of an SLI.

Add your own summary points here:

_____

_____

_____

WORKING WITH STUDENTS WHO SPEAK SPANISH-INFLUENCED ENGLISH

General Considerations

Globally, Spanish is spoken as a first language by approximately 322 to 358 million speakers (Grimes, 2003). Hispanics are the fastest-growing racial/ethnic group in the United States. In the last ten years, the US Hispanic population has grown 58 percent; today, Hispanics make up 12.1 percent of the US population, and 35 percent of them are under 18 years

CASES TO CONSIDER

At a local high school, I was confronted with a hard-of-hearing Spanish-speaking seventeen-year-old whose family had come from Mexico one year ago. The school asked me to evaluate his language skills and provided a cordial Spanish-speaking interpreter to assist me. Approximately five minutes into the testing session, she stopped and said that she was from Argentina and that some of the vocabulary words on one of the tests were unfamiliar to her. What would you have done at that point? What steps would you have taken?

_____

_____

_____

There are many varieties of Spanish, and this can impact service delivery to Spanish-speaking students.

CONNECT & EXTEND

Detailed information about cultural and linguistic characteristics of Spanish-speaking children is available in Brice, A.E. (2002). *The Hispanic child: Speech, language, culture and education.* Boston, MA: Allyn & Bacon.

of age (US Bureau of the Census, 2000). Many varieties of Spanish are spoken in the United States. The two major Spanish dialects in the United States are southwestern (e.g., Mexican) and Caribbean (e.g., Puerto Rican and Cuban). Many variations occur within and between these two major Spanish dialects. Variations of Spanish spoken in countries such as Spain, Brazil, and Guatemala are reflected in phonology, syntax, morphology, and semantics. SLPs must constantly keep these variations in mind when assessing and treating Spanish-speaking students (Goldstein, 2000).

The 23rd Annual Report to Congress on the Implementation of IDEA (Individuals with Disabilities Education Act) indicated that a significant number of students with limited English proficiency have concomitant disabilities, and that these students are at even greater risk for negative educational outcomes. In addition, this report stated that 12.7 percent of students with speech and language impairments were Latinos (US Department of Education, 2001). Thus, it is important to be aware that many Spanish-speaking children may have legitimate communication disorders. However, sometimes Spanish-speaking students are referred by classroom teachers for SLI when in reality, the students are merely manifesting characteristics of Spanish-influenced English. Table 4.3 describes language differences commonly observed among Spanish speakers. This information is useful in differentiating a language difference from SLI in a Spanish-speaking student.

Characteristics of Communication

Spanish-speaking children may differ greatly in their communication style depending upon many factors such as length of residence in the United States, educational level of

TABLE 4.3 Language Differences Commonly Observed Among Spanish Speakers

Language Characteristics	*Sample English Utterances*
1. Adjective comes after noun.	The house green.
2. *'s* is often omitted in plurals and possessives.	The girl book is . . . Juan hat is red.
3. Past tense *-ed* is often omitted.	We walk yesterday.
4. Double negatives are required.	I don't have no more.
5. Superiority is demonstrated by using *más*.	This cake is more big.
6. The adverb often follows the verb.	He drives very fast his motorcycle.

Used with permission. From Roseberry-McKibbin, C. (2008) *Multicultural students with special language needs: Practical strategies for assessment and intervention* (3rd edition), Oceanside, CA: Academic Communication Associates, Inc.

the parents, gender, language transfer between Spanish and English, and others (Brice, 2002; Jackson-Maldonado, 2004). However, SLPs can be aware of certain common characteristics so that misdiagnoses are not made.

First, rules of **proxemics**, or the use of space in conversations, differ between Hispanics and mainstream American speakers. Many Hispanics tend to stand or sit quite close to their conversation partners. When children talk to adults, they may often look down or away as a sign of respect, thus breaking the mainstream eye contact rule of "look at me when I talk to you" (Zuniga, 2004).

In addition, children are often not expected to participate in adult conversations out of respect; conversations are usually held with siblings or peers instead. I have heard mainstream professionals comment that Hispanic children are "so quiet" and "don't participate." I also have found it challenging to engage Hispanic children in conversation during speech-language testing when they do not know me. It is important to not misdiagnose these children as having expressive language delays.

> Hispanic students manifest some differences in communication style. These may include lack of eye contact with adults as well as reluctance to talk with adults out of respect.

Expressive language among Hispanic children is influenced by other factors as well. In many Hispanic homes, parents do not relate actions to words by verbalizing about ongoing events. Adults do not usually ask children to repeat facts or foretell what they will do. Madding (1999), in her research with Mexican mothers, found that many of them taught their children politeness and respect, but did not prioritize the teaching of prekindergarten concepts such as shapes, colors, or letters. The mothers considered this to be the school's responsibility. Garcia, Mendez Perez, and Ortiz (2000) also stated that Mexican American mothers may be more likely to view their role as "mothering" rather than "teaching."

A study by Mendez Perez (2000) examined the beliefs and attitudes of Spanish-speaking Mexican American mothers whose young children had disabilities. Mendez Perez found that the mothers in her study did not expect their children to speak until the age of three; thus, they were not especially concerned about their children's communication problems. The mothers believed that their children would eventually "catch up," and they did not associate limited verbal skills with disabilities. The mothers in this study viewed themselves as active participants in their children's language learning.

More research with Spanish-speaking mothers is needed, and this research should extend to (among other things) mothers from Cuban, Central American, South American, and Caribbean backgrounds. Bliss, McCabe, and Mahecha (2001) found that some Spanish-speaking children, especially from Central America or the Caribbean, came from homes where narratives deemphasized sequencing and action events. SLPs must keep all these variables in mind so that Spanish-speaking children are not misdiagnosed as SLI when in fact their communication style reflects their linguistic and cultural background.

Hammer, Miccio, and Wagstaff (2003) studied the developing bilingual skills of Spanish-speaking preschool children in a US community. They found that some of these children learned English in a *sequential* fashion (described in Chapter 3), where they had been exposed to English through things like trips to the grocery store, television, and other excursions into the English-speaking community. However, even though these children had been exposed to English, they had not been placed in situations where they had to communicate in English. For example, they had not been asked to follow directions, speak, or interact in English with members of their community until they attended preschool at three years of age.

The *simultaneous* learners had been systematically exposed to English and Spanish from birth and had been required to answer questions, follow directions, and interact with family and community members in English and in Spanish. Hammer et al. (2003) pointed out that professionals cannot assume that mere exposure to English (as in the case of the sequential learners) is the same thing as being both exposed to and required to interact in English (simultaneous learners). Children who have learned English and Spanish simultaneously may find it easier to fit in, at least initially, in environments such as school where only English is spoken.

Another variable to keep in mind is that some Hispanic students live in migrant families. More than 70 percent of all migrant farmworkers here in the United States are Spanish speaking. Here in California, we have hundreds of students from migrant farm families. I have had several Hispanic university students who told me stories about how as children, they would travel from town to town, working the fields with their parents. When they were seven or eight years old, they would pick strawberries for hours in 100-plus degree weather. Their lives primarily centered on survival, and education was not a high priority.

> For migrant Hispanic students, school attendance is an issue that can impact linguistic and academic progress.

Fifty percent of United States migrant farm children leave school before ninth grade (Bennett, 2003). A challenge for me as a public school SLP providing services to students from migrant families is that the students often leave school in the middle of the year; they may be back months later, or they may not. These types of students face linguistic and academic challenges because their lifestyle makes school attendance sporadic.

SUMMARY

- Hispanics are the fastest-growing ethnic/racial group in the United States. A large percentage of the Hispanic population is under eighteen years of age.
- Spanish-speaking students, when speaking English, may show signs of transfer from Spanish. For example, in Spanish, the adjective comes after the noun (as in "the horse brown" instead of "the brown horse").
- SLPs must be aware of cultural communication differences that can lead to a false diagnosis of SLI. For instance, many Hispanic children are taught to be silent in the presence of unfamiliar adults and to not make eye contact.
- Hispanic students from migrant homes may have sporadic school attendance that impacts their linguistic and academic development.

Add your own summary points here:

_____

_____

_____

WORKING WITH STUDENTS WHO SPEAK ENGLISH INFLUENCED BY ASIAN LANGUAGES

General Considerations

The variation in Asian languages makes it extremely difficult to generalize about the characteristics of "Asian-influenced" English. The reader is referred to sources that describe these characteristics by specific language groups in greater detail (e.g., Cheng, 1991, 2002; Hwa-Froelich, Hodson, & Edwards, 2002). In this section, general considerations are discussed and specific "generic" characteristics of Asian-influenced English are presented.

In the United States today, some of the most widely spoken Asian languages are Tagalog, Chinese (both Mandarin and Cantonese), Khmer, Korean, Vietnamese, and Japanese. Some of these major groups have languages and dialects within them. In the Philippines, where I was raised by missionary parents, one could travel ten miles to the next barrio and not be able to understand the residents of that barrio. I mentioned earlier that my sisters and I learned Tagalog (the national language), Hiligaynon (the language of the region), and Odionganon (the language of the town of Odiongan where we lived). These were all separate languages.

CONNECT & EXTEND

For an extensive description of Asian languages and Asian-influenced English, see Cheng, L.L. (2002). Asian and Pacific American cultures. In D.E. Battle (Ed.), *Communication disorders in multicultural populations* (3rd ed.) (pp. 71–112). Woburn, MA: Butterworth-Heinemann.

> There is great variety in Asian languages. Most Asian languages have dialects.

There may also be dialects within each language. I remember being asked to assess a Hmong-speaking fifth-grader. When the interpreter arrived and began conversing with the girl, the interpreter said she was unsure of the eventual testing results because she spoke White Hmong and the girl spoke Green Hmong. Thankfully, the assessment was satisfactorily completed because there was enough overlap between the two Hmong dialects for mutual intelligibility.

Some Asian languages are **tonal**. Each tone change represents a meaning change and is phonemic in nature (Fung & Roseberry-McKibbin, 1999; Wong, Schwartz, & Jenkins, 2005). For example, in the Chinese language of Mandarin, the word "ma" can mean *curse, scold, flax*, or *horse* depending on the tone used. Tones that affect meaning, or **tonemes**, are plentiful in some languages. Northern Vietnamese has six tonemes, and Cantonese has seven tonemes. Korean, Khmer (spoken in Cambodia), and Japanese are not tonal languages.

Some Asian languages, such as Laotian, Vietnamese, and Chinese are almost exclusively monosyllabic. Other languages, such as Tagalog and Thai, have words containing many syllables. For example, the Tagalog word *pakikisama* means good will or harmony between people. Vietnamese and Chinese do not contain consonant blends, and some languages are spoken with slight nasality. Some languages such as Japanese, Tagalog, and Indonesian do not have specific gender pronouns such as "she" and "he"; everything is referred to as "it." Many Asian languages do not have inflectional markers such as plurals and past-tense endings.

I have found that teachers often refer Asian children for speech-language screenings for "grammar" errors. If SLPs are not familiar with language differences commonly observed among children from Asian backgrounds, these children may be misdiagnosed as having speech-language disorders. Table 4.4 reflects some characteristics of Asian-influenced English production.

Earlier in this chapter, we discussed the importance of being culturally competent, which involves, among other things, being sensitive to our CLD children and their families. Part of this sensitivity, in my opinion, is knowing about the names of our clients. We need to know how to pronounce these names—sometimes an adventure in itself—and we also benefit from knowing background information about names. I remember one experience at a local high school. I was to assess a student named T. Nguyen. I went to the school office to look up her records. To my shock, in this large high school, there were 30-plus students with the last name of Nguyen! I would have benefited from knowing that approximately 52 percent of Vietnamese individuals have the family name "Nguyen." Table 4.5 gives information about Asian names to assist the reader in this area so that errors are not made.

Characteristics of Communication

Families from Asian countries differ vastly in their communication styles. However, some common tendencies have been noted and are briefly discussed here. First, some Asian children are taught that they need to say "yes" and agree with the speaker no matter how they

TABLE 4.4 Language Differences Commonly Observed Among Asian Speakers

Language Characteristics	Sample English Utterances
Omission of plurals	Here are two piece of toast. I got five finger on each hand.
Omission of copula	He going home now. They eating.
Omission of possessive	I have Phuong pencil. Mom food is cold.
Omission of past-tense morpheme	We cook dinner yesterday. Last night she walk home.
Past-tense double marking	He didn't went by himself.
Double negative	They don't have no books.
Subject-verb-object relationship differences/omissions	I messed up it. He like.
Misordering of interrogatives	You are going now?
Misuse or omission of prepositions	She is in home. He goes to school 8:00.
Misuse of pronouns	She husband is coming. She said her wife is here.
Omission and/or overgeneralization of articles	Boy is sick. He went the home.
Incorrect use of comparatives	This book is gooder than that book.
Omission of conjunctions	You_____I going to the beach.
Omission lack of inflection on auxiliary "do"	She_____not take it. He do not have enough.
Omission, lack of inflection on forms of "have"	She have no money. We_____been the store.

Used with permission. From Roseberry-McKibbin, C. (2008) *Multicultural students with special language needs: Practical strategies for assessment and intervention* (3rd edition), Oceanside, CA: Academic Communication Associates, Inc.

> Many Asian children are taught to be quiet and re-spectful with authority figures. They are also taught to not question authority figures.

feel or think. In the Philippines, children always agreed with adults to show respect, even if they had no intention of doing what the adult asked. Sue and Sue (2003) discuss the fact that in some parts of the Philippines, if you want to say "no," you say a weak and hesitant "yes." It is the job of the listener to pick up on the *way* you said "yes," and assume that you really meant "no."

Most Asian children are taught not to make eye contact with adults, because this is considered disrespectful. Many children are

TABLE 4.5   Information about Asian Family Names

Characteristics of names most often given to members of various Asian populations are summarized below.

Cambodian	Names consist of two parts. Family name precedes personal name. Middle names are rare.
Chinese	Names consist of two parts. Family name precedes personal name. Most Chinese names consist of only one syllable. Common Chinese names: Chan, Chang, Chiang, Chin, Chow, Chung, Lee, Louie, Lum, Wong, Woo.
Hmong	Most names consist of two parts. Family name precedes personal name. Common Hmong family names: Chang, Chue, Fang, Her, Khang, Kue, Lor, Lee, Moua, Thao, Vang, Vue, Xiong, Yang.
Indonesian	Names consist of two parts. Many are polysyllabic and thus quite lengthy by American standards (e.g., "Pranawahadi"). Many Indonesians have Muslim names.
Japanese	Most names consist of two parts. Family name precedes personal name. To be polite when interacting with an authority figure, "san" is added to the end of the individual's last name. Japanese names often consist of more than one syllable. Common Japanese surnames: Kawaguchi, Nakamura, Tanaka, Watanabe, Yamamoto.
Korean	Most names consist of a family name that precedes a two-part personal name. Common Korean surnames are Kim, Park, Lee.
Laotian	Family name precedes personal name. Names may consist of more than one syllable, and some are quite lengthy by American standards (e.g., Souphanouvong).
Thai	Personal name precedes the surname. Some names are quite long (e.g., Suvarnarami).
Vietnamese	Names consist of three components: family, middle, and given names. The family name is followed by the middle name and personal name respectively. The name, Nguyen Van Thieu, for example, begins with the family name "Nguyen" and ends with "Thieu," the name that the individual is called by family members and friends. Approximately 52% of Vietnamese individuals have the family name "Nguyen"; 31% have the family name "Tran." Other common family names are Pham, Le, Ngo, Do, Dao, Vu, Hoang, Dang, Dinh, and Duong.

Information included in this table was obtained from the *Asian American Handbook* (1991). Used with permission. From Roseberry-McKibbin, C. (2008) *Multicultural students with special language needs: Practical strategies for assessment and intervention* (3rd edition), Oceanside, CA: Academic Communication Associates, Inc.

taught to be "seen and not heard." Authority figures are never questioned. Modesty and humility are highly valued, and cooperation is much more the norm than competition. Many children are not encouraged to question or criticize; rather, rote memorization and agreement with authority figures is encouraged.

CASES TO CONSIDER

I was asked to assess Fong, a twelve-year-old speaker of Mien who was being considered for placement in a Communicatively Handicapped classroom. I went to Fong's classroom, introduced myself, and brought her to my speech room. I attempted to draw Fong into conversation about various games, toys, and books. She would not look at me or speak to me. What would have been a good next step in this situation? How could I have helped Fong become more comfortable with me so that she would give me the expressive language sample that I needed to gather?

_____

_____

_____

Many Asian children learn that outward emotional expressions such as body movements and facial expressions are discouraged except for extreme situations (Sue & Sue, 2003). It is easy for SLPs to misdiagnose these children as being "passive," having expressive language problems, pragmatics problems, and difficulties with problem-solving and critical thinking skills. However, the children are merely behaving as they were taught to. Table 4.6 summarizes cultural variants that are characteristic of children from diverse cultures, including Asian cultures. These variants must be considered as SLPs provide service to CLD students.

SUMMARY

- Asian languages may have many dialects within each language group. These may or may not be mutually intelligible.
- Some Asian languages are tonal; tonemes are tone changes that change the meaning of words.
- Some Asian languages are monosyllabic, and some are polysyllabic.
- Many Asian children are taught to be modest, humble, and silent in the presence of adults. They may be encouraged to conform to what adults want them to know rather than question information and think critically.

Add your own summary points here:

_____

_____

_____

TABLE 4.6 Cultural Variants That May Influence Assessment

Concept	Other Cultures*	Majority US Culture
Achievement	Cooperation and group spirit. Accept status quo. Manual labor respected.	Emphasis on competition and success. Define self by accomplishments. *To the victor go the spoils.*
Age	Elders are revered. Growing old is desirable.	Youth is valued.
Communication	Respectful, avoid eye contact, loudness for anger, Silence means boredom. Nonlinguistic and paralinguistic cues important.	Casual, direct eye contact, loud voice acceptable. Silence means attentiveness. Emphasize verbal skills.
Control	Fate.	Free will, control over destiny.
Education	Formal for few. Entrance into mainstream society. Elders, peers, and siblings are teachers. Active, physical learning. Spontaneous, intuitive. Testing not integral.	Universal, formal, verbal, key to social mobility. Teacher is authority. Classroom passivity rewarded. Reflective, analytical. Tests are part of learning.
Family	Extended, kinship important, more varied, elder or parent centered. Male or female dominated.	Nuclear, small, contractual partnership, child centered.
Gender/role	Males independent, pampered. Females have many home responsibilities.	Relative equality.
Individuality	Humility, anonymity, deference to group.	Individual makes own life. Stress self-reliance.
Materialism	Excessive accumulation is bad, status ascribed.	Acquisition, symbol of success and power.
Social interaction	Contact, physical closeness. Kinship more important than friends.	Noncontact, large interpartner distance. Large group of friends desired.
Time	Enjoy the present, can't change future. Little concept of wasting time. Flexible.	Governed by clock and calendar, punctual, value speed, future oriented. Time is money. Scheduled.

*No specific culture.

Compiled from Chamberlain & Medinos-Landurand (1991); Goldman & McDermott (1987). From Robert E. Owens Jr. *Language disorders. A functional approach to assessment and intervention 4e.* Published by Allyn 8 Bacon, Boston, MA. Copyright © 2005 by Pearson Education. Reprinted by permission of the publisher.

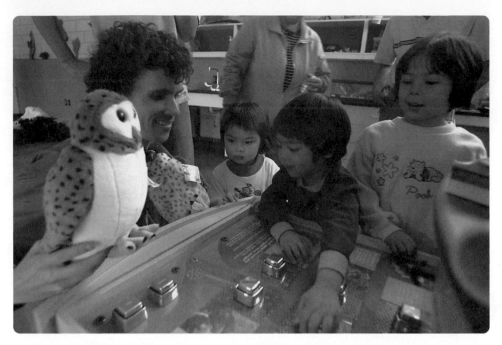

A culturally competent professional practices appropriate, relevant, and sensitive assessment and intervention strategies when serving CLD students.

CHAPTER HIGHLIGHTS

- It is important for SLPs to be culturally competent. Part of cultural competence involves recognizing the impact of different variables on the behavior of members of various cultures.
- SLPs can improve their cultural competence in practical ways. Some of these include reading, teaming up with persons from a local cultural community, and asking families to share important aspects of their culture.
- Immigrant and refugee families have unique needs and situations that may impact students' school performance. These needs and situations include poverty, lack of familiarity with English, and varying degrees of acculturation.
- Internationally adopted children may experience some difficulties in acculturation to the United States. These are compounded by other challenges such as language delays and possible delays in other areas.
- Some families have strong religious beliefs that impact their belief in and receptivity to intervention. If a family believes that a child's disability is caused by God or fate, they might not believe that intervention is desired or warranted.
- If a child has a disability, the family might believe that nontraditional forms of intervention are warranted. These can include herbal remedies, religious ceremonies, and treatment by a medicine person.

- Some students speak English that is influenced by their first language of African American English, Spanish, or an Asian language. These children may manifest language characteristics that are signs of a difference, not SLI.
- Children who speak African American English have grammatical characteristics that differ from those of Mainstream American English. They also may have unique communication styles that include such aspects as nontraditional turn-taking and narrative differences.
- Spanish-speaking children have communication style characteristics that differ from mainstream English. For example, they may not look an adult in the eye; they may also not converse readily with an unfamiliar adult out of respect.
- Asian languages are greatly varied. Many languages have a number of dialects. Some Asian languages are tonal; tone changes represent meaning changes.
- Some children from Asian language backgrounds may have been taught to be "seen and not heard." Thus, they may not question authority or volunteer in class because this is viewed as disrespectful.
- When working with children from diverse linguistic and cultural backgrounds, SLPs must always consider the impact of culture, immigrant/refugee status, religious values, and influence of the primary language on English production.

Add your own chapter highlights here:

_____

_____

_____

_____

STUDY AND REVIEW QUESTIONS

ESSAY

1. What is cultural competence? Describe how you can increase your cultural competence.

2. Immigrants to the United States generally experience one of four types of acculturation. Describe these four types.

3. What types of challenges are faced by children who are internationally adopted?

4. Describe how a CLD family's religious beliefs can impact their views of disabilities and their receptivity to language intervention.

5. Briefly describe two communication characteristics each of African American English–speaking, Spanish-speaking, and Asian language–speaking children that could be mistaken for signs of SLI.

FILL-IN-THE-BLANK

6. The concept of _____ refers to the view that in the United States, we all live together, but the distinguishing characteristics of each group are preserved and valued.

7. _____ poverty refers to a short-term circumstance for a family resulting from events such as moving to a new country where the parents' professional credentials are not accepted.

8. In the _____ level of acculturation, individuals adapt to the new culture but lose some parameters of their culture of origin.

9. Among some African Americans, the communication pattern of _____ occurs where listeners echo back part of the speaker's utterance.

10. _____ is a dynamic set of values and belief systems that shape the behavior of individuals from various groups and communities.

MULTIPLE CHOICE

11. Ways to become a culturally competent SLP include
    a. Evaluating your own values and assumptions
    b. Reading as much as you can about the family's cultural and linguistic background
    c. Not asking family members or interpreters questions about their culture because these questions might be considered prying
    d. a, b
    e. a, b, c

12. A teacher has referred Juan Lopez to you. His family is originally from Mexico. Juan has been in US schools for two years and is now in third grade. He is doing well academically given his status as an English Language Learner. However, his teacher thinks that he has an SLI. She tells you that "Juan makes mistakes in his English grammar; I think he needs speech-language therapy." You conduct a quick screening with Juan to see if you think he just has a language difference—normal transfer from Spanish to English—or an SLI. Which of the following utterances would NOT be typical for a student from a Spanish-speaking background? Which one of these utterances might possibly be an indicator of SLI, not just a normal language difference?
    a. He don't have no more of that.
    b. Yesterday my mom cook dinner for us.
    c. The dinner, it not be as good as was last Saturday.
    d. The teacher book is on her desk.
    e. The man drives very fast his car.

13. You are working with a kindergarten child, Ryan, whose family is from China. The Zhangs came to the United States three years ago. The parents have accented but very fluent English. As part of gathering information about Ryan and his family, you find out that in the home, both Mandarin and English are spoken. The Zhangs put Ryan in an English-speaking preschool one year prior to kindergarten. They made friends with some of the other parents, and frequently socialize with Americans. They also have many friends in their Chinese community. The Zhangs tell you that at Ryan's recent

birthday party, they had almost an equal number of Chinese and American friends. In your opinion, what kind of acculturation do the Zhangs have to US culture?

   a. Bicultural
   b. Traditional
   c. Marginal
   d. Acculturated
   e. None of the above

14. Which of these utterances would be typical for a TD child who speaks African American English?

   a. I been had the chicken pox when I was three years old.
   b. You is a good teacher.
   c. My daddy done fixed our car after it broke down.
   d. b, c
   e. a, b, c

15. In the past year, there has been a large influx of Southeast Asian children in the school where you work. The classroom teachers have been referring many of these children to you for assessment because they feel that the children have SLI. Which of the following would be a *legitimate* reason for a teacher to refer a Southeast Asian child to you?

   a. The child says things like "There are only two slide on playground."
   b. The child says things like "Yesterday, we walktid home be."
   c. The child makes little eye contact with adults, especially authority figures such as teachers.
   d. The child appears not to be proficient in critical thinking tasks.
   e. The child says things like "My mommy is in home with my brother."

See Answers to Study and Review Questions, page 465.

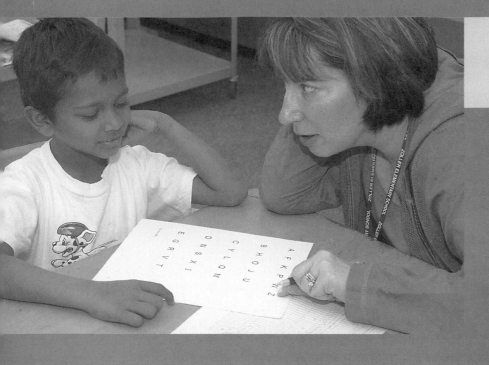

Assessment of Children with Language Impairments: Basic Principles

CASE STUDY

Mary Anne M. was an experienced kindergarten teacher. For the past thirty years, she had taught a wide range of children from upper-middle-class to low-income backgrounds. Mary Anne worked at an elementary school of 1,200 children. In her district, children represented more than eighty different languages; at her elementary school, one-third of the children came to school speaking a language other than English. Mary Anne had grown accustomed to teaching culturally and linguistically diverse (CLD) children and had learned to allow them time to gain English skills.

Many of them had not been in preschool, and she was accustomed to giving them the year of kindergarten to "catch up" with their peers in various areas.

But Abdul was different. A beautiful little boy with wide brown eyes and a sweet smile, Abdul was not learning as quickly as the majority of CLD children Mary Anne had taught in the past thirty years. As the other CLD children began to speak some English and make friends, Abdul remained silent and alone. While the other CLD children began to write their names and even print the alphabet, Abdul struggled to copy basic shapes. When Mary Anne asked the children to get their lunch cards and line up at the door, all the children did it except Abdul, who didn't seem to comprehend this basic routine even three months after school had started.

Mary Anne didn't want to be too preliminary in referring Abdul for a special education evaluation. She had taken extra coursework in the area of teaching CLD children and remembered that these children are often overreferred for special education. But at the end of the school year, Abdul was clearly far behind all his classmates—even the other CLD children. His mother asked Mary Anne if he could stay in kindergarten one more year. Mary Anne agreed, but she felt that it was important to at least bring Abdul's situation to the attention of the school Student Study Team. This team comprised the principal, speech-language phathologist (SLP), resource specialist, psychologist, and several teachers. The team's purpose was to discuss students who were having inordinate difficulty in the classroom and recommend ways to help these students be more successful. After some discussion, the team decided that Abdul needed to be screened for possible learning problems that went beyond his status as an English Language Learner. The SLP (this author) agreed to administer a full evaluation in both English and Urdu (his primary language) and share the results with the team.

To begin the evaluation, I met with Abdul's mother, Mrs. H. Mrs. H. shared that she and her husband were immigrants from Pakistan; Abdul and his brother were born in the United States. Mrs. H. had some difficulties with her pregnancy with Abdul, and several tests were performed to examine the status of the fetus. Testing in Mrs. H.'s second trimester revealed that Abdul had only one kidney and some other major problems; hospital personnel recommended that Mrs. H. terminate the pregnancy. Mrs. H., a Muslim, did not

agree with their recommendation and chose to carry Abdul for as long as she could. When Abdul was born prematurely at seven months' gestation, he had to spend weeks in the neonatal intensive care unit and he underwent several surgeries during his first year of life.

Mrs. H. told me that she was concerned because although Abdul was a happy child, he had not spoken his first word in Urdu until he was two-and-a-half years old. Even at the age of five, Abdul spoke in simple, three- or four-word utterances in Urdu and often echoed what he heard. He did not appear to understand even basic directions in Urdu at home. "Abdul's older brother did much better than this," she said. "In comparison to his older brother, Abdul has developed so much more slowly."

With the assistance of an interpreter, I attempted to informally assess Abdul's basic language and processing skills in Urdu. But he generally shook his head and smiled; when he answered, it was usually in English. The interpreter made continuous efforts to encourage Abdul to answer questions in his first language of Urdu. Abdul occasionally answered in Urdu, often answered in English, and frequently echoed the interpreter's exact words.

At the end of the evaluation, the interpreter said that Abdul appeared to have inordinate difficulty understanding what he heard and expressing himself, even in Urdu. His English wasn't much better. I brought this information back to the team, and Abdul was enrolled in speech-language therapy. It took me and my colleagues a whole year to teach Abdul basic prepositions and to have him state his chronological age correctly. His progress in therapy has been extremely slow. At this time, several years later, Abdul is being considered for placement in a classroom for special learners because he continues to perform much lower academically than his peers—even CLD peers.

INTRODUCTION

In this chapter and the rest of the book, we will be taking a closer look at "Monday morning" or practical suggestions for working with children with language impairments, so let's review the term *evidence-based practice,* which we have referred to earlier in the book. The American Speech-Language-Hearing Association (ASHA, 2005) reminds us that the goal of evidence-based practice is the integration of clinical expertise, client values, and best current evidence that helps us to provide quality services to the individuals we serve. Ultimately, the goal of evidence-based practice is ". . . a dynamic integration of ever-evolving clinical expertise and external evidence in day-to-day practice" (p. 1). As we discuss assessment, we need to keep in mind that ideally, any assessment of children's language skills should embody the principles of evidence-based practice.

Assessing children's language skills is one of the key activities of most SLPs who work with children. Assessment differs from diagnosis. **Assessment** (or evaluation) refers to the process of arriving at a diagnosis. A **diagnosis** is an understanding of the child's problem, or the identification of a disorder by analyzing the symptoms presented and, when possible, their underlying causes. Assessing a child's language skills is a process of observing and measuring the child's receptive and expressive language to determine 1) whether a clinically significant problem exists, 2) the nature and extent of the problem, and 3) what course of action needs to be taken to help the child if a problem does exist (Roseberry-McKibbin & Hegde, 2006).

Essentially, the SLP is making a decision about whether a child's language is developing normally or whether the child has a specific language impairment (SLI) or a language impairment related to another condition such as a developmental delay (explained in more detail in Chapter 9). In this chapter, I have referred to children with SLI in order to keep terminology consistent with the first four chapters; however, these assessment principles are widely applicable to children with language impairments related to conditions explained in subsequent chapters. Subsequent chapters will contain more detailed information about assessing the language of children with associated conditions such as autism, fetal alcohol syndrome, and others. The purpose of this chapter is to explore foundational assessment principles as they apply to testing the language of all children, both monolingual and CLD.

> Assessment refers to the process of arriving at a diagnosis.

With CLD children, the SLP is usually distinguishing whether or not the child has actual SLI or just a **language difference** due to the influence of the first language or to the processes of second language acquisition. In Chapter 3, we said that certain aspects of second language acquisition can impact a child's language in ways that make her appear that she has SLI; it is important to be familiar with these aspects so that CLD Children are not mistakenly diagnosed as SLI. In addition, as explained in Chapter 4, many typically developing (TD) CLD students speak English with patterns that reflect the influence of their first language. These students do not have SLI; they are TD learners whose English patterns reflect L1 (language 1) influences.

In order to assess children and arrive at a diagnosis, ideally SLPs use a combination of five tasks or procedures: 1) screening, 2) gathering of a case history, 3) evaluation of related areas such as hearing, 4) standardized measures, and 5) nonstandardized or informal

TEAM APPROACH TO COMPREHENSIVE ASSESSMENT

ASSESSMENT WHEEL FOR MULTICULTURAL STUDENTS

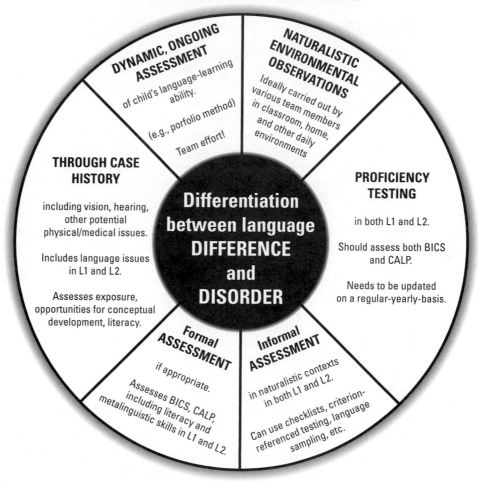

FIGURE 5.1

Used with permission. From Roseberry-McKibbin, C. (2008). *Multicultural students with special language needs: Practical strategies for assessment and intervention* (3rd edition), Oceanside, CA: Academic Communication Associates, Inc.

assessment measures such as language samples. Sometimes SLPs also evaluate a child's information processing skills, as these skills have been shown to be highly correlated with the presence of SLI. Lastly, with some CLD students, SLPs assess language with the assistance of interpreters who speak the students' primary language. The assessment wheel (Figure 5.1) illustrates the process that should ideally take place when evaluating a CLD child for the presence of SLI.

PRELIMINARY COMPONENTS OF AN ASSESSMENT

Screening

Screening refers to the process of quickly and efficiently obtaining a general view of the child's language skills. In screening, the SLP decides if 1) more, in-depth assessment is needed or 2) the child's language skills appear to be developing in a typical fashion and no further assessment is needed at this time. Published screening measures are available; however, many SLPs (including me) use simple activities such as conversational samples and reading books to obtain a general overview of children's language skills. In most public school settings, the SLP does not legally need to obtain parent consent for a screening.

In some school districts, SLPs automatically screen all kindergarteners for potential speech and language problems. In my district, we do not do this for several reasons. Many kindergarteners come to school before they have turned five; they do not speak English at home and have never been to preschool. Screening these children at the beginning of kindergarten would undoubtedly lead to many overreferrals for in-depth, comprehensive assessment for possible SLI. In many cases, by the end of kindergarten, most of these children are performing in a satisfactory way in the classroom. If they are not performing satisfactorily, they may be referred for screening at the end of the year or even in subsequent grades.

> The purpose of screening is to quickly and efficiently obtain a general view of a child's language skills and decide if more in-depth assessment is needed.

Screening should also include hearing screening. One second-grade teacher referred an African American student, Jasmine, to me for in-depth language testing. The teacher was concerned about Jasmine's classroom performance and overall academic skills. Jasmine did an excellent job on the language tests I gave her, and most of her scores were above average. Jasmine's school records indicated that she had passed a school group hearing screening that was administered by the school nurse. I decided to read the records more thoroughly and I found an audiogram from a hospital audiologist. The school nurse had made a mistake. Jasmine was almost completely deaf in her left ear. I made several suggestions to the classroom teacher, who said, "Oh—sit her front and center in the classroom? I hadn't thought of that! Great idea—thanks!" The new seating position helped Jasmine immensely, and her work improved. The case of Jasmine illustrates how important it is for hearing screening to yield accurate results.

In summary, screening is a quick and efficient way to determine whether a child needs more in-depth, comprehensive evaluation for SLI or whether the child is normally functioning and does not need any further evaluation. SLPs can automatically screen children, especially at the kindergarten level, or just screen children who are specifically referred by teachers or parents. If the results of a screening indicate that a child needs an in-depth evaluation, then the SLP needs to start that evaluation with the case history.

Case History

It is very important to gather a case history when a child is going to have an in-depth language evaluation. The case history yields detailed information that helps the SLP understand

CONNECT & EXTEND

Detailed case history questions and forms are available in Shipley, K.G., & McAfee, J. (2004). *Assessment in speech-language pathology: A resource manual* (2nd ed.). San Diego: Singular/Del Mar as well as in Haynes, W.O., & Pindzola, R.H. (2004). *Diagnosis and evaluation in speech pathology* (6th ed.). Boston, MA: Allyn & Bacon.

the child, his communication disorder, and the impact of associated variables such as hearing loss. Textbooks written specifically on the topic of assessment often have in-depth case history forms and a more detailed description of questions that need to be asked (e.g., Haynes & Pindzola, 2004; Shipley & McAfee, 2004). Generally speaking, the SLP gathers information in the following areas (Roseberry-McKibbin & Hegde, 2006):

- Description of the communication disorder (e.g., from the parent's and/or teacher's point of view)
- Information about whether the child's language behavior is considered to be within or outside the norms for that particular cultural and linguistic community
- Prior assessment and treatment for the language problem
- Family constellation and communication patterns (e.g., does anyone else in the family have a communication disorder?)
- Prenatal, birth, and developmental history
- Medical history (especially hearing loss)
- Patterns of language use in the home (e.g., does the family speak a language other than English? What languages are spoken by whom? Has the child had English exposure prior to school? Does the child have a strong oral and literacy foundation in L1? etc.)
- Educational history (I have found it very useful to look in the child's cumulative file for information and school records). This seems easy enough, but it is often overlooked as a rich source of information that can be very helpful in a diagnosis of SLI versus language difference, as illustrated by the case study of Alejandra V. below.

CASES TO CONSIDER

I received a referral for Alejandra V., a cheerful Mexican girl in a fourth-grade classroom. The teacher was concerned because Alejandra was functioning in the "low-average" range academically in the all-English classroom. I engaged Alejandra in a series of informal tasks and found that Alejandra expressed herself well and comprehended everything that was said to her. She read a book fluently in English. A few quick measures of Alejandra's information-processing skills revealed that these were within normal limits for her age. I went to her school file and found that she had been in predominantly Spanish-speaking classrooms up until about nine months ago, when the family moved and Alejandra transferred to my school, where all classes are conducted in English. Alejandra's teachers in kindergarten through third grade had said that she was very successful in the classroom in the previous school district. Based on this brief description, do you

(continued)

think Alejandra probably had SLI or was just still in the process of learning English? Explain your answer. What would you tell the classroom teacher?

_____

_____

_____

In the public schools, each child has a "cum file," as mentioned earlier. This cum (or cumulative) file contains information about the child such as health history, report cards, teacher comments, results of vision and hearing screenings, and other important information. I have found that a most helpful part of gathering a case history is examining the contents of a child's cum file to see if there are any notations of problems or patterns on report cards. For example, a teacher recently referred a child to me for language problems. Before I screened this girl, Karen, I went to her cum file. Her mother had written a note that there was a restraining order against Karen's father. In addition, the mother wrote, "I am disabled. My children all have special education needs. Is it possible that all my children could be put on the same track [for a year-round school]?" This was potentially important information, as Karen's language problems possibly were related more to her environment than to SLI.

Sometimes it is beneficial to read students' report cards and see if there are any patterns to areas of difficulty over the years, or if there is a pattern in teachers' comments. Many times, if a student has a genuine SLI, there will be teacher notes on report cards each year such as "Pablo tries hard, but has difficulty following directions" or "Marcos struggles to express himself verbally and often cannot find the word he is looking for." The SLP who reads a student's cum file as part of the gathering of the case history often has many questions answered by merely taking ten to fifteen minutes to read through the contents of the file. This should be done before the student's parent(s) are interviewed.

Sometimes it is necessary to conduct a case history interview with an interpreter present to talk with the parent(s). SLPs who do not take this step risk making major mistakes in assessment and diagnosis. For example, I was asked to assess the language skills of Adam X., a Hmong-speaking high school freshman. He was referred for testing for possible SLI because he was failing biology. In biology class, he sat in the back of the room and the teacher used few or no visuals. A psychological evaluation, conducted all in English,

POINTS TO PONDER Describe three components of a thorough case history.

_____

_____

_____

CASES TO CONSIDER

I was asked to evaluate the language skills of Sarah S., a monolingual English-speaking five-year-old girl entering kindergarten at my school. Sarah's biological mother had abused alcohol and drugs throughout her pregnancies with each of her five children. The mother was abusive to Sarah and her siblings, and they were removed from her custody and placed in foster care. By the age of five, Sarah had been in six different foster homes. She had a history of bed-wetting, tantrums, middle ear infections, and other medical and emotional problems. What do you think is the impact of the above variables on Sarah's language skills? Do you suspect that Sarah might have SLI or other language problems influenced by her life circumstances? Describe the type of language problems that you think a child like Sarah might have.

_____

_____

_____

> When SLPs are gathering case histories regarding CLD students, they may need to use the services of interpreters.

indicated that this Hmong-dominant student had a substantial gap between nonverbal and verbal performance, with nonverbal performance almost 30 points higher than verbal performance.

Based on the results of this assessment, the psychologist recommended that Adam be placed in a self-contained classroom for SLI students for all four years of high school. During my assessment session with Adam, I was fortunate to have a Hmong interpreter who was able to call the home and speak to a relative about Adam's health and language history. The interpreter found out that Adam was almost completely deaf in his right ear. That certainly helped to explain the F in biology! Adam did very well on language testing in Hmong and was not placed in special education. He did start participating in a non–special education study skills group at the high school to help him catch up on some academic content that he had missed.

The Preevaluation Process: Evaluating Environmental, Linguistic, and Cultural Variables That Influence Children's Language Skills

With all children, it is important to examine variables that impact their language performance. Before actual assessment takes place, clinicians need to gather a case history as described above. Then they need to take several other steps: 1) obtain a comprehensive teacher evaluation of the student's classroom performance, 2) conduct one or more classroom observations of the student, 3) assess the student's language proficiency in L1 and L2 (language 2), 4) examine the student's school records as previously mentioned, and 5) ascertain whether or not there are medical, emotional, or social variables that are impacting the student's language and academic performance (e.g., medications) (Brice & Roseberry-McKibbin, 1999).

For example, I worked with a girl named Sarah, who had been placed in a variety of foster homes; the impact of this lifestyle on her language development needed to be considered as illustrated in the case study on page 145.

There are several ways for a clinician to obtain a comprehensive teacher evaluation of a student's classroom performance. One is to informally interview the teacher. Another is to ask the teacher to fill out a questionnaire and return it. A third way is to formally interview the teacher using a questionnaire; in other words, use an interview plus a questionnaire. This way is often ideal because it provides structure and helps the SLP not to forget any questions.

The Bilingual Classroom Communication Profile (see Table 5.1) is one example of a questionnaire that can be used with a classroom teacher to create a comprehensive background picture of the child's language performance. This profile can also be used with parents, classroom aides, interpreters, and others who are familiar with the child's performance. Sometimes I have used one form and three different colors of ink—for example, blue

> The Bilingual Classroom Communication Profile is a questionnaire that can be used with adults who are familiar with a child's performance in various areas.

for the teacher, red for the mother, and green for the classroom aide or interpreter. Though the finished product is quite colorful, I can quickly ascertain patterns or "common threads" throughout the interviewees' responses. For example, with many CLD children who have a true SLI, everyone interviewed will state that the child has difficulty expressing herself in both her first language and English; they will also frequently report that she has difficulty remembering what she is told. SLPs can ascertain the influence of a number of variables on a child's language performance, including the impact of cultural and linguistic phenomena.

Chapters 3 and 4 covered in detail how children's language is impacted by such factors as second-language acquisition phenomena and cultural variables. Chapter 3 described the impact of normal second-language acquisition phenomena such as the silent period, codeswitching, and transfer from L1 to English. Chapter 3 also showed the importance of ascertaining a child's language proficiency in both English and the first language; this is a crucial step to take with CLD children before they are actually assessed for SLI.

When language proficiency is being assessed, several steps need to be taken (Roseberry-McKibbin, 2008):

1. Determine the student's **primary language** (the one she learned first and used most frequently in the early stages of language development)
2. Determine the student's **dominant language** (the language spoken most proficiently by the student at this time)
3. Determine oral and written proficiency or skill levels in each language the child speaks

After school personnel have assessed the CLD student's language proficiency, they will better understand which language(s) should be used in assessment. The Individuals with Disabilities Education Act (IDEA, 2004) mandates that testing and evaluation materials must be provided and administered in the language or other mode of communication in which the child is most proficient. For some children, English is now their most proficient language. Other children may still be dominant in their primary language, and thus the assessment will need to be conducted in this language.

TABLE 5.1   Description of the Bilingual Classroom Communication Profile (BCCP)[1]

- **Background Information**—The first step in using the BCCP is to collect information about the student's background:
  1. Names of individuals residing in the home with the student and their relationship to the student.
  2. Countries where student has resided. The time period of residence should be recorded for each country listed.
  3. First language or languages learned by the student.
  4. Language used most often by the student both at home and at school.
  5. Individuals who are responsible for caring for the student. The name, relationship to student, and language(s) spoken by each of these individuals should be recorded.
  6. Date and circumstances in which the student was first exposed to English.
  7. Previous schools attended, location of these schools, and dates of attendance.

- **Health information**—Specific health concerns and the results of hearing and vision screening tests are recorded.

- **Instructional Strategies**—Special programs in the regular classroom that are available to students (e.g., tutors, ESL, etc) and classroom modification made to accommodate the student (e.g., preferential seating, special materials used, etc.) are noted.

- **Classroom language Use**—The student's performance in this section of the BCCP is evaluated by asking the teacher to respond "Yes," "No," or "Don't Know" to each item. Performance is evaluated separately in English and in the home language.
  1. Answers simple questions about everyday activities
  2. Communicates basic needs to others
  3. Interacts appropriately and successfully with peers
  4. Tells a simple story, keeping the sequence and basic facts accurate
  5. Communicates ideas and directions in an appropriate sequence
  6. Describes familiar objects and events
  7. Maintains a conversation appropriately

- **School Social Interaction Problems**—A plus (+) is recorded on the record form for each statement that describes the child accurately, and a minus (−) is recorded for each statement that is false. Responses should be based on observations of the student during interactions with peers from a similar cultural and linguistic background.
  1. Communicates ineffectively with peers in both English and the home language
  2. Often plays alone
  3. Is ridiculed or teased by others
  4. Is often excluded from activities by peers
  5. Does not get along well with peers

- **Language and Learning Problems**—The teacher indicates areas of concern by responding "Yes," "No," or "Don't Know" to each item on the record form.
  Items 1–10 in this section provide an "overall performance summary."
  1. Appears to have difficulty communicating in English
  2. Appears to have difficulty communicating in the primary language
  3. Has difficulty learning when instruction is provided in English

(continued)

[1]Used with permission. From Roseberry-McKibbin, C. (2008) *Multicultural students with special language needs: Practical strategies for assessment and intervention* (3rd edition), Oceanside, CA: Academic Communication Associates, Inc.

TABLE 5.1   Description of the Bilingual Classroom Communication Profile (BCCP)[1] (*continued*)

4. Has difficulty learning when instruction is provided in the primary language
5. Acquires new skills in English more slowly than peers
6. Acquires new skills in the primary language more slowly than peers
7. Shows academic achievement significantly below his/her academic English language proficiency, as assessed by an ESL or bilingual professional
8. Is not learning as quickly as peers who have had similar language experiences and opportunities for learning
9. Has a family history of learning problems or special education concerns
10. Parents state that student learns language more slowly than siblings

Items 11 through 26 are used to pinpoint specific problems observed.
11. Rarely initiates verbal interaction with peers
12. Used gestures and other nonverbal communication (on a regular basis) rather than speech to communicate
13. Is slow to respond to questions and/or classroom instructions
14. Is not able to stay on a topic, conversation appears to wander
15. Often gives inappropriate responses
16. Appears to have difficulty remembering things
17. Does not take others' needs or preferences into account
18. Has difficulty conveying thoughts in a clear, organized manner
19. Appears disorganized much of the time
20. Appears confused much of the time
21. Has difficulty paying attention even when material is understandable and presented using a variety of modalities
22. Has difficulty following basic classroom directions
23. Has difficulty following everyday classroom routines
24. Requires more prompts and repetition than peers to learn new information
25. Requires a more structured program of instruction than peers
26. Has gross and/or fine motor problems

- **Environmental Influences and Language Development**—The teacher indicates areas of concern by responding "Yes," "No," or "Don't Know" to each item on the record form.
  1. Has the student had frequent exposure to literacy-related materials (e.g., books) in the primary language?
  2. Has the student had sufficient exposure to the primary language to acquire a well-developed vocabulary in that language?
  3. Was the student a fluent speaker of the primary language when he/she was first exposed to English?
  4. Have the student's parents been encouraged to speak and/or read in the primary language at home?
  5. Has the student's primary language been maintained in school through bilingual education, tutoring, or other language maintenance activities?
  6. Does the student show an interest in interacting in his/her primary language?
  7. Has a loss of proficiency in the primary language occurred because of limited opportunities for continued use of language?
  8. Does the student have frequent opportunities to speak English during interactions with peers at school?
  9. Has the student had frequent opportunities to visit libraries, museums, and other places in the community where opportunities for language enrichment and learning are available?

TABLE 5.1   Description of the Bilingual Classroom Communication Profile (BCCP)[1] (*continued*)

> **10.** Has the student had frequent, long-term opportunities to interact with fluent English speakers outside of the school environment?
>
> - **Impressions from Classroom Observations**—The teacher is asked to respond to questions designed to elicit descriptive information about the child's performance.
>   1. To what extent does the student have difficulty learning in school because of limited proficiency in English?
>   2. Do you feel that this student requires a different type of instructional program that other students who have had similar cultural and linguistic experiences? Please explain.
>   3. Briefly summarize the communication and learning problems observed in the school setting.

Many children need to be assessed in both the primary language and English so that a full profile of their skills can be obtained (Bedore, Peña, Garcia, & Cortez, 2005; Roseberry-McKibbin, 2003). This is especially true if the child is experiencing language loss in L1 (described in Chapter 3) and is still in the process of gaining English proficiency (Anderson, 2004). I have informally found that in assessment, combining the child's responses in L1 and English into a total score often gives the most complete description of the child's language skills. This method of combining scores was described in a study by Bedore, Peña, Garcia, and Cortez (2005), who showed that **conceptual scoring**, or scoring meaningful responses regardless of the language the responses were produced in, yielded optimal scores for Spanish-speaking children. Bedore et al. recommended that SLPs consider conceptual scoring when assessing the language skills of bilingual children.

Chapter 4 described variables such as cultural practices and religious beliefs that could impact children's language development in ways that are very important in the assessment process. For example, a child from a CLD family who believes that children are to be seen and not heard might show slow progress in English oral language development. This slow progress would not be due to SLI, but rather to the family's cultural belief system. It is crucial to keep all these environmental, linguistic, and cultural variables in mind during preevaluation. When these variables have been examined and accounted for, then formal assessment can begin. Many clinicians begin formal assessment with standardized tests.

 SUMMARY

- The purpose of a language screening is to ascertain whether 1) more, in-depth assessment is needed or 2) the child's language skills appear to be typically developing and no further assessment is needed at this time.
- The case history yields detailed information that helps the SLP understand the child, his communication disorder, and the impact of associated variables such as hearing loss.

(*continued*)

- In the preevaluation process, the SLP evaluates environmental, linguistic, and cultural variables that influence a child's language skills.
- The following steps are included in the preevaluation process:1) obtain a comprehensive teacher evaluation of the student's classroom performance, 2) conduct one or more classroom observations of the student, 3) assess the student's language proficiency in L1 and L2, 4) examine the student's school record, and 5) ascertain whether or not there are medical, emotional, or social variables that are impacting the student's language and academic performance.

Add your own summary points here:

_____

_____

_____

STANDARDIZED TESTS

Definitions

Standardized or **formal** tests can be used to assess children's language skills. A test can be standardized without being **norm-referenced** (defined below); however, most standardized tests (though not all) are norm-referenced. In this section, when I use the term *standardized tests,* I am assuming that these are norm-referenced. Standardized, norm-referenced tests give clinicians a quantitative means of comparing a child's performance to the performance of large groups of children in a similar age category. Haynes and Pindzola (2004, p. 51) describe these tests as follows:

> In developing norm-referenced tests, the designers have created some tasks they feel are relevant (valid) and have administered the instrument to large groups of subjects who hopefully represent the population on whom the test is to be used. From these large-scale administrations, the designers are able to calculate normative data that reflect the performance of the large sample. When an individual is given the test, his or her score is compared to the performance of the normative sample and it is determined how this person performed relative to the large group. The purpose of norm-referenced tests is to determine if an individual obtains a score similar to the group average or, if not, how far away from average the score is. Generally, if the individual scored within 1.5 to 2 standard deviations above or below the mean, he or she is said to reflect performance within "normal limits." If the score was more than 2 standard deviations above or below the mean, the performance is said to be exceptional, since only about 5% of the normative population scored in a similar manner. Thus, norm-referenced tests have the major purpose of determining if there is a problem, or a significant enough difference from standard performance to warrant concern with regard to normalcy.

Many SLPs prefer to use standardized tests because they yield psychometrically based, quantitative measures such as percentile rank, standard deviation from the mean,

> Not all standardized tests are norm-referenced; however, most are.

and language age. A child's language age refers to his level of language skill in relation to his chronological age. For example, a TD child who is 6:6 years of age should have a language age of approximately 6:6 years. His language skills are commensurate with his chronological age. Federal and state laws may require these kinds of quantitative measures to place a child into special education in the public school system. However, as will be explained later, the law does actually allow the use of nonstandardized measures for children from CLD populations if standardized measures are found to be inappropriate.

Test Validity

When SLPs select standardized tests to measure children's language abilities, they need to consider test validity and reliability. **Test validity** asks, "Does the test measure what it says it measures?" For example, for many years, the Peabody Picture Vocabulary Test-Revised (PPVT-R) purported to measure intelligence. This was not valid, because the test measured only one skill: receptive vocabulary, one very small part of intelligence. Thus, people came to view the PPVT-R as being invalid as a measure of intelligence. However, the PPVT-R was considered to be a valid measure of receptive one-word vocabulary skills. To-

> When using standardized tests, it is important to examine four kinds of validity: construct, concurrent, predictive, and content.

day, the PPVT-3 (Dunn & Dunn, 1997) is considered by some experts to be a valid measure of receptive vocabulary skills in African American as well as White children (e.g., Craig & Washington, 1999).

SLPs need to look at several types of test validity when considering using standardized tests with the children they serve. These are construct, concurrent, predictive, and content validity. **Construct validity** refers to the degree to which test scores are consistent with theoretical constructs or concepts. Construct validity includes any quantitative or qualitative information that supports the test maker's theory or model underlying the test. Most experts view construct validity as the linchpin of test development; some believe that a lack of construct validity is a serious problem for many of language tests that are currently on the market (Haynes & Pindzola, 2004).

Concurrent validity refers to the degree to which a new test correlates with an established test of known validity. For example, as mentioned, the popular PPVT-3 is an established test of known validity for measuring single-word receptive vocabulary skills. The new EVT (Expressive Vocabulary Test; Williams, 2001) has been said to correlate highly with the PPVT-3; thus, concurrent validity has been established for the EVT.

Predictive validity refers to a test's accuracy in predicting future performance on a related task. For example, on the Clinical Evaluation of Language Fundamentals-4 (CELF-4; Semel, Wiig, & Secord, 2003), a major goal of the *Concepts and Directions* subtest is to predict how well a child will follow directions in the classroom. (Author's note: In my personal experience, this subtest has excellent predictive validity.) In another example, many universities use GRE (Graduate Record Examination) scores as a criterion for admission into their graduate programs, believing that GRE scores will accurately predict a student's success in graduate school.

POINTS TO PONDER Compare and contrast construct, concurrent, content, and predictive validity as parameters of standardized tests.

_____

_____

_____

Content validity is a measure of a test's validity based on a complete examination of all test items to determine if 1) the items are relevant to measuring what the test purports to measure and 2) the items adequately sample the full range of skills being measured. For example, let's say that a standardized test called the Comprehensive Assessment of Morphological Skills (CAMS) uses nothing but fill-in-the-blank items ("Here is one shoe; here are two _____"). The test only measures each bound morpheme once. This test has poor content validity because a) it uses only one response format and b) the child has only one opportunity to show knowledge of the morpheme being tested.

Test Reliability

When considering using standardized tests, SLPs also need to look at test reliability. **Reliability** refers to the stability or consistency with which the same event is repeatedly measured. Reliable scores are consistent across repeated measurements (Roseberry-McKibbin & Hegde, 2006). An example close to the hearts of many readers is the weighing of oneself. If you get on the scale one morning, it may say 135 pounds. If you get on it ten minutes later (assuming you haven't eaten anything), the scale should still say 135 pounds. This scale is reliable. However, if you get on the scale ten minutes later (you still haven't eaten anything) and it says 129 pounds, the scale is unreliable (although you may be very happy!).

> Reliability refers to the consistency of repeated measurements under similar conditions.

When we assess children, several factors influence the reliability of our testing. First, there can be an instrumentation or equipment error—this is especially true in audiology, where equipment can malfunction or respond inappropriately due to lack of calibration. Second, there may be an examiner error. The examiner may be distracted or tired and may not administer a test according to the procedures indicated in the manual. When the air conditioning at my school malfunctioned last year and it was almost 90 degrees in the speech room, I had to force myself to administer tests in a reliable manner!

Fluctuations in the examinee's behavior are a third influence on test reliability. For example, a child may do well on parts of a test in the morning when she is fresh and do more poorly in the afternoon when she is tired and ready to go home. I had a humbling experience with this type of situation recently, explained in the case of Tracy C on page 153.

Different types of reliability are associated with different types of measurements. **Interjudge reliability** looks at how two different raters score the same set of behaviors. For example, a child might speak for five minutes, talking about a movie he just saw. An SLP

CASES TO CONSIDER

Tracy C., a Cantonese-speaking eight-year-old girl, was recently referred for a speech-language assessment to determine if she had an SLI. My colleague Shelley started a test with Tracy, who was in a good mood and highly responsive. Tracy's scores were good on the subtests Shelley administered. In a situation that was not too ideal (one can always serve as a bad example!), I was requested by school personnel to come to the school to finish the assessment a week later. Wanting to be helpful, I agreed to do so with the assistance of a Cantonese interpreter. At that time, Tracy had gone off-track (my district is on a year-round school system), and her mother brought her in to finish the testing. The Cantonese interpreter was there too, helping me assess Tracy's skills in her first language.

It was one of those "what can go wrong will go wrong" sessions. Tracy was very unhappy to have her vacation interrupted. Her mother, dressed in a formal business suit, told me she only had one hour to be there and requested that the testing be finished as fast as possible. During the evaluation, Tracy's mother sat one foot away from Tracy and me at the table. The mother's cell phone kept ringing and she kept answering and having short conversations loudly, in Cantonese, while I was trying to efficiently finish the assessment. She looked constantly at her watch. Tracy looked balefully at me and the interpreter throughout the assessment and spoke very little in either Cantonese or English. Needless to say, her subtest scores were quite poor that day. What were the threats to the reliability and validity of the tests in this situation? What went wrong? (A question with a much briefer answer might be: what went right?) What should have been done differently?

_____

_____

_____

might count fourteen times in this sample that the child did not use present progressive -*ing*. A different SLP might listen to a sample of the same conversation and count thirteen times that the child did not use the -*ing* appropriately. Because both SLPs reach almost the same conclusion, interjudge reliability is quite high in this case.

Split-half reliability refers to a test's internal consistency. Split-half reliability is determined by comparing scores on one half of a test with scores on the other half of the test (assuming the two halves of the test measure the same skill). **Test-retest reliability** refers to the consistency of measures when the same test is administered more than once to the same children or groups of children.

Potential Misuses of Standardized Tests

Clinicians often use the results of standardized tests to create therapy objectives. There are a number of problems with this; the major ones will be discussed briefly here (McCauley & Swisher, 1984; Roseberry-McKibbin & Hegde, 2006). First, standardized tests alone may not identify all the problems that need to be addressed in therapy. Second, these tests serve something like headlines in a newspaper: they give a quick summary of the language problem but don't describe the problem fully (McCauley & Swisher, 1984). Third, most standardized tests sample each behavior only a few times; perhaps even just once. If the child misses an item that evaluates a particular form or skill, therapy objectives are often created on this basis; in reality, the child may actually have intact skill in this area.

For example, a clinician might be evaluating a child's use of past tense *-ed*. The one item to evaluate this might be "Today we walk to the store; yesterday we _____ to the store." The child might get distracted; she might not understand the concept of fill-in-the-blank; she might be preoccupied. She might not say "walked" and give an incorrect answer instead. On this basis, a therapy goal might be "The child will use the regular past tense *-ed* in conversation with 80 percent accuracy."

> SLPs must be careful not to misuse standardized tests by assuming that these tests describe a child's problems fully.

Now, imagine the SLP's surprise as she goes out to the playground during recess and hears the child tell her friends, "Hey! You jumped rope already! It's my turn! And you turned the rope last time; next time, I get to do it." What happened? Clearly the child knew and used past tense *-ed* correctly; it just was not sampled enough times in enough contexts for the SLP to obtain a complete picture of the child's knowledge of this form.

SUMMARY

- Standardized, norm-referenced tests give clinicians a quantitative means of comparing a child's performance to the performance of large groups of children in a similar age category.
- Validity asks if a test measures what it says it measures. There are four types of validity to consider when evaluating a standardized test: construct, predictive, current, and content.
- Reliability refers to the stability or consistency with which the same event is repeatedly measured. There are three types of reliability to consider when evaluating a standardized test: interjudge, test-retest, and split-half.

Add your own summary points here:

_____

_____

_____

CONSIDERATIONS FOR STANDARDIZED LANGUAGE TESTS WITH CLD STUDENTS

Formal Test Assumptions

When using standardized, norm-referenced tests to assess CLD students, many clinicians do not consider that these tests have been developed from a middle-class, literate, Western framework. Researchers have explained the assumptions that underlie these tests

(Kayser, 1989; Lund & Duchan, 1993; Roseberry-McKibbin, 2008). When a formal test is administered, it is assumed that the child will

- feel comfortable enough with the examiner in the testing situation to perform optimally and to the best of his ability
- understand the test tasks (e.g., fill-in-the-blank, describe a picture)
- follow the cooperative principle by performing to the best of his ability and trying to provide relevant answers
- attempt to respond even if the test tasks do not make sense

These assumptions do not hold true for many CLD students. Children from some cultures believe that children are supposed to be silent in the presence of adults, especially unfamiliar ones (Genesee et al., 2004). Some female students may not feel comfortable with male examiners, and vice versa. A male psychologist friend of mine tried to assess a Hmong fifth-grade girl, who was so uncomfortable with him that he was not able to obtain valid results from his testing. The same girl performed very well for me, with whom she spoke quite comfortably and freely.

> Most formal, standardized tests have been developed based on a middle-class, Western framework that may not be appropriate for CLD students.

Sometimes students have cultural customs that are incompatible with the demands of standardized tests. For example, standardized test tasks often encourage children to guess and to try tasks with little demonstration. In addition, many subtests of standardized tests do not allow the examiner to repeat items; children have to listen to items once and then perform accurately. Neha (2003), a Native American SLP, described her experiences working with Navajo children. She stated that (p. 5)

> . . . I noticed that Navajo children observed an activity completely before performing it themselves. After the explanation of activities, many of them refrained from asking questions, even if they did not understand the directions. I found myself having to repeat an entire set of directions and asking them if they understood or requesting them to clarify parts I needed to repeat.

Clearly, some Navajo children might have difficulty with standardized tests that require them to guess and remember information the first time it is heard. Probably these children have not been represented in the norming group for that test.

A clinician who uses a normed, standardized test assumes that the child being tested has the same characteristics as the norming group. An acquaintance of mine used a standardized test with a CLD child. The test was normed on a group of monolingual, English-speaking Midwestern children from middle-class homes. The CLD child was born in California into a Vietnamese-speaking low-income home. Clearly, that was a flagrant misuse of a standardized test. SLPs need to always be careful to read the test manual and find out the characteristics of the norming population (e.g., White, middle class, Midwestern) and ask, "Is this child I am testing represented in the norming population?" If the answer is no, that test should not be used with that child. There are many potential sources of bias in standardized tests, especially when these tests are used with CLD children.

Sources of Bias in Standardized Tests with CLD Students

SLPs nationwide have become increasingly sensitive to the inappropriateness of many standardized tests for CLD students (Crowley, 2003; Roseberry-McKibbin et al., 2005). This includes students who speak African American English. Some standardized tests are appropriate for these students (Craig & Washington, 1999; Craig et al., 2004), but some are not. Many authors have pointed out standardized tests' biases against students who speak African American English (van Keulen et al., 1998; Terrell & Jackson, 2002; Thomas-Tate et al., 2004).

> Sources of potential bias when standardized tests are used with CLD students include cultural-linguistic, value, format, and examiner bias.

For example, a test of grammatical competency might have items such as "Listen to this sentence. Tell me if it is correct or incorrect. *The man, he be goin' to the store.*" The answer would be "incorrect"; however, this sentence is consistent with the rules of AAE. An AAE speaker who answered "correct" would be marked wrong on that item. Johnson (2005) showed that standardized tests that contain third-person singular -*s* in either production or comprehension items may be biased against children who speak AAE. A new instrument on the market was created specifically for AAE speakers, and it can be adapted for other children as well. It is called the Diagnostic Evaluation of Language Variation (Seymour, Roeper, De Villiers, & De Villiers, 2003).

Many authors have discussed sources of bias in standardized tests with CLD students (Brice, 2001; Goldstein, 2000; Roseberry-McKibbin, 2008; van Keulen et al., 1998; Windsor & Kohnert, 2004; Wyatt, 2002). These sources are summarized below.

Cultural-linguistic bias. Cultural-linguistic bias (also called **content bias**) occurs when the examiner uses activities and items that do not correspond with the child's experiential base or background. For example, Amish children in Kansas might not be able to label electrical appliances on a vocabulary test. A Filipino immigrant child might not be able to answer questions about a story involving ice-skating because in the Philippines, there are two seasons: rainy and dry. The temperature rarely goes below 80 degrees.

I came to the United States to live permanently at the age of seventeen after being raised in the Philippines and had an experience somewhat relevant to this point. I obtained my Ph.D. from Northwestern University in Chicago. My friends, during the second winter of my Ph.D. program, told me what a snow angel was and how to make one. So one evening I went out and, trying to fit in with my American peers, made a snow angel. The next day, my friends were excited to hear that I had had this landmark cultural American experience. But they were most chagrined to hear that the only unpleasant aspect of this experience was that my face got very cold. I didn't know that you make snow angels on your back! Needless to say, that mistake was not made again.

> Cultural-linguistic bias occurs when the examiner uses activities and items that do not correspond with the child's experiential base or background.

Value bias. This occurs when test items assume a value system that is different from the child's. Wyatt (2002) gives the example of an African American child who is asked on a standardized test, "Why should you brush your teeth?" The only acceptable, correct answer is "because you can get cavities if you don't." However, an African

American child might say, "Cause my momma tell me to." This answer, which is consistent with the African American child's value system, would be scored as incorrect.

Format bias. Format bias (also called **situational bias** by some authors) refers to the use of testing procedures, materials, or both that are less familiar to some children. For example, an examiner might say to a child, "Tell me everything you can about an apple." An Asian child raised in a home where children are expected to maintain respectful silence around adults might do poorly on a test that contained these kinds of items. In some cultures, children are rarely asked known-information questions. If the clinician knows that this is a picture of a lamp and says, "What's this?" some children will not answer because the answer is obvious; the clinician already knows that this is a lamp, so why answer the question? In addition, some young CLD children are not placed into day care; they remain close to family and friends until they enter school. For example, Malaysians often prefer to have their children cared for by a close friend or family member rather than placed into formal day care settings (Lian & Abdullah, 2001). It would be intimidating for a Malaysian child from this background to speak freely with an unfamiliar adult.

As we have discussed, in mainstream US culture, we are accustomed to children verbally displaying their knowledge—even to relative strangers (Genesee et al., 2004). Children (like my son) in mainstream US culture are routinely encouraged to "Tell Grandma and Grandpa what you did in vacation Bible school this week" or to share experiences with teachers and classmates in front of the class. In my son's public elementary school, children who come to the front of the class to recite are routinely rewarded with "Beaver Bucks," the school's reinforcement system. At the end of each month, there is a "store" where children redeem their Beaver Bucks for prizes. My son, who is rather shy, routinely gets smaller toys than the more outgoing, verbal children who enjoy telling a whole group what they know. In the same way, CLD children may be penalized on tests where the format of the items requires them to perform in ways that are not familiar or comfortable to them.

> Format bias refers to the use of testing procedures, materials, or both that are less familiar to some children.

Examiner bias. Examiners may be biased in how they administer tests and/or interpret test results. For example, most monolingual English-speaking examiners value direct eye contact during conversational speech. CLD students who look away from the examiner because this is culturally appropriate would most likely be penalized on tests of

POINTS TO PONDER Describe two types of bias that may be present when using a standardized test with a CLD student.

_____

_____

_____

pragmatics skills. In another example, boys from certain Eastern European countries are often raised more permissively than girls and are not required to sit and follow instructions for long periods of time. These boys can easily be judged as having clinically significant problems with following directions and comprehending spoken language, when in fact they are behaving in culturally appropriate ways (Domyancic, personal communication, April 7, 2000).

Modifying Standardized Tests for CLD Students

I am frequently asked, "If standardized tests are so inappropriate for use with CLD students, why use them at all? Why not just use solely informal assessment?" That question is a good one. The answer is that it is probably ideal to use primarily, if not entirely, informal assessment procedures and materials with CLD students. However, the reality is that most SLPs feel uncomfortable doing this. Many SLPs have shared with me over the years that in their particular school districts, they were seriously pressured to use standardized tests with all children, even though federal law does not technically mandate this (as we shall see later). In addition, most SLPs are more comfortable with standardized tests than they are with informal, nonstandardized means of assessment. The practice of using standardized tests with CLD students is a little bit like paying taxes: you don't like it, but it is not going to go away any time soon.

> Although it is not ideal to use standardized tests with CLD students, there are ways to modify these tests so that they are less biased.

Because of this, many authors have made recommendations for modifying standardized tests for use with CLD children (Gopaul-McNichol & Armour-Thomas, 2002; Roseberry-McKibbin, 2003, 2008; Wilson, Wilson, & Coleman, 2000; van Keulen et al. 1998; Wyatt, 2002). These recommendations are summarized below:

1. Allow students extra time to respond.
2. Provide instructions in both English and the student's first language.
3. Explain or rephrase confusing instructions.
4. Give extra practice items, examples, and demonstrations.
5. Repeat items if necessary.
6. Omit biased items that students are likely to miss.
7. Continue testing even after the ceiling has been reached.
8. Devote more than one session to the testing.
9. Have a trusted, familiar adult such as a parent or an interpreter administer test items under the clinician's supervision.
10. If students give "wrong" answers, ask them to explain the answers and write down the explanations. Score these answers as correct if they are appropriate from the viewpoint of the student's linguistic and cultural background. Record all responses. For example, I asked an eighth-grader from Uzbekistan (in the former USSR) to label a picture (the "right" response was *capitol*). When the boy said "the Kremlin" he was given credit for this response.
11. Use a multiple scoring system to show 1) the child's answers in English, 2) the child's answers in her first language, and 3) the child's combined answers in both languages (Bedore et al., 2005).

CLD students often demonstrate language proficiency in L1 in certain content areas and proficiency in L2 (English) in other areas (Gutierrez-Clellen et al., 2000). For example, a student may know "home vocabulary" (e.g., furniture, foods) best in L1 and school vocabulary (e.g., colors, shapes, numbers) best in L2. As previously stated, a combined score of both L1 and English answers usually gives the most comprehensive picture of the child's knowledge.

 SUMMARY

- When using standardized, normed (formal) tests to assess CLD students, many clinicians do not consider the fact that these tests have been developed in a middle-class, literate, Western framework that may not be appropriate.
- Many sources of potential bias exist when standardized tests are used with CLD students: cultural-linguistic, value, format, and examiner.
- SLPs can modify standardized tests for use with CLD students to reduce bias.

Add your own summary points here:

_____

_____

_____

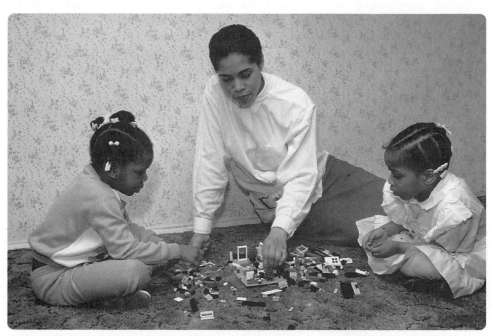

When evaluating the language skills of CLD students, it is ideal to analyze their interactions in natural communication situations with peers from a similar cultural and linguistic background.

LANGUAGE SAMPLES

Introduction

Many experts recommend that SLPs gather and analyze a **spontaneous language sample** from a child as part of the overall assessment process. This is true for monolingual as well as CLD students. When gathering the sample, the SLP talks with the child and tries to draw him out to talk as much as possible. The goal is to evaluate parameters of language based on the language the child uses during these interactions. Ideally, language samples should be **representative**. They should give the SLP a picture of what the child's language is like in different daily situations in the "real world" context.

> A spontaneous language sample should represent a child's daily use of language in different daily situations.

Experts give very specific strategies for precise analysis of language samples. General suggestions are presented below, and readers are encouraged to utilize other sources for more specific details (Gutierrez-Clellen et al., 2000; Nelson, 1998; Owens, 2004; Paul, 2001).

CONNECT & EXTEND

A very helpful book for learning how to analyze language samples is Bliss's (2002) *Discourse impairments: Assessment and intervention applications*. Boston, MA: Allyn & Bacon. Many case studies and examples are provided so the reader can practice analyzing language samples of children with SLI, autism, and other profiles.

Strategies for Collecting Language Samples

• *Make sure that the situation is comfortable and culturally congruent for the child.* SLPs must remember that, as we said in Chapter 2, parents in some cultures do not encourage young children to interact with adults. Genesee et al. (2004) described how they tried to gather language samples from Inuit children in the northern part of Canada, thinking that this would be a good way of analyzing these children's language skills. Genesee et al. constructed the situation to have Inuit-speaking children talk with Inuit-speaking teachers. The authors described how " . . . we had made one very significant oversight in setting up this procedure. Inuit children are not accustomed to, nor are they comfortable with, talking to adults. The end result was that the language samples collected by the teachers contained very limited language and were very misleading" (p. 35). Genesee et al. recommended that for children from cultures such as these, language samples might best be gathered by listening to children talk with other children. In their study, when they had the Inuit subjects talk with other children, the subjects used grammatical structures and vocabulary that were much more complicated than they had used when talking to the teachers.

• *Use a variety of conversational partners.* As we just said, often spontaneous conversational samples are gathered in a situation where an adult questions a child. Although this can yield helpful information about a child's language skills, it is not enough. Much more can be learned if the SLP collects language samples of the child interacting with peers, family members, or both.

• *If the child's primary language is not English, obtain the services of a bilingual SLP or other knowledgeable speaker of the L1 to help collect and analyze the language sample.*

Ideally, at least two knowledgeable native speakers of the L1 should help collect, transcribe, and analyze the sample.

- *Collect language samples in different settings over a period of time.* When the SLP collects language samples from a child in different locations over the course of several days, she is able to obtain a more representative picture of the child's expressive language skills than if she just collects the sample in the speech room in one sitting.

- *Analyze both form and content.* It is important to analyze the student's syntactic and morphological skills in the primary language, English, or both. However, it is important to evaluate the student's vocabulary and pragmatics skills in both languages also. A question I often ask is "Is this student able to competently communicate *meaning*?" When students can competently communicate meaning, even if they have some grammatical errors, usually they do not have SLI. The example of Meuy on page 162 illustrates a student who is communicating meaning despite grammatical errors.

- *Remember that grammatical errors in English are sometimes the result of transfer from the student's primary language.* For example, Spanish-speaking Araceli said to me, "I like very, very much speech." This utterance reflects the influence of Spanish syntax, not a sign of SLI.

- *Use interesting, culturally relevant books, toys, and pictures to elicit language.* Have students describe and discuss what they see.

- *Ask students to talk about the steps required to complete a task* such as fixing a bike, cooking a certain dish, or playing a favorite game like kickball. Look for ability to describe the task with adequate detail and sequencing skills.

- *Ask students to describe their favorite movies or TV shows.* I have often obtained detailed descriptions of cartoons from students.

- *Give the student story picture cards and have him sequence them and tell the story.* Students with SLI frequently have difficulty sequencing a story and telling it appropriately. Recent research has shown that having students generate stories can be more effective than other methods for eliciting long utterances during a language sample (Southwood & Russell, 2004).

- *Present problem situations—either verbally or in picture form—and ask the student to describe how to solve the problem.* Make sure these problem situations are relevant to the student's background experience. For example, my school is located in a low-income area where safety is an issue for many students. I have asked questions like "What would you do if . . ." and had students problem-solve the situations verbally. One nine-year-old boy said that if a stranger came when he was alone in the apartment, he would get his mom's gun that she had taught him how to fire. Though not the answer I expected, this was unfortunately relevant to the boy's personal experience.

Language samples can be gathered through many methods, such as using picture cards and playing games.

There are many ways to evaluate language samples. Formal programs can be used to obtain detailed analyses of monolingual English-speaking students' language content, form, and use. Sometimes

CASES TO CONSIDER

I was asked to assess the language skills of Meuy, a 10-year-old Mien-speaking student who was suspected of having an SLI. During the course of a language sample, Meuy said to me, "In Seattle I did go to a party. They make egg roll and they bake some corn muffin . . . and we had turkey and bread stuffing and mashed potato and gravies. I make the mashed potato and they make the turkey . . . we all help. They say if they don't help, they don't get some." List the grammatical errors that Meuy made. Was she able to communicate meaning adequately? Explain your answer. Do you think, based on this very small sample, that Meuy was a student who had an SLI?

_____

_____

_____

CONNECT & EXTEND

Thorough descriptions of formal and informal language sampling techniques and programs are provided by Owens, R.E. (2004). *Language disorders: A functional approach to assessment and intervention* (4th ed.). Boston, MA: Allyn & Bacon.

When evaluating a CLD child's language sample for form, contrastive analysis between English and the first language can be used to assess the presence of first language transfer to English. A professional who speaks the child's first language can analyze form in that language.

clinicians evaluate language samples informally. Owens (2004) describes in detail both formal and informal methods for language sample analysis. The next section presents two informal ways to evaluate a language sample: through 1) evaluating language use and 2) calculating mean length of utterance.

Informal Strategies for Evaluating Morphology and Syntax

Evaluating a student's language form involves analyzing skills in phonology, morphology, and syntax (Owens, 2004). In this section, the analysis of morphology and syntax will be discussed. First, evaluation of a CLD student's syntax and morphology is unique to each situation depending on the student's L1 and degree of proficiency in L1 and English. I analyze CLD students' language form in English through the contrastive analysis with L1 that was discussed in Chapter 4.

To review, the SLP looks at the child's English utterances and analyzes whether or not English "errors" can be traced to the influence of L1. For example, in some Asian languages such as Mien (spoken by Meuy in the case study), the pronouns *he, she, it* are not differentiated; speakers only use *it.* Thus, if a child from a Mien background pointed to a picture of a girl and said "Look! It's riding a bike!" this would be considered an error due to transfer from L1, not a sign of SLI. When evaluating the CLD student's form in the first language, the SLP needs the assistance of a knowledgeable speaker of that language (ideally a bilingual SLP).

If a monolingual English-speaking child is being evaluated, the clinician can calculate her mean length of utterance (MLU), or the average length of morphemes in the child's utterances. MLU is generally considered to be an accurate indicator of language complexity up until the child is around four years old (Owens, 2004). It is usually calculated in morphemes through the following method:

$$\text{MLU} = \frac{\text{number of morphemes}}{\text{number of utterances}}$$

Thus, for example, let's say a child spoke 100 utterances that contained a total of 250 morphemes:

$$\frac{250 \text{ morphemes}}{100 \text{ utterances}}$$

The child's overall MLU would be 2.5. The clinician can compare the individual child's MLU to norms expected for the child's chronological age (see Chapter 2). For example, in Chapter 2, we said that by four to five years of age, a child's MLU is between 4.5 and 7.0. If the child in this example is four years old, then her MLU indicates that she is delayed and is performing more like a two-year-old. This child will probably need intervention to increase her morphological and syntactic skills.

You will recall that in Table 2.4, Brown's morphemes were discussed. One way to evaluate a child's syntactic and morphological development is by assessing the presence or absence of Brown's fourteen grammatical morphemes according to the child's chronological age. For example, we said that the contractible auxiliary (e.g., *Daddy is going* or *Dad's going*) is mastered between thirty and fifty months of age. If this four-year-old child does not evidence any use of contractible auxiliary at all, then we might assume that she has not mastered this construction; this can be an example of a morphological delay.

Language samples can also be analyzed with a type-token ratio (TTR), which is calculated as follows:

$$\text{TTR} = \frac{\text{number of different words in a sample}}{\text{total number of words in a sample}}$$

TTR represents the variety of different words that a child can use expressively. In order to calculate TTR, the SLP first counts the total number of words in a sample (even if they are repeated). This total becomes the denominator. The SLP then calculates each different word in the sample. For instance, if the child used the word "Mommy" fifteen times, it would only count once. The number of different words used becomes the numerator. For children three to eight years of age, the TTR is typically 1:2. The total number of words spoken by the child during the language sample is approximately twice the number of different words in the sample (Johnson, 1996). An example follows:

$$\text{TTR} = \frac{50 \text{ different words in a sample}}{100 \text{ total words a sample}}$$

The TTR in this case is 1:2, indicating that the child's performance is within normal limits.

POINTS TO PONDER What are the differences between evaluating language form and evaluating language use? Describe.

_____

_____

_____

Informal Evaluation of Language Use

With both monolingual and CLD students, it is very important to analyze student interactions in natural communication situations with peers from similar linguistic and cultural backgrounds. The goal is to evaluate the student's semantic and pragmatics skills and ascertain if she is an effective communicator in her day-to-day environment. If CLD students are evaluated based on their interactions with mainstream monolingual English-speaking peers, the SLP can make diagnostic errors. Research has shown that mainstream monolingual English-speaking children, even as young as three years of age, may not readily respond to children who are not yet fluent English speakers (Rice, Sell, & Hadley, 1991). Thus, CLD students need to be compared to their peers from similar cultural and linguistic backgrounds.

> When evaluating a CLD student's language use, be sure to compare her to peers from a similar cultural and linguistic background.

When my son Mark was in preschool, a monolingual Mandarin-speaking boy, Ryan, entered the preschool. Mark liked Ryan very much, but came home and said that "Ryan doesn't talk; I can't be his friend." Eventually things worked out very well as Ryan learned more English and Mark learned to be more accommodating. However, it was very interesting to personally see that an intelligent, intact non-English speaking child was almost rejected by my own four-year-old son in preschool because of his lack of English facility. Again, it is important to judge CLD students by their use of language with similar peers.

In Chapter 1, we discussed Fey's (1986) model of conversational assertiveness and responsiveness. If the SLP suspects that a child—monolingual English-speaking or CLD—has an SLI, he can utilize this model when observing a child's interactions with peers as well as observing other language-use patterns that typify many SLI children (Roseberry-McKibbin, 2008):

- The student replaces speech with gestures and communicates nonverbally when it would be more appropriate to talk
- Peers indicate that they have difficulty understanding the student
- The student expresses basic needs inadequately (e.g., cannot even communicate that she has to go to the bathroom)

- When peers initiate interactions, the student often does not respond
- The student rarely initiates verbal interaction with peers
- When asked a question or engaged in conversation, the student gives inappropriate responses
- The student has difficulty conveying thoughts in an organized, sequential manner that listeners can understand and make sense of
- The student has difficulty appropriately maintaining a topic
- Nonverbal aspects of language are inappropriate (for example, the student does not use appropriate gestures or facial expressions)
- The student has difficulty with **presuppositions** (providing background information that the listener needs to understand the topic of conversation)
- The student has difficulty with turn-taking skills; either she interrupts inappropriately or is passive and does not take her conversational turn when she should
- The student needs to have information repeated, even when the information is expressed clearly and is thus easy for the student to comprehend

 SUMMARY

- SLPs can gather and analyze a spontaneous language sample from a child as part of the overall assessment process. The goal is to evaluate parameters of language based on the language the child uses during interactions in various situations. Ideally, language samples should be representative.
- Language samples can be gathered through many methods, such as using picture cards, playing games, and observing interactions with peers from similar cultural and linguistic backgrounds.
- When evaluating a CLD child's language sample for form, a professional who speaks the child's first language can analyze form in that language. Contrastive analysis between English and the first language can be used to assess the presence of first language transfer to English.
- When the language samples of monolingual English-speaking children are evaluated for form, SLPs commonly use techniques such as calculating mean length of utterance and type-token ratio.
- Language samples can also be informally evaluated in terms of the student's language use. Essentially, the SLP is evaluating how successfully the child communicates in various settings with various people in her environment.

Add your own summary points here:

_____

_____

_____

OTHER ALTERNATIVES TO STANDARDIZED ASSESSMENT

Introduction

Statistics indicate that CLD students are overrepresented in special education programs around the United States. For example, Hispanic children represent a large and rapidly growing CLD group in special education; African American children are overrepresented in programs for those with emotional disturbances and mental retardation (Drew & Hardman, 2004). At the other end of the spectrum, disproportionately few CLD students are represented in programs for the gifted and talented (Gollnick & Chinn, 2002). There are many reasons for this highly unfortunate situation; one reason relevant to us as SLPs is that it is such a challenge to CLD children's language skills in a reliable, valid, nonbiased manner (Roseberry-McKibbin et al., 2005).

It is important that our field and related fields (such as psychology) continue to work to develop nonbiased assessment instruments and methods for detecting SLI in CLD children. We have discussed federal law IDEA (2004); this law specifically places a greater emphasis on decreasing the numbers of CLD students in special education. As of July 2005, states were required to keep track of how many "minority" students were being identified for special education, and states will be required to provide coordinated, comprehensive early intervention programs for children in groups that are determined to be overrepresented (Klotz & Nealis, 2005).

> The development of standardized tests "tailored" to various linguistic populations is problematic for many reasons, such as dialectal variety within various languages.

In relation to having access to nonbiased assessment instruments, SLPs have wished that norm-referenced, standardized tests could be developed for CLD students. However, as Seymour and Valles (1998) point out, this would be virtually impossible due to the tremendous linguistic diversity among CLD students. In addition, many languages have dialectal variations. Truly, it would be very difficult to create valid, reliable standardized tests for each language and each dialect in any given geographic location.

In addition, even tests that are supposedly tailored for certain populations may be problematic (Peña & Kester, 2004). For example, Restrepo and Silverman (2001) evaluated the validity of the Spanish edition of the Preschool Language Scale-3 (PLS-3; Zimmerman, Steiner, & Pond, 1993) for use in evaluating the expressive and receptive language skills of young Spanish-speaking children. Restrepo and Silverman examined the Spanish PLS-3 in light of rigorous psychometric criteria. They found that the test met very few of the criteria. They also found that there were problems with the test's construct and content validity. They used the Spanish PLS-3 to assess typically developing Spanish-speaking children and found that as a group, the children performed approximately 1.5 standard deviations below the mean. Clearly, creating tests geared toward specific CLD groups is not "the answer" that most SLPs are looking for.

> Methods for alternative assessment can be used effectively with monolingual English-speaking children as well as CLD children.

Since the early 1980s and before, researchers and clinicians have discussed the lack of adequately developed alternatives to norm-referenced testing (McCauley & Swisher, 1984). Because of the difficulties of using standardized tests with CLD students, many researchers and clinicians have explored alternatives that are more appropriate for CLD students. It needs to be noted that many of these alternatives can be used with monolingual English-speaking students also, especially to supplement the results of standardized tests. These alternatives are described below, especially as they apply to fulfilling legal requirements.

Legal Considerations in Assessing CLD Students

Recent federal legislation (IDEA, 2004) and other laws have emphasized prevention of inappropriate identification and mislabeling of CLD students. Public school districts can be in violation of federal law if too many of their minority students are referred for special education services (Crowley, 2004). The key points of federal law are summarized here (for a fuller description of federal legislation pertaining to the assessment of CLD students, the reader is referred to Gopaul-McNichol & Armour-Thomas, 2002; Moore-Brown & Montgomery, 2001; Roseberry-McKibbin, 2008; Silliman & Diehl, 2002; van Keulen et al., 1998):

> **CONNECT & EXTEND**
>
> Federal law requirements for assessment of language skills in public school children are described in depth in Moore-Brown, B., & Montgomery, J.K. (2001). *Making a difference for America's children.* Eau Claire, WI: Thinking Publications.

1. All children, regardless of handicap, are entitled to a free and appropriate education.
2. Testing and evaluation procedures and materials must be selected and administered in a nondiscriminatory manner.
3. Testing and evaluation materials must be provided and administered in the language or other mode of communication in which the child is most proficient.
4. Accommodations may include alternative forms of assessment and evaluation.
5. Tests must be administered to a child with a motor, speech, hearing, visual, or other communication disability, or to a bilingual child, so as to reflect accurately the child's ability in the area tested, rather than the child's impaired communication skill or limited English language skill.
6. No single procedure may be used as the sole criterion for determining an appropriate educational program and placement for a child; multiple measures must be used.

Federal law is very clear that biased assessment materials and procedures should not be used with CLD children. The law is also clear that it is acceptable to use alternative procedures with CLD students. Kratcoski (1998, pp. 3–10) said that

> Evaluations and assessments in school settings have traditionally involved the use of standardized tests . . . to adhere to state and federal regulations. . . . According to federal regulations, the present level of performance must be presented in terms of objective measurable evaluations 'to the extent possible' (U.S. Department of Education, 1980, p. 20). [But] the provisions of P.L. 94-142 IDEA do not mandate specific assessment tools *or even require that standardized measures are used* . . . tools must display equity, validity, and nondiscrimination . . . and they stipulate a team assessment approach that incorporates multimeasure decisions, and evaluation based on specific educational needs, and a look at the whole child. . . . Traditionally, many SLPs have used standardized tests . . . operating from the belief that a *quantitative standard score is mandated by federal law. . . . However, the*

> According to federal law, it is legal to use informal nonstandardized measures for assessment provided these measures are nonbiased and are presented for a team decision.

law does not exclude subjective or qualitative measures . . . it leaves the choice of measurement tools and criteria to the educator. (excerpts quoted from pp. 3–10; italics are this author's)

Because it is legal to use subjective, qualitative, informal tools to assess language skills, and clinicians are not required to use formal standardized measures, it is important for clinicians to be aware of other assessment options. Several options are summarized below (Brice, 2002; Gutierrez-Clellen & Peña, 2001; Roseberry-McKibbin, 2003; Peña, 2003). Table 5.2 describes assessment alternatives for Hispanic students; these may be utilized with students from other CLD backgrounds.

Dynamic Assessment

CONNECT & EXTEND

Alternative assessment techniques are illustrated with live examples in a video by Roseberry-McKibbin, C. (2003). *Assessment of bilingual learners: Language difference or language disorder?* Rockville Pike, MD: American Speech-Language-Hearing Association.

Often when SLPs assess students, they use **static assessment**, which involves measuring the student's skills at one point in time to make a judgment about whether there is a language difference or an SLI. A child's current level of performance in a given area is determined relative to the performance of her peers. So, for example, if Josefina Q. is referred for testing, she would come to the SLP's office and be given several normed, standardized tests—usually in one sitting. The tests would be scored by the SLP, and a diagnosis would be made on this basis. However, a problem with this is that static assessment does not look at a child's ability to learn; it just looks at what she knows on any given day.

Dynamic assessment evaluates a student's ability to learn when provided with instruction. Instead of asking what the student already knows, the SLP asks *how* the student learns. The dynamic assessment model is characterized by a test-teach-retest format that observes a child's ability to learn. In dynamic assessment, the SLP looks at the student's **modifiability**, which involves the child's responsiveness to instruction, his ability to transfer learning to new situations, and the amount of examiner effort that was required during the assessment (Peña, Iglesias, & Lidz, 2001).

> Dynamic assessment, which evaluates a student's ability to learn when provided with instruction, is preferable to static assessment, which measures a student's language knowledge at one point in time.

When using dynamic assessment with a CLD student, SLPs can ask, *In comparison to typically developing culturally and linguistically similar peers:*

- Was this particular student slow to learn new information?
- Did he have more difficulty learning it?
- Did this particular student require more structure and individualized attention than similar peers?
- Did this student require instructional strategies that differed from those that had been used effectively with similar peers?

If the answer to most or all of those questions is "yes," then the SLP will probably conclude that the child has an SLI. This conclusion, based on dynamic assessment, results

TABLE 5.2   Assessment Alternatives

Procedure	Pro	Con
1. Standardize existing tests on English Language Learner (ELL) Hispanic students.	1. Tests with appropriate local norms may be valid measures of language for bilingual Hispanic students.	1. New norms may be created that are lower than those of the original population. The test may be biased in its use of standard English and format. The new norms will not change this.
2. Modify or revise tests that will make them appropriate for ELL. Hispanic students.	2. The modified tests with appropriate local norms may be valid measures of language for bilingual Hispanic students. The modified tests may be quicker to develop than new tests.	2. If done incorrectly, the test may become invalid. Results using original (not local) norms should not be reported.
3. Use a language sample when assessing an ELL Hispanic student's language.	3. The language sample may yield representative results of the child's true language abilities. Samples can be taken in a variety of contexts and in both languages.	3. The sample will have to be taken in both languages/dialects. Developmental data for the other language/dialect may not be available. Procedures to elicit the sample may be biased.
4. Use criterion-referenced tests.	4. The criterion-referenced measures may yield more adequate results, i.e., freer of norm-referenced biases. The criterion can be SLP or teacher selected. Criteria may be adjusted to reflect cultural and linguistic factors.	4. Is the criterion developmentally appropriate? Is the criterion culturally appropriate in that the child has had sufficient exposure/motivation to attain mastery?
5. Refrain from using all normed tests that have not been corrected for bias for use with ELL Hispanic students.	5. Results from the tests can be converted into criterion-referenced results; e.g., the child scored 17/20 on the oral vocabulary subtest revealing 70% correctness.	5. School districts like the use of standardized tests for eligibility placement criteria.
6. Develop new tests.	6. New tests with appropriate local norms may be valid measures of language for bilingual Hispanic students.	6. The new test may be appropriate only for a limited segment of the population. Test development involves many resources (time, effort, and money).
7. Test in both languages/dialects and use a combined scoring method.	7. The results can be compared to determine if a stronger language exists. Additionally, test items that are identical can be double-scored.	7. Time consuming and many of the problems above still exist.

(*continued*)

TABLE 5.2   Assessment Alternatives (*continued*)

Procedure	Pro	Con
8. Conduct classroom-based ethnographic observations; obtain three separate points of reference (triangulation).	8. A true picture of performance and classroom expectations may emerge. The SLP and teacher may conference and discuss the student's performance.	8. Time consuming. No normed comparisons; descriptive information that school districts may not accept.
9. Teach test items and periodically retest (dynamic assessment).	9. A true picture of performance may emerge over a period of time. The standard for measurement is based on learning and not static results.	9. Time consuming.
10. Use teacher interviews, questionnaires.	10. Teachers may observe behaviors not seen by the SLP. An opportunity to confer with the teacher may result.	10. Time consuming. Nonnormative data that does not yield standard scores.
11. Confer with other professionals from a similar cultural and linguistic background.	11. The other professionals may shed insight into cultural or language factors unknown to the SLP.	11. Time consuming; other professionals from the child's culture may not be readily available.

from the evidence that the child has difficulty in her *ability to learn* overall. This difficulty affects a child's learning in any language.

As one example of the effectiveness of dynamic assessment with CLD children, we will briefly discuss a study by Ukrainetz, Harpell, Walsh, and Coyle (2000). These researchers studied two groups of Native American children. One group was from a Shoshone background, and the other group was from an Arapahoe background. Based on teacher reports and examiner observation of these children in the classroom setting, the children were labeled as "weaker" or "stronger" language learners. All children participated in a dynamic assessment procedure. Findings of the study showed that differences between pre- and post-test performance and modifiability scores were consistently greater in the "stronger" language group. Ukrainetz et al. suggested that dynamic assessment might be considered as one valid and reliable way to differentiate language differences from language impairments in CLD children.

Assessment of Information Processing Skills

In Chapter 1, we said that research has suggested that students with SLI have difficulty retaining the sequential order of information and that they have specific difficulties on tasks that require verbatim, immediate ordered recall. For example, SLI students have difficulty repeating back lists of nonwords, real words, and digits. They have an especially hard time repeating back lists of nonwords (Munson, Kurtz, & Windsor, 2005). They also have difficulty recalling sentences. The research of Dollaghan and Campbell (1998) was mentioned in Chapter 1 and will be reviewed briefly again. These researchers developed procedures designed to measure language processing capacity (e.g., repeating nonsense words) and found that these procedures had good potential to be used with CLD students in differentiating language differences from actual SLI.

In an earlier study, Campbell, Dollaghan, Needleman, and Janosky (1997) examined the use of knowledge-based and processing-dependent language assessment measures with 156 randomly selected twelve-year-old boys. Parents of all participants in this study reported that English was the primary language spoken in the home. Thirty-one percent of the subjects were White, and 69 percent of the subjects came from CLD groups (Asian American, African American, and Native American). The investigators administered a knowledge-dependent measure that especially tapped vocabulary knowledge. They also administered several processing-dependent measures (e.g., nonword repetition) to all the subjects.

Results of this study showed that there were no significant differences in the scores of the White and CLD students on the processing-dependent measures. However, on the knowledge-dependent measure, CLD students scored significantly lower than White students. Campbell et al. (1997) concluded that knowledge-based measures have the potential to be more biased against CLD students than processing-dependent measures and suggested that clinicians consider processing-dependent measures as a nonbiased alternative for CLD students.

> Information processing tasks have been shown to be a valid and reliable indicator of potential SLI in both monolingual and CLD children.

A study of monolingual English-speaking and bilingual English- and Spanish-speaking children by Kohnert and Windsor (2004) also found that processing-dependent measures have excellent potential for nonbiased assessment of CLD learners. Processing-dependent measures with Spanish-speaking children with SLI have been recommended by Restrepo and Gutierrez-Clellen (2004). In Chapter 1, we also cited the research of Hwa-Froelich and Matsuo (2005), which showed that performance on language processing tasks could provide valuable information for clinicians attempting to differentiate language differences from SLI in Vietnamese-speaking children.

Laing and Kamhi (2003, p. 51) said that

> The use of processing-dependent dynamic measures with ELL (English Language Learner) populations is appealing for a number of reasons. They are not biased toward life experience, socialization practices, or literacy knowledge, and they are quick and easy to administer. . . . It is very advantageous to use assessment measures that do not rely on a child's prior experience or world knowledge. . . . Performance on nonword repetition and working memory measures has been found to be highly correlated with language impairment and second-language vocabulary acquisition in adults and children. When children perform poorly on processing-dependent measures, there is a high likelihood that they will have some type of language-learning difficulty.

Jacobs and Coufal (2001) conducted a pilot study where they examined the efficacy of a computerized language screening instrument for use with CLD children. The results of the study indicated that

. . . the single measurement of expressive morphology in processing-dependent, language-learning tasks may be a powerful method for efficiently and accurately identifying language learning impairment in multicultural populations of children. This subtest required the child to both learn and express a novel linguistic rule . . . (p. 73)

CONNECT & EXTEND

A computerized language screening instrument for use with CLD students is described in the research of Jacobs, E.L., & Coufal, K.L. (2001). A computerized screening instrument of language learnability. *Communication Disorders Quarterly, 22*(2), 67–75.

Jacobs and Coufal concluded that processing-dependent language-learning tasks have excellent potential to discriminate language differences from SLI in CLD students.

I have experimented with processing-dependent measures with CLD children for the last several years. These measures are extremely useful because, as Laing and Kamhi (2003) state, they do not rely on a child's prior experience or world knowledge. A major problem with standardized, formal tests is that they do rely, often heavily, on a student's prior experience and world knowledge. A child might come from a background where there was excellent stimulation and adequate language learning experiences, but there was a mismatch between the child's background and the school's expectations.

For example, some immigrant students come from countries where they excelled in school but did not have the kinds of experiences assumed by American schools. In other situations, a child may have normal language-learning ability but come from a background where she did not receive adequate stimulation in the home (as discussed in more detail later). These kinds of students may do poorly on standardized tests because they have not been exposed to the information assumed by the tests, not because they have an SLI.

I worked with LaVera T., a first-grade African American student who had been identified as SLI by another clinician. As I worked with LaVera, it became clear that she was a bright little girl with excellent language-learning skills. It was discovered that in LaVera's home, there were twelve children, one father, and three different mothers. LaVera had never been to preschool prior to kindergarten. I suspect that had LaVera originally been evaluated using processing-dependent measures that ruled out her background situation, she would never have qualified for speech-language therapy. Again, processing-dependent measures are an excellent tool for differentiating language differences from SLI in CLD children (Kohnert, 2004). However, as Haynes and Pindzola (2004) caution, these measures alone are not sufficient; they should be used in conjunction with other measures. In addition, clinicians who work with bilingual children must remember that there may be differences in their processing skills depending on their current stage of bilingual development (Gutierrez-Clellen, Calderon, & Ellis Weismer, 2004).

Assessment of Narrative Skills

Many authors recommend that an evaluation of children's language skills include an assessment of their ability to retell stories and construct narratives (e.g. Gutierrez-Clellen, 2004; Wong, W-S Au, & Stokes, 2004). As we have said before, when the SLP evaluates a student's narrative skills, she must be sure to take cultural narrative differences into account (Bliss et al., 2001; Gutierrez-Clellen & Quinn, 1993). For instance, in some cultures, there is no "moral to the story." African American children's narrative styles may differ from mainstream styles in that these children may tell stories with structured discourse on several linked topics and a lack of consideration for detail as discussed in Chapter 4 (Terrell & Jackson, 2002; van Keulen et al., 1998). Again, the SLP must be sensitive to cultural differences in narrative styles.

With this in mind, SLPs can evaluate students' narrative skills by asking the following questions (Roseberry-McKibbin, 2008):

- Does the student include all the major details of the story?
- Is the information in the story comprehensible to the listener?
- Does the student organize the story in a way that is easily understood?
- Does the student make relevant or irrelevant comments when telling the story?

> Culturally sensitive narrative assessment is an excellent way to evaluate a CLD student for the possible presence of SLI.

Again, the SLP must consider the student's cultural and linguistic background as a backdrop to assess narrative skills. Students with SLI have great difficulty with narrative skills. If a CLD student is being evaluated, it can be most helpful to have the input of two or more native speakers of the student's L1 to evaluate the student's narrative abilities from a linguistically and culturally sensitive point of view.

Portfolio Assessment

A portfolio is a container (e.g., a notebook, folder, or box) that holds information about and materials created by a student. Portfolios are valuable because if student work samples are collected over time, a team of professionals can evaluate the student's progress in one or more areas.

> In portfolio assessment, samples of a student's work are evaluated over time to assess progress and student learning ability.

In the same way, SLPs can use the portfolio method of assessment to analyze children's oral and written language progress over time. The SLP along with the classroom teacher can collect audiotapes of language samples in L1 and English and can collect other types of oral and written language products. Then these can be evaluated over a period of time, usually a period of months, to see if the

POINTS TO PONDER Describe two methods of alternative assessment that can be used with CLD students who are suspected of having an SLI.

_____

_____

_____

student is progressing at an acceptable rate. If the student is progressing a great deal more slowly than expected, then it is possible that she has SLI. CLD students' progress can be evaluated as compared to that of peers from a similar cultural and linguistic background.

Use of Interpreters in Assessing CLD Students

When SLPs assess the language skills of CLD students, they often use interpreters. If a CLD student's strongest or dominant language is the first language or L1, the law mandates that testing must be carried out in that language. A recent national survey (Roseberry-McKibbin et al., 2005) that we mentioned earlier in the book found that only 12.5 percent of 1,736 public school SLPs surveyed spoke a language other than English with enough fluency to provide services in that language. Thus, many SLPs used interpreters to assist in assessment with CLD students.

The role of an interpreter may include many tasks, such as translating forms, interviewing parents, administering tests, translating for parents and teachers, and so forth. When utilizing interpreters, SLPs must be sure that they (Langdon & Cheng, 2002; Roseberry-McKibbin, 2008):

- Train the interpreters for their role
- Ensure that interpreters understand their ethical responsibilities
- Ensure that interpreters are able to relate well to members of their cultural group
- Provide interpreters with background information about the students who are going to be tested
- Show interpreters how to use tests and make sure interpreters are comfortable with testing

> Appropriately trained interpreters can be invaluable to the process of assessing CLD students in their first language.

- Remain present during all testing conducted with an interpreter so it can be assured that the interpreter is administering the tests and recording results accurately
- Spend an adequate amount of time with interpreters after students leave to debrief and talk about assessment findings

Lastly, I have found that it is important to show appreciation to interpreters for their services. Many interpreters (at least in my district) work very hard and are underpaid. I know that assessment of CLD children would be impossible without the support of my interpreters, and I try to thank them always and let them know how valuable they are to the assessment process. They appreciate being appreciated.

SUMMARY

- According to federal law, testing and evaluation procedures and materials must be selected and administered in a nondiscriminatory manner and must be provided and administered in the language or other mode of communication in which the child is most proficient.

- Dynamic assessment evaluates a student's ability to learn when provided with instruction. In dynamic assessment, the SLP looks at the student's modifiability.
- Assessment of information-processing skills has potential to validly and reliably distinguish language differences from SLI in CLD students.
- Many experts recommend the assessment of students' narrative skills as another way to determine the potential presence of SLI.
- In portfolio assessment, samples of a student's work are collected over time and analyzed to see how much and how well the student is learning.
- Well-trained interpreters are often critical in assessment situations where a CLD student needs to be evaluated in his first language.

Add your own summary points here:

_____

_____

_____

CLD STUDENTS: LANGUAGE DIFFERENCE OR LANGUAGE IMPAIRMENT?

Introduction

When CLD students struggle in school, teachers often refer them for special education testing—including speech-language assessment. Generally, the teachers are wondering if these students have SLI or just language differences. In Chapter 1, we discussed characteristics of students with SLI. In this chapter, we have examined basic principles of language assessment as they apply to both monolingual and CLD students. Clinicians must remember that in order to diagnose a CLD student with actual SLI, it must be proven that the student has an underlying difficulty learning any language—L1 and English.

CLD students should not be labeled as SLI if "problems" are observed only in English and not in L1. SLI is a disability that affects the child's learning of any language. Exposure to two languages is *not* a cause of a disability; as we stated in Chapter 3, proficient bilingualism is an advantage. If a student has a genuine SLI, difficulties will be observed in both L1 and in English.

> When a CLD student is being assessed for a possible SLI, the Diagnostic Pie is a useful way to conceptualize the role of environment in his language performance.

When assessing a CLD student for a possible SLI, it is very important to rule out the impact of environment as well as a mismatch between the child's background and the school's expectations. The Diagnostic Pie (Figure 5.2) is a simple conceptual framework that clinicians can use to help distinguish language differences from SLI in CLD students who are learning English as a second or third language (Roseberry-McKibbin, 2008).

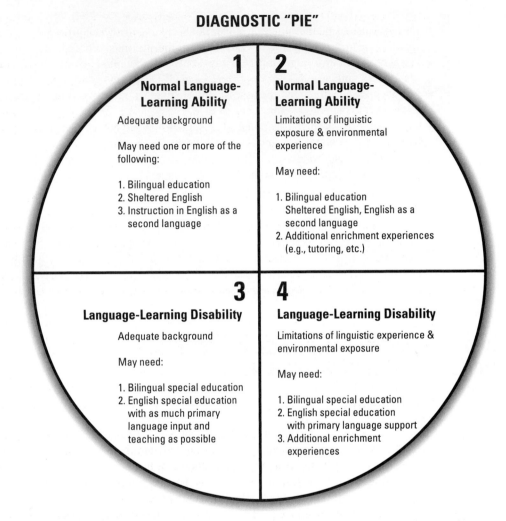

DIAGNOSTIC "PIE"

1
Normal Language-Learning Ability

Adequate background

May need one or more of the following:

1. Bilingual education
2. Sheltered English
3. Instruction in English as a second language

2
Normal Language-Learning Ability

Limitations of linguistic exposure & environmental experience

May need:

1. Bilingual education
   Sheltered English, English as a second language
2. Additional enrichment experiences (e.g., tutoring, etc.)

3
Language-Learning Disability

Adequate background

May need:

1. Bilingual special education
2. English special education with as much primary language input and teaching as possible

4
Language-Learning Disability

Limitations of linguistic experience & environmental exposure

May need:

1. Bilingual special education
2. English special education with primary language support
3. Additional enrichment experiences

FIGURE 5.2

Used with permission. From Roseberry-McKibbin, C. (2008). *Multicultural students with special language needs: Practical strategies for assessment and intervention* (3rd edition), Oceanside, CA: Academic Communication Associates, Inc.

The Diagnostic Pie

Students who fall into Quadrant 1 of the Diagnostic Pie have no abnormalities in their language-learning ability. They come from backgrounds where there has been adequate stimulation and language-learning experience, but their background does not match the school's expectations.

I was one of these students. When we moved to the Philippines as I was turning six years old, my parents placed me in first grade at Jose Abad Santos Memorial School in

Manila, the capital. I was a full year younger than most of the children, did not speak Tagalog, and was one of the only white children in the school. I had been successful in US kindergarten but was unable to keep up with the curriculum in my new Filipino school. To this day, I am thankful that no one diagnosed me as having an SLI! My mother homeschooled me intensively to help me catch up and put me back in Filipino public school in third grade, where I was successful.

In the United States, Quadrant 1 students do not need special education services. They frequently need bilingual education, instruction in English as a second language, or **Sheltered English** programs. In Sheltered English programs, students learn academic content (e.g., math, science, social studies) in simple, comprehensible English that is accompanied by many visual stimuli and hands-on activities. These programs have been extremely successful in supporting students from a wide variety of CLD backgrounds.

Students in Quadrant 2 of the Diagnostic Pie have normal language-learning ability. However, they come from backgrounds where they may have experienced some limitations in cognitive-linguistic stimulation and school-type experiences. I've worked with many children like this—both CLD and monolingual English-speaking children—from low-income homes where they did not have the advantages of being read to, being taken places like the zoo, and having oral and written language experiences to prepare them for kindergarten.

As the mother of a child who just finished kindergarten, I am overwhelmed with what is expected of children entering elementary school in the early twenty-first century. You may remember a day when kindergarten consisted of painting, playing, singing, taking a nap, and learning shapes and colors. As we said in Chapter 2, these days, kindergarteners in states such as California are expected to begin school knowing most basic concepts, including the alphabet. My son was expected to begin writing sentences and reading small books before he was halfway through his kindergarten year.

CLD students who begin school with limitations of linguistic exposure and environmental experience may increasingly flounder under today's rigorous academic requirements. Rather than being diagnosed with SLI and placed into special education, these students frequently need bilingual education or Sheltered English (whichever is available) as well as enrichment experiences such as tutoring or special after-school enrichment programs. When given learning opportunities, these students demonstrate good gains and are able to generally keep pace with their monolingual English-speaking peers.

> Students in Quadrants 1 and 2 of the Diagnostic Pie do not have SLI; they have mismatches between their environment/background and the school's expectations.

Students in Quadrant 3 of the Diagnostic Pie come from backgrounds in which they have had adequate language stimulation and exposure. Many times, parents have given these students as much support as possible at home, and the students still do not succeed in school. In other cases, the school has provided substantial additional support over time to assist these students in developing language and academic skills (e.g., tutoring, after-school enrichment programs, English as a second language services). Despite all this extra support, the students continue to show learning difficulties and stand out as being slower than similar CLD peers to learn new information. These students usually have an SLI and need special education services as well as primary language support.

CASES TO CONSIDER

Hello Celeste,

My name is Donna, and my daughter Sasha is seven years old. I adopted her from a Romanian orphanage when she was four years old. She was neglected, had parasites, and years of malnutrition. Shortly after arriving in Connecticut, she was diagnosed as having a language disorder and was placed in special education. However, I cannot get the school to give her English as a second language services or any other additional support. My health insurance company won't provide any additional speech services. Please help me. I don't know how else to fight for my daughter. Can you suggest anything?

What would you say to this mother? What else can you recommend that will help support Sasha? (See Chapter 4 for a description of the needs of internationally adopted children.)

_____

_____

_____

Children in Quadrant 4 of the Diagnostic Pie have environmental/background limitations as well as SLI. They need special education services, primary language support, and additional enrichment experiences. They can usually benefit from all the enrichment and special education support the school has to offer. As I was writing this chapter, I received the e-mail above from a mother on the East Coast. Some of the details have been changed for purposes of confidentiality, but I share this case as an example of a child in Quadrant 4 of the Diagnostic Pie.

 SUMMARY

- If "language problems" are observed only in English and not in L1, CLD students should not be labeled as SLI.
- SLI is a disability that affects the child's ability to learn any language. Exposure to two languages is *not* a cause of disability.
- If a student has a genuine SLI, difficulties will be observed both L1 and English.
- When assessing a CLD student for a possible of SLI, it is very important to rule out the impact of environment as well as a mismatch between the child's background and the school's expectations.
- The Diagnostic Pie provides a simple conceptual framework that clinicians can use to help distinguish language differences from SLI in CLD students who are learning English as a second or third language.

Add your own summary points here:

_____

_____

_____

CHAPTER HIGHLIGHTS

- Assessing a child's language skills is a process of observing and measuring a child's receptive and expressive language to determine 1) whether a clinically significant problem exists, 2) the nature and extent of the problem, and 3) what course of action needs to be taken to help the child if a problem does exist. In the case of CLD students, the goal is to distinguish a language difference from an SLI.

- Before an in-depth assessment takes place, the SLP conducts a screening to see if more in-depth testing is even needed. If it is, then the SLP gathers a case history and conducts a thorough preevaluation process.

- Children's language skills can be assessed through **standardized** or **formal** tests. A test can be standardized without being **norm-referenced**; however, most standardized tests (though not all) are norm-referenced. Standardized, norm-referenced tests give clinicians a quantitative means of comparing a child's performance to the performance of large groups of children in a similar age category.

- Standardized tests are broadly evaluated by two parameters: validity and reliability. Validity asks: does this test actually measure what it says it is measuring? There are several different kinds of validity. Reliability refers to the stability or consistency with which the same event is repeatedly measured. Reliable scores are consistent across repeated measurements.

- If we choose to use standardized tests with CLD students, we have to be aware of formal test assumptions and potential forms of bias. These forms include cultural-linguistic bias, value bias, format bias, and examiner bias. There are ways to modify standardized tests so that they are less biased if used to assess CLD students.

- In order to evaluate a child's use of spontaneous language in various contexts, we can gather and analyze a language sample. It should be representative. Common informal methods of evaluating a monolingual English-speaking child's language form include calculating mean length of utterance, type-token ratio, or both.

- To evaluate the English skills of a CLD student, the SLP must use contrastive analysis to ascertain whether the child's grammatical errors reflect the presence of SLI or just transfer from the first language. A professional who speaks the child's first language fluently can help to assess the child's content, form, and use in the first language.

- Besides the language sample, other legal, informal alternatives to standardized assessment are available. They can be used with monolingual English-speaking children and are especially appropriate for CLD children.

- Assessment alternatives include dynamic assessment, assessment of information-processing skills, assessment of narrative skills, and portfolio assessment. An interpreter who speaks the child's first language can be of great assistance in assessment.
- CLD students should not be labeled as having an SLI if "problems" are observed only in English and not in L1. SLI affects the child's ability to learn any language. If a student has a genuine SLI, difficulties will be observed in both L1 and in English.
- When assessing a CLD student for a possible SLI, it is very important to rule out the impact of environment as well as a mismatch between the child's background and the school's expectations. The Diagnostic Pie is a simple conceptual framework that clinicians can use to help distinguish language differences from SLI in CLD students who are learning English as a second or third language.

Add your own chapter highlights here:

_____

_____

_____

_____

STUDY AND REVIEW QUESTIONS

ESSAY

1. Discuss the components of a preevaluation process. Before we conduct an in-depth assessment of a child's language skills, why is it so important to go through this type of process?

2. What is the purpose of standardized, norm-referenced tests? What are some possible misuses of these tests?

3. Describe strategies for collecting a language sample from a child. How can we informally evaluate her language use?

4. Discuss legal considerations that we need to keep in mind as we assess CLD students. What does the law say we must do when we assess these students?

5. Describe the Diagnostic Pie. How do we define SLI in a CLD student?

FILL-IN-THE-BLANK

6. _____ assessment measures a student's skills at one point in time to make a judgment about whether she has a language difference or an SLI.

7. A test with _____ or _____ bias uses testing materials, procedures, or both that are less familiar to some children.

8. _____ reliability looks at how two different raters score the same set of behaviors.

9. The process of _____ involves quickly and efficiently obtaining a general view of a child's language skills.

10. The _____ validity of a new test refers to the degree to which it correlates with an established test of known validity.

MULTIPLE CHOICE

11. You are evaluating a standardized, norm-referenced test for possible use with SLI students in your school district. Upon reading the manual, you find that there is little or no qualitative or quantitative information that supports the test maker's theory or model underlying the test. The test could be said to have poor

   a. Face validity
   b. Construct validity
   c. Concurrent validity
   d. Predictive validity
   e. Split-half reliability

12. Mario N., a Spanish-speaking student, has come to kindergarten at your school. After the first three months of kindergarten, he is "picking up" according to the teacher but is not yet performing at a level commensurate with that of his monolingual English-speaking peers. When you screen Mario, with the help of a Spanish-speaking interpreter, you find that in Spanish he has good information-processing skills. The interpreter says that Mario has no difficulty conveying meaning or following directions in Spanish. When you inquire into Mario's background, you find out that he is the youngest in a family with six children. His parents are migrant farmworkers and have moved frequently. Mario has no preschool background. What quadrant of the Diagnostic Pie would Mario probably fit into?

   a. Quadrant 1
   b. Quadrant 2
   c. Quadrant 3
   d. Quadrant 4
   e. None of the above

13. Acceptable ways to modify an English standardized test for a CLD child would include

   I. Explaining or rephrasing confusing directions
   II. Devoting more than one session to the assessment
   III. Having an interpreter translate items into the child's first language, then using the norms to evaluate the child
   IV. Omitting biased items that the child is likely to miss
   V. Allowing the student extra time to respond

   a. I, II, IV, V
   b. All of the above
   c. I, III, V
   d. II, III, IV
   e. I, III, IV, V

14. You were assigned to evaluate the skills of Aubtin, a Farsi-speaking boy from Iran. Because you had no standardized tests in Farsi, you used alternative forms of assessment with assistance from a competent Farsi-speaking interpreter. As part of the assessment, you had Aubtin repeat back digits and words in Farsi. You were assessing

   a. Narrative skills
   b. Language use
   c. Morphosyntactic skills
   d. Information-processing skills
   e. His ability to be patient

15. What is one thing that you do *not* want to do when you utilize an interpreter during an assessment session?

   a. Ensure that he understands his ethical responsibilities
   b. Provide him with background information about the student who is going to be tested
   c. Leave the room for a ten- to fifteen-minute break during the assessment so he won't feel like you are breathing down his neck
   d. Show him how to use the tests and make sure he is comfortable with them
   e. Train him for his role

See Answers to Study and Review Questions, page 465.

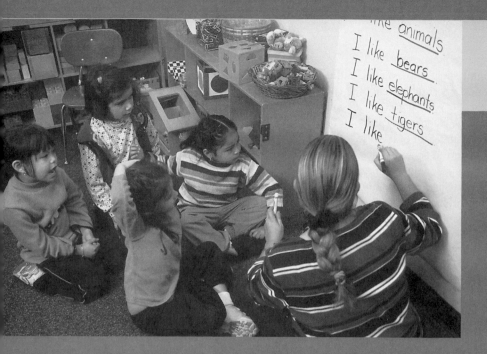

Intervention for Children with Language Impairments: General Principles and Strategies

CASE STUDY

Francisco, a shy, charming kindergartener with a wide grin, was from a migrant Hispanic family in the south Sacramento area. Francisco's classroom teacher referred him to me in November for an assessment. She was concerned because although he was very well behaved and courteous, he did not seem to be "keeping pace" academically with his classmates in his all-English classroom.

As we discussed in Chapter 5, part of any thorough evaluation is gathering a thorough case history. I found out that Francisco was born in south Sacramento to a Mexican couple who already had

four children. The family struggled financially and lived in a trailer with five children, two parents, and two grandparents. Only Spanish was spoken in the home. Francisco had never been to preschool. There were no books in the home. He had never held a pencil before. His parents were nonliterate in Spanish.

With the assistance of a Spanish-speaking professional, I evaluated Francisco in both English and Spanish, focusing most heavily on Spanish as it was his dominant language. He achieved low scores even in Spanish. I was reluctant to label

Francisco with specific language impairment (SLI) because of his environmental situation. I wanted him to have more time and exposure to school and school-related materials.

The other speech-language pathologist (SLP) and I decided on the following strategy. For the rest of kindergarten, Francisco received special assistance in the classroom from an aide. He also met several times a week with a Spanish-speaking teacher so that we could continue to build his Spanish skills. Francisco showed some improvements, but eventually he was retained in first grade because his parents demanded it. They would not allow him to go on to second grade because he was far behind academically, even compared to Spanish-speaking Mexican peers.

We reassessed Francisco in both English and Spanish, because it was clear that his linguistic and academic skills had not "caught up," even as compared to those of similar peers. Results of a comprehensive assessment at the end of his

second year of first grade showed that Francisco did indeed have an SLI and needed intervention.

We placed Francisco in a combination of individual and small-group therapy. We worked closely with the classroom teacher to connect therapy to the second-grade curriculum. Because Francisco was still quite shy, we used token reinforcers to encourage him to verbalize. We also used techniques such as expanding his language during therapy sessions to build his sentence length and complexity. Unfortunately, due to lack of a Spanish-speaking SLP, all therapy was conducted in English. However, we made sure that Francisco still continued to meet with a Spanish-speaking professional on a weekly basis in hopes that his Spanish would be maintained and that he would not experience language loss in Spanish. We worked on Francisco's social and academic language skills, using literacy materials to help him build his academic language.

INTRODUCTION

When we conduct therapy or intervention with children with language impairments (LI) our goal is to support them in developing their potential to express and comprehend language as normally as possible in social and academic situations. There are different approaches to language intervention, and there are a variety of ways in which SLPs can structure intervention depending on children's individual needs. Many SLPs use various types of reinforcement in language intervention to motivate LI children to communicate.

SLPs have at their disposal a wide array of intervention techniques to promote children's language skills. A very important component of intervention is facilitation of generalization (habituation to other settings and persons) of language skills learned in intervention sessions. To help children generalize language skills outside of the therapy room, SLPs work with significant others. These significant others include caregivers/family members, classroom teachers, and others.

When SLPs conduct intervention with CLD children with LI, it is important to be sensitive to which of the children's languages will be used in therapy. SLPs should also display sensitivity to students' cultures. It is very important to involve families of CLD students in therapy as much as possible, remembering that some families might not be familiar with English and/or the American school system. In these cases, SLPs can make an additional effort to reach out to and include the families as much as possible so that they are included in intervention efforts.

GENERAL PRINCIPLES OF INTERVENTION FOR CHILDREN WITH LANGUAGE IMPAIRMENTS

Introduction

In Chapter 1, we defined SLI as a language impairment that is not associated with any other condition such as autism. To review, SLI is referred to by some researchers as a *primary language impairment.* Language impairment can also be *secondary condition* when it can be accounted for by another primary condition such as hearing impairment, neurological impairment, autism, and other types of problems (Law, Garrett, & Nye, 2004; Windsor & Kohnert, 2004). In addition, children may have language problems associated with environmental factors such as maternal use of drugs and alcohol (described in Chapter 10), or language problems associated with other factors such as hearing and/or vision impairment (described in Chapter 11). This chapter, because it addresses general and foundational principles of intervention, refers to all these children as having "language impairments." Thus, in this chapter, I have used the term LI to refer to these children. In subsequent chapters, more specific intervention techniques are described for specific populations; in this chapter, foundational and underlying principles are described as an introduction to more specific techniques.

> Children may have language impairments due to associated conditions such as fetal alcohol syndrome, autism, and others. Some children may also have an impairment that is specific to language with no associated condition.

Purposes of Intervention

What is the purpose of **intervention** (also called **therapy** or **treatment**) for children with LI? Generally speaking, the goal is for the child to express and comprehend language as normally as possible in academic and social situations. Children must function in many areas of society: the home, the playground, the school, and others. We try to help children achieve their communication potential in all situations. Some children have very great potential for improvement; for others, as we shall see in subsequent chapters, the potential is somewhat more limited.

Paul (2001; based on Olswang and Bain, 1991) described four purposes of language intervention:

> The ultimate goal of intervention is for the child to express and comprehend language as normally as possible in academic and social situations.

- *Change or eliminate the underlying problem.* This rarely happens. Many times parents want to know if their child will "outgrow" the LI. With rare exceptions, the answer is "no."

• *Change the disorder by teaching the child specific language behaviors.* For example, if a child eliminates plural and past-tense forms, teach him to use these appropriately. If the child's vocabulary is limited, teach him new words.

• *Teach the child compensatory strategies instead of specific language behaviors.* For example, if a student has a word retrieval problem (difficulty remembering and using a word she already knows in a specific situation), the SLP would not necessarily teach her to come up with specific vocabulary words on command (e.g., "This is a picture of a ___"). Rather, the student would be taught how to use word retrieval strategies at the conversational level so that specific vocabulary words would be remembered during discourse. The approach of teaching compensatory strategies often works best for older students who will probably always have some deficits.

• *Try to change the child's environment, not the child.* For example, if a student has a language impairment associated with attention deficit hyperactivity disorder (described in Chapter 10), it might make sense to put that student in a small, calm, well-ordered classroom rather than a large, noisy one. The student would probably perform much better under the latter condition.

Often, SLPs use a combination of the above to help the child's language skills be as normal as possible in light of the demands of her cultural and linguistic communities. It is important to remember that the concept of "normal" or "typical" communication differs from culture to culture. When we conduct language intervention with all students, including culturally and linguistically diverse (CLD) students, we want to help them 1) interact successfully with those from their cultural and linguistic background and 2) interact successfully in mainstream society.

I attended an American Speech-Language-Hearing Association (ASHA) seminar years ago where a Hispanic speaker talked passionately about these goals. He said that if we train a child to communicate successfully in his own cultural and linguistic milieu, that's a good thing; but how about mainstream society? The speaker argued that CLD children must learn to communicate successfully in both venues: their own communities and mainstream society. For if CLD children do not communicate successfully in mainstream society, their vocational and financial opportunities as adults will probably be quite limited. It is our goal for all children who receive language intervention to communicate successfully with persons from their individual communities and to communicate successfully with others in mainstream society (Genesee et al., 2004).

> CLD students need to learn to communicate successfully within their own communities and also within mainstream society.

Children must communicate successfully at the oral and written language levels. This will be covered in much greater depth in later chapters; however, it is critical to note at the outset of any discussion of intervention that we are not looking at just successful speaking and listening; we are looking at successful reading and writing as well. Historically, SLPs have not always conducted intervention at the written language level. However, ASHA (2000) has definitively stated that SLPs must address written as well as oral language in order to help children be successful. A language impairment generally impacts both oral and written language; we must not address one without addressing the other (Gillam & Ukrainetz, 2006).

Basic Approaches to Language Intervention

As we delve deeper into the topic of language intervention, it should be noted that there are many approaches to intervention. In this section, we will consider two commonly described approaches: developmental and functional. The **developmental** or **normative approach** involves the SLP basing intervention targets on language development norms. Essentially, the SLP ascertains where a particular child is at developmentally and then follows language development guidelines in planning goals. For example, let's say an eight-year-old child does not accurately use basic pronouns *he, she, it* and *her, his*. Because these pronouns are accurately used by most five-year-olds, the SLP would make accurate use of a goal of intervention. In another example, let's say that a five-year-old is unable to tell a simple, understandable story. Typically developing (TD) children are generally able to do this by three years of age. The SLP might make a treatment goal to have the child tell a simple story in sequence.

Kuder (2003) and Owens (2004) make the point that it is helpful to use language developmental norms in planning therapy. However, they also point out that children with disabilities do not develop language in the same way that TD children do. For instance, children with Asperger syndrome (a form of high-functioning autism) develop language very differently than do TD children—more will be said about that in Chapter 9. Because of this reality, many clinicians and researchers have turned to the **functional approach**—an approach to intervention where children are taught specific skills that they need in their present environment and/or an environment that they will be entering. For example, a student might be taught how to interact successfully with a greater variety of conversational partners because she is going to enter junior high school soon. The functional approach may hold greater promise for CLD students, especially because we do not have developmental language norms that are appropriate for use with these students.

> Two common approaches to language intervention are the developmental/normative approach and the functional approach.

Kuder (2003) suggested that it is possible to combine developmental and functional approaches to language intervention. With younger children, it can be useful to ascertain which children are at risk for LI because they have not met appropriate developmental language milestones in a timely fashion. Remembering that language developmental norms are influenced by culture (Chapter 2), SLPs can very generally use language development guidelines to help them plan effective therapy for young children.

POINTS TO PONDER Describe the developmental/normative and functional approaches to intervention. For which types of children would you use each?

_____

_____

_____

For example, in Chapter 5, I discussed Abdul, a five-year-old kindergartener who did not speak in Urdu until he was two-and-a-half years old; he also echoed much of what he heard. At age five, he still only spoke in three- or four-word utterances in Urdu and used even shorter utterances in English. He did not comprehend basic instructions in either language. You will recall that Abdul's mother asked that he repeat kindergarten, and he was also placed onto the speech-language caseload for services.

The developmental approach to intervention for Abdul would suggest that appropriate intervention targets include expanding his mean length of utterance in both English and Urdu, reducing his use of echolalia, and helping him comprehend simple directions in both languages. The functional approach to intervention would involve adding treatment goals to help Abdul succeed in kindergarten—for example, labeling basic shapes and colors, counting to 100, recognizing the alphabet, and writing his name.

Using the developmental approach for older students is often less successful; they can benefit mostly from intervention approaches that focus on skills needed immediately in their current environments (Kuder, 2003). These include academic and social skills. SLPs must especially target language behaviors that create social penalties for students. For example, students who interrupt their peers frequently and are insensitive to peers' verbal and nonverbal cues are likely to be rejected and have few friends.

In Chapter 1, I mentioned that I was asked to evaluate the pragmatic skills of a thirteen-year-old student with Asperger syndrome. Previous reports indicated that Brian was insensitive to peers, monopolized conversations, and used nonverbal cues and gestures inappropriately. Because Brian is going into junior high school next year, his parents want him to fit in with his peers as much as possible, and they are very interested in having Brian improve his pragmatics skills.

Rather than going back to my developmental language milestones list, I evaluated a number of verbal and nonverbal pragmatics skills that will impact Brian's relationships next year—especially with his peers. To give a very concrete example, Brian shared about a big fish he had recently caught (and no, it didn't get away). I gave him a high-five; this tall, strong thirteen-year-old karate expert returned my high-five so hard that he almost knocked me off my feet. His mom flinched; as I nursed my stinging hand, I just smiled and said, "The assessment has begun!"

> Developmental approaches to intervention are often more appropriate for younger LI children, while functional approaches are appropriate for older children. Many clinicians use a combination of both.

I think we all would agree that if Brian gave a high-five like that to another thirteen-year-old boy, it would definitely create a social penalty for him. Part of therapy for Brian will involve incorporating work on a more appropriate way to deliver a high-five—a nonverbal behavior that is important for teenagers to master as part of being socially acceptable to their peer group. Table 6.1 is an example of a self-evaluation form that students can complete—alone or with assistance—to become more aware of their social language skills.

Structure of Therapy Sessions

The ways that therapy sessions can be structured are as limitless as the clinician's imagination. First, the clinician must consider whether the student will receive individual or group therapy. In some settings, such as university clinics and private practices, clinicians may offer therapy in a one-on-one format. However, in public schools, children are generally seen

TABLE 6.1   A Communication Skills Quiz for Students

Student's Name:_____ Date:_____

___ **1.** I greet people when I see them by smiling and saying "hi."
___ **2.** I listen to people without interrupting.
___ **3.** I apologize when I have to interrupt.
___ **4.** I try to be interested in what people say.
___ **5.** I try to take time to listen when people want to talk to me.
___ **6.** When people ask me questions, I try to answer as best I can.
___ **7.** When I talk, I try to talk as clearly as possible so other people will understand me.
___ **8.** During conversations, I take turns talking.
___ **9.** During conversations, I try to talk about what other people are talking about instead of bringing up new things in the middle of someone else's sentence.
___**10.** If I don't understand what someone says, I ask the person to please repeat what was said.
___**11.** If someone doesn't understand me, I repeat myself more clearly.
___**12.** I try to look at people when I talk to them.

Used with permission. From Roseberry-McKibbin, C. (2008) *Multicultural students with special language needs: Practical strategies for assessment and intervention* (3rd edition), Oceanside, CA: Academic Communication Associates, Inc.

in groups. (This chapter and Chapter 12 describe in detail the various service delivery models available to students in kindergarten through twelfth grades.) Many clinicians use three basic structures as guidelines when planning therapy sessions for LI students as individuals or as groups (Pena-Brooks & Hegde, 2000):

> In therapy, SLPs may use drill, drill play, or play.

Drill involves a highly efficient, structured response mode
Drill play is similar to drill, except that there is a motivational and fun event for the student(s)
Play—work on treatment stimuli occurs as a natural part of play activities

Let's take an example of how this might look with an actual student. Let's say that our student, Anita, is learning how to use possessive -*s* correctly.

Drill

Clinician: Anita, I am going to show you some pictures. You tell me what you see in each picture. Let me do the first one. "That is Kate's ball." Now you try the next one.

Anita: That is the dog's bone.

Clinician: Nice job—here's the next one. Tell me what you see here.

Anita: That is the man's car.

Clinician: Good—tell me what you see here.

Anita: That is the lady's purse.

Clinician: Good! Tell me what you see here.

Anita: That is the girl's ball.

Drill Play

> *Clinician:*   We are going to play Candy Land. When you land near a character, tell me what he or she has. Be sure to use your special -*s*. Ready?
>
> *Clinician:*   Oh, look! You landed near Lord Licorice! What does he have?
>
> *Anita:*   That is Lord Licorice's castle.
>
> *Clinician:*   Super! Now it's my turn.
>
> *Clinician (a little later in the game):*   Anita, you landed near Jolly. What does he have?
>
> *Anita:*   Those are Jolly's gumdrops.
>
> *Clinician:*   Good job using your -*s*. Now (later in the game) you are beside Grandma Nutt. What does she have?
>
> *Anita:*   That is Grandma Nutt's peanut brittle house.

Play

> *Clinician:*   Anita, I brought a dollhouse today. Let's play with it.
>
> *Clinician:*   The mommy is going into the living room. She is getting her purse. Whose purse is it?
>
> *Anita:*   That's the mommy's purse.
>
> *Clinician:*   Yes. Now . . . (more play occurs; Anita puts the toy dog by his doghouse)
>
> *Clinician:*   Hey, what's this?
>
> *Anita:*   That's the dog's house.

In my work with children, I have found that many of them enjoy drill play. They like the feeling that they are accomplishing a specific goal, and they enjoy having a good time doing it. However, in my university clinic, we just finished working with a six-year-old boy who told us that he didn't like our games; he just wanted to do drill work. As the old saying goes, "Different strokes for different folks."

With some children, I have effectively used a mixed approach. I have told them that if they do solid drill (e.g., give me thirty productions of a target such as possessive -*s*), they will get three minutes of just play with no work. I use a happy-face sheet (shown on page 193) to keep track of the number of productions they make. They will usually drill very diligently in order to get a "break."

Using Reinforcement in Language Therapy

Positive reinforcement is a powerful way to help LI children improve their language skills. **Positive reinforcers** are events that increase the frequency of a response when made contingent upon that response. Put differently, a positive reinforcer is a consequence that follows a response and thus increases the frequency of that response (Pena-Brooks & Hegde, 2000). Consider the following example:

> *Child:*   (points to a puzzle piece)
>
> *Clinician:*   Do you want that puzzle piece?
>
> (Child nods)

> Positive reinforcers are events that increase the frequency of a response when made contingent upon that response.

Clinician: OK—say, "I want the puzzle piece."

Child: I want the puzzle piece.

Clinician: Great! Here it is!

In this example, the child is more likely to verbalize a request the next time because in this instance, verbalization of his wants got him what he desired.

Primary positive reinforcers are biological in nature and don't rely on past learning or conditioning. Food and water are primary reinforcers. Food is quite effective with children who are very young, nonverbal, developmentally delayed, or behaviorally resistant. Here is an example from my own work with Clint, a student with a low IQ:

Me: Clint, tell me what this picture is.

Clint: (refuses to talk)

Me: Clint, if you tell me what this is, you will get an M&M.

Clint: Horse.

Me: Great job! Here's an M&M.

Although primary reinforcers can be very effective in certain situations, they have their limitations. They are vulnerable to the **satiation effect**—the child gets full and stops working for the reinforcer. In addition, food is not a natural reinforcer; when Clint is in the "real world," no one is going to pop an M&M into his mouth every time he uses language appropriately. Because of its lack of naturalness, food as a reinforcer may not promote generalization and maintenance of treatment targets.

> Primary reinforcers are biological in nature; secondary reinforcers have cultural or social benefits.

Secondary positive reinforcers are events or actions that increase the occurrence of a behavior. These reinforcers have cultural or social benefits. They depend on past learning and conditioning. For example, most children have learned that a smile means that the other person is happy with them. There are several kinds of secondary reinforcers (Pena-Brooks & Hegde, 2000):

• **Social reinforcers**—verbal praise, touch, eye contact. Clinicians must use this wisely with CLD students. For example, in some Native American tribes, being praised in front of others is embarrassing; the goal is to blend into the group. A Native American student (in a group therapy setting) who was told, "Fabulous job! That's right! I'm so proud of you!" would not experience this verbal praise as a social reinforcer. She might be extremely embarrassed and become unwilling to speak again.

• **Conditioned generalized reinforcers**—These are secondary reinforcers that depend on past experience or conditioning. This type of reinforcement has also been called a **token economy**; children get something in return for complying with what the SLP wants. Children get to earn something. For example, I often use plastic happy-face chips that children may redeem for stickers. I also have a chart on the wall of the therapy room. Children get stars for cooperative behavior during therapy. When they have earned a certain number of stars, they get to go to the silver prize box. Some children may not tolerate waiting to win a prize "down the road"; this delayed reinforcement may be too frustrating for them. They need immediate reinforcement, where they receive something immediately for doing as the SLP asks. I use a combination of both immediate and delayed reinforcement. I save the silver box prizes for several weeks of compliance but give stickers much more frequently. I find that this combination works well for most of the children I serve.

• **Informative feedback**—This type of conditioned reinforcer gives a child specific information about her performance. For example, I worked with Maria, a Spanish-speaking LI child who was very reluctant to speak in either English or Spanish. One of my goals was to have her use three or four descriptors for common objects, so I would use my whiteboard and make a hash mark for each descriptor she used. I accompanied this with verbal praise. (I also used happy-face chips.)

> *Me:* Maria, tell me about this.
>
> *Maria:* It's a watch.
>
> *Me:* OK (hash mark), you told me one thing. Now I need you to tell me two or three more things about it.
>
> *Maria:* It is black.
>
> *Me:* (hash mark) Maria, that's great! You have told me two things! Now I need one or two more. What else can you tell me?
>
> *Maria:* Well . . . it has a second hand.
>
> *Me:* (hash mark) Maria, look—you told me three things! One-two-three! You told me that this is a watch, that it is black, and that it has a second hand.

> Verbal and nonverbal formative feedback give children specific information about their performance.

Informative feedback can be **verbal**, as in the example above. **Nonverbal informative feedback** can be provided in the form of charts and graphs. This works best for older students. However, I have used my "happy-face sheet" successfully with children as young as three years of age. I have included a miniature example of this on page 193. In reality, I have a laminated orange construction paper sheet with stickers across the top. When the child responds correctly, I draw a happy face in a box with a felt-tip pen. (Therapy hint: *You* do the drawing; otherwise this can take forever. Children will draw beards, jewelry, hats . . . you get the picture.) Children love this and will work really hard to fill the sheet with happy faces. I have 100 spaces on the sheet, and even young children will work hard to fill up the whole sheet. It's cheap, fun, and easy!

Schedules of Reinforcement

How frequently do you reinforce a child for correct responses? After every response? After 100 responses? There are two primary types of reinforcement schedules: continuous and intermittent.

In the early stages of therapy, when we are trying to establish certain language behaviors, we use **continuous reinforcement** by rewarding every single one of the student's

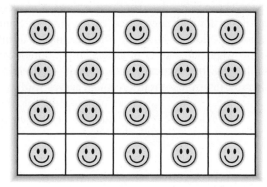

In a continuous reinforcement schedule, we reward every response; in an intermittent schedule, only some responses are reinforced.

responses. Continuous reinforcement is usually very effective. However, it does not match the real world. In the child's everyday environment, she will not receive reinforcement for every accurate response or behavior that she displays. Thus, when behaviors are somewhat established, it is necessary to change to an **intermittent schedule of reinforcement** where only some, but not all, responses are reinforced. There are several types of intermittent reinforcement schedules.

In a **fixed-ratio (FR) schedule**, the student has to give a certain set number of correct responses before getting a reinforcer. For example, in a 1:4 FR schedule, the student might get a happy face after labeling four word cards accurately. In a 1:20 FR schedule, the student would need to label twenty word cards accurately to get a happy face.

In the latter stages of therapy, a **variable ratio (VR) schedule** is used. Clinicians can predetermine an average number of responses to reinforce, but this is time consuming. Thus, many clinicians use a modified VR schedule where they intermittently reinforce the student's responses. Let's say a student has been working on using the correct form of irregular plurals (e.g., *feet, mice*). The student, in the final stages of treatment, might be asked to play a game with the clinician where he was only reinforced occasionally for using these correct forms—and he didn't know when the reinforcement was coming. The VR schedule is very powerful and most closely matches the real world.

POINTS TO PONDER Compare and contrast continuous and intermittent reinforcement. In what situations are each of these appropriate?

_____

_____

_____

Now, I am too cheap to gamble, but the few times I have actually chosen to blow ten dollars, I've played the slot machines (does the daughter of Baptist missionaries dare admit this in a textbook?). Slot machines are prime examples of intermittent reinforcement. You just never know when that shower of nickels might rain down into your bucket, so you keep playing and hoping. Intermittent reinforcement is extremely powerful. Again, in the later stages of therapy, intermittent reinforcement serves well to help treatment targets become habitual. After these targets have been habituated in the therapy setting, it is time to help them carry over or generalize into the student's outside environment.

 SUMMARY

- The developmental or normative approach involves the SLP basing intervention targets on developmental norms. The functional approach to intervention involves teaching specific skills that students need in their present environment and/or an environment that they will be entering.
- In therapy sessions, the SLP may use drill, drill play, or play to teach treatment targets.
- SLPs may use primary or secondary positive reinforcers to encourage the language behaviors they desire from children.
- When delivering reinforcement, two basic types of schedules can be used: continuous and intermittent.
- Two types of intermittent reinforcement schedules are fixed ratio and variable ratio.

Add your own summary points here:

_____

_____

_____

CONNECT & EXTEND

Foundational principles of language intervention are extensively described by Paul, R. (2001). *Language disorders from infancy through adolescence & assessment and intervention* (2nd ed.). St. Louis, MO: Mosby.

SPECIFIC TREATMENT TECHNIQUES

As we discussed in Chapter 1, children with language problems are a heterogeneous group. A variety of intervention techniques can be used with LI children in general from different backgrounds depending on their needs. Basic, widely applicable techniques are described here (Fey, Long, & Finestack, 2003; Hegde, 2001b; Paul, 2001; Roseberry-McKibbin & Hegde, 2006).

Incidental Teaching

This method uses verbal interactions that arise naturally out of everyday situations to teach functional communication skills. The child selects the activity, situation, or conversation topic, and the clinician works language goals into it. For example, a clinician might be working on the "*is verb-ing*" construction with a child. If the child chooses to play with a Fisher Price farm, the clinician can say things like "Oh, look! The cow *is walking* over to the fence. Now the farmer *is driving* after him. Now, can you tell me what's happening here?"

Incidental teaching, a natural approach to intervention, is excellent for caregivers because it works well in their daily routine.

Incidental teaching is an excellent method to teach to caregivers, because they can usually work it into their normal daily activities. The mother of the child above could be taught to use the nightly bathtime, for example, to say things like "Look—now *I'm washing* your hair! Oooh—the duck *is floating* over here. And the boat *is sailing* after it."

Focused Stimulation

If the child needs to work on a particular structure, the clinician repeatedly models that structure in hopes of encouraging the child to use the structure. Usually this is done during a play activity that the clinician has prearranged for the express purpose of modeling the target structure. For example, if the child needs to work on appropriate use of past tense *-ed*, the clinician might use a dollhouse to create a story: "Look, the lady just *stepped* onto the porch. The girl *petted* the dog, and the boy *walked* into the house. I just saw that the daddy *cooked* dinner. The family *watched* TV after dinner for a while, and then *brushed* their teeth. Look—you took the mommy, and she just *climbed* up the stairs."

If the child says the target structure incorrectly, the clinician does not overtly correct the child but rather models the correct response:

> *Child:* The girl brush teeth before bed.
> *Clinician:* Yes, the girl brushed her teeth before bed.

Self-Talk

In this approach, the clinician describes her own activities as she plays with the child. Self-talk is often used in conjunction with focused stimulation. Self-talk can be very useful as a technique to use with children who are unwilling to interact with the clinician. For example, if the treatment target is plural *-s*, the clinician can say, "I am putting some chairs in the dollhouse living room. Oh, and there are pretty curtains too. I will make the parents sit in the living room and look at books. Now I will have the children do homework on their computers."

Parallel Talk

When using this technique, the clinician plays with the child and comments on the objects the child is interested in and about what the child is doing in general. The clinician provides a running commentary on the child's actions. For example, if the child is playing with an ocean stickerboard, the clinician can say, "Oh—there goes the shark! You are moving him toward the diver. The diver is in the seaweed. Uh-oh—I wonder if the shark will eat the diver!"

I have found that both parallel and self-talk work well with children who are not ready to talk. Children may be unwilling to talk in therapy for a number of reasons. In Chapter 3, we discussed the silent period that many CLD children go through as they learn a new language. We said that it is important to respect this silent period and not force children to talk before they are ready. Yet in therapy, one has to do something to support language development. Parallel talk is very successful in these cases.

I have also had some children who were selectively mute for various reasons. **Selective mutism** is a psychiatric disorder in which a child who is capable of talking refuses to do so, except maybe to a certain small group of familiar people (Nelson, 1998). It often occurs in conjunction with anxiety disorders and is usually viewed as an emotional or psychiatric disorder (Paul, 2001). Some selectively mute children I have worked with were refugees who had seen horrific trauma in their home countries. Others had experienced trauma in their homes in the United States. Parallel talk (and focused stimulation) can be successful language intervention techniques with children such as these.

Expansion

If a child makes an incomplete or telegraphic utterance, the clinician expands it into a more grammatically complete utterance.

> *Child:*   Truck drive.
>
> *Clinician:*   Yes, the truck is driving.

The clinician does not add any extra semantic information to the child's utterance; she just models the child's sentence with added grammatical information.

CASES TO CONSIDER

Loan X., a third-grade refugee student from Southeast Asia, was selectively mute. She was placed into speech-language services and also received psychological counseling. What types of intervention techniques would you use with Loan? Why?

_____

_____

_____

Extension

The clinician comments on the child's utterances and adds new information to them. In an expansion as described above, grammatical information is added to make the sentence complete. In an extension, both grammatical and semantic information are added:

> *Child:*   Truck drive.
> *Clinician:*   I see the red truck driving down the freeway and it's going fast!

In expansion, the clinician adds grammatical information to the child's utterance. In extension, the SLP adds both grammatical and semantic information to the child's utterance.

When my son Mark was very small, I used many extensions of his utterances when we were together. His expressive language became so advanced that when he was 2 years old, he said, "I need to put on my shoes and socks because the stones will hurt my feet" (re: going barefoot into the yard). Today, his expressive language continues to be so advanced that it attracts others' attention. It has been fun to see the effects of the extension technique with my own son as well as with the students I work with clinically.

Mand-Model

The mand-model is a variation of incidental teaching that uses a play-oriented setting to teach language through typical adult-child interactions. The clinician uses attractive games, toys, books, or all of these and designs a naturalistic play situation. Then he establishes joint attention with the child to a particular item such as a game.

Next, the clinician mands a response from the child by requesting her to do something. For example, if they are playing Candy Land, the clinician might say, "Tell me what color gingerbread man you want to be." If the child says, "green," the clinician might say "OK, say, 'I want the green gingerbread man.'" The child is praised for accurate responses and is then given the green gingerbread man.

This technique has also been called (perhaps more commonly) **elicited imitation**. In another example, the clinician tells the child, "Say, 'I moved to Candy Castle.'" The child has to reply, "I moved to Candy Castle." The child is rewarded for imitating the clinician.

I have found the mand-model technique to be most effective with children who are accustomed to successfully using gestures to get what they want. I remember five-year-old Kevin K., who was indulged at home by his mother and older siblings. When Kevin wanted something, he'd point to it and look soulfully at me. I taught him to say, "May I please have the _____?"

SLPs must be culturally sensitive in using this technique with children from some cultural groups where children are taught to be quiet and respectful. I remember one CLD student with LI who was so quiet that I actually had to give her tokens for speaking at my request. In these situations, I talk to children about the "home way" and the "school way." I tell them that at home, it is appropriate to be quiet and not ask for things. But at school, the rule is that you have to speak up for what you want. In many situations, with CLD students, I teach them to be bicultural in their language use; again, we discuss the home

> **POINTS TO PONDER** Describe three specific language intervention techniques that would be appropriate for CLD students with LI who tend to be somewhat verbally reticent.
>
> _____
>
> _____
>
> _____

way and the school way. This has been most effective as a method for accepting students' individual cultural customs and also teaching them how to fit in successfully in mainstream American schools where they are expected to be verbally assertive.

Recasting

When SLPs are helping children learn to use more complex grammatical forms, recasting is an excellent technique. Here, the clinician expands the child's utterance into a different type of utterance. The clinician changes the modality or voice of the sentence rather than simply adding grammatical or semantic information. For example:

> In the technique of recasting, the clinician changes the voice or modality of the child's sentence.

Child: The doggy is barking. (declarative)

Clinician: Is the doggy barking? (change to interrogative or question)

Child: Doggy barking at cat.

Clinician: The cat is being barked at by the dog. (change to passive voice)

Joint Routines

Joint routines involved repetitive, routinized activities that are often used with young children for language stimulation. For example, many children love peek-a-boo or patty-cake. Clinicians can also create their own routines and encourage children to use the words and phrases along with them when the routines are memorized. This helps children expand their language use.

Joint Book Reading

Clinicians who use this technique use systematic storybook reading to stimulate language in children. When clinicians and children read a book together, they can practice and repeat certain words and phrases. You may have heard of the famous joint book routine of "Brown bear, brown bear, what do you see? I see a _____ looking at me." This is an example of joint book reading in which the clinician uses a predictable pattern to help fill in words.

Clinicians can also use books that are not predictable but that are read so often, children can eventually fill in the words from memory. Though a simple task, this helps children achieve a sense of story grammar, enhance their vocabularies, and develop phonological awareness skills that are foundational to reading (Goldsworthy, 2001).

Whole Language

Most professionals think of the whole language approach as it applies to reading and writing. The whole language approach holds that for children, learning written language should be like learning oral language. Supporters of the whole language approach believe that children learn to read and write in the same way they learn to talk: through being immersed in a literate environment, communicating through print, and getting supportive feedback from adults.

In whole language, the focus is on acquiring meaning. The SLP does not teach specific subskills or language components. So, for example, the SLP would help a child learn to read by using children's literature rather than basal readers. Writing would be taught by helping the child communicate in print when she needed to do so (e.g., writing a thank-you note to someone for a birthday present). The child would not be directly taught specific subskills such as spelling and punctuation in a predetermined order. These would only be addressed as the need arose in the child's natural attempts to communicate meaning in writing. No workbooks!

Paul (2001) stated that whole language approaches to oral language intervention can make a contribution to children's language-learning progress and serve as part of a battery of language intervention techniques. However, used in their strictest sense, these approaches do not allow the use of extrinsic reinforcement, sequential skill teaching, dividing language into component skills, or formal structure—and many LI children need these things.

> In whole language, the focus is on children's acquisition of meaning. The SLP does not teach specific subskills or language components.

When I think of using the whole language approach with LI children—for written or oral language—I always feel like I do not want to "throw out the baby with the bath water." I have personally found that many LI children profit greatly from sequential skill teaching and extrinsic reinforcement, for example. However, I have found that LI CLD students often profit, especially in the initial stages of therapy, from a focus on communicating meaning with little to no emphasis on dividing language into component skills.

Let's say that a CLD student with an LI is in the early stages of learning English. This shy Filipino student, Nelda, rarely speaks in class, in therapy, or on the playground. My primary goal would be to help her communicate meaning in words—no matter how incorrect her grammar—as a first step in treatment. Later, as her English became more fluent, I might address more discrete components of language such as grammar. But I have found that if I address discrete components too early in the therapy process, some CLD students may "shut down" and stop trying to communicate. Consider the following scenario:

Nelda: (points to a doll she wants)

Clinician: Can you tell me in words what you want?

Nelda: (points again)

Clinician: Nelda, I need to hear words.

Nelda: Want doll over there.

Clinician: Okay, Nelda, but first you have to say, "I want the doll over there."

Nelda: Want the doll over there.

Clinician: No, I need to hear "I want the doll over there."

Nelda: I want doll over there.

Clinician: No, that won't do it. Let's try again. Say, "I want the doll over there."

Nelda: (shuts down, begins to fidget)

Now . . . has Nelda been encouraged to verbalize? Was she rewarded when she talked instead of pointed? What has she learned from the above interaction? She has learned that using words is not enough—she has to say them perfectly. This is too difficult for her in the early stages of language therapy. I have learned this the hard way with CLD students: if we focus too much on discrete language components in early stages of intervention, especially if the students are in or just exiting the silent period, we do more harm than good. My goal is always to encourage these students to use words to communicate meaning even if their morphology and syntax are not perfect. In the beginning, this is good enough. The whole language concept of communicating meaning is relevant in these types of situations.

> In the sabotage technique, the clinician can disrupt the environment and routines within that environment.

Using Sabotage

An excellent article by Fey et al. (2003) states that clinicians need to manipulate the therapy context so that children can have the most possible opportunities to practice treatment targets. Fey and his colleagues say that there are different ways to do this, and that "in many, the clinician takes on the role of the saboteur, disrupting the physical environment and routines within the environment" (p. 8). For example, the clinician can withhold objects a child wants (till the child verbalizes that he wants it), misplace objects, use objects in unusual ways, and even sabotage familiar verbal routines. Fey et al. recommend that puppets or dolls can be used to get "mixed up" so the child has to correct them.

For example, if the SLP is working on the correct use of irregular plurals, the puppet can say, "Hey! Don't step on my foots!" The child then has to tell the puppet the right way to say that. When I work with children, I will often tell them that they are the "teacher" and they have to "catch" me. I let them take tokens (such as plastic happy faces) away from me when I make mistakes. So I might be playing with a child and say, "Here come some gooses! The gooses want food!" If the child "catches" my error, I say, "Oh—uh-oh. You have to take away one of my happy faces! (sob, sob) What *should* I have said?" The child gleefully says, "The *geese* want food."

There are other ways to sabotage the situation as recommended by Fey et al. (2003). I was asked to evaluate a monolingual English-speaking four-year-old who absolutely would not talk to me. So I said, "Hey diddle diddle, the dog in the fiddle, the fork jumped over the moon.

The little plate laughed to see such sport, and the spoon ran away with the cow." His lip quivered, and when he finally could not take any more of me butchering this nursery rhyme, he blurted out, "No! No! That's not it!" Giving him my most astounded innocent look, I expressed shock and then asked him to tell me how it should go. He did so, and rapport was established.

A former professor of mine used to discuss the "broken toy" technique. Children are always curious to know why something is broken and how it got that way. Puzzles with missing pieces are a variant of this. Towers of blocks can also work well. Once when I was really desperate to engage a recalcitrant preschool boy who clung voraciously to his mother, I built a very tall, tempting tower of blocks. It looked as though it would teeter over at any second. I looked at Tyrone and said, "Tyrone, there is no way in the world that you can knock this down. I know you can't do it." Now, the tower was about five feet away from Tyrone, meaning that he would have to leave his mother's side to get to it. I watched as the battle waged in his head, and finally he left mom, ran over, and gleefully kicked the tower down. Oh, the mess! Together we built another tower, and he was willing to engage with me for an extended time.

Sometimes it seems virtually impossible to engage a child's attention and to get her motivated. One "sabotage" technique I have used with virtually 100 percent success is the "play and ignore" technique. I get a very tempting, cool toy or activity the child wants. If she still will not engage with me, I ignore her and sit in a corner and play with the toy by myself. I will have a seemingly wonderful time without her. Without fail, she will eventually come around to see what she is missing. I have used this with great success in group therapy also. Once, I had a stickerboard that I just knew this group of fourth-grade boys would love. As I got ready to use it for my expressive language activity, one boy looked at me defiantly and said, "Dude, there's no way I'm doin' this." "No problem," I said calmly. "You can just sit there and watch the rest of us." After about two minutes of seeing the great time he was missing, the boy joined me and the three other students in the activity.

CONNECT & EXTEND

Specific and detailed instructions for increasing the grammatical skills of children with SLI are available in Fey, M.E., Long, S.H., & Finestack, L.H. (2003). Ten principles of grammar facilitation for children with specific language impairment. *American Journal of Speech-Language Pathology, 12,* 3–15.

Modifying Linguistic Input

The *way* that we as SLPs talk to our children in language intervention is as important as the specific treatment activities that we conduct. I remember starting as a twenty-three-year-old brand-new clinician in my first job. I worked in a low-income school district with many CLD students, and knew I was going to save the world. During therapy sessions, to provide "language stimulation," I would speak quickly, with few pauses, in long and complex sentences. For some strange reason, the children did not understand what I was saying. I'm not very proud of this, but I guess that in university, I somehow missed the fact that I needed to change the way I talked when I conducted therapy with LI children.

Those who work with LI children need to modify their linguistic input to facilitate comprehension. This is especially critical if these children are CLD.

The following suggestions are relevant for all those who interact with students with language disorders, especially CLD students with LI. (We will revisit some of these ideas in Chapter 12). Remember

POINTS TO PONDER You go to observe the fifth-grade class of a CLD student who has an LI and tells you that she does not understand what the teacher says. You see that the teacher speaks rapidly, says most things only once, and uses virtually no visuals. What can you do to help?

_____

_____

_____

that CLD students with LI are trying to master two linguistic codes with an underlying system that is inadequate for even one, and thus these suggestions can be utilized by SLPs, teachers, family members, and others who work with LI students from all backgrounds (Roseberry-McKibbin, 2001, 2008; Paul, 2001).

• *Slow down your rate of speech.* Pause frequently. Research shows that students with LI often learn more efficiently if they hear input that is slower than normal.

• *Repeat information many times.* My father, a minister, says that the average adult forgets 95 percent of what he hears within 72 hours of hearing it. If this is true for normally functioning adults, think of how often LI children need to hear information in order to retain it!

• *Rephrase and restate information.* For example, the SLP could say: "We will share, do a worksheet, and then play a game. So today, it's sharing, worksheet, and a game."

• *Use a multimodal approach to instruction.* When information is presented auditorily, accompany it with visuals such as pictures, maps, diagrams, writing on the board, gestures, and facial expressions. Many of my LI children learn best visually. Some are tactile learners. One Urdu-speaking boy with severe language problems learned best when I taught him signs to accompany new vocabulary words he was learning.

• *Use short sentences; reduce sentence length and complexity.* Ideally, the SLP should use sentences that are just slightly longer and more complex than the child is capable of producing.

• *Emphasize target words through increased volume and stress.* Research has shown that LI children will more easily learn words that are louder and somewhat exaggerated. CLD students especially benefit from this technique. For example, if the SLP is teaching the use of "the" to a student with telegraphic speech: You said you wanted **the** ball. **The** ball is over here. **The** ball is red. Look at **the** red ball!

• *Enunciate words clearly, especially for CLD students.* Some immigrant students, for example, don't know what "jeet" is, as in "Good morning—jeet breakfast?" Many of my older English Language Learners have told me that they are extremely confused by the way Americans coarticulate words. This is especially true if they have grown up in countries where British English is used. Thus, if you say "Izeebizee?" about a man who is busy, you may get a blank stare.

- *Make sure that listening conditions in the classroom are favorable.* Even TD CLD students may have extra difficulty if there is a poor signal-to-noise ratio and the teacher is speaking rapidly using decontextualized language. Processing information in a second language under less-than-ideal conditions is a risk factor for second language learners; it is even more of a risk factor for those who have LI (Nelson, Kohnert, Sabur, & Shaw, 2005; Windsor & Kohnert, 2004).

Table 6.2 is an example of a checklist that can be used by professionals—SLPs, teachers, and others—who work with CLD students to assess whether or not they are modifying their linguistic input.

TABLE 6.2 Working With Linguistically And Culturally Diverse Students: The Interventionist's Self-Evaluation Checklist

Do I	*Almost Always*	*Some-times*	*Very Rarely*	*Never*
1. Use a multimodal approach to teaching material?				
2. Review previous material?				
3. Make input comprehensible by slowing down, pausing, and speaking clearly?				
4. Rephrase and restate information?				
5. Check frequently for comprehension?		ʻ		
6. Focus on teaching meaning rather than focusing on teaching correct grammar?				
7. Avoid putting students on the spot by demanding that they talk immediately?				
8. Give extra time for processing information?				
9. Attempt to reduce students' anxieties and give them extra attention when possible?				
10. Encourage students' use and development of their primary language?				
11. Encourage students to interject their own cultural experiences and backgrounds into learning situations?				
12. Expose all my students to multicultural activities and materials on a regular basis?				
13. Include parents and community members from different cultural backgrounds in my teaching?				

Used with permission. From Roseberry-McKibbin, C. (2008) *Multicultural students with special language needs: Practical strategies for assessment and intervention* (3rd edition), Oceanside, CA: Academic Communication Associates, Inc.

SUMMARY

- The incidental teaching approach to treatment involves working language intervention into everyday situations.
- In the technique of focused stimulation the clinician repeatedly models a structure in hopes of encouraging the child to use that structure.
- A clinician can use self-talk and parallel talk to comment on her own and the child's actions in therapy.
- Expansions and extensions add information to the child's utterances.
- Recasting changes the child's utterance into a different form or voice.
- Clinicians may use joint routines and joint book reading to stimulate language production.
- Whole language encourages holistic communication of meaning; component parts of language are not specifically addressed.
- Clinicians can sabotage treatment in a number of creative ways to encourage children to use language.
- SLPs and others who work with LI students must modify their linguistic input to increase LI children's comprehension of what they hear.

Add your own summary points here:

_____

_____

_____

FACILITATING GENERALIZATION OF TREATMENT TARGETS TO OTHER SETTINGS

Introduction

Most SLPs believe that one of the greatest challenges in conducting successful intervention is to get children to use intervention targets outside the therapy room. Many clinicians have had children perform very accurately in the clinic setting, only to have these children walk out the door and lapse back into their old ways. In order to help children **generalize** or habituate their treatment targets to settings outside the clinic, SLPs need to consider varying **stimuli**, **settings**, and **interlocutors**.

Varying the stimuli involves using different materials to achieve the same treatment goal. For example, with Anita whom we discussed earlier, the clinician used picture cards, Candy Land, and a dollhouse. Many beginning clinicians make the mistake of using just a certain set of cards, or a certain game, to teach language targets. The trouble with this is that the child associates the treatment target with just that one activity or item. When it comes to using different materials, the more variety the better: children will generalize

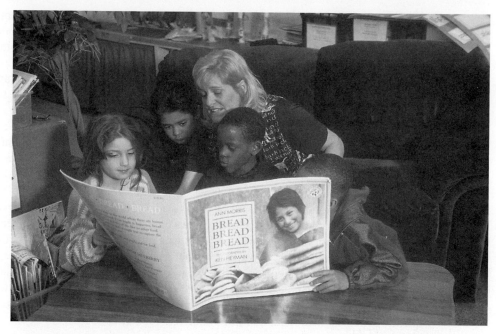

Speech language pathologists can go into regular education classrooms and demonstrate language stimulation techniques that are beneficial to all children.

> Children will generalize treatment targets better if the clinician varies stimuli, settings, and interlocutors.

more successfully if they are exposed to a variety of materials and activities that work toward achieving the same goal.

Students also profit from using treatment targets in different **settings**. With Anita in the case described above, the SLP could take her outside the therapy room to use her possessive -*s* on the playground, in the school cafeteria, at the bus stop after school, and with the school secretary at the front desk. I try to do this type of thing in my public school job when possible; students generalize treatment targets much more quickly when I vary the settings in which the targets are produced. It is also important to have different interlocutors or conversational partners for the student to interact with. Anita used her possessive -*s* just with the clinician. But she will generalize more quickly if she uses it with other children, her teacher, and family members.

Connecting with Significant Others in the Child's Environment: General Principles

I once attended a workshop where the speaker showed us a simple visual that reinforced this fact: a child has 100 waking hours a week. If she spends two hours in therapy with an SLP, that is only 2 percent of her week. Ninety-eight percent of her week is spent in settings outside the clinic. If we do not enlist the assistance of those in her environment to enhance her language skills, very little progress will occur! In Chapters 7 through 13, we will discuss in more detail how SLPs can and should interact with significant others in the environment of a child who is receiving language intervention. In this brief introduction, we will look at the importance of connecting and working with these significant others in various settings outside the therapy room.

First and most obviously, it is crucial to work closely with a child's caregivers to train them how to facilitate language at home. We often assume that we will be working with a child's mother; however, in some cultures, we might be interacting with a variety of other family members (Roseberry-McKibbin, 2008; van Kleeck, 1994). For example, in Samoan culture, caretaking of children rotates between relatives; at any one time, a different relative might be currently "in charge" of a child. This could be the mother, an aunt, a grandparent, or even an older sibling. Thus, we must never assume that our work with families is primarily restricted to work with the child's mother.

As I have worked in the field of speech-language pathology over the years, I have witnessed more and more children being raised by their grandparents. This phenomenon is occurring for a variety of reasons, and SLPs nationwide are finding that more often than not, it is a grandparent with whom they are connecting, not a father or mother. I have profound respect for grandparents who make many sacrifices to take on "second families"; no relaxing at the fishing hole with the RV for them. Children may also be in a foster situation; some on my caseload are. This presents unique challenges as foster parents are frequently extremely busy, with multiple children to look after.

CASES TO CONSIDER

I worked with Cody S., a Hispanic kindergartener whose dominant language was English. He was being raised by his grandma, Dolores. Cody was born to Dolores' sixteen-year-old daughter who was in jail for drug use when we met. Cody had multiple needs: he was severely unintelligible, delayed in language skills, and had gross and fine-motor difficulties. In addition, he was quite overweight. I'll never forget the meeting the school personnel had with Dolores. This tiny fifty-six-year-old woman was surrounded by me, the resource specialist, principal, nurse, psychologist, and several other school personnel. We shared our assessment findings with Dolores and tried to give her constructive suggestions to help Cody in the home. Dolores broke down crying. She said she worked the night shift at a factory so she could be available for Cody in the daytime. She had no time for him, and even less money. She was a widow, barely able to feed herself and Cody, much less follow through on suggestions at home. Assuming you were the SLP, what suggestions might you have given Dolores for enhancing Cody's language skills that she could actually use given her circumstances? List and briefly describe.

_____

_____

_____

Suggestions for Working with Caregivers

We have talked in this book about working with caregivers, and basic principles are introduced here as applied to a wide variety of children with LI (Hegde, 2001a):

- Evaluate the caregivers' educational level, motivation, and availability of time to follow through with your instructions for language stimulation
- Design a language instruction program for the child
- Test your program yourself in the clinical setting to make sure it works
- Have the caregivers observe you doing the activities
- Train the caregivers to use the techniques appropriately
- Have the caregivers carry out the techniques while you observe
- Give feedback to help the caregivers refine their skills
- Train the caregivers to keep records so you can evaluate progress
- Give caregivers clear, simple instructions as well as videotaped samples of effective treatment techniques
- Periodically assess the caregivers and children's interactions in the home
- Suggest modifications and move to a higher level of training as appropriate

In my career, I have worked with children of every background, from those living with millionaire parents to those living in their cars. I have found that not all caregivers are able to work with me at the level suggested above. Sometimes, I have merely given a caregiver one simple suggestion that I know he is able to act on within the circumstances of his life.

> Clinicians may work with caregivers who include grandparents, foster parents, and day-care workers as well as biological parents.

A former student of mine was meeting with a migrant Hispanic family to share suggestions that they could implement with their LI child at home. She and the rest of the team felt very pleased with themselves as they shared detailed, specific, successful academic and language strategies with the family. The family was given pages of information and suggestions. The family nodded politely for an hour. At the end of the hour, the father said, "We live in our car. Can you help us understand how to implement your suggestions under these conditions?" This illustrates the point that before we make recommendations, we must know the circumstances and life situations of our children's caregivers. We must tailor our recommendations to their ability to carry out these recommendations.

CONNECT & EXTEND

An example of a model that was used successfully to train child-care providers to improve children's language can be found in Girolametto, L., Weitzman, E., & Greenberg, J. (2003). Training day care staff to facilitate children's language. *American Journal of Speech-Language Pathology, 12,* 299–311.

In this day and age, children's caregivers increasingly include day-care providers. Many children in the United States spend eight or more hours a day with day-care providers—it is not uncommon for children to be in day care forty to fifty hours a week or more. Some SLPs do not have access to the day-care providers of the LI children they serve. However, other SLPs do have this access. Research suggests that day-care providers can be trained to effectively facilitate language development in children; SLPs can consider this option as they attempt to involve key people in LI children's environments (Girolametto, Weitzman, & Greenberg, 2003). We will discuss this more in Chapter 7.

Suggestions for Working with Classroom Teachers

SLPs also need to work with classroom teachers; this is described in detail in Chapter 12. For purposes of introduction in this chapter, basic principles are described as a foundation for further, more detailed information.

Students with LI spend 30 hours or more a week in classroom settings. If they do not have opportunities to practice appropriate language and receive language stimulation in the classroom, valuable time is wasted. SLPs must work with teachers to ensure that classroom time is maximized. The following suggestions are made for collaboration between classroom teachers and SLPs to help LI students become more successful in both social and academic language skills (Merritt & Culatta, 1998; Kuder, 2003):

1. *Help teachers be conscious of calling upon students who don't regularly volunteer.* Many CLD students especially are quiet in class and do not volunteer. Teachers need to attempt to draw these students out by calling on them and encouraging them to interact.

2. *Help teachers learn to respond in ways that promote continued talk.* For example:

Hiroki: My mommy and daddy and I went to Chicago.

Kindergarten teacher: Wow! That sounds like fun. Tell us about some of the places you visited.

An example of a way to discourage continued talk would be:

Hiroki: My mommy and daddy and I went to Chicago.

Teacher: That's nice. Welcome back. Tricia, please go sharpen your pencil.

3. *Help teachers learn to arrange the physical setting of the classroom so that it promotes talking and interaction.* Individual desks and carrels do help students focus for certain tasks, but they discourage interaction. For purposes of enhancing students' interaction with one another, teachers can provide learning centers, interactive classroom displays, and large tables for group work.

> Teachers can be taught simple, effective techniques for stimulating children's language development in the classroom setting.

4. *Help teachers learn to provide opportunities for children to use language and interact during the learning process.* For example, if the class is learning about the ocean, children who have been to the ocean can be encouraged to share these experiences with the class. When children are learning new concepts in a subject like math, they can be encouraged to rehearse their strategies out loud. My son's kindergarten teacher always asked for volunteers to come and read sentences on the whiteboard; these sentences were related to the theme for the month (e.g., the ocean or the solar system).

5. *Help teachers understand the importance of giving all students opportunities to practice various forms of language.* For example, students need to gain facility with making requests, negotiating, problem solving, explaining concepts to others, and so forth. Students need many opportunities to practice these kinds of language acts in the classroom setting (Brice & Montgomery, 1996).

When I give workshops and discuss the importance of working in collaboration with classroom teachers, my audience members almost always ask me *how* to do this. Teachers are busy; they frequently feel overwhelmed. Most teachers I work with in my job in the public schools are stretched to the maximum; I don't dare ask them to do one more thing. Yet I know that if a child's language goals are not reinforced in the classroom, his chances of progressing are extremely minimal. Here, I offer some practical suggestions that have helped me enlist the aid of busy, overworked classroom teachers to help LI children in the classroom:

1. *Ask them to do things that seem easy to do.* In Chapter 5, I talked about Jasmine, who was found to be deaf in her left ear. I asked her second-grade teacher to please seat Jasmine front and center. The teacher was receptive and grateful for the idea; Jasmine now sits front and center and is doing much better in class.

2. *Explain why you are asking what you are asking.* Strange as this sounds, SLPs and other busy special-education personnel often do not explain to teachers *why* they want something done for a particular child. Psychology would suggest that people are much more likely to comply with a request when they know *why* you want something.

3. *Show the teacher how implementing your suggestions can help a child's standardized achievement test scores become higher.* In the United States, today, public school personnel such as teachers and administrators face intense pressure to have children produce high achievement-test scores. Principals in my area can lose their jobs if their schools do not achieve certain standards. At one point, in my district, the administration was thinking of offering bonuses to teachers whose classes achieved certain test scores. I deplore this, but it is reality. If you are asking a teacher to help a student achieve language intervention goals in the classroom, point out how these extra efforts can raise the child's achievement test scores.

4. *If it is relevant, help the teacher understand how implementing your suggestions can help other students in the class, not just this particular student.* For example, we talked in Chapter 1 about how students with LI often have difficulty remembering what they hear. Let's say you are recommending that the teacher slow down her instructions, use more visuals, and repeat instructions two or three times. That's a lot to ask of a teacher. But if you can point out that this will benefit many other children in the classroom and help them be more successful, the teacher is more likely to cooperate with you.

> In order to enlist the support of classroom teachers to implement helpful techniques for LI students, demonstrate the techniques and explain why you are recommending them.

5. *Come into the classroom and demonstrate recommended techniques for the teacher.* We described ways to modify linguistic input; the SLP can go into a classroom and teach a lesson using these techniques so the teacher can see how to use them.

6. *Invite the teacher to observe you working in therapy with the child.* Sometimes teachers can create ten- to fifteen-minute breaks in their classroom schedules to come and observe you (during recess, for example). They appreciate being able to observe, and they learn much more by watching you than by just being handed a list of suggestions.

 SUMMARY

- Language intervention in a vacuum is almost never successful. SLPs must involve other adults in the child's life to promote generalization of treatment targets.
- When working with children's caregivers, SLPs need to assess caregivers' ability to carry out tasks and allow caregivers to observe therapy. SLPs should watch caregivers use the suggested techniques and give them appropriate feedback.
- When working with classroom teachers, remember to make suggestions easy to implement. Allow teachers to watch you implement the suggestions you are making.
- Always provide teachers with a rationale for why you are asking them to implement your suggestions in the classroom setting.

Add your own summary points here:

_____

_____

_____

SPECIAL CONSIDERATIONS FOR CLD CHILDREN WITH LANGUAGE IMPAIRMENTS

Introduction

When a CLD student is diagnosed with a language problem such as an LI, she must receive intervention. Many questions come to mind. What type of program does she need? What will be the language of therapy? How can the SLP tailor intervention especially to her? What about working with her family? The first decision to be made when a CLD student is diagnosed with an LI is the language in which intervention will take place.

Language of Intervention

When a CLD student is placed into special education and receives speech-language therapy, a major consideration is the extent to which the student's first language (L1) and English will be used in therapy. Several factors should be considered in making this decision (Brice & Roseberry-McKibbin, 2001; Genesee et al., 2004; Roseberry-McKibbin, 2008).

CONNECT & EXTEND

A persuasive case for using a child's first language in intervention is made by Gutierrez-Clellen, V.F. (1999). Language choice in intervention with bilingual children. *American Journal of Speech-Language Pathology, 8* (4), 291–302.

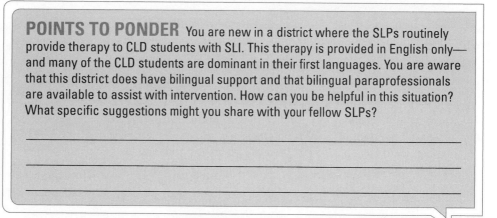

POINTS TO PONDER You are new in a district where the SLPs routinely provide therapy to CLD students with SLI. This therapy is provided in English only—and many of the CLD students are dominant in their first languages. You are aware that this district does have bilingual support and that bilingual paraprofessionals are available to assist with intervention. How can you be helpful in this situation? What specific suggestions might you share with your fellow SLPs?

_____

_____

_____

- *What is the student's proficiency level in the L1 and in English?* These skills can be ascertained by observing the student's language usage in functional speaking contexts and by testing language proficiency. Researchers recommend that if the student is dominant or more proficient in L1 (language 1, or the language first learned by the child), intervention conducted in L1 will usually be most effective (Goldstein, 2000; Gutierrez-Clellen, 1999; Kayser, 2002; Kiernan & Swisher, 1990; Perozzi & Sanchez, 1992). It is especially beneficial to introduce new concepts in L1 first and reinforce them in English. When a concept has been acquired in the primary language first, it will be easier to learn in English.

- *What language is used in the home?* If the student's L1 is not developed or reinforced in the school setting, the student may lose the ability to effectively communicate in the home with family members.

> If a CLD student is dominant in her first language, it is most advantageous to conduct intervention in that language.

- *What resources are available for conducting intervention in the primary language?* It is ideal if an SLP who speaks the student's L1 fluently is available to conduct therapy. However, often the SLP is a monolingual speaker of English. In these cases, it is ideal if the SLP can work collaboratively with personnel such as interpreters or bilingual paraprofessionals who speak the child's L1 fluently (Kohnert, Yim, Nett, Kan, & Duran, 2005). If these personnel are not available, therapy must be conducted in English. This is not the ideal, but often it is the reality.

Program Placement Alternatives

Probably the most key variable dictating program placement for a CLD student with an LI is the availability of services at that student's school. Some families may have money to seek additional resources; however, most families do not have money for additional resources, and so the student with LI receives intervention through his public school district. In Chapter 12, we will explore school-based intervention options in more detail. For the time being, we will briefly examine a few general suggestions.

CASES TO CONSIDER

Nga N. was a Vietnamese teenager in the Newcomers' Sheltered English classroom in one of our local high schools. This classroom provided academic instruction for a variety of CLD high school–age students who had just arrived in the United States within the last six to twelve months. Nga's aunt reported that Nga had been diagnosed in Vietnam as "mentally retarded." With the help of the Vietnamese interpreter, I assessed Nga's skills in both English and Vietnamese, and she qualified for speech-language services. The SLP on the high school campus did not speak any Vietnamese; Nga spoke no English. The interpreter, Mr. Ly, was willing and able to come to the high school several days a week to work with Nga in Vietnamese. What type of service delivery model would you suggest in this situation? What would work best to help Nga be an effective communicator?

_____

_____

_____

For CLD students who are dominant in L1, it is ideal if they can be in a bilingual regular or special education classroom that supports both English (their L2, or second language) and L1 development (Brice & Roseberry-McKibbin, 2001). In this situation, speech-language therapy ideally is provided by an SLP who speaks the child's L1 fluently. This is rarely the case. There are many other options along a continuum of services, but in general, CLD students are in English-speaking regular or special education classes; there may be support from an SLP who usually speaks only English. In my district we have worked collaboratively with an L1 interpreter who helps us attain intervention goals in the primary language. We are fortunate indeed to obtain the services of such personnel, but it is rare that this happens. When it does, the student benefits greatly as illustrated in the case of Nga N above.

Incorporating Principles of Multiculturalism into Treatment Activities

Whether an SLP is bilingual or monolingual English-speaking, she can incorporate activities and materials into therapy to help CLD students feel accepted and supported. I speak primarily English and a smattering of four other languages (*smattering* being the operative word here). Thus, when I work with my CLD students, I am not able to work with them in their primary languages; however, there are activities and materials I can use to help these students feel supported and accepted.

• *Show interest in the student's home country, language, and culture.* Many of my students travel back and forth from Mexico. I like to ask them to share stories of their travels. I also have a globe in my room. I can help students see where they and/or their families have come from originally. I was once working with three students; I asked them to tell me about their ancestors. Gabriel shared that her ancestors were from China, Korea, and Africa. Dominique proudly announced that his ancestors were from Africa. Little blonde, blue-eyed Ricky thought hard for a minute, and then proclaimed, "And I'm from Sacramento!"

> Clinicians can support CLD students by incorporating multicultural activities and materials into therapy sessions.

- *Learn a few words in the student's first language*; you'd be surprised how hard this can be. I once tried to take a course in Mandarin. I lasted about half an hour. It is humbling and eye opening to have students teach you how to accurately pronounce words in their languages, especially languages like Mandarin and Russian. But students love to share, and they love being the "teacher." Tell them that you think it's cool to speak another language. Make bilingualism feel (to students) as special as it is.

- *Display objects and pictures depicting various cultural groups*. Make sure the materials you use in therapy represent a variety of people, not just blue-eyed blondes. Make sure multicultural materials are used regularly in your therapy all year long.

- *Use thematic units that incorporate information about various cultural groups*. For example, during Black History Month, you can build therapy activities around this theme.

- *Read stories about leaders and role models from various cultural backgrounds*. In California, a Mexican leader named César Chávez is highly respected for his advocacy for migrant farmworkers. Find leaders and role models relevant to your students and read stories about them.

- *Avoid stereotyping*. For example, showing pictures of Native Americans only in wigwams with long feather headdresses is stereotyping. It is also stereotyping to show only pictures of non-Anglos who live in poverty. Sometimes I download pictures from the Internet to use in therapy. It is surprising to see that even some of these pictures are very stereotyped in their depiction of adults and children from CLD backgrounds.

POINTS TO PONDER You are a monolingual English-speaking clinician who serves students from a variety of CLD backgrounds. What are three ways you could incorporate multicultural activities and materials into your therapy sessions?

_____

_____

_____

Suggestions for Therapy with CLD Students with LI

Many of the therapy ideas that are relevant for use with monolingual English-speaking students are relevant for CLD students. However, there are a few extra considerations when working with CLD students with LI:

- *As previously stated, try to arrange for intervention to occur in L1 for those students who are dominant in L1* (Genesee et al., 2004; Kohnert et al., 2005; Restrepo & Gutierrez-Clellen, 2004).

- *If you conduct therapy in English, make sure that you match treatment activities and goals to the student's stage of English acquisition.* Table 6.3 shows specific ways to match intervention to second-language acquisition stages. Notice that CLD students who are acquiring English take some time to be ready for more sophisticated or advanced activities in English. I have found it valuable to share this table with classroom teachers, who often expect more of CLD students than they are ready to produce.

- *Frequently check to make sure that students are understanding you.* CLD students with LI may have some difficulty comprehending what you are saying. Be sure that students are "with you." One good way to do this, besides asking questions, is to ask them to summarize what you just said.

- *Make vocabulary acquisition a treatment priority.* As a part-time public school clinician in a district where more than 80 languages are represented, I provide services for many CLD students with LI. I do not have access to support personnel who speak all these students' languages. Thus, I and my colleagues provide therapy all in English. While far from ideal, this is the reality, and I have found that helping these students learn English vocabulary is a very high priority. My colleagues and I focus especially on 1) vocabulary of the classroom and 2) social vocabulary. When teaching vocabulary to CLD students with LI, it's important to remember that they need much repetition to learn the words. Gray (2003) states that some children with LI may require twice the practice opportunities and exposures to learn new words in comparison to typically developing peers, and her study examined the language skills of monolingual children. If monolingual LI children required this much exposure and repetition to learn new vocabulary words, CLD LI children surely would require even more exposure and repetition in order to acquire new vocabulary words.

- *When working with CLD students who are in the early stages of learning English, present receptive vocabulary activities first.* Research in second language acquisition shows that students often learn vocabulary words more readily when these words are presented receptively first and then followed up with expressive activities.

- *Help students learn to use visualization to remember what they hear.* I have found that many of my CLD students with LI who have auditory memory problems perform much better when they are taught to visualize what they are hearing. I tell them to think of their minds as TV screens and actively make pictures as people are talking. There are formal programs that

TABLE 6.3   Matching Intervention to Second-Language (L2) Acquisition Stages

Stage I Preproduction (First 3 months of L2 exposure)	Stage II Early Production (3–6 months)	Stage III Speech Emergence (6 months–2 years)	Stage IV Intermediate Fluency (2–3 years)
Student Characteristics			
• Silent period • Focusing on comprehension	• Focusing on comprehension • Using 1–3-word phrases • May be using routines/formulas (e.g., "gimme five")	• Increased comprehension • Using simple sentences • Expanding vocabulary • Continued grammatical errors	• Improved comprehension • Adequate face-to-face conversational proficiency • More extensive vocabulary • Few grammatical errors
Goals: *Oral Responses*			
• *Yes-no* responses in English • One-word answers	• 1–3-word responses • Naming/labeling items • Choral responses • Answering questios: *either/or, who/what/where, sentence completion*	• Recalling • Telling/retelling • Describing/explaining • Comparing • Sequencing • Carrying on dialogues	• Predicting • Narrating • Describing/explaining • Summarizing • Giving opinions • Debating/defending
Goals: *Visual/Written Responses*			
• Drawing/painting • Graphic designs • Copying	• Drawing/painting, graphic designs • Copying • Grouping and labeling • Simple Rebus responses	• Written responses • Drawing, painting, graphics	• Creative writing (e.g., stories) • Essays, summaries • Drawing, painting, graphics • Comprehensible written tests
Goals: *Physical Responses*			
• Pointing • Circling, underlining • Choosing among items • Matching objects/pictures	• Pointing • Selecting • Matching • Constructing • Mime/acting out responses	• Demonstrating • Creating/constructing • Role playing/acting • Cooperative group tasks	• Demonstrating • Creating/constructing • Role playing • Cooperative group work • Videotaped presentations

Used with permission. From Hearne, J.D. (2000). *Teaching second language learners with learning disabilities.* Oceanside, CA: Academic Communication Associates, Inc.

In intervention with CLD children with LI, targeting vocabulary is a very high priority. Receptive vocabulary should be targeted first, followed by expressive vocabulary.

CONNECT & EXTEND

A sequenced, detailed program for helping students learn to visualize is provided in Bell, N. (1991). *Visualizing and verbalizing for language comprehension and thinking.* Paso Robles, CA: Academy of Reading Publications.

In intervention with CLD students, help them learn vocabulary, pragmatics, and literacy skills.

can be used to help students learn to actively visualize as an adjunct to listening (e.g., Bell, 1991).

• *Help students, especially those new to the American public school system, to become familiar with American public school routines and expectations.* A friend of mine used to work with newly immigrated junior high students. They would ask to go to the bathroom, and Margaret would give them passes. Half an hour would go by, and the students would not be back to class. Margaret would find them on the playground, not knowing that they were expected to come back to class immediately. Clinicians need to help these kinds of students learn routines and expectations of US schools.

• *Help students learn pragmatics skills that will assist them in succeeding in US schools and society.* My goal for my CLD students with LI is to help them become bicultural in their pragmatics skills: able to fluidly and successfully fit in pragmatically with both their communities and US mainstream society. We want students to continue to integrate successfully in their own communities; yet we do these students a great disservice if we do not help them fit into mainstream US society. I so clearly remember coming to live in the United States permanently with my family when I was seventeen years old. When people had birthdays, I'd congratulate them and ask them how old they were. If they proudly showed me some new item they'd purchased, I asked them how much it had cost. Oh, the shocked looks and rejection I experienced for these faux pas! Yet in the Philippines, these kinds of "personal" questions are both routine and expected. Again, we want to help students be successfully bicultural in their pragmatics skills.

• *Support students in acquiring basic literacy skills.* This topic is addressed in other chapters in greater depth. For now, we will note that some CLD students come from homes where parents are nonliterate in L1 and English. I have worked with many of these students, who come to kindergarten not even knowing how to turn the pages of a book. We can incorporate many literacy activities into therapy to support these students.

• *Help students with academic English and curriculum materials so that they will succeed in school.* More will be said about this in subsequent chapters. However, I introduce it here because many CLD students with LI have substantial difficulty with school curriculum requirements. I try to use classroom materials in therapy. For example, if Mario's class is learning about the solar system, I use stickerboards and games about the solar system for my therapy activities. If Trang's class is reading about dinosaurs, I read about dinosaurs in language therapy.

• *Take an active role in helping facilitate extra, non–special education support for CLD students.* For instance, the elementary school where I work has a very active after-school Homework Club. Because our school of 1,200 children has such a high proportion of low-income students, we also receive extra state and federal funds for programs that provide even more support for students who are struggling academically but do not qualify for special education. Sometimes it's so easy for a school-based SLP to have the attitude—even subconsciously—that if a child does not qualify for speech-language services, "He's not my problem." But I have found that with a little extra effort, I can help teachers and parents think creatively about non–special education support services that will provide extra support that many CLD students greatly need.

For example, earlier today a kindergarten teacher asked me to screen the language skills of Reontay N., a cute CLD five-year-old who is academically not keeping up with his peers. Both Reontay's parents were killed in a car accident when he was four years old; he currently lives with an aunt and uncle. It was decided that Reontay's language skills are commensurate with his chronological age; however, grief counseling will be implemented to support Reontay as he deals with difficult life circumstances.

Involving the Families of CLD Students with LI

One unfortunate phenomenon I have encountered is that many parents of CLD students believe that school personnel will scold them for speaking a language other than English in the home. I have had parents actually lie to me, saying they speak only English at home, because they are afraid I will be upset if I hear that they are speaking their primary language with their children. As we have emphasized before, is critical for SLPs and other personnel who work with parents of CLD students with LI to emphasize that being bilingual is a great asset in our society. We need to stress to parents that fluent bilingualism is highly desirable.

> Parents of CLD students need to speak with their children in the language in which they are most fluent. Professionals should never tell these parents to speak only English with their children.

Unfortunately, many educators will tell parents to speak only English at home. It is very hard for me to remain calm about this advice. In Chapter 3, we discussed the advantages of fluent bilingualism. Parents need to speak to their children in the language in which they (the parents) are most fluent. Parents need to provide rich linguistic models for their children.

I will never forget Jessie M., a third-grader with an LI. His parents were from Mexico. Mom's English was quite fluent; Dad's was rudimentary and showed many patterns of grammatical transfer from Spanish. Somewhere along the line, Dad had been told to speak only English to Jessie. He obediently did this, and Jessie told me, "My mom speaks English one way, my dad speaks it another way, and my teacher speaks it even a different way" (the classroom teacher was Dutch). Jessie's father was providing him with a nonstandard English model that was doing far more harm than good. It is *always* best for children to hear grammatically sound, semantically rich language models instead of models that have many errors and are quite basic.

In a related vein, often educators and other professionals will counsel parents of CLD children with SLI to use only one language with the child. The rationale behind this recommendation is that because the child has an LI, she will be confused by a dual language environment. However, research has shown that this is not the case; children with LI can and do learn two languages effectively, and being bilingual is not a disadvantage (Genesee et al., 2004; Gutierrez-Clellen, 1999; Paradis, Crago, Genesee, & Rice,

2003). "Cutting off" a child from one of her languages can have a negative impact in many areas. It can decrease her ability to communicate with family members, alter her ethnic identity, and limit her educational and career opportunities. Thus, SLPs should not recommend that bilingual parents of LI children speak to these children in only one language. Again, research has shown that LI children can and do learn two languages despite their LI status.

It is crucial to encourage families to work with the SLP and other special-education team members in a collaborative manner. However, some CLD families may not want to do this because they feel that the child's education is the school's responsibility. We have said that in many countries, the teacher is the authority figure, and parents respect this boundary. They would consider it rude and out of line to make suggestions or have input into their child's education. SLPs who work with these kinds of families need to sensitively share that in the United States, parents are expected to be part of the team, and their input is welcome. How can SLPs help parents be more involved in their children's education—both regular and special education? Here are some suggestions:

- *When meeting with parents at the school site or conducting home visits, bring samples of the student's work to show.*

- *Help parents understand the academic/curricular expectations of US schools.* Parents who have not been educated in the United States (like me) may have very little idea

> Help parents of CLD students understand what US schools expect of them and their children.

of what actually goes on in their children's classrooms. Because I was raised in the Philippines, I have had a steep learning curve in terms of finding out what is expected of my son in US schools. I have been very fortunate to volunteer in his classroom on a regular basis. If a parent has time to do this, it can be revealing, helpful, and very rewarding and can help parents understand what is expected of their children in US classrooms.

- *Help parents understand common US school routines such as waiting in line, volunteering to speak in class, and eating lunch in a cafeteria.* In an example that is probably stretching this point, I was surprised to find that at Mark's school, we are not allowed to walk on the grass. Being raised in an island country (where I rarely wore shoes), I never would have thought of something like this.

- *Relatedly, help parents understand their role in helping their children with homework.* I have been so shocked to find that in kindergarten, my son has a half-hour to an hour of homework a night—and I am expected to help him with all of it. Not that I mind, but when my family and I lived in the Philippines, my sisters and I did not have homework (at least on the islands my family and I lived on during those years). We worked very hard in school, but our schoolwork was the teacher's responsibility, not the parents'. Parents accustomed to this situation need to become oriented to US school expectations of their role in actively helping children with homework.

- If parents are nonliterate, encourage them to engage in literacy-related activities such as (H. Kayser, personal communication, 7/7/04; Roseberry-McKibbin, 2008):

CASES TO CONSIDER

I recently met with the mother of Jacky C., a very bright and active first-grader from a Cantonese-speaking home. He was referred for a language screening. Results of the screening revealed that Jacky's language learning ability was within normal limits. He definitely did not have an LI; however, because of his status as an English Language Learner, he was somewhat academically behind his classmates. I met with his mother Bao, an immigrant from Hong Kong, who cried for the better part of an hour as I handed her tissue after tissue. She said that her husband was not supportive at home and that he let Jacky stay up till all hours watching TV. She had a full-time job outside the home and was exhausted when she got home at the end of a long day. Her English, she said, was not even good enough to help Jacky with his homework at the first-grade level. She said that she felt so much despair, she did not know where to turn. What advice and support would you give her? What recommendations might you make to help Jacky enhance his academic performance?

_____

_____

_____

- look at wordless books with their children and discuss the stories
- take children to the local library to look at and check out books[*]
- find quality, inexpensive books at such places as the library, flea markets, and garage sales (these things are virtually nonexistent in many developing countries)
- come to literacy events at the school, such as book fairs
- avail themselves of local adult English classes
- provide writing tools (e.g., pencils, crayons, markers) and paper for children to play with

It is privilege to work with the families of CLD students. I have often found that the parents of these students have made great sacrifices to create better lives for their children than they themselves had. As we said in Chapter 3, many parents are struggling to provide their children with the basics of life, such as food, shelter, and clothing. They work in low-paying jobs and work two jobs (per parent) to support their families. I have come to have profound respect for these families, the challenges they face, and their desire to help their children succeed in a new country.

---

[*]The local library where I live is small, but they have a number of special programs. One is called Reading with Delilah. Delilah is a trained dog, and the child reads to Delilah along with an adult facilitator. My own son just loves this. Many libraries have special programs and services such as this that are free. You can share these options with parents, who do not have to be literate themselves in order to avail their children of these programs.

SUMMARY

- If a student is dominant or more proficient in L1, intervention conducted in L1 will usually be most effective. It is especially beneficial to introduce new concepts in L1 first and reinforce them in English. When a concept has been acquired in the primary language first, it will be easier to learn in English.
- Clinicians can incorporate multicultural materials into therapy sessions. They can show interest in CLD students' languages and cultures.
- In therapy with CLD students with LI, learning vocabulary is a high priority.
- Clinicians can involve the families of CLD students in therapy and also help these families learn routines and expectations of US schools.

Add your own summary points here:

_____

_____

_____

CHAPTER HIGHLIGHTS

- The overall purpose of language intervention is to help LI children express and comprehend language as normally as possible in academic and social situations.
- The developmental or normative approach to language intervention involves basing intervention targets on language developmental norms. In the functional approach, the SLP teaches LI children specific skills that they need or will need in their environments.
- In therapy sessions, SLPs can use drill, drill play, or play to teach language targets.
- Most SLPs use positive reinforcers to increase the occurrence of correct language targets during therapy sessions. These may be primary or secondary reinforcers used on a continuous or variable-ratio reinforcement schedule.
- Many specific therapy techniques can be used with LI children. These include incidental teaching, focused stimulation, self-talk, parallel talk, expansions, extensions, mand-model, recasts, joint routines, joint book reading, whole language, and sabotage techniques.
- SLPs and others who work with LI children need to modify their linguistic input so that the children understand what they hear. Among the number of ways to do this, are slowing down the rate of speech and repeating information several times.
- A major goal of intervention is to help LI children generalize treatment targets outside the therapy room. To do this, clinicians can use a variety of stimuli, settings, and interlocutors.
- It is crucial for SLPs to connect with LI children's caregivers and teachers and encourage them to use language stimulation techniques in the home and classroom settings.

- For the CLD student with LI who is dominant in his first language, it is ideal to conduct therapy in that language.
- Clinicians can incorporate multicultural materials and activities into therapy. Clinicians can also prioritize teaching vocabulary—both social and academic—to CLD students with LI.
- It is important to help CLD students with LI and their families to understand common routines and expectations in US schools.
- Parents should be encouraged to communicate with their children in whatever language they are most fluent in. It is critical for them to provide good language models for their children.

Add your own chapter highlights here:

_____

_____

_____

_____

STUDY AND REVIEW QUESTIONS

ESSAY

1. Describe two basic approaches to language intervention. For what populations of children would each approach be appropriate? Why?

2. Describe three language treatment techniques that you could use with a child who was reluctant to talk.

3. Why is it important to work with caregivers and teachers? Describe some ideas for enlisting their support in helping generalize children's language treatment targets into outside environments.

4. Discuss the role of reinforcement in language intervention. What are the two primary types of reinforcement? Discuss reinforcement schedules and when you might use each type.

5. Discuss considerations in providing intervention for CLD students with LI. How can we incorporate multicultural materials into treatment activities? How can we involve these students' families?

FILL-IN-THE-BLANK

6. Primary positive reinforcers are vulnerable to the _____ effect, which occurs when the child gets full and stops working for the reinforcers.

7. In the approach of _____ talk, the clinician describes the child's activities and comments on what the child is doing.

8. In the treatment technique of _____, the clinician elicits a response from the child (e.g., "Joey, say, "I have a red marker."")

9. When teaching vocabulary to CLD students with LI, it is best to start with _____ activities.

10. If a clinician reinforced a child once after every four responses, this would be a _____ ratio schedule of reinforcement.

MULTIPLE CHOICE

11. A child says, "doggy brown!" and the clinician says, "Yes, that is a brown doggy with a red collar on." The clinician has just use the technique of

   a. Expansion
   b. Extension
   c. Incidental teaching
   d. Mand-model
   e. Recast

12. A clinician is working with a child to learn the names of classroom items. In the therapy session, she sits with him and says, "Okay—every time you see a new card, I want you to tell me what it is. What's this? (answer) Good. What's this? (answer) Nice job. What's this? She uses nothing but a stack of picture cards. This could be called

   a. Incidental teaching
   b. Joint routines
   c. Drill
   d. Drill play
   e. Play

13. You are working with a child adopted from an Eastern European orphanage. He has undergone a great deal of trauma in his past, and his American adoptive parents want him to have therapy focusing on language stimulation. The boy is very quiet and does not like to verbalize. He does love computers, so you use a reinforcement program where the computer shows him each time he has answered a question accurately. The computer also creates a chart so he can see his progress. For reinforcement, you are using

   a. Token reinforcers
   b. Primary reinforcers
   c. Social reinforcers
   d. Conditioned generalized reinforcers
   e. Informative feedback

14. Which one of these is NOT a way that we might recommend for modifying linguistic input to enhance the comprehension of LI students?

   a. Use sentences with reduced length and complexity
   b. Enunciate words clearly

    c. Use pauses

    d. Say every word in a very slow, exaggerated manner

    e. Rephrase and restate information

15. A child says, "The police chased the bad guy," and the SLP says, "Yes, the bad guy was chased by the police." This is an example of

    a. Recast

    b. Extension

    c. Mand-model

    d. Self-talk

    e. Joint routines

See Answers to Study and Review Questions, page 465.

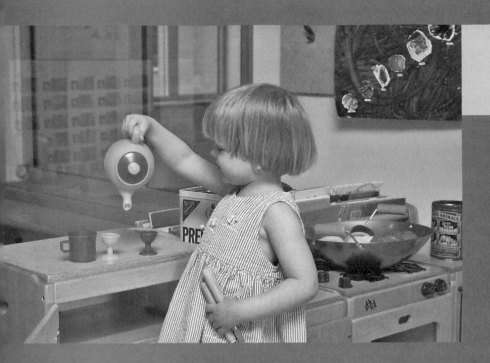

Language Impairment in Toddlers and Preschoolers

Three-year-old Aimee L.'s parents brought her to us at the university clinic because they were concerned about "how she pronounces her sounds." When we first saw Aimee, the first thing we noticed was that she was quite small for her age. She was accompanied by her parents, Mr. and Mrs. L., and her five-year-old sister Amanda. As we talked with Mr. and Mrs. L., we discovered that there were many more issues than just articulation. Aimee did not say her first words in Arabic until she was two years old. She was born prematurely. Eating was a major issue; Mr. and Mrs. L. shared that it took Aimee about one hour to eat

a pita bread sandwich. She had had feeding problems in infancy. We noticed that when Aimee walked, she appeared somewhat uncoordinated. She was still in diapers, and her self-help skills appeared delayed.

Mr. L. shared that they had not sought help for Aimee up till this time because they thought she might be healed through a miracle. He said that a family member in the Middle East had brought a key to the tomb of Jesus, rubbed the key on the door of the tomb, and put the key into the mouth of a family member with a speech problem. The family member was instantly "cured."

Mr. L. had hoped that Aimee might spontaneously "recover" from her problems and be cured in a similar fashion, but she clearly had not. Thus, Mr. and Mrs. L. thought that they would begin the assessment process with a speech and language evaluation.

It became apparent during the evaluation that Aimee was generally nonverbal. I asked her parents if her reticence was due to the unfamiliar situation, or if this behavior was typical of the home. They said that Aimee "is always like this." We took Aimee outside to the playground, hoping that swinging and playing on the equipment might help her to verbalize more. These activities did not help, and we ultimately were forced to end the assessment due to Aimee's general lack of cooperation; also, our assessment hour was almost over.

By this time, it was fairly clear that Aimee had many more issues than the family realized. Her parents were so anxious, and my heart went out to them because I knew that they had hoped that she only had problems with articulation. I referred them to a local regional center for a comprehensive evaluation by a multidisciplinary team of professionals. I also called the pediatrician. He said that he had not noticed any delays or problems with Aimee in the times that she had visited him. Trying to cover my shock, I tried to be as diplomatic as possible in asking him if he agreed with my recommendation that Aimee's parents take her to the regional center for a comprehensive evaluation. Thankfully, the pediatrician agreed and said that he would reinforce my recommendation when the family came back to see him.

INTRODUCTION

Background Facts

Delays in communication development are probably the most common symptom of developmental disability in children under three years old and affect approximately 5 to 10 percent of those children (Rossetti, 2001). In previous chapters, we have said that specific language impairment (SLI) is a language impairment that is not associated with any other condition such as autism, Down syndrome, and others. Children with SLI have a developmental disorder of language ability in the absence of significant comorbid (accompanying) intellectual, neurological, or sensory difficulties (La Paro, Justice, Skibbe, & Pianta, 2004).

We also said that children may have language impairments associated with conditions such as autism, Down syndrome, hearing loss, traumatic brain injury, and others. These language impairments are discussed in more detail in other chapters. In Chapter 6, I used the term *LI (language impaired)* to refer to all children who do not develop language normally because they have an SLI or because they have an associated condition. In this chapter, I will also use the term LI for several reasons.

First, when children are young, it is often difficult to differentiate between SLI and LI due to established risk factors or factors that place children at risk (described later). Second, it has increasingly been my experience as a speech-language pathologist (SLP) in the public schools that for many children, language problems co-occur with other problems, and it is difficult to diagnose SLI. For example, I serve children born into low-income homes to mothers who have ingested drugs and alcohol while pregnant and are also abusive to the children. Many of the children have had middle ear infections and have spent the first five years of their lives in front of the TV.

Personally, I agree with the statements of Law et al. (2004), whom we cited in Chapter 1. Law et al. stated that LI can occur as either a primary condition (as in the case of SLI) or a secondary condition, where it can be accounted for by another condition such as autism, neurological impairment, and others. We quoted Law et al. (p. 924) as saying that " . . . The term specific language impairment is sometimes used, but *exactly how specific such a condition is remains debatable given the reported comorbidity* . . . " (italics mine). I see fewer and fewer children whom I could genuinely describe as "SLI." Most of the children I serve experience multiple factors that put them at risk for language impairments. Thus, again, as in Chapter 6, I will use the general term *language impaired*.

The third reason I am using the term *LI* is that many of this chapter's suggestions for assessment and intervention apply both to children with SLI and to children with language impairments accompanying conditions such as cerebral palsy, Down syndrome, and other "obvious" diagnosed factors. The strategies I am suggesting in this chapter are applicable across a wide range of toddlers and preschool children who are having difficulties developing language skills.

Established Risk Factors for Developing Language Impairment

Young children may have LIs secondary to established risk factors or conditions that put them at risk for LI. Established risk factors, which are generally diagnosed and known to professional teams, are as follows (Roseberry-McKibbin & Hegde, 2006; Rossetti, 2001; Weitzner-Lin, 2004):

- genetic syndromes (e.g., Down syndrome)
- congenital malformations (e.g., spina bifida, cleft palate)
- sensory disorders (e.g., visual impairment, hearing loss)
- atypical developmental disorders (e.g., autism)
- neurological disorders (e.g., cerebral palsy)
- chronic illnesses (e.g., cystic fibrosis, diabetes)
- metabolic disorders (e.g., pituitary diseases, Tay-Sachs disease)
- severe toxic exposure (e.g., fetal alcohol syndrome, lead poisoning)
- severe infectious diseases (e.g., encephalitis, meningitis, HIV)

Again, toddlers and preschoolers may have diagnosed problems such as those above that are accompanied by LI.

Conditions That Put Children at Risk for Developing Language Impairment

Sometimes children appear to be developing normally during the first months of life in terms of language and other skills. However, there may be some conditions that place them at risk for developing LI. These conditions include environmental factors, genetic background, and some disease-related conditions (Rossetti, 2001; Roseberry-McKibbin & Hegde, 2006).

- chronic middle-ear infections
- serious prenatal and natal complications, including fetal anoxia (oxygen deprivation at birth), smallness for gestation age (< tenth percentile), and low birth weight (<1,500 grams)
- signs of early behavior disorders (e.g., tantrums, irritability, withdrawal)
- chronic or severe physical or mental illness or mental retardation in caregivers
- family history of predisposing medical or genetic conditions (e.g., mother had gestational diabetes)
- chronically dysfunctional interaction between family members (e.g., parents frequently argue violently; father abuses mother)
- serious questions raised by a parent, other caregiver, or professional about the child's development
- isolation of the child or prolonged separation of the child from the primary caregiver or parent
- caregiver or parental substance abuse

> There are both established risk factors for developing LI and conditions that put children at risk for developing LI.

- parental education below ninth grade; parental unemployment or chronic welfare dependency
- dangerous or unstable living conditions (e.g., homelessness)
- lack of health insurance; inadequate prenatal care; overall poor health care

Again, seemingly typically developing (TD) children may be at risk for LI due to the presence of one or more of the above-listed conditions.

SUMMARY

- The term *language impaired* is used to refer to all children who do not develop language normally for one or more reasons.
- Children may have LIs secondary to established risk factors or conditions that put them at risk for LIs. These include genetic syndromes, neurological disorders, and others.
- Children may appear to be TD in the early months of life. However, they may experience conditions that put them at risk for developing LIs. These conditions include chronic middle-ear infections, severe family dysfunction, isolation of the child, and others.

Add your summary points here:

_____

_____

_____

CHARACTERISTICS OF TODDLERS AND PRESCHOOLERS WITH LANGUAGE IMPAIRMENTS

Precursors to Language Development

As we have stated, children with LI are a heterogeneous group. Thus, toddlers and preschoolers with language problems will show different profiles. However, there are some general precursors to language development that SLPs can be aware of. If a young child is showing difficulty with these precursors, there is an increased chance that she will eventually be diagnosed with an LI.

First, the child needs to recognize and attend to environmental change. This is a major precursor to language development. Second, the child needs to be aware that she can be an agent of change in her environment (McLaughlin, 2006). For example, she needs to know that if she is hungry, she can cry or point to food and vocalize, and someone will feed her. If a child does not view herself as an agent of change, she will be unlikely to learn that language is one of the most effective means that she can use to produce change (Reed, 2005).

> Important precursors to language development include the child's ability to attend to environmental change, his awareness that he can be an agent of change in his environment, and the ability to engage in reciprocal interactions and routines and establish joint reference with adults.

A third important precursor to language development is the ability to engage in reciprocal interactions and routines and establish joint reference with adults (Delgado, Mundy, Crowson, Markus, Yale, & Schwartz, 2002). For example, preschoolers with LI seem to have difficulty playing games like patty-cake and other give-and-take routines. In addition, toddlers and preschoolers with LI may communicate more via gestures and vocalizations than by verbal means.

Other "red flags" shown by some very young children who are later diagnosed with LI include reduced amount of babbling and less complex babbling, difficulty establishing eye contact, and difficulty establishing mutual gaze and joint reference. You will recall from Chapter 2 that joint reference refers to a situation where the child and another person are both paying attention to the same object or event.

> **POINTS TO PONDER** Describe important precursors to language development in children. Why is it important to be aware of these precursors?
>
> _____
>
> _____
>
> _____

Young children with LI frequently have difficulty with play skills (Wetherby, Allen, Cleary, Kublin, & Goldstein, 2002). They may exhibit unusually aggressive or uncooperative behaviors or they may passively watch others play or engage in isolated or parallel play beyond the appropriate developmental level. Other children often avoid these children. In addition, young children with LI may show atypical behavior in the area of symbolic play, a very important precursor to language skills. We will recall that *symbolic play* refers to a child using one object to represent another. For example, a child might pick up a stick and pretend it is a gun; another child might take a Kleenex and use it as a doll's blanket. Children with LI often underutilize symbolic play.

Linguistic Characteristics of Young Children with Language Impairments

In Chapter 1 we extensively discussed linguistic characteristics of children with SLI. Many of these characteristics are also typical of young children with LI that may be the result of SLI or an LI associated with another condition.

Children with LI often have problems with their grammatical skills (Beverly & Williams, 2004). As we said in Chapter 1, these include problems with syntax and morphology. Problems with syntax include using sentences that are not complex enough for the child's age level, use of shorter sentences than one might expect, use of single words or phrases in place of sentences, and a limited variety of syntactic structures. Problems with morphology may include difficulty with bound morphemes such as -*ed* (liv*ed*) (e.g., Leonard, Deevy, Miller, Rauf, Charest, & Kurtz, 2003; Rice, Tomblin, Hoffman, Richman, & Marquis, 2004), -*est* (biggest), and overgeneralization of certain forms past the appropriate developmental point (e.g., *digged* for *dug*, *mans* for *men*).

Many children with LI have impaired pragmatics skills (Brinton & Fujiki, 1999; La Paro et al., 2004). They frequently have difficulty initiating conversations, turn-taking, maintaining eye contact, and so forth. These difficulties with pragmatics skills often lead to social problems for young LI children. Research has shown that even children as young as three years of age will often reject peers whom they view as "different" (Rice et al., 1991; Rice, Hadley, & Alexander, 1993).

There is also some evidence to show that preschoolers with LI have difficulties with narrative skills. In comparison to the narratives of TD children, the narratives of preschoolers with LI tend to contain less information and be less mature. Reed (2005, p. 118) states that

> Production of narratives generally challenges most aspects of a language-impaired child's language system so that difficulties with one aspect of language may overload the child in such a way that other aspects of language break down or the whole system breaks down. For this reason, preschoolers who to the "naked ear" may appear to have adequate conversational language skills or who score within normal limits on standardized language tests may evidence even quite severe language problems when they are asked to relate narratives.

The quality of LI preschoolers' narrative skills is a major predicting factor for their later success in school (McCabe & Bliss, 2003; Stothard, Snowling, Bishop,

Linguistic difficulties of young children with LI include problems with narratives, grammatical skills, and pragmatics skills.

Chipchase, & Kaplan, 1998). According to Kaderavek and Sulzby (2000), narrative ability is one of the best predictors of school success for children with LI and learning disability. Paul and Smith (1993) found that the narrative skills of four-year-olds were one of the best predictors of later school outcomes for children who were at risk for language and academic problems. Bishop and Edmundson (1987) found that children's performance on a narrative task was the single best predictor of literacy functioning at five-and-a-half years of age.

A study by Fazio, Naremore, and Connell (1996) examined skills of low-income children in kindergarten through second grade who were at risk for SLI. They found that the best kindergarten predictors of children who were eventually assigned to remedial education were rote memory problems and diminished storytelling skills. Tabors, Snow, and Dickinson (2001) followed children enrolled in Head Start from the time they were three years old until they were in seventh grade. These children were from the New England area of the United States and included Hispanic, African American, and North European American children. Tabors et al. found that the children's narrative production in kindergarten was one of four measures that significantly correlated with receptive vocabulary and reading comprehension in fourth grade and in seventh grade.

With regard to development of semantic skills, we will recall from Chapter 2 that most children say their first words at approximately twelve months of age. If a child says his first word significantly later than twelve months of age, this can be an indication of LI. Children with LI are not only slower to say their first words than TD children, but they are slow to add lots of words to their vocabularies. They are also slower to use two-word combinations than TD children.

Another key "red flag" for possible LI is preference for using gestures instead of vocalizations, especially after eighteen months of age. Remember, at eighteen months of age, a child should have an expressive vocabulary of fifty words and should begin putting two words together; an otherwise healthy, normal child who does not do this may have a clinically significant LI.

Late Talkers

As a clinician, I often hear parents of toddlers say, "He doesn't say anything, but he seems to understand everything I say! And I know he's bright!" Such children may have an LI characterized by normal receptive language and late-to-develop expressive language. Experts describe these children as late talkers or "late bloomers" (e.g., Dale, Price, Bishop, & Plomin, 2004; Haynes & Pindzola, 2004). These are children who reach two years of age with significantly delayed expressive language despite normal auditory, cognitive, structural abilities. They also have normal language comprehension skills.

We will recall that at two years (twenty-four months of age), children should have between 200 and 300 words in their expressive vocabularies and should be regularly using two-word combinations (McLaughlin, 2006). "Late bloomers" usually have an expressive vocabulary of less than fifty words and do not use any two-word phrases. Some experts suggest that approximately 50 percent of these children will "catch up" and exhibit normal

> Some children are "late talkers." They may have accompanying receptive language problems, or they may have normal receptive language skills.

expressive language by three years of age. However, the other 50 percent will be at risk for having a language delay that persists beyond three years of age (Kouri, 2003). According to Rescorla, Dahlsgaard, and Roberts (2000), most toddlers with an expressive language delay only will perform within the average range by the time they are four or five years of age. However, late talkers with both receptive and expressive delays are more likely to be diagnosed in preschool as having LIs (Rescorla & Achenbach, 2002).

Rescorla (2002) showed that although late talkers with normal receptive language generally have a better outcome than toddlers with both receptive and expressive language delays, they may have some subtle problems in elementary school. Rescorla's research showed that late talkers with normal receptive skills, in comparison to TD peers, had significantly poorer reading/spelling skills at ages eight and nine although they performed "within average range" on national measures. Rescorla suggested that parents and professionals should be aware that although these late talkers may eventually perform within normal limits on most language measures, an early expressive language delay may indicate " . . . some subclinical weakness in the component skills that serve language and reading" (p. 370).

Based on the results of her research, Rescorla suggested that late talkers or other children with mild residual learning problems might significantly underperform in comparison to their TD peers while appearing to be within average range by national standards. Thus, Rescorla recommended that for late talkers, even those with normal receptive language skills, it might be a good idea to give them extra exposure to activities and games that strengthen verbal memory, phonological discrimination, grammatical processing, and word retrieval.

In a more recent study, Rescorla (2005) examined language and reading outcomes at thirteen years of age in thirty-eight children who had been identified as late talkers when they were between twenty-four and thirty-one months of age. The children all came from middle- to upper-class socioeconomic status families and had adequate hearing, receptive language, and nonverbal skills. These children were compared with a group of twenty-five TD children who were matched on age, socioeconomic status, and nonverbal ability.

At age thirteen, the late talkers and TD children were compared on standardized language and reading tasks. The late talkers performed within average range on these tasks;

CONNECT & EXTEND

Detailed longitudinal research regarding late talkers is found in Rescorla, L. (2005). Age 13 language and reading outcomes in late-talking toddlers. *Journal of Speech, Language, and Hearing Research, 48,* 459–472.

however, they scored significantly lower than their TD age-matched peers on aggregate measures of verbal memory, vocabulary, grammar, and reading comprehension. The conclusions of this study generally agreed with those of Rescorla (2002): relative to TD peers from the same backgrounds, late talkers may (in adolescence) have continuing weaknesses in verbal memory, reading comprehension, grammar, and vocabulary even while performing in the average range by national standards in most language skills by the time they enter high school. Rescorla (2005) made recommendations similar to those in her 2002 study: possibly, if we provide late talkers with activities to improve phonological discrimination, language processing, verbal memory, and word retrieval skills, we may be able to prevent future weaknesses in language relative to TD children from a similar background.

Girolametto, Wiigs, Smyth, Weitzman, and Pearce (2001) examined the higher-level language abilities of a group of five-year-old children who had been diagnosed earlier in their lives as late talkers. All the children and their mothers had participated in a language program that trained parents to stimulate language development in naturalistic contexts when the children were between two and three years old. For children who continued to have slow language gains, there was direct and focused intervention. Girolametto et al. found that at age five, scores on standardized tests of language development indicated that most of the late-talking children had caught up with TD, age-matched peers in expressive vocabulary and grammar. However, weaknesses remained in a number of areas of higher-level language (e.g., narrative tasks, short-term auditory memory skills). Girolametto et al. suggested that late talkers continue to be monitored into elementary school—especially in areas such as narrative discourse.

> It is important for SLPs to monitor children who have normal receptive language skills and delayed expressive skills and to provide early language stimulation for these children.

Clearly, SLPs need to be aware of early "red flags" that might indicate that a young child has a clinically significant LI. It is my professional experience that many parents are told by their family pediatricians to not worry about signs of LI in their young children. The parents are reassured that the children will "outgrow" their problems, and the children thus do not receive much-needed early intervention that can be so effective in preventing greater difficulties later on.

 SUMMARY

- There are several important precursors to language development: the ability to recognize and attend to environmental change, a child's awareness that she can be an agent of change in her environment, and the ability to engage in reciprocal interactions and routines and establish joint reference with adults.
- Young children with LI show difficulty with play skills and have grammatical problems. They also show difficulties in the areas of pragmatics and narrative skills.
- In terms of skills in semantics, children with LI are slower to say their first words and word combinations, and are slow to add words to their vocabularies.
- Some young children are labeled "late bloomers" or "late talkers." Research has suggested that even late talkers with normal receptive language skills may be at risk for later, subtle language problems.

Add your own summary points here:

_____

_____

_____

ASSESSMENT OF TODDLERS AND PRESCHOOLERS WITH LANGUAGE IMPAIRMENTS

General Principles

Assessment of and intervention for younger children has become increasingly visible in the past decade. Reasons for this include 1) state and federal laws and 2) increased survival of medically fragile infants. Public Law 99-457 (Preschool Amendments to the Education of the Handicapped Act, 1986) has provided incentives at state and federal levels for SLPs to identify and treat infants, toddlers, and preschoolers who have LI. There are greater numbers of these children today, partially because medically fragile infants are surviving instead of dying as they did in past decades (Rossetti, 2001). Thus, it is important for SLPs to be aware of general principles of assessment, described below, as well as specific techniques for assessment, described later.

First, SLPs need to *make a family-centered communication assessment in both home and clinical settings.* We need to assess the family's resources, communication patterns, strengths and weaknesses, and overall family constellation. In addition, we should remember that "an effective assessment is based on concerns as specified by the family" (Weitzner-Lin, 2004, p. 23). It is easy for SLPs with heavy caseloads to not take the time to really find out what families' specific concerns are; however, ultimately it is worth it to take this time; when families feel listened to and understood from the beginning, they will often be more cooperative in carrying out treatment plans. This is especially true for families from culturally and linguistically diverse (CLD) backgrounds (e.g., Mokuau & Tau'ili, 2004; Santos & Chan, 2004; Jacob, 2004).

Second, we must *begin assessment as early in the child's life as possible and repeat assessments throughout the childhood period.* With young children, it's never just a "one-shot deal." As children grow, they need to be reassessed on a regular basis. A third general principle of assessment is that we must *work on a multidisciplinary team with other professionals.* Public Law 99-457 requires that a multidisciplinary team conduct an assessment of infants, toddlers, and preschoolers with disabilities. These teams often include such members as SLPs, social workers, psychologists, educators, physical therapists, occupational therapists, physicians, nurses, and day-care staff. We need to make decisions as a team regarding assessment materials, methods, and how assessment results will be used.

> Federal law mandates that SLPs work on multidisciplinary teams to provide early and ongoing, culturally sensitive assessment for children at risk for language impairments.

Fourth, it is critical to *involve individuals from the child and family's culture when possible.* As we shall say several times in this chapter, families are often most comfortable when there is at least one team member from their cultural and linguistic background (Chan & Lee, 2004; Sharifzadeh, 2004). This person, called a **cultural mediator**, can act as a "go-between" for clinicians and family members, helping them understand and work successfully with one another. Assessments are most successful when the SLP is open to the family's cultural style and is willing to tailor assessment and intervention to the family's practices and beliefs (Hammer et al., 2004).

CASES TO CONSIDER

I was asked to assess the language skills of Trinh H., a young Vietnamese boy who "wasn't progressing in preschool." The team told me that Trinh had been working regularly with a Vietnamese interpreter who was trying to help him. The interpreter, who had a great deal of experience in the district, said that Trinh stood out as "very slow to learn" and the interpreter was quite concerned about Trinh's lack of ability to retain material. The teacher asked me to evaluate Trinh to see if he just had a language difference based on his first language of Vietnamese, or if he might have an LI.

As I prepared to conduct an assessment, I gathered a case history with the help of the Vietnamese interpreter, who spoke with Trinh's parents on my behalf. I found out that Trinh's mother had gestational diabetes, which went uncontrolled during her whole pregnancy with him. The gestational diabetes was so bad that Trinh's mother went blind after giving birth to him. The family had no health insurance, so prenatal care was nonexistent. When Trinh was two years old, he had fallen off the family car roof (apparently someone had set him up there) and hit his head quite hard. Given just this case history, do you think Trinh's difficulties in learning can be explained solely by the fact that he speaks Vietnamese? Or, given the case history, do you think Trinh might have a genuine LI? Explain. What will be your next steps in the assessment process?

A fifth general principle of assessment is that we must *conduct interviews and gather an extensive case history*. We need to include such areas as maternal health during pregnancy, circumstances of the birth, and early development patterns of the child in such areas as gross and fine-motor development, feeding patterns, communication skills, self-help skills, and others. It is important for SLPs to remember, however, that some CLD families might take offense at being asked such personal questions as circumstances surrounding childbirth, the child's development, and other questions that are a routine part of case histories (Sharifzadeh, 2004). In these cases, a cultural mediator might be needed to serve as the informant or liaison between the family and the SLP (Shipley & Roseberry-McKibbin, 2006; Weitzner-Lin, 2004). Many CLD families I have worked with have been far more comfortable talking with a person from their own cultural and linguistic background than with me.

A sixth general assessment principle is to *evaluate caregiver-child interaction patterns*. Some formal, published instruments can be used for this. These instruments offer suggestions and guidance for observing young children and caregivers in naturalistic situations. Haynes and Pindzola (2004, p. 91) state that

> . . . the caregiver's model as it presently exists may not be conducive to language development and should be changed. The only way to determine the quality of this relationship

is through the observation of caregiver-child interaction. Evaluating and working with caregiver-child interaction is especially important when dealing with infants and toddlers who are at "high risk" for language disorder. Providing the best-quality stimulation for these children will go a long way toward preventing, or at least reducing, the severity of potential language disorders . . .

Among other things, these instruments help assess the child's mood, general affect, and responsiveness and how the caregiver handles and provides stimulation to the child. For example, does the caregiver hold the child a great deal, or does she seldom touch him?

> Clinicians need to evaluate child-caregiver interactions, keeping in mind that different cultures have different interaction styles that must be considered.

It is crucial to remember that in some cultures, there is a great deal of physical warmth and affection between parents (especially mothers) and young children (e.g., Sharifzadeh, 2004; Zuniga, 2004). I have heard mainstream US clinicians say things like, "Wow, she really babies that kid." Such statements are culturally insensitive and inappropriate. In some cultures, for example, children routinely sit on their mothers' laps until they are five or six years of age.

An important aspect of the interaction between children and their caregivers that should be evaluated is book sharing. In mainstream US culture, many caregivers read books with their children from birth onward. There are several formal protocols for evaluating shared book reading between caregivers and their children; some experts recommend evaluating caregiver-child joint book reading activities and strategies used by caregivers during these times (e.g., Kaderavek & Sulzby, 1998; Rabidoux & Macdonald, 2000).

A seventh general assessment principle is to *make sure that the child's hearing has been thoroughly tested*. Although newborn hearing screenings are now mandatory, it is still important for children's hearing to be assessed on a regular basis. This is especially true when children have repeated middle-ear infections; these repeated infections can predispose children to speech and language impairments.

Eighth, we must *use multiple measures in assessment of young children with potential language impairments*. Public Law 99-457 requires that professionals in public schools who evaluate young children incorporate multiple measures as well as multiple sources of information. This means that a child is not just given one or two tests and then diagnosed. Again, multiple measures are required by law.

CONNECT & EXTEND

Specific suggestions for early literacy screening are detailed in Justice, L.M., Invernizzi, M.A., & Meier, J.D. (2002). Designing and implementing an early literacy screening protocol: Suggestions for the SLP. *Language, Speech, and Hearing Services in Schools, 33,* 84–101.

A ninth general assessment principle is that we must *make sure that assessment is nondiscriminatory and appropriate for the child's and family's linguistic and cultural background*. Public Law 99-457 mandates that assessment procedures are administered to the child or the parents in their native language (or whatever language the family prefers to use) and that the materials used in the assessment not be discriminatory.

Lastly, we need to *conduct thorough and early evaluations for at-risk children to prevent future problems with both oral and written language* (Justice, Invernizzi, & Meier, 2002). As we have said elsewhere in this book, many children identified as LI due to oral

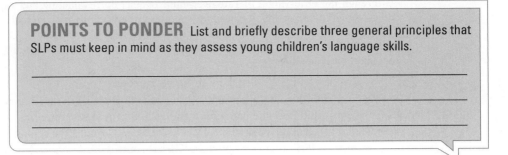

POINTS TO PONDER List and briefly describe three general principles that SLPs must keep in mind as they assess young children's language skills.

language problems in early childhood go on to demonstrate problems with written language later (Catts, 1991; Goldsworthy, 2003; Hallahan, Lloyd, Kauffman, Weiss, & Martinez, 2005). Thus, it is critical for clinicians to evaluate preliteracy skills (described in detail later in this chapter) as well as oral language skills.

Specific Strategies for Assessment

We have just described some general principles for assessing young children with LI; now we will briefly discuss some specific techniques that SLPs can use for evaluation.

Many SLPs assess children's narrative skills. We previously discussed the fact that when young children have difficulties with narratives, they often have later difficulty in school. Thus, it is very important to evaluate the narrative skills of preschoolers, because these can be predictive of LI (Hemphill, Uccelli, Winner, Chang, & Bellinger, 2002). Bliss (2003) provides specific suggestions and strategies for assessing the narrative skills of children.

Many SLPs observe children's play activities as a means of assessment. SLPs can observe the child engaged in play with one or several children or with a caregiver. In Chapter 2, we talked about developmental milestones of play for appropriate ages. The SLP can use these types of milestones to guide her assessment of whether the child is at an appropriate age level with play skills. Assessment of toddlers' symbolic play has become increasingly prevalent because it has been found to correlate with language development in children with and without language delays (Snyder & Scherer, 2004). Rossetti (2001) and Westby (1980) provide specific details on how to assess play and what behaviors to look for.

Play-based assessment (which may occur in a therapy room or in the child's home) is usually characterized by an informal atmosphere, freedom to explore, and the use of toys. The child takes the lead and the examiner follows his lead. The examiner adapts to the

---

CONNECT & EXTEND

Specific strategies for assessing children's narrative skills are detailed in Bliss, L.S. (2003). Discourse impairments: Assessment and intervention applications. Boston: Allyn & Bacon.

Play-based assessment, conducted in an informal atmosphere, allows the clinician to assess the child's functional communication skills.

child and does not prioritize administering tests in a certain order within a given time frame. The examiner is able to better assess the child's functional communication skills, and directions for intervention are based on what the child is able to do, not on test scores. Usually parents are part of the assessment process, and thus the examiner is able to discuss the child's performance with them and ascertain whether or not the child's behaviors are representative of his daily functioning in different environments.

Observation is a critical part of play-based assessment because it often provides information about how the young child uses language to achieve communicative outcomes. When we observe young children's language skills, it is often ideal to have the child interact with a familiar person such as her mother, because the interaction with the familiar person will probably be most representative of how the child communicates in "real life" (Weitzner-Lin, 2004).

Sometimes observations don't yield all the information a clinician wants about the child's language skills. In these situations, the clinician who is using play-based assessment can try to elicit various structures from the child. Researchers have suggested **communicative temptations** for this purpose (Weitzner-Lin, 2004; Wetherby & Prizant, 1998). Communicative temptations are elicitation tasks that increase the likelihood that the child will produce the behavior that the clinician is looking for. They are best used with children between the prelinguistic stage and two years of age. For example, let's say that the clinician wants to know if the child uses greetings like "hi." She might hide a stuffed animal under the table, knock, and then bring out the animal and have it greet the child. The clinician might need to repeat this several times in order to assess whether or not the child uses any type of greeting in response.

When the SLP is playing with the child (assuming the child is willing to talk), she can also gather a language sample and calculate the child's mean length of utterance to evaluate grammatical skills. One of the most common measures used in a basic language evaluation is the MLU (mean length of utterance) count, which we have discussed elsewhere in the book. In children up to four years of age, there is a general correlation between MLU and chronological age; also, MLU is a better predictor of language development than is chronological age (Brown, 1973; Miller, 1981). However, MLU is a subjective measure, and Muma (1998) has shown that sampling error rates are very high unless one analyzes samples of 200 to 400 utterances. Most SLPs would find this prohibitive due to time constraints.

> Wetherby and Prizant's Communication and Symbolic Behavior Scales allow the clinician to examine a number of parameters that have predictive value in terms of children's communication development.

In the assessment of young children, it is very common to use communication and symbolic behavior scales. These scales usually have several components: a parent questionnaire, observation of unstructured play activities, and direct sampling of nonverbal and verbal communication (Nelson, 1998). The clinician can videotape the child if she wants to and review the tape later. Parents can watch the tape with the clinician and provide feedback as to the representativeness of the behavior. In other words, does the child's behavior during the assessment reflect how he usually behaves in other settings?

Wetherby and Prizant (1992) developed the Communication and Symbolic Behavior Scales when they found that many standardized tests for young children did not look at some important parameters.

These parameters, which they included in their Communication and Symbolic Behavior Scales, were shown to have predictive value in terms of children's communication development (e.g., Yoder, Warren, & McCathren, 1998). The parameters were 1) evaluating social-affective signaling, 2) assessing communicative functions, 3) analyzing preverbal communication, 4) profiling communicative, social, and symbolic abilities, 5) directly assessing a child's communication in spontaneous child-initiated interactions, and 6) using caregivers as active participants and as informants in the evaluation (Haynes & Pindzola, 2004).

Because there are few standardized instruments available for assessing children under three years old, many SLPs use parent report instruments (Westerlund, Berglund, & Eriksson, 2006). Most instruments for these young children include developmental scales or questionnaires that help structure the parents' and/or clinicians' observations of various behaviors (Roseberry-McKibbin & Hegde, 2006). Parent/caregiver report is an increasingly popular evaluation technique, with advantages for assessing toddlers especially because toddlers' behavior can make them challenging to assess in a valid and reliable manner. In terms of providing a general evaluation of early developing skills, it is more cost effective than behavioral assessments. In addition, these reports can sample behaviors outside of the clinic and reflect the child's skills in a broad range of contexts.

One study did caution, however, that on one parent report instrument, parents with less education tended to overestimate their children's language abilities while parents with more education tended to underestimate their children's language abilities (Wetherby, Allen, Cleary, Kublin, & Goldstein, 2002). Conti-Ramsden, Simkin, and Pickles (2006) found that parents were more accurate in describing children's expressive language problems than in describing their receptive language problems. But even keeping this research in mind, more SLPs are using parent/caregiver report as part of an evaluation battery for young children (Marchman & Martinez-Sussmann, 2002; Thal, O'Hanlon, Clemmons, & Fralin, 1999).

There are published instruments for parent report. Often, they include vocabulary checklists in which parents review lists of words commonly used by young children and check off the words their child can comprehend and/or produce. Productive vocabulary skills are a key index of language ability at age two (Van Hulle, Goldsmith, & Lemery, 2004), and thus it is recommended that SLPs assess these skills in young children through parent report and other measures.

For example, the Language Development Survey (Rescorla, 1989; Rescorla & Alley, 2001) is an inexpensive, simple screening tool for identifying language delay in toddlers. The Language Development Survey is easy to score, requires only fifth-grade reading skills, and can be completed by parents in about ten minutes. Rescorla and Achenbach (2002) reported, based on the results of their study, that the Language Development Survey has potential to be used with CLD children and their families as well as children and families from low-income backgrounds. Rescorla, Berstein Ratner, Jusczyk, and Jusczyk (2005) also found that the Language Development Survey correlates with longer measures such as the MacArthur-Bates Communicative Development Inventories: Words and Sentences (Fenson, Dale, Reznick, Bates, Thal, & Hartung, 1992).

The MacArthur Communicative Development Inventories are another widely used parent report measure (Fenson et al., 1992). They

> For assessing young children's language skills, widely used parent report measures include the Language Development Survey and the MacArthur Communicative Development Inventories.

have been translated into a number of languages, including Spanish (Jackson-Maldonado, Bates, & Thal, 1992), and research has shown that they can be successfully used with Spanish-speaking parents to help assess toddlers who have potential LI (Heilmann, Ellis Weismer, Evans, & Hollar, 2005; Marchman & Martinez-Sussmann, 2002; Thal, Jackson-Maldonado, & Acosta, 2000). Today, more SLPs are using parent questionnaires to evaluate emergent literacy as well as oral language (e.g., Boudreau, 2005).

Clinicians can evaluate phonological awareness skills and other skills relevant to written language through both formal and informal measures. Justice et al. (2002) give a number of practical suggestions for informal assessment of preliteracy skills.

Teacher report questionnaires may also be used for assessment. However, SLPs must be careful because teachers may be biased with regard to CLD children. For example, in one study that we mentioned in Chapter 1, Hwa-Froelich and Westby (2003) found that in a Head Start program, the teachers did not believe that any of the Asian children had language learning problems because these children were so respectful, obedient, and well behaved. Basically, the teachers believed that because the children did not misbehave, they did not have language learning problems. Any difficulties evidenced by the Asian children were attributed to their status as English Language Learners. SLPs need to provide in-service training for early childhood education teachers so that they can make culturally appropriate referrals of children with potential LI.

A last major mode of assessment for young children is published instruments that provide norms. Haynes and Pindzola (2004) stated that with the enactment of federal legislation mandating services for children from birth to five years of age in the public schools, test developers have increased their efforts to devise assessment instruments for preschoolers. Haynes and Pindzola divided preschool tests that deal with communication into two categories. First, there are large test batteries that include communication or language as one aspect of the assessment. These large test batteries are designed to assess all areas: cognition, personal-social behavior, gross and fine-motor skills, adaptive behavior, and communication skills. Thus, language skills are included as a part of these batteries; the assessment, though superficial, can at least guide the clinician toward a decision about whether more testing of language skills is necessary.

The second category of tests for preschoolers' communication skills is those that focus specifically on communication and language (for example, the Preschool Language Scale:4; Zimmerman, Steiner, & Pond, 2002). Many of these instruments are formal; that is, they are standardized and norm-referenced, which can be helpful for public school SLPs who are frequently asked to provide specific scores to qualify children for services. However, SLPs must remember that many of these formal measures are inappropriate with young children from CLD backgrounds (Restrepo & Silverman, 2001). The ERIC Clearinghouse on Assessment and Evaluation provides detailed information on available, current tests that are appropriate for young children, including CLD children with potential communication disorders.

> SLPs can assess children's language with published instruments; these include 1) large test batteries that include language as one aspect of assessment and 2) tests that focus specifically on communication and language.

CONNECT & EXTEND

Eric Clearinghouse on Assessment and Evaluation provides a current, updated list of tests with reviews and descriptions. The clearinghouse can be accessed at http://ericae.net/main.htm.

Formal tests have some other drawbacks (Rossetti, 2001; Weitzner-Lin, 2004). They are not generally designed to guide planning for intervention, and they offer a limited view of how the child communicates in naturalistic contexts. In addition, most formal tests leave very little allowance for adaptation to individual children. And since many young children are too young to truly cooperate with a structured format, the results of the test may not be reliable or valid indicators of their abilities. Most young children have very limited experience with taking standardized tests. If they do not perform well, part of their poor performance might be an artifact of lack of familiarity with the testing situation itself.

Another problem with formal tests is that in this situation, the child comes to an unfamiliar environment and focuses on formal, standardized test materials. The child is in response mode (e.g., pointing to pictures) and usually does not initiate interaction. The child is alone with an unfamiliar adult where communication is restricted; the emphasis is on "getting the tests over with." The examiner controls the interaction. Formal tests often do not assess functional, daily communication skills in the child's natural settings, and children may be labeled "untestable" if they do not respond well to the formal tests that the examiner attempts to administer during the session. Parents are generally not part of the assessment process (Weitzner-Lin, 2004).

 SUMMARY

- Due to changes in federal laws, visibility and importance of assessment and intervention for young children has increased. One major factor impacting service delivery to young children is the increased survival rate of medically fragile infants.
- When assessing young children, it is important to involve families and to use culturally and linguistically appropriate and sensitive methods. It is critical to gather a thorough case history and work on a multidisciplinary team with other professionals. Multiple assessment measures must be used.
- One very successful assessment technique for young children is to observe their play. Formal and informal evaluation methods can be used. It is important to assess narrative skills, as these are important predictors of LI.
- Parent report measures have become increasingly popular. Teacher report measures may also be used, although caution is warranted with CLD children whose teachers are not culturally sensitive and aware.
- Published, formal instruments provide norms that can be very helpful for school-based SLPs especially. However, these instruments may be inappropriate for use with CLD children.

Add your own summary points here:

_____

_____

_____

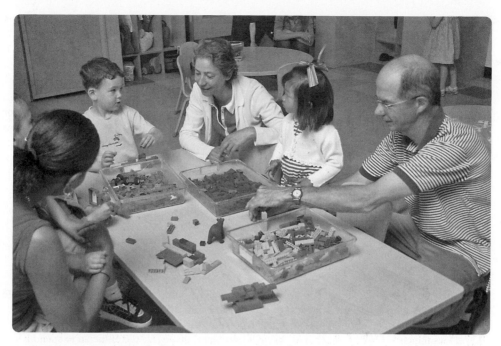

Young CLD children with language impairments need the adults around them to facilitate language interaction opportunities with peers.

INTERVENTION FOR TODDLERS AND PRESCHOOLERS WITH LANGUAGE IMPAIRMENT

General Principles

Experts agree that in terms of intervention for children with LI, the earlier the better (e.g., Reed, 2005; Rescorla, 2005; Weiss, 2002, Weitzner-Lin, 2004). Generally, intervention for young children with LI can take three forms: direct, indirect, or both. In **direct intervention**, the SLP conducts therapy with the child. In **indirect intervention**, the SLP trains others (e.g., parents, preschool teachers) to carry out intervention in naturalistic settings such as the home and preschool classroom. Sometimes the SLP conducts intervention with the child herself and also trains those in the child's environment to use specific techniques to stimulate the child's language development.

> Young children with LI may be served through direct intervention, indirect intervention, or a combination thereof.

One overarching principle that SLPs must remember regarding language intervention for young children is that it should closely approximate the natural process of communication. As Weitzner-Lin (2004, p. 95) says:

TABLE 7.1   Information Needed to Develop Appropriate Language Intervention Plans for Young Children

Background Factors

1. Is the intervention appropriate for the child's cultural and linguistic background?
2. Do the child's caregivers agree with and support the intervention plan?
3. Have the child's caregivers expressed interest in participating in their child's language intervention program?
4. Do they have the necessary resources to participate? (e.g., a car to get to therapy; paper, crayons, books at home)
5. How much time do the caregivers have to devote to follow through at home?
6. Are the caregivers willing to modify their style of interaction with the child to facilitate improvement in the child's language skills?
7. Do the caregivers believe that it is important for young children to communicate independently? Is it important, in the child's culture, for children to be verbally competent?

Child Factors

8. Is the child willing to separate from the caregiver to work with the clinician?
9. Is the child cooperative and able to comply with structured tasks?
10. How long can the child focus on any given intervention activity? Two minutes? Five minutes? Ten minutes?
11. Does the child show any awareness of his language disorder?
12. Does he show frustration in his attempts to communicate?
13. Does the child have accompanying behavior problems that cause the clinician to spend a large portion of therapy time trying to engage his cooperation rather than focusing on language intervention?

From Deena K. Bemstein and Ellenmorris Tiegerman-Farber. Language and communication disorders in children, 5 ed. Published by Allyn & Bacon, Boston, MA. Copyright © 2002 by Pearson Education. Adapted by permission of the publisher.

. . . language is not learned in a vacuum but rather during dynamic interactions with responsive partners. Communication and language develop in a social context to achieve largely social ends. . . . Communication occurs in natural contexts for naturally occurring reasons (intents). When working with young children, the early interventionist should remember to focus on communicative exchanges as they occur naturally in everyday environments. The major focus should be to provide the child with a communication system that is effective, efficient, and flexible. . . . The ultimate goal of intervention is age-appropriate communication.

Weiss (2002) also gives some considerations for planning intervention for young children; these are summarized in Table 7.1.

CASES TO CONSIDER

Joshua K. was a three-year-old from a monolingual English-speaking home. He had never been to preschool. He showed a substantial LI that impacted both receptive and expressive language. Joshua's mother was young, and the family had little money. Joshua had a baby brother whom the mother always brought to language therapy because she could not obtain a babysitter. In the university clinic, where I had been assigned to supervise Joshua's therapy with a graduate student, it was originally thought that Joshua would profit from one-on-one intervention designed to improve his language skills. We used a naturalistic intervention model involving toys and other items we thought would be interesting to Joshua.

After the first two or three sessions, it became clear to us that Joshua was accustomed to a very nonstructured life at home. From the mother's report, it appeared that the home life was somewhat haphazard. We were unable to get Joshua to sit in a chair for more than several seconds. Even when we tried to play with him on the floor, Joshua could not focus on an activity for more than one to two minutes. We used blocks, cars, and other appropriate and attractive materials for little boys; nothing worked. My clinic director observed therapy one day and commented that Joshua just seemed to be "bouncing off the walls."

Was this therapy setting appropriate for Joshua? Why or why not? What type of language intervention might be best for Joshua?

_____

_____

_____

Indirect Intervention: Working with Caregivers and Preschool Teachers

As Reed (2005) points out, toddlers and preschoolers spend most of their time interacting with parents/caregivers. Thus, one of the best uses of the SLP's time is to provide training and education for these people in the children's natural environments. The training and education should focus on two objectives: 1) enhancing the child's environment to facilitate change in the child's language and 2) helping the caregivers respond within that environment in a manner that is most optimal for facilitating language change (La Paro et al., 2004; Reed, 2005; Rossetti, 2001). This can often be accomplished through training caregivers and other adults who interact with young children with LI to use **milieu teaching** techniques. (Note: The SLP can use any of these techniques in direct intervention.)

POINTS TO PONDER Describe the concept of indirect intervention. Why is it important? What are two practical suggestions for utilizing indirect intervention with young children with LI?

_____

_____

_____

We will remember from previous chapters that the SLP must always keep in mind that members of other cultures believe intervention is the job of professionals, not the family (Chan & Lee, 2004; Santos & Chan, 2004; Sharifzadeh, 2004). Some CLD families may be very uncomfortable when asked to be involved in milieu teaching techniques; SLPs must work sensitively and appropriately in this situation to help the family feel comfortable.

> Because young children spend so much time with caregivers in natural environments, we can train these caregivers in milieu teaching techniques.

Milieu teaching involves organizing the child's environment with desirable activities and objects that they must request or comment upon in order to receive these activities and objects (Paul, 2001). Here, we will look more closely at milieu teaching techniques and how they can be successfully used with toddlers and preschoolers with LI (Robinson & Robb, 2002).

In the technique of **responsive interaction**, the adult works within environments that are arranged to engage the child in relevant activities (for example, playing with a dollhouse). The adult follows the child's lead and establishes joint attention; for example, when the child selects the dollhouse to play with, the adult focuses on the dollhouse too. Then, the adult follows the child's lead and comments, requests, and expands the child's attention within the context of play and social interactions.

For example, the child might pick up a chair and put it in the living room of the dollhouse. The adult can *comment*, "The brown chair is in the living room now." Then the adult can ask (*question*), "I wonder who is going to sit on the chair? Is the mommy going to sit on the chair?" Let's say the child says "no"; the adult can say, "The mommy is not going to sit on the chair (*comment*). Who will sit on the chair?" (*question*) (Note: When I worked with preschoolers with LI, I used a dollhouse; the children especially loved dropping small toys down the chimney and seeing where the toys would land. Much interaction was generated from the chimney, although that was not its original purpose!)

The milieu teaching technique of **incidental teaching** (discussed in Chapter 6) requires the adult (caregiver or SLP) to carefully observe the child and identify "teachable moments." For example, if the child reaches for a cookie, the adult can say, "You want a cookie to eat," thus engaging the child's attention and providing a label for what she is doing. As with responsive interaction, incidental teaching requires that the adult establish joint attention with the child and follow her lead (Robinson & Robb, 2002).

In another example of incidental teaching, when my son Mark was two years old, we could look out the window into our yard and see squirrels chasing each other. If he was the first to see the squirrels, he would point and call out in great excitement, "Kwerl, Mommy! Kwerl!" I would go to look at the squirrels (establish joint attention) and say something like, "Yes! Wow! Those two brown squirrels are chasing each other around the oak tree." In this way, I was establishing joint attention with Mark, following his lead, and labeling what he was seeing.

Adults who interact with children in natural settings must be encouraged not to force verbal output and to learn to use periods of silence during communicative exchanges. As someone who did not grow up in the United States, I have observed that most Americans are uncomfortable with silence and will rush to fill it. Many American caregivers and professionals believe that periods of silence during intervention should be avoided. However, in many instances, silence is followed by increased communicative attempts on the child's part (Tabors, 1997; Weitzner-Lin, 2004). If the adult bombards the child with verbalizations, the child can become overwhelmed and reluctant to take conversational turns (Rossetti, 2001). Also, among some groups such as Arabs, conversational silences are accepted and even expected (Sharifzadeh, 2004). SLPs who work with children from these groups must remember that continuously verbally bombarding them during therapy sessions may be incompatible with the expectations of the culture.

It is ideal if adults, during their interactions with young children, can avoid yes/no questions as much as possible. When the child responds with a yes/no answer, opportunity for turn-taking is restricted. As Rossetti (2001, p. 241) says, yes/no questions are "the death of communication exchanges." Instead of asking yes/no questions, adults can ask wh- questions such as "why . . . " or "how . . . " or they can use lead-in phrases such as "Tell me about. . . . "

It is ideal if SLPs can go into children's homes and videotape interactions between children and family members. These videotapes can be viewed later by the caregivers and the SLPs so that parents have direct, visible feedback about their interaction patterns with their child. Parents can give their opinions about the interactions, and they can be asked for suggestions as to how they can improve communication with their child. They can also be asked to identify what is currently working successfully. After this, the SLP can give his input. The SLP can then videotape the parents at a later date as they are implementing the specific suggestions that were previously discussed. In this way, parents are given continuous feedback and support for improving their communication with their children and interacting in ways that will most optimally facilitate language growth (McNeilly & Coleman, 2000; Watson & Weitzman, 2000).

More SLPs are providing services to children in their preschool classrooms. As part of these services, SLPs are training preschool teachers in strategies for language facilitation. As de Rivera, Girolametto, Greenberg, and Weitzman (2005) point out, training teachers can extend the SLP's services by enhancing the teachers' skills and ultimately freeing up some of the SLP's time. Some formal programs can be used for teacher training (such as the Hanen program mentioned in "Connect and Extend" at the left).

SLPs can also use informal methods to train preschool teachers in promoting children's language development. De Rivera et al. (2005) found that preschool children used significantly more multiword responses following topic-continuing and open-ended questions used by their teachers. Based on these results, de Rivera et al. specifically recommended that SLPs help preschool teachers to use more open-ended and topic-continuing questions to enhance children's language skills. For example, instead of asking "closed questions" such

When working with young children, we must allow periods of silence and avoid yes/no questions; the latter restrict a child's opportunities for turn-taking.

CONNECT & EXTEND

The Hanen Centre in Ontario, Canada, has a series of practical books and videotapes that can be used with parents of young children with language impairments. Some of the materials have been translated into different languages for CLD families. To learn more, contact The Hanen Centre, 1075 Bay Street Suite 515, Toronto, Ontario, Canada. You can also contact them at http://www.hanen.org

Research has shown that preschool teachers can be trained effectively to provide language stimulation for children in the preschool setting.

as "Do you want juice or milk?" teachers can ask open-ended questions like "What would you like to drink?" Examples of topic-continuing questions might be

> *Child:* I saw *Sesame Street* yesterday.
>
> *Teacher:* That's great! Did you see Big Bird?
>
> *Child:* No, I didn't see Big Bird, but I saw Kermit.
>
> *Teacher:* What was Kermit doing on the show?

You might think that preschool teachers automatically use these kinds of questions, but in fact, research has shown that many do not (O'Brien & Bi, 1995; Wittmer & Honig, 1991). I was privileged to volunteer in my son's preschool and can personally vouch for the fact that the teachers are quite busy, with many children to attend to. It is harder than one might think for a preschool teacher to truly stop and ask open-ended and topic-continuing questions of children. SLPs who encourage preschool teachers to ask these types of questions might demonstrate how easy and quick it is to incorporate them into existing daily preschool routines such as washing hands before lunch, circle time, recess, and others.

SLPs can also work with preschool teachers and day-care providers to train them in facilitating successful peer interactions for children with LI. Girolametto, Weitzman, and Greenberg (2004) showed that day-care providers can be successfully trained to do this. In the study by Girolametto et al., the day-care providers were given an in-service addressing methods for developing peer-interaction skills in preschool children and setting up peer interactions through verbal supports. For example, a caregiver might specifically prompt a child to play with a peer or might praise the child for interacting with a peer.

Girolametto et al. showed that children in the experimental group (those whose day-care providers had been trained) increased their frequency of peer-directed utterances during certain types of play. These results are encouraging, because today so many children spend much of their time in day-care settings. SLPs can provide simple suggestions or even in-services for day-care providers to teach them practical methods for helping young children with LI integrate more with their peers.

Increasing Oral Language Skills: Direct Intervention Techniques

Weitzner-Lin (2004) suggested that language intervention with young children is often successful in a context of play. The SLP can arrange activities so that targeted outcomes occur naturally. For example, if the SLP wants to work on greetings and leavetakings (*hi* and *bye*), she can use puppets or dolls in a play house to model and encourage use of these structures.

Robinson and Robb (2002) discuss several naturalistic communication intervention techniques that have been successfully used to increase the oral language skills of young children with LI. They state that (p. 156)

Naturalistic approaches to language and communication are based on the assumptions that (1) young children learn to communicate using speech and language in a variety of daily routines and activities with caregivers; and (2) intervention is best conducted within the context of familiar environments. . . . Naturalistic approaches to language intervention have their basis in "incidental teaching" techniques that rely primarily on a time-delay procedure (withholding desired items briefly) in order to elicit further communicative attempts with children with developmental delays . . . [these approaches have been called] milieu approaches . . . [there are] several common elements, including incidental teaching, social routines, turntaking, and environmental arrangement.

It is important for SLPs to intervene early to help toddlers and preschoolers with LI learn to socialize competently and successfully with their peers. Much has been written about intervention for young children with LI who have difficulties with pragmatics/social skills. These children are at increased risk of being viewed negatively by their peers; many of these children also do not have reciprocal friendships (Nungesser & Watkins, 2005). In one study, the researchers looked specifically at the difficulties that children with LI have

> A number of direct intervention techniques can be used to increase oral language skills of young children. Among other things, these techniques should focus on helping young children with LI socialize competently and successfully with their peers.

with entering peer groups and initiating play. They found that for their young subjects, these aspects of pragmatics skills were enhanced through picture symbols that visually depicted social rules. For example, Rule/Step 1 included a picture of a stick figure that said "walk" (the step was "walk over to your friend"). Step 2 had a simple picture depicting the rule "watch your friend." The picture for Step 3 depicted "get a toy like your friend is using." The Step 4 picture depicted "do the same thing as your friend," while Step 5 showed "tell an idea." The study showed that the LI children became more successful in their peer interactions as a result of the picture symbols depicting social rules (Beilinson & Olswang, 2003).

Rossetti (2001) suggested simple language-expression activities for young LI children. One is to encourage the child to play with words and noises. I used to work with a three-year-old who was practically nonverbal; however, she loved making animal noises in response to toy animals that I had in the "zoo" and on the "farm." We can also encourage the child to say "hi" and "bye." In addition, the child can be encouraged to name familiar objects and people in his environment as well as answer basic questions. It is very helpful if the child can answer such simple questions as "What do you want to eat?" "Are you sleepy?" "Where is Daddy?"

Another reason it is important to address oral language skills in young children is that research has shown that children's oral language skills in preschool are predictive of their later literacy development (e.g., Nathan, Stackhouse, Goulandris, & Snowling, 2004). The following section describes techniques to enhance development of early literacy skills.

Increasing Emergent Literacy Skills:
Direct Intervention Techniques

Emergent literacy is a term used to describe the concepts, behaviors, and skills of young children that precede and develop into conventional literacy. Emergent literacy is the foundation for later reading and writing. For most children, the foundation of emergent literacy is acquired from approximately birth to six years of age, or the time preceding formal reading

> It is important to address emergent literacy skills, which comprise two different but highly interrelated areas of development: phonological awareness and print awareness.

instruction. Emergent literacy comprises two different but highly interrelated areas of development: phonological awareness and print awareness (Justice, Chow, Capellini, Flanigan, & Colton, 2003). Print or written language awareness "describes the implicit and explicit knowledge children acquire concerning the fundamental properties of print, such as the relationship between print and speech and the functions and forms of particular language units (e.g., letters, words, punctuation marks)" (Justice et al., 2003, p. 320). Both print awareness and phonological awareness are critical to later literacy, and children with LI are at risk for problems in both of these areas.

One successful strategy for enhancing children's emergent literacy skills is **print referencing** (Justice & Ezell, 2004; Justice, Skibbe, & Ezell, 2006). Print referencing is an evidence-based strategy that SLPs and others can use to enhance the emergent literacy skills of young children. It refers to an adult's use of verbal or nonverbal cues to direct a child's attention to the functions, features, and forms of written language during shared storybook reading.

Examples of such cues are as follows (using the book *The Big Red Dog* as an example): 1) the adult can *track print*; for example, he can say, "The title of this book is *The Big Red Dog*" as he tracks his finger under the title; 2) the adult can *ask a question about the print*; for example, "Which word do you think says *bark*?" and have the child point to the word he thinks says *bark*; 3) the adult can also *comment about print*; for example, "The author of this book is Jan Hopkins" (the adult points to the two words). Empirical evidence has shown that print referencing is an excellent way to facilitate children's written-language awareness skills, and that print referencing can be applied to children from CLD as well as low-income backgrounds (e.g., Justice & Ezell, 2001; Justice & Ezell, 2002).

Using storybooks to increase emergent literacy skills (including vocabulary skills) in young children can be very effective. For example, Justice, Meier, and Walpole (2005) carried out a study where they used storybooks to foster vocabulary growth with at-risk kindergarteners who had low vocabulary knowledge. In the study, the adults who read books to children used a vocabulary-word elaboration strategy that was shown to be effective. There were three steps: 1) read the words in context, 2) define the word, and 3) use the word in a supportive context. For example (Justice et al., p. 23):

1. Adult reads text: "They came down to a *marsh* where they saw a muskrat cleaning his house."
2. Adult provides definition: "A *marsh* is a very wet place where there are wetlands covered with grasses."
3. Adult uses word in supportive context: "Like, we took a boat through the *marsh* and we saw lots of birds and alligators."

Again, for at-risk young children with low vocabulary skills, this strategy proved to be effective for vocabulary enrichment.

Paul (2001) gave a variety of suggestions for caregivers and preschool teachers to promote emergent literacy skills in young children. Paul's ideas are especially relevant for families who may be too busy to set aside specific times for emergent literacy activities during the day. The following activities can be worked into the daily routines of busy parents.

First, Paul emphasized that books should contain simple pictures that can be described or labeled with just a few words. Caregivers can "read" these simple books with their children whenever they find themselves with a few extra moments—for example, while waiting at the bus stop or in the doctor's office. Caregivers can also draw attention to and talk about print. For example, they can show the child their shopping list or read various signs (e.g., at the grocery store, at the dentist's office). At the breakfast table, caregivers can even read words on cereal boxes! Caregivers can also have children "write" thank-you notes and letters to others, even if these notes and letters are just scribbles.

Preschool teachers can have "literacy artifacts" in their classrooms such as magnetic drawing boards, stapled paper books for writing and drawing, crayons, and others. SLPs can encourage preschool teachers to display print around the classroom at the children's eye level. For example, teachers can have calendars, letters of the alphabet, small posters with print, and other things that will help enhance children's awareness of print. Chapter 10 has a list of written language attainments/preliteracy skills that children should have reached by six years of age.

In terms of preliteracy skills, Fey, Windsor, and Warren (1995) and Kaderavek and Boucher (2006) give an important caution to clinicians. According to these experts, studies suggest that a significant factor in a child's learning to read is his motivation to read. Forcing children who are not interested in reading materials to participate in shared book-reading activities when they would rather do something else may have negative effects.

If children with LI seem uninterested in shared book reading, caregivers and clinicians may need to modify their style of reading and telling stories. Fey et al. suggested that adults can modify by 1) getting the child actively involved through choral reading, completion of cloze sentences (e.g., "The sun shines during the _____"), open-ended questions, and story retelling, 2) providing feedback in the form of sentence recasts, requests for clarification, and integration of story content, and 3) focusing joint attention on a mutually pleasurable story experience. Kaderavek and Boucher (2006) recommended that for young children who are highly active, adults can use books that are short, dramatic, and manipulative (e.g., that have flaps, movable parts, or buttons to press that make noises or music). These methods will probably have the greatest impact when they are incorporated into a more comprehensive language intervention program.

Preliteracy skills develop at home and/or at preschool. As we have been saying, many young children who are diagnosed with oral language impairments in preschool are diagnosed with written language impairments in elementary school (Catts & Kamhi, 1999; Van Kleeck, Vander Woude, & Hammett, 2006). Numerous studies have shown that for preschoolers with LI, nearly half have written language difficulties into the school years (Aram, Ekelman, & Nation, 1984; Catts, Fey, Tomblin, & Zhang, 2002; Snowling, Bishop, & Stothard, 2000). Thus, it is critical that SLPs target preliteracy skills in the preschool population. In addition to targeting print awareness, SLPs can target phonological awareness (Fey et al., 1995).

> Phonological awareness is the ability to consciously reflect upon and manipulate the sound component of language.

You will remember that phonological awareness is the ability to consciously reflect upon and manipulate the sound component of language. The child with adequate phonological awareness can analyze the structure of an utterance as distinct from its meaning (Segers &

Verhoeven, 2004). For example, a child might know that a *dog* is a furry animal that barks. She would be demonstrating phonological awareness skills if she told you that the word *dog* has one syllable, begins with the /d/ sound, and ends with the /g/ sound. This child has analyzed the structure of the word *dog*.

We will remember that the promotion of literacy has been emphasized by the American Speech-Language-Hearing Association (ASHA, 2000), and as we shall discuss again in Chapter 8, phonological awareness skills are a very important precursor to reading (Gillon, 2000, 2004; Rvachew, Ohberg, Grawburg, & Heyding, 2003). Ideally, we would target phonological awareness in the preschool years to prevent delays in acquiring reading skills during the elementary school years (Rvachew et al., 2003).

Techniques to develop phonological awareness skills in children have been detailed in other sources (e.g., Blachman, 1991; Gillam & van Kleeck, 1996; Gillon, 2004; Goldsworthy, 2003; Hadley, Simmerman, Long, & Luna, 2000; Roseberry-McKibbin, 2001). Several of these techniques are summarized here based on the above-listed sources. The clinician can teach the child to

1. Count the number of words in a sentence
2. Identify the number of syllables in a word
3. Identify the number of sounds in a word
4. Identify words that rhyme
5. Demonstrate sound-blending skills (e.g., the SLP says "c-a-t; what word is that?")
6. Identify the first sound in a word (e.g., "Jose, what is the first sound in the word *dog*?")
7. Identify the last sound in the word (e.g., "Maria, what is the last sound in the word *car*?")

SLPs can use fun activities to help children develop their phonological awareness skills. Rhythm sticks and clapping can emphasize the number of sounds or syllables in words. Clinicians can also use rhymes; Dr. Seuss books are excellent for this purpose. Children can recite rhymes, act them out, and even sing the rhymes. As rhymes are sung, recited, or read, children can clap or shake a shaker for each word or syllable they hear. These are just a few of the many ideas available for increasing children's phonological awareness skills (Roseberry-McKibbin, 2006). As a clinician, I have discovered that the younger the child, the more she enjoys things like music and rhythm sticks. The goal is to actively involve the child and to make phonological awareness activities fun!

Hallahan et al. (2005) discuss the fact that using appropriate technology for increasing phonological awareness and emergent literacy skills overall can very valuable to young children, even those with mild disabilities. One option is **computer-assisted instruction (CAI)** where a computer is used to present instructional tasks. The child must always be assisted by a professional, of course, but as we will discuss again in Chapter 8, SLPs should be aware that there are many software programs available for intervention. As one example, some clinicians use Earobics (Cognitive Concepts, 1997–2003), a program on a CD with colorful, interactive games that work on skills such as auditory attention and sequential memory, sound-symbol correspondence, overall phonological awareness skills, and others.

CONNECT & EXTEND

A very thorough resource for those who wish to learn more about phonological awareness is Gillon, G.T. (2004). *Phonological awareness: From research to practice.* New York: Guilford Publications, Inc.

Serving Toddlers and Preschoolers in the Public School Setting

According to Public Law 99-457 (1986), preschool programs must be a part of the full spectrum of education offered by public schools. All states are required to assure a free and appropriate public education for every eligible child between three and five years of age. For infants and toddlers (birth to two years old), a new program called Part H was created to support states in developing and implementing early intervention services. Under Part H, each state now provides services for infants and toddlers with disabilities.

Part H specifies that programs include the following services:

- Special instruction, training, and counseling for families; this includes home visits
- Occupational and physical therapy
- Speech-language pathology services
- Psychological testing and counseling
- Coordination of services
- Early identification, screening, and assessment devices
- Medical services necessary for diagnostic and evaluation purposes only
- Health services necessary for the infant or toddler to benefit from other early intervention services

> Federal law has specific mandates for provision of free and appropriate services for children from birth to five years of age.

Each state has a *child-find* system set up to locate young children who are at risk and refer them to the local education agency for preschool services (Hardman et al., 2006; Nelson, 1998). Referrals may come from doctors, social workers, parents, preschool teachers, and others. When a young child is referred, generally a multidisciplinary team conducts an assessment to see if the child is eligible for special education services under the guidelines of federal law. If the child is found eligible, then a specific plan is developed for her that delineates specific services to be provided.

If a young child is found to have a speech-language disorder, services may be provided in various settings such as a special daily preschool for children with disabilities, a day-care center, the typical preschool the child currently attends, a typical public school (kindergarten through sixth grade), or in the child's home. For these young children, the special education team develops an Individual Family Service Plan (IFSP). The IFSP lists all the necessary services, the location of the services, the person responsible for providing each service,

> **POINTS TO PONDER!** Summarize what the federal law says about providing services to young children with LI in public school settings.
>
> _____
>
> _____
>
> _____

and the responsibilities that will be assumed by the child's caregivers (Moore-Brown & Montgomery, 2001; Weitzner-Lin, 2004).

In this book, I emphasize the importance of working with the families of children with language impairments. This work can be viewed through the lens of **family systems theory** (Luterman, 2001). Family systems theory emphasizes that clinicians should view clients as individuals and also as members of a family system that can be defined by 1) relationships between family members, 2) relationships between the family and school and/or the family and work; 3) the legal system, social policy, and public attitudes that influence people with disabilities, and 4) the family's social support network (e.g., other family members, friends, churches, and other organizations). When working with CLD children and their families, a family systems theory perspective is particularly relevant.

 ## SUMMARY

- When we provide intervention for young children, we can think in terms of direct intervention, indirect intervention, or both.
- Toddlers and preschoolers spend most of their time with caregivers. Thus, speech-language pathologists should train these caregivers (parents, preschool teachers) to use effective language stimulation techniques such as those found in the milieu teaching model.
- Direct intervention techniques to increase children's oral language skills include those that we discussed in Chapter 6 as well as naturalistic communication intervention strategies such as encouraging children to play with words and noises.
- As we work directly with increasing emergent literacy skills in young children, we can use strategies such as print referencing and phonological awareness activities. Computer-assisted instruction can be utilized.
- Federal law states that clinicians who work in public schools must follow the mandates of Part H, which specifically delineates services that programs are expected to provide for young children with disabilities.

Add your own summary points here:

_____

_____

_____

ADDITIONAL CONSIDERATIONS FOR CLD CHILDREN AND THEIR CAREGIVERS

Working with Families

We have discussed the fact that children and other family members must be viewed as part of a larger family system; when working with CLD families, we must remember that working within this larger family system is critical to success (Hanson, 2004). When we make recommendations to families for working with their LI children in the home, it is important that we are sensitive to the language and culture of the home (Brice, 2002; Hammer & Weiss, 2000; Roseberry-McKibbin, 2008; Weiss, 2002).

In previous chapters, we discussed and gave examples of how caregivers from various CLD backgrounds interact with their children. The ways that they interact are often different from what many SLPs would consider "mainstream," and we must be careful never to imply to families that their way of doing things is wrong or inadequate. For example, we might think that parents who do not encourage their children to speak as much as possible are doing things "wrong." Van Kleeck (1994, p. 69) addresses this issue:

> Parent programs focused on parent-child interactions often have as either an explicit or implicit goal that parents should try to encourage the child to communicate as frequently as possible. This aligns well with the mainstream culture generally valuing a relatively high degree of verbosity in children. Indeed, an entire line of social science research views reticence as a social deficiency. . . . For example, as compared to their more talkative peers, reticent children are viewed by their teachers as significantly less likely to do well in all academic areas, and less likely to have positive relationships with other students. . . . Indeed, quietness in the classroom may lead to a speech-language pathology referral.

Van Kleeck goes on to remind us that in contrast to mainstream culture, many cultures value quietness in children. For example, American Indians value a child's ability to observe and wait silently (Joe & Malach, 2004). Many Asian parents also value quietness in children (Chan & Lee, 2004). In a recent study, Johnston and Wong (2002) surveyed English-speaking North American and Chinese mothers regarding their discourse practices with their children. They found that there were clear differences between the two groups. The Chinese mothers were much less likely to report that they often talked with their children about nonshared events of the day, allowed their children to converse with adults who were non–family members, and prompt their children for personal narratives. Doing activities such as these would potentially treat the child as an equal conversational partner and thus reflect an expectation that the child would exhibit early verbal competence as well as independence.

These are not the child-raising goals of many Chinese parents, who value social interdependence (as opposed to independence) and hold only modest performance expectations for preschool-age children (Chan & Lee, 2004; Fung & Roseberry-McKibbin, 1999; Chao, 1995; Wang, 2001). Johnston and Wong (2002) also found that only 30 percent of the Chinese mothers reported that they frequently read books to their young children. Chinese mothers disagreed more strongly than the Western mothers that children learn through play and agreed more strongly that children learn best with instruction (e.g., use of flashcards).

Based upon the results of their survey, Johnston and Wong made several recommendations for professionals who work with Chinese families, and these recommendations can be extrapolated to some other CLD groups as well. First, when a currently recommended Western practice (e.g., reading with children) is not found in a particular

CONNECT & EXTEND

An excellent, readable article about being culturally sensitive when working with parents of LI children was written by van Kleeck, A. (1994). Potential cultural bias in training parents as conversational partners with their children who have delays in language development. *American Journal of Speech-Language Pathology, 3,* 67–78.

Mainstream US clinicians expect children to be very verbal and act as conversational partners with adults. However, these values are incompatible with those of some CLD families.

culture, professionals can recommend "functional equivalents." For example, for families who do not have a tradition of reading books to their children when they are young, clinicians might recommend using family photo albums or oral storytelling in place of reading. Second, SLPs may recommend that Chinese parents create explicit language lessons for their children rather than embed their language teaching in play as Western experts usually recommend.

Earlier in this book, we discussed research by Hammer et al. (2004) about working with Mexican American families. Hammer et al. stated that many of these families believe that the role of the school and the home should not interfere with each other. Many Mexican American families believe that they are being helpful by maintaining a respectful distance from the educational system. Hammer et al. concluded that Hispanic families in general are very interested in and supportive of their children's education and they believe that they should not interfere with the educational process.

I have found that families from other CLD backgrounds often believe and behave in a similar manner. I have attempted to use cultural mediators in these cases to help the families understand that in the United States, we welcome and encourage family involvement. To put it informally, this has sometimes been a "hard sell." I have attempted to maintain a balance between respecting families' beliefs and encouraging them to participate in their children's speech-language intervention. Many times, I have ended up just recommending that they read with their children as much as possible. Most families have seemed comfortable with this (if the parents themselves were literate).

As we have said, and will reiterate in Chapter 8, SLPs need to support parents in carrying out literacy activities in the home. Specific suggestions for helping CLD families to do this are given in Chapter 8; for right now, we will say that research has conclusively shown that the home environment is one of the most important variables contributing to the development of literacy skills (Fritjers, Barron, & Brunello, 2000; Justice et al., 2002; Snow, Burns, & Griffin, 1998).

Roberts, Jurgens, and Burchinal (2005) conducted a study examining how four specific measures of home literacy practices and a global measure of the quality and responsiveness of the home environment during the preschool years predicted children's language and emergent literacy skills between the ages of three and five. The subjects were seventy-two African American children and primary caregivers (mostly mothers) from low-income families. When the children were between eighteen months and five years of age, their mothers were interviewed annually about how often they read to their children and how much the children enjoyed being read to. The researchers also observed the mothers reading with their children; in addition, the researchers observed the overall quality and responsiveness of the home environment.

Roberts et al. (2005) concluded that the global measure of overall responsiveness and support of the home environment was the strongest predictor of the children's language and early literacy skills. In other words, the overall environment of the home was more important to children's overall language and literacy skills than specific literacy/ reading strategies employed by the mothers. Thus, we can conclude from this study that although it is important to help parents learn specific strategies for promoting emergent literacy, it may be as or more important for us to help parents learn to provide a home environment that is organized, emotionally and verbally responsive, accepting of children's behavior, and characterized by maternal involvement as well as availability of materials

SLPs must help CLD families to carry out in the home literacy activities that are culturally congruent.

that provide academic and language stimulation. More research is needed to support the findings of this one study.

Paul (2001) gives some specific suggestions for working with CLD families to encourage them to enhance emergent literacy skills in their young children with LI. Like Johnston and Wong, she points out that many families are more comfortable telling stories orally than reading to their children. In these cases, we can encourage parents to tell as many stories as possible and to retell them frequently. We can encourage parents to read books to their children in their first languages if such books are available. As we said before, we can also encourage parents to access the local library for culturally relevant books, where they can point out pictures and discuss these pictures with their children.

All in all, it is recommended that clinicians create training programs that fit the family—programs that are culturally congruent with the family being served. Clinicians can do this by carefully observing the family to see which interactions are successful and which lead to frustration (McNeilly & Coleman, 2000). Clinicians can build on the successful interactive strategies that the family is already using, thus reinforcing what the family is doing right (van Kleeck, 1994). For interactions that lead to frustration, clinicians can problem-solve with families and ask for the families' input regarding what they think might be helpful. Once trust and positive interaction are established between the clinician and family, the clinician can present suggestions and ask for the family's input about the suggestions.

From my experience in working with families, I think that many SLPs (including me!) are guilty of telling families what to do without gathering their input about what we are suggesting. Because we are frequently in a hurry, we hand the family ideas—verbally, on paper, or both—and rush through the suggestions without really pausing to make the families an integral part of the interaction. We don't take the time and care to find out if what we are suggesting is culturally congruent for our CLD families, or even possible for families to implement given their circumstances. I talked in a previous chapter about a former student of mine who was working with a migrant Hispanic family. After an hour of hearing suggestions, they told the team that they lived in their car and asked how (given their circumstances) they might implement the many ideas that the team had given them. We don't want to make that mistake!

As we work with CLD families, we need to remember that families of children with any type of disability are under more stress than other families (Hardman et al., 2006; Rossetti, 2001; Shipley & Roseberry-McKibbin, 2006). When a child is born with a recognizable disability, families often experience shock. They can also feel anger, confusion, anxiety, and bewilderment. As Hardman et al. state, the level of impact varies, but for most parents, an event such as this creates a family crisis of considerable magnitude. For parents who speak little or no English and are struggling with acculturating to the United States, their difficulties are greatly compounded (Lynch, 2004; Zuniga, 2004). You have probably been in a medical situation where you felt confused by the maze of paperwork and negotiations needed to get services you need. Imagine how a CLD family must feel, especially if they do not speak English and have limited financial resources. They need SLPs to be empathetic and supportive.

One way that SLPs can be empathetic and supportive is to emphasize the positive and interact in a personable manner. Many CLD families expect the professional to be somewhat like a friend (Chan & Lee, 2004; Shipley & Roseberry-McKibbin, 2006;

Sharifzadeh, 2004; Zuniga, 2004). The SLP can take advantage of this (within professional boundaries, of course) and show an interest in the family as a whole rather than just in the child who is being assessed and/or treated. For example, I like to ask parents about the child's siblings and, if time allows, a little bit about how the family came to the United States and how they like it here. I have learned a great deal by doing this, and the families I have worked with have been very appreciative of my interest. Of course, not all families may want to chat; we have to interact with families on an individual, case-by-case basis.

I have found that many CLD families appreciate hearing that their child is well-behaved, obedient, and respectful (if this is indeed the case!). Even if a child has a relatively severe LI, clinicians can still find many good things to say about the child, and families appreciate hearing it. I frequently find that when I am sharing the results of my diagnostic reports and recommendations for treatment, it is highly effective to begin with a statement like "I really enjoyed working with Anaak. She was respectful, hardworking, and had a great attitude. You must be very proud of her! Let me share with you what I found during my assessment of her language skills."

> Though there are exceptions, many CLD families appreciate it when the SLP is warm and friendly and takes an interest in the family as a whole.

McNeilly and Coleman (2000) state that we can empower families by giving them information. However, we need to remember that some families may be reluctant to participate in early intervention services. "For some, there is a high degree of shame associated with receiving certain types of services, especially if those services are offered through government agencies such as the health department or social services. Some people may have religious convictions that make them hesitant to participate in services offered by various agencies" (McNeilly & Coleman, 2000, pp. 85–86).

Hwa-Froelich and Westby (2003; mentioned earlier) found in their study of Southeast Asian children in Head Start programs that the parents believed 1) invisible learning problems are not a disability, 2) children with severe disabilities are not able to contribute to the family and thus should be provided with lifelong care; and 3) if children perform poorly at school, they and their families lose face. Thus, for these parents, it was better to stay at home than to go to school and lose face. SLPs and other professionals need to be aware of these beliefs and be aware that they may be unable to support families without the services of cultural mediators (defined earlier).

When professional teams encounter challenges in working with CLD families, it can be helpful to utilize the services of a cultural mediator. Roles and responsibilities of the cultural mediator include acting as a liaison between parents and members of the team, being an advocate for the family, and serving as a source of information from the parents to the team. In addition, the cultural mediator can serve as a community link between staff and parents to ensure that parents are part of the team and that their needs are voiced. Cultural mediators often also serve as interpreters during assessments and meetings with parents, and they may translate written documents for the parents (McNeilly & Coleman, 2000). Cultural mediators can be of great assistance when SLPs conduct home visits. Guidelines for home visits with CLD children and their families are given in Table 7.2.

> A cultural mediator can contribute greatly to the SLP's success in interacting with CLD families.

TABLE 7.2   Guidelines for Professionals: Home Visits with CLD Families

Family Structure

Family Composition

> Who are the members of the family system?
> Who are the primary decision makers?
> Is decision-making individual or group oriented?
> What is the family hierarchy with regard to status? Is status related to age, gender, or both?
> Do family members all live in the same household?
> Are there several generations living under one roof?

Primary Caregivers

> Who is the primary caregiver?
> Does the primary caregiver role rotate between members of the household?
> Who participates in the caregiving?
> Are siblings involved in caregiving?
> What is the amount of care given by the mother versus other family members?
> How much time does the child spend away from the primary caregiver?
> Is there any conflict between the child's caregivers regarding child-care practices?

Child-Rearing Practices

> What are the family's eating practices?
> What does the family believe about breast-feeding? About bottle feeding?
> Does the child sleep with the parents or other family members?
> Is there an established bedtime?
> Does the child take a nap during the day? If so, how often and for how long?
> What are the boundaries of acceptable child behavior?
> What form does discipline take?
> Who carries out the discipline?
> If a child cries, how long does he cry before someone responds?
> How does the caregiver calm down the crying child?

Language and Communication Styles

> What language(s) are spoken in the home?
> Who speaks which languages?
> What language do adults use to speak to each other? To the children?
> What are considered typical first words for a child to speak in the family's language?
> Do any family members speak English? If so, how proficiently?
> Are the adults in the family literate in their native language? In English?
> Does the family generally interact in a loud or quiet manner?
> Does the family share feelings easily?
> When a visitor comes to the home, does the family want social "chit chat" before getting down to business?
> What is the best communication style for team members to use in regard to pace of conversation, eye contact, and distance between speakers?

(continued)

TABLE 7.2 Guidelines for Professionals: Home Visits with CLD Families (*continued*)

Other

> How do members of the family gain access to and utilize social services?
>
> What are the healing systems used by this family's culture?
>
> How do members of the family typically interact with members of the teaching and medical professions?
>
> What are the family's rituals and routines? (e.g., church or temple attendance each Sunday, dinner together each evening)

Based on Lynch, 2004; McNeilly & Coleman, 2000; Roseberry-McKibbin, 2008; Weitzner-Lin, 2004

As I've said before, I have frequently been humbled by seeing the critical role that cultural mediators play in my own work setting. Sometimes I have done my very best to work with a family and had limited success until the cultural mediator showed up. Professionals need to be humble and open to help from these team members; often, we cannot do our jobs without them. The case below illustrates this point.

CASES TO CONSIDER

Trong N. was a young Vietnamese boy with an SLI and fluency problems. I evaluated him and wanted to place him on my caseload as he qualified for services. Because my schedule was so very busy (I was trying to do my own job plus that of another SLP who was out on sick leave), I tried to catch Trong's father when he picked Trong up from school to have him sign the individualized education plan (IEP). The teacher pointed out Mr. N. to me, and when I approached him and tried to obtain his signature, I was met with a suspicious stare from a parent who spoke very little English. As best I could, I explained the IEP to Mr. N., but he frowned and shook his head, refusing to sign the IEP.

As I reflected on my lack of sensitivity and rushed behavior in this situation, I realized that I might be more successful if I took the time to obtain the services of the Vietnamese interpreter, Ms. Chang, to be a cultural mediator for me. Ms. Chang called Mr. N. and invited him to a private meeting. The three of us sat down, and Ms. Chang explained my evaluation findings and recommendations in Vietnamese. Ms. Chang and Mr. N. had a lengthy conversation in Vietnamese, where I saw Mr. N. begin to visibly relax and even start to smile. He willingly signed the IEP and left campus a happy man.

Ms. Chang told me that five years before, Trong's mother had deserted her family of a husband and five children. Mr. N. had lived on welfare ever since with his children, and understandably was under a great deal of pressure. He was afraid to sign any papers because he was afraid they would reflect badly on him and his son. But after hearing a full explanation of the evaluation and speech-language services being offered to Trong, he was "thrilled" (in Ms. Chang's words) that his son was going to get help.

> What did I do wrong in the first place? (Perhaps a better question—what *didn't* I do wrong?) In what ways was I insensitive to Mr. N's needs? How could I have handled this situation differently?
>
> _____
>
> _____
>
> _____

In addition to asking the questions in Table 7.2, the clinician can also keep the following guidelines in mind. First, emphasize to parents that being bilingual is a great asset to their child. As I've said before, I have worked with so many families who have been told by school personnel to "speak only English at home." This deplorable advice is not only detrimental for children whose caregivers speak a different language, but it also undermines a family's self-confidence.

I have worked with so many parents who were vastly relieved to hear that using their primary language with their children was advantageous. If parents speak only English when they are not comfortable with it, their interactions with their children will be less rich in the vocabulary and extended discourse that children need to develop language skills as fully as possible (Genesee et al., 2004; Kohnert et al., 2005). Wong Fillmore (1991, p. 343) wrote

> What is lost when children and families can't communicate easily with one another? What is lost is no less than the means by which parents socialize their children: When parents are unable to talk to their children, they cannot easily convey to them their values, beliefs, understandings, or wisdom about how to cope with their experiences. . . . When parents lose the means for socializing and influencing their children, rifts develop and families lose the intimacy that comes from shared beliefs and understandings.

In addition to reinforcing use of the primary language at home, SLPs can also bring some of the child's completed work to show parents as well as pictures of the children participating in preschool activities. For parents who do not have transportation to visit their child's preschool, it is a great gift to see their child actively engaged in the preschool environment. If parents can see some of their child's work, such as pictures or crafts, they often feel more engaged and involved in what is happening at the preschool. Parents who feel more involved and engaged in their child's preschool experience are more likely to cooperate with SLPs' and teachers' recommendations for home carryover assignments and/or environmental modifications.

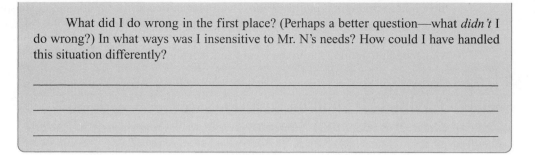

SLPs should emphasize to CLD parents that it is advantageous to speak the primary language to the child in the home; additionally, families appreciate being put in touch with support networks of people from their own backgrounds.

Many families also appreciate being put in touch with support networks, especially those composed of people from their own cultural and linguistic background. In Chapter 6, I told the story of the Chinese immigrant mother whom I was unable to comfort or communicate success-fully with despite my best efforts; however, when she saw the Chinese interpreter come into the therapy room, she lit up, smiled, and was extremely receptive to the interpreter, who ended up inviting her to the local Chinese church.

Serving CLD Children with LI in Day Care or Preschool Settings

Earlier in this chapter, we talked about intervention occuring in the day care or preschool set-ting. It would be ideal, as we have discussed previously, if intervention for CLD children with LI could occur in their first language (Kohnert et al., 2005). However, the reality for many CLD children is that their parents place them in monolingual English-speaking preschools and thus, they must face the challenge of learning to interact successfully with peers in a lan-guage that is unfamiliar to them. CLD children with LI in preschool settings can pose a spe-cial challenge for SLPs and classroom teachers (Damico & Damico, 1993; Weiss, 2002).

Teachers and SLPs cannot just assume that CLD children who are LI will automati-cally engage in beneficial interactions with TD mainstream English speakers. Rather, these children will need the adults around them to facilitate language interaction opportunities with peers. Genesee et al. (2004) recommended that if CLD children are not fully socialized with mainstream children, they should be given assistance and support in acquiring the cul-tural understanding and social skills that they need to make friends and function effectively in mainstream settings. Other researchers (e.g., Tabors, 1997; Weiss 2002;) have specifically recommended that when a CLD child with LI asks or tells the adult something, the adult can redirect the child to a TD mainstream child in the classroom. The adult can also teach the child specific strategies for speaking to a TD peer. This technique can be used with CLD children with LI or even with TD CLD preschool children who are learning English.

For example, let's take the case of Ryan Z., my son Mark's best friend in Montessori preschool, whom I have mentioned earlier in the book. Ryan, who came to Montessori speaking only Mandarin, might come and tug on the teacher's arm and point to the bath-room. The teacher could say, "Ryan, go ask your friend Mark to go to the bathroom with you. Walk up to him and say, 'Mark, bathroom,' and take his hand." In this way, Ryan would be encouraged to interact with a peer and also learn a strategy for gaining the peer's atten-tion. SLPs and preschool teachers can do a number of things to help these children succeed in the English-speaking preschool setting.

> CLD children with LI will need extra support to inte-grate with peers in the pre-school setting. These chil-dren can be taught specific strategies for suc-cessful peer interaction.

Tabors (1997) coordinated the Harvard Language Diversity Project, a research activity of the New England Quality Research Center on Head Start. Tabors' research yielded some excellent, prac-tical, evidence-based strategies for providing additional support to preschool children who are learning English as a second language. We said earlier that even young children tend to not interact with peers whom they somehow perceive as different; unfortunately, some preschool monolingual English-speaking children tend to reject peers who are learning English because these English Language Learners often interact little if at all. As Tabors (p. 110) stated, this probably happened in her study because " . . . the English-speaking children probably believed that the second-language children's unresponsiveness to their social advances was meant as rejection rather than an inability to understand." The monolingual English-speaking children may interpret the CLD children's lack of communication as a general lack of interest and thus tend to not choose the CLD children as playmates for games and other activities.

To support CLD children in this situation, Tabors recommended that teachers give these children some immediate, routine phrases to initiate conversation with peers. For example, even young children in the very early stages of English language learning can be taught to say, "Hi, how are you?" or "See ya!" When children are taught these routine phrases, they immediately open themselves up to more language exposure and interaction with other children.

A second strategy that preschool teachers can use is to ask parents of CLD children to teach them a few key words in the children's home language. The research of Tabors and her colleagues showed that it was most helpful for CLD preschoolers during the first few weeks of preschool if the teachers could say words like *listen, eat*, and *bathroom* in the children's first languages. This gave the CLD preschoolers a sense of connection with the teachers and also helped the children learn the preschool routines more quickly.

A third strategy successfully used by teachers of CLD children was to give the children a great deal of verbal "space" for the first few weeks. The teachers smiled at the children and welcomed them, but did not overwhelm the children by calling on them right away or issuing directives to them (which the children wouldn't understand anyway). When the teachers eventually did start addressing the children directly, they "doubled the message" by accompanying their words with an action, gesture, or directed gaze. This gave the children some redundance and enhanced their comprehension of what the teachers were communicating.

Tabors (1997) stated that in her research, it was found that one of the most helpful strategies used by preschool teachers of CLD children was the establishment of a consistent set of routines. These routines could be learned very easily by children who spoke little or no English, because the routines were simple and were used daily. The routines included things like cleanup, snack time, outside play, circle time, putting toys away, and others that allowed the CLD children to immediately act like members of the group. During routines such as singing, it was found that many CLD children "opened up" for the first time as they sang songs in their second language of English.

Another strategy that helped the CLD children fit into the group faster and thus socialize more was that the teachers always structured small group activities to include a mix of CLD and monolingual-English-speaking children. This was very helpful to the CLD children because they did not have to negotiate entry into the groups; they were automatically included. Once included in the activities, they had opportunities to interact with the other children and also opportunities to be exposed to English.

We have said earlier that a major challenge for some CLD children with LI who enter a school situation is that they have not been read to at home. When they enter preschool and teachers read in their second language, it can be difficult for them to pay attention and receive any benefit from being read to. Tabors' research found that there were several practical strategies that helped book-reading time become more productive for CLD children.

First, teachers had more success in maintaining the children's attention when they kept book-reading time short. Second, it was found that predictable books worked very well because they had simplified and highly repetitive text that made it easy for the CLD children to

> Preschool teachers can help CLD children to integrate successfully into the classroom setting in many ways. They can establish a consistent set of routines, structure small-group activities appropriately, and help book-reading time to be productive.

CONNECT & EXTEND

Dr. Patton Tabors from Harvard University has many practical suggestions for working with preschool CLD children in her 1997 book *One child, two languages: A guide for preschool educators of children learning English as a second language.* Baltimore, MD: Paul H. Brookes Publishing Co.

become engaged. For example, a predictable book might start off by saying, "ten little monkeys sitting in a tree—teasing Mr. Alligator—can't catch me! Along comes Mr. Alligator, quiet as can be, and SNAPS that monkey right out of that tree!" Then on the next page, "nine little monkeys sitting in a tree . . . ," etc. It was also helpful to read the books many times so that the CLD children got more information and vocabulary each time they listened to stories. When they were somewhat familiar with a story, the CLD children were encouraged to "read" the story to other children. This increased their confidence with reading.

We talked earlier in this chapter about having preschool teachers redirect children's questions and comments to peers. Tabors and her colleagues at Harvard found that this was an excellent technique for helping their CLD children increase peer interactions. For example, if a CLD child came to a teacher wanting to share a toy with another child, the teacher would say something like, "OK, Shauntaye, I want you to go over to Nathan and say, 'May I play with the truck too?'" The teacher then stayed close by to make sure that the CLD child successfully completed the interaction.

Tabors (1997) and her colleagues successfully integrated the parents of the CLD children into the preschool setting and increased their involvement by allowing them to volunteer for simple tasks (e.g., pouring juice, cleaning up the paint area) that did not require knowledge of English. They also had the parents demonstrate a skill or talent such as dancing a folk dance with a costume from the home country, cooking a native dish for all the children, and others. One mother came and taught all the preschool children how to use chopsticks. Chopsticks were subsequently incorporated permanently into the playhouse area.

SUMMARY

- As we have frequently stated, it is very important to work with families of young children with LI. This is particularly important for CLD children, who are considered to be members of a family system.
- Some CLD families have values that differ from those of mainstream US clinicians. For example, some families value quietness in children and do not value verbosity. Other families believe that it is disrespectful for them to become "too involved" in their child's program. Utilization of cultural mediators can be important in such cases.
- Many families are under a great deal of stress, and we must be sensitive to this. It is important in our interactions with these families to "emphasize the positive" and to provide as much support as possible to empower families.
- Part of this empowerment is to emphasize that using the first or primary language in the home is ideal for children. Another idea for empowering families is to put them in touch with support networks of people from their own backgrounds.

- CLD children with LI in preschool settings need support from their teachers. Preschool teachers can utilize many practical strategies to provide this support.

Add your own summary points here:

_____

_____

_____

CASES TO CONSIDER

Phong H. was referred to me by his preschool teacher, who was concerned about his language development and his classroom skills. I found out that Phong's family only spoke Vietnamese at home; they did not read or write in Vietnamese. Phong had few friends, even among the other Vietnamese students. He could not even communicate basic needs, such as the need to go to the bathroom. Mr. L., the Vietnamese interpreter who had worked with Phong, said that Phong appeared "slow" in his Vietnamese development. With Mr. L.'s help, I conducted an assessment of Phong's language skills and found, among other things, that even in Vietnamese, Phong's utterances were very short. When Mr. L. read Phong a simple story in Vietnamese and had Phong retell the story, Phong was disorganized, omitted many major details, and was unable to tell the story sequentially. He demonstrated very low vocabulary skills in Vietnamese and had difficulty following simple directions (Phong's father, Mr. H., confirmed that this was representative of Phong's communicative behavior at home also). Other assessment tasks confirmed the presence of an LI.

When Mr. H. came to pick Phong up, I was able (with the interpreter's help) to find out more information about his concerns regarding Phong (I had not been able to talk with him before the evaluation, unfortunately, but this is often typical when parents are busy). Mr. H. shared that when his wife became pregnant with Phong, she was diagnosed with an ovarian cyst shortly thereafter. No one knew that she was pregnant, and she was given a general anesthetic while the cyst was surgically removed. After this, she took strong medications for several weeks to control her pain.

Approximately ten weeks into the pregnancy, Mrs. H. realized that she was pregnant. Mr. H. said that he had always been worried that the baby would be "slow." According to Mr. H., when Phong was a toddler, "Phong don't say much words in Vietnamese. He slow to walk too." He shared that Phong's younger brother was "much faster than Phong" in both speech and motor skills. He said that "At home, when I tell Phong to do something, he ignore me; I have to tell him four or five times. I think he just disobedient."

With the interpreter's help, I shared my testing results with Mr. H. I told him how much I had enjoyed working with his son, and emphasized that Phong was very

(continued)

cooperative during testing. I said that I would like to see him several times a week for speech-language therapy, and Mr. H. agreed to this. I recommended that Mr. H. and his wife talk with Phong at home as much as possible and encourage Phong to verbalize more. He said that he and his wife worked several (low-paying) jobs and were very tired; plus, in the area of Vietnam where he was raised, parents did not conduct language stimulation activities with their young children.

I told Mr. H. that he and his wife did not have to take extra time out of their schedules to do special, additional activities with Phong. I shared some milieu teaching techniques, and asked Mr. H. if he or his wife could look at one book with Phong each day and discuss it in Vietnamese. He said he thought that could work. I also told Mr. H. that rather than being disobedient, Phong might not be comprehending the directions that he heard. We discussed ways for Phong's parents to simplify directions so that Phong could comprehend them.

Toward the end of our meeting, Mr. H. said that several professionals had told him and his wife to speak only English at home and not speak in Vietnamese to their children so the boys would learn English faster. The interpreter and I explained that this was completely erroneous advice, and said that Phong was very fortunate to have the opportunity to be raised bilingual. We stressed that if Phong was a bilingual Vietnamese-English-speaking adult, he would be eminently desirable to employers. Mr. H. understood this, and was quite relieved to learn that it was not only okay, but was optimal for him and his wife to talk to Phong and his brother in Vietnamese.

Are there any other recommendations I could have made to Mr. H.? Describe any other ideas you think might have been relevant in this situation.

_____

_____

_____

CHAPTER HIGHLIGHTS

- Children may have LI secondary to established risk factors such as genetic syndromes, neurological disorders, and others that are known to professional teams. They may also appear to be TD early in life, but be at risk for developing LI due to conditions such as serious prenatal and/or natal complications, a chronically dysfunctional home, and others.
- Important precursors to language development include the ability to recognize and attend to environmental change, awareness on the child's part that he can be an agent of change in his environment, and the ability to engage in reciprocal interactions and routines and establish joint reference with adults.
- Young children with LI have difficulty in all areas of language. Late bloomers/late talkers often have normal receptive language skills but delayed expressive language skills. Research suggests that even though many of these children may go on to perform within normal limits on standardized tests of language and academic

development, they may still have subtle language deficits that place them at a disadvantage compared to TD peers from similar backgrounds.

- Service delivery to infants and young children with LI and/or other challenges has taken on increased visibility in the last decade. This is due to two major factors: the increased survival rate of premature infants and more specific federal legislation mandating services for these children.

- SLPs must keep some general considerations in mind when evaluating young children with potential LI. These include beginning assessment early and repeating it throughout the childhood period, working with multidisciplinary teams, making sure assessment procedures and materials are culturally and linguistically appropriate, and others.

- Specific strategies for evaluating young children with potential LI include observing their play activities, using communication and symbolic behavior scales, assessing narrative skills, using parent and teacher report measures, and using published instruments that provide norms. Clinicians can also gather language samples and calculate mean length of utterance (MLU). It is important to evaluate preliteracy skills.

- Clinicians may provide direct intervention, indirect intervention, or a combination of both for young children with LI. When utilizing indirect intervention, clinicians can train caregivers and preschool teachers. When utilizing direct intervention, clinicians can use a combination of specific techniques designed to stimulate oral language and emergent literacy skills.

- When working with young CLD children with LI and their families, it is crucial to remember that some families have different oral and literacy values than mainstream US clinicians do. We must honor these values and work in culturally congruent ways to assist families in supporting their children's language development in the home.

- Young CLD children with LI who attend preschool or day care can be supported in a number of ways. Many of these ways involve helping the children integrate successfully with peers and communicate effectively with them.

Add your own chapter highlights here:

_____

_____

_____

_____

STUDY AND REVIEW QUESTIONS

ESSAY

1. Describe established risk factors and conditions that put children at risk for developing LI.

2. Research describes "late talkers." Many of these children have normal receptive language skills but are delayed in their expressive language skills. What has research shown about long-term outcomes for these children when compared with matched, TD peers?

3. Describe three specific strategies for evaluating the language skills of a young child with potential LI.

4. Why is it important to work with the caregivers and teachers of young children with LI? How can we do this in a manner that is appropriate to the child's and family's cultural and linguistic background?

5. Let's imagine that you are an SLP assigned to several preschools that serve a number of CLD children with LI. List and briefly describe three things that you can do to support these children.

FILL-IN-THE-BLANK

6. A person who acts as a "go-between" for CLD families and mainstream professionals is called a(n) _____.

7. Rescorla's _____ is an inexpensive, simple screening tool for identifying language delay in toddlers.

8. In _____, the SLP herself conducts therapy with the child.

9. The term _____ refers to the ability to consciously reflect upon and manipulate the sound component of language.

10. The law that specifies that preschool programs must be a part of the full spectrum of education offered by public schools is _____.

MULTIPLE CHOICE

11. Which of the following are true of the language skills of preschoolers?
    a. The quality of their narrative skills is a major predicting factor for their later success in school.
    b. Preschoolers with LI often are slower to use two-word combinations than TD children.
    c. Late talkers with normal receptive language skills will eventually be on par with their TD peers in all aspects of language development.
    d. a, b
    e. a, b, c

12. You have been asked to assess the language skills of a two-year-old who was referred to you by her pediatrician. The child says very few words, and the pediatrician and parents are concerned that she may have an LI. You decide to use an instrument reputed to contain tasks and parameters that have predictive value in terms of children's communication development. These tasks and parameters include evaluating social-affective signaling, assessing communicative functions, analyzing preverbal communication, profiling communicative, social, and symbolic activities, directly assessing a child's communication in spontaneous child-initiated interactions, and using caregivers as active participants and as informants in the evaluation. This instrument is called the
    a. Preschool Language Scale: 4
    b. Language Development Survey

    c. Communication and Symbolic Behavior Scales

    d. Test of Language Development: Preschool

    e. Sequenced Inventory of Communication Development

13. You are working with the family of Roberto S., a bilingual Spanish-English–speaking four-year-old with LI. His parents are most comfortable speaking Spanish to him in the home, and he attends an all-English-speaking preschool. You encourage Roberto's parents to work with him at home in Spanish, and they are very willing to do whatever they can to support his language development. You model for them the technique of _____, which requires them to carefully observe Roberto and identify teachable moments.

    a. Incidental teaching

    b. Emergent literacy teaching

    c. Phonological awareness instruction

    d. Adult-directed interaction

    e. Child-directed interaction

14. You observe a conscientious preschool teacher with a number of LI children in her class. She uses storybooks, comments about print, uses vocabulary elaboration strategies, and has a number of books and other literacy artifacts in her classroom. Which term *best describes* the type of skills that this teacher is promoting?

    a. Pragmatics skills

    b. Emergent literacy skills

    c. Morphological skills

    d. Phonological skills

    e. Syntactic skills

15. Ehua F. is a three-year-old girl from a Mandarin-speaking home. Her parents are from Beijing, China, and came to the United States six years ago. They are highly educated, and Ehua is their only child. You "inherit" Ehua on your preschool caseload; she and her parents moved to your city from a city where Ehua was diagnosed as having an LI. Which one of the following suggestions would you probably *not* give Ehua's parents because it would be culturally incongruent for them?

    a. Use a great deal of play activities in the home to promote Ehua's language skills.

    b. Use oral storytelling as frequently as possible.

    c. Create explicit language lessons for Ehua.

    d. Use family photo albums with pictures of relatives and friends as a point of conversation.

    e. Use formal materials such as flashcards to help build Ehua's language skills.

See Answers to Study and Review Questions, page 465.

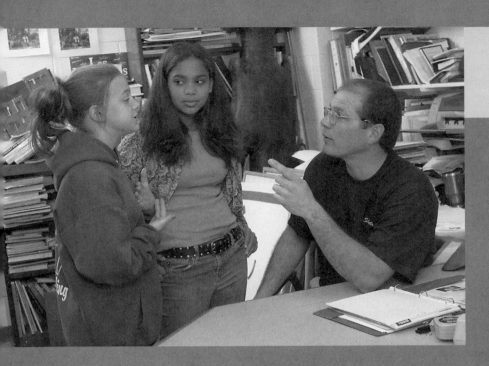

Language in School-Age Students and Adolescents with Learning Disabilities

CASE STUDY

The school personnel were baffled. Tanveer D., a handsome and outgoing fourth-grader, was struggling quite a bit in school. He had excellent conversational skills in English and was popular with other children, but according to the resource specialist, the teacher had said that "reading, writing, and spelling just aren't clicking." Tanveer's writing appeared to be quite immature for his age. His letters were large and unevenly formed. He was unable to read even basic sight words.

When I was called in to assess Tanveer, I found that the family spoke Urdu in the home and

had traveled back and forth from Pakistan extensively during Tanveer's lifetime. He had missed a great deal of school in both the United States and Pakistan due to illness. The Urdu interpreter who had been working with Tanveer said that he was "slow to catch on" even in Urdu for academic tasks. However, she stated that his conversational skills in Urdu appeared to be equivalent with those of his peers.

Because of Tanveer's inconsistent school attendance and his status as an English Language Learner, I and the other special-education team members were very reluctant to give him any type of special-education label. However, he clearly needed extra support in the form of academic assistance. The resource specialist, who specialized in intervention for students with written and academic language problems, provided extra support in the form of *neverstreaming* to see if this would help Tanveer perform better in the classroom. My school district has a special, legal arrangement with the state of California called neverstreaming. In the neverstreaming model, a student with difficulties may receive short-term intervention without an official special-education label or Individualized Education Plan. We often use the neverstreaming model with English Language Learner students such as Tanveer, whom we want to provide with extra support without giving them a label such as *learning disabled*, *speech-language impaired*, or others.

Despite being neverstreamed for resource services, Tanveer did not improve in his academic skills. He continued to struggle greatly with written language. Eventually, it was discovered through extensive testing by different specialists that Tanveer had dyslexia, a reading disorder. He was placed formally into a self-contained special education classroom where he could receive the intensive assistance that he needed to succeed in school.

INTRODUCTION

Learning Disability: Definition, Identification, and General Characteristics

Literature is replete with varying definitions of **learning disability** (e.g., Bender, 2004; Hallahan et al., 2005; Long, 2005). Woolfolk (2004) summarizes the term learning disability (LD) as describing a student who 1) has normal hearing and vision, 2) does not have emotional problems, mental retardation, or educational disadvantages, and yet 3) struggles with writing, spelling, and reading.

Of the six million students enrolled in special education across the United States, approximately half are identified as having a specific learning disability (President's Commission on Excellence in Special Education, 2002). According to the National Joint Committee on Learning Disabilities (1997)

> Learning disabilities is a general term that refers to a heterogeneous group of disorders manifested by significant difficulties in the acquisition and use of listening, speaking, reading, writing, reasoning, or mathematical skills. These disorders are intrinsic to the individual, presumed to be due to central nervous system dysfunction, and may occur across the life span. Problems in self-regulatory behaviors, social perception, and social interaction may exist with learning disabilities but do not, by themselves, constitute a learning disability.

Basically, for the student with LD, deficits in reading, writing, and spelling negatively impact other academic areas such as math and science (Paul, 2001). Table 8.1 lists common characteristics of students with LD.

TABLE 8.1   Characteristics of Students with Learning Disabilities

General Characteristics

- Boys demonstrate LD more than girls; in classes for students with LD, boys outnumber girls three or four to one.
- Most students with LD are identified during grades three or four, and most receive related services throughout their school years.
- Most students with LD have average or above average intelligence and potential.
- Student's achievement in school is not commensurate with age and grade-level expectancies, even when she is provided with appropriate learning experiences. Ninety percent of students have a discrepancy between intellectual ability and reading achievement.
- There is an uneven pattern of development in intellectual, academic, and/or social skills.
- Many students with LD perform acceptably in math even though they have significant difficulty with reading, writing, and spelling.
- A pattern of behavior problems is often evident.
- Attention problems and high levels of distractibility are common during learning tasks. Younger students with LD may fidget or move around too frequently.
- Students with LD frequently have difficulties with organization.
- Many students with LD have difficulty copying material from the blackboard or performing other tasks involving copying designs.

The student may have difficulties in one or more of the following areas:

- *Listening skills*—receptive problems, inability to comprehend what is heard
- *Oral expression*—inability to express thoughts or feelings in an appropriate, organized manner
- *Reading*—limited decoding skills and poor comprehension of what is read
- *Written language*—difficulties with spelling, grammar rules, mechanics, and usage
- *Mathematics*—difficulties with calculation, reasoning, and problem-solving; difficulties with basic operations such as addition, subtraction, multiplication, and division

The student may have difficulty and may appear "learning disabled" when he is not; rather, he may have experienced one or more of the following situations:

- Poor school attendance
- Inappropriate or inadequate instruction
- Mismatch between the student's environmental, cultural, and/or linguistic background and the instruction he is receiving in school

Learning disabilities do not exist if the student's problems can be attributed entirely to any of the following (alone or in combination):

- Emotional disturbance
- Hearing loss
- Vision problems
- Motor problems
- Mental problems
- English Language Learner status

Adapted from Bender, W.N. (2004) *Learning disabilities: Characteristics, identification, and teaching strategies* (5th ed.). Boston: Allyn & Bacon, and Hearne, D. (2000). *Teaching second language learners with learning disabilities: Strategies for effective practice*. Oceanside, CA: Academic Communication Associates.

Oral and Written Language: The Relationship

Many traditional speech-language pathologists (SLPs) have avoided working specifically on written language problems in students with LD. We will discuss this in more depth later. However, for right now, we will note that this trend is changing because professionals are seeing commonalities that underlie both oral and written language impairment.

As we have said, researchers agree that a number of children who are identified as having oral language impairments when they are young (e.g., preschool age) will later be identified as having written language impairments when they are in school (Bishop & Adams, 1990; Goldsworthy, 2003; Mody, 2004; Snowling et al., 2000). Lewis, Freebairn, and Taylor (2000) stated that 40 to 100 percent of children with early speech and language disorders have persistent language problems, and 50 to 75 percent will have difficulties with academics.

> SLPs are becoming increasingly involved in serving students with impairments in written language skills.

Kavanagh (1991) reminds us that spoken and written language are no longer viewed as parallel processes in different modalities or as separate skills. Goldsworthy (2003) describes the reciprocity between oral and written language, and Dickinson and McCabe (1991) have suggested that the acquisition of language be viewed as a "French braid" of multiple strands that interact rather then a sequential process where we first have oral language, then written language. Because of the strong relationship between oral and written language, SLPs have an integral role to play in supporting students with written language problems—students with LD.

Because the vast majority of students with LD have difficulty with reading, sometimes researchers refer to these students as being "reading impaired." Students with LD/reading impairment often have an accompanying oral language impairment (Bishop et al., 2003; Kuder, 2003; Mody, 2004). This makes it imperative that SLPs be involved in providing service delivery to these students. Long (2005, p. 143) states that

> Although the majority position at this time appears to be that language disorders and learning disabilities represent different points on a developmental continuum, several cautions are warranted. First, the position should not be misinterpreted to mean that all students with learning disabilities are also language impaired. Research on subtypes of learning disabilities . . . suggests that most but not all students with learning disabilities are deficient in some language skill or skills. Second, students with learning disabilities who have no history of spoken language impairment are not immune to language-learning deficits. Thus, students might be able to perform adequately during the preschool years when only oral language is required, but find themselves overmatched once they are asked to read and write. Third, it is possible that there are subgroups among students with language-learning disabilities. The suggestion has also been made that the labels language disorder and learning disability are applied differentially by professionals, even though they have no formal guidelines for doing so.

Gilger and Wise (2004) discuss the terms *language impairment* and *reading impairment*. Their definition of language impairment agrees with the one that we defined as *specific language impairment* in Chapter 1: the failure to develop normal expressive and/or receptive language skills that cannot be explained by deficits in nonverbal IQ, neurological impairment, or environmental or emotional problems. Gilger and Wise define developmental reading impairment as an unexpected difficulty learning to read and spell

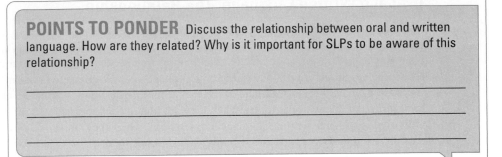

POINTS TO PONDER Discuss the relationship between oral and written language. How are they related? Why is it important for SLPs to be aware of this relationship?

despite adequate opportunity and intelligence and without demonstrable psychiatric, neurological, or sensory factors that could explain the problem. They discuss an underlying genetic component to both language and reading impairment, and state that (pp. 27–28)

> . . . it is critical to recognize that we are really talking about the genes that control the structure and function of the brain areas responsible for variations in language and reading. . . . Although the etiologic relationship between language impairment and reading impairment is unclear, the two disorders may have a common neuropsychological basis, perhaps reflected in phonology-related deficits, and the neurology of oral and written language is known to have similarities. . . . Roughly 50% of students with language impairments go on to develop reading impairments (Catts, Fey, Zhang, & Tomblin, 2002).

> Both oral and written language impairments may have a genetic base and often co-occur in students.

In Chapter 1, we mentioned a study by Flax et al. (2003). They reported on the results of two family aggregation studies that looked at the occurrence and co-occurrence of oral language impairments (e.g., specific language impairment) and reading impairments. They found that there was a pattern of frequent co-occurrence of language impairments and reading impairments in families. Like Gilger and Wise (2004), Flax et al. concluded that oral language and reading impairments probably have a genetic base and often co-occur in individuals. They emphasized the fact that early oral language impairments in students have been found to affect written and/or oral language abilities throughout the life span, creating challenges into adolescence and adulthood.

CONNECT & EXTEND

A detailed description of genetic bases for oral and written language impairment can be found in Gilger and Wise (2004), Genetic correlates of language and literacy impairments. In Stone, Silliman, Ehren, and Apel (Eds.), *Handbook of language and literacy* (pp. 25–48). New York: The Guilford Press.

Flax et al. summarized the results of studies that indicate that oral language impairments and reading impairments may not actually be separate disorders; rather, both disorders may share some common core elements that impact their co-occurrence in many individuals, with patterns of deficit changing as the individual develops. Thus, in sum, it seems safe to say that oral language and reading problems often co-occur in students and aggregate within families (Flax et al., 2003; Gilger & Wise, 2004; Koster, Been, Krikhaar, Zwarts, Diepstra, & Van Leeuwen, 2005; Rice, Haney, & Wexler, 1998).

Federal Laws Impacting Service Delivery to Students with Learning Disabilities

Some professionals do not like the term *learning disabled* because they feel it is pejorative; they prefer the term *learning different*. However, others (such as the Learning Disabilities Association of America (www.ldanatl.org) are concerned that without the specific label of learning disability, students will not receive the services they need (Morrison, 2003). It is my experience that in order to receive services through the public schools, students do need to be specifically identified as learning disabled according to state and federal guidelines.

CONNECT & EXTEND

An informative Web site with detailed information regarding LD is www.ldanatl.org.

Historically, most school districts have used a discrepancy model to identify students as having an LD. In order to be eligible for special education services, a student must have a "significant discrepancy" between potential (usually measured by IQ testing) and achievement (generally measured by one or more standardized tests of school performance). IQ must be significantly higher than achievement. This model has been criticized by experts (e.g., Bender, 2004; Goldsworthy, 2003; Hallahan et al., 2005; Paul, 2001; Parkay & Stanford, 2004; Woolfolk, 2004) for several reasons.

First, as Nelson (1998) said, even if a student doesn't have a "significant discrepancy," she still may need intervention. Goldsworthy (2003) discussed these types of students as those who "fall through the cracks." These students do not score low enough in achievement tests to have a "significant discrepancy," so they do not qualify for any extra support. However, they still struggle in school. The National Institute of Child Health and Human Development (NICHD; 2000, p. 1) says that "even people with a mild reading impairment do not read much for fun. For them, reading requires so much effort that they have little energy left for understanding what they have just read." And it is common knowledge that to succeed in school, good reading skills are critical.

Second, another problem with the discrepancy model is that it is challenging to measure IQ. When IQ tests are administered to LD students, they perform unevenly across tasks. Yet their sum total IQ score is used to decide whether or not they are truly LD or not. The sum total IQ does not accurately represent a student's strengths and weaknesses in various areas. It is especially difficult to measure IQ in culturally and linguistically diverse (CLD) students because most IQ tests are standardized on monolingual, English-speaking students. Many experts have criticized the practice of using IQ tests with CLD students to determine the presence or absence of an LD (Bender, 2004; Commission on Excellence in Special Education, 2001; Hyun & Fowler, 1995; Leung, 1996). For this and other reasons, federal law was revised so that assessment of students for special-education services in general would be less biased.

> Public schools have traditionally identified students as having a learning disability based on a large discrepancy between potential (IQ) and actual achievement.

On December 3, 2004, President Bush signed into law the Individuals with Disabilities Education Improvement Act of 2004 (Public Law 108-446). There were some changes that substantially impacted the way the term *learning disability* is defined according to federal law. The new reforms allow local education agencies to eliminate the IQ-achievement discrepancy gap, stating that local education agencies will not be required to consider whether or not a child has a severe discrepancy between intellectual ability and achievement.

In addition, the new law places greater emphasis on the use of prereferral services to prevent unnecessary referrals to special education and to minimize overidentification of children. School districts will now be permitted to use up to 15 percent of their federal funds annually, combined with other funds, to develop and implement coordinated early-intervention services. There is a special focus on children in kindergarten through third grades who have not been technically identified as needing special education but who may need additional support to succeed in the general-education environment. There is a particular focus on early intervention for students who are having difficulty developing their basic reading skills.

The newly reauthorized law also emphasizes that CLD students are often overrepresented in special education, and individual states will be asked to account for this situation if it is true for them. The law indicates that states will not only be required to keep track of how many "minority" students are being identified for special education, but they will also be required to provide coordinated, comprehensive, early intervention programs for students in groups that are overrepresented.

It will be interesting to see, in the next few years, how various states throughout the country will respond to the recently updated law that has eliminated the need for the discrepancy model in identifying LD in students. Some states may choose to continue using this model in order to manage caseload sizes. I have talked with professionals who are afraid that if the discrepancy model is no longer used to identify LD students for services, the proverbial floodgates will open and they will be asked to serve many more students than they have time to serve. Basically, individual states will have to decide whether or not to keep using the discrepancy model.

Another federal law impacting services to students with LD is the No Child Left Behind Act (U.S. Department of Education, 2002), which attempts to address inequities that are summarized below. Silliman, Wilkinson, & Brea-Spahn, (2004, p. 99) state that

> This sharp increase in enrollment [in American public schools] coexists with a crisis of illiteracy in America, which is particularly regrettable given the changed sociodemographic characteristics of American classrooms. A growing achievement gap exists among (1) minority and nonminority students, (2) those from poorer versus richer families, (3) those whose native language is English, in contrast to those whose first language is not English, and (4) those identified for special education services versus those in regular education.

> The No Child Left Behind Act tries to minimize performance inequities between mainstream students and those who perform poorly in school for various reasons.

The No Child Left Behind Act attempts to address these inequities in several ways. First, it requires students with disabilities to participate in state accountability systems for reading and math in grades three through eight. In other words, students with disabilities must take standardized state achievement tests along with their typically developing (TD) peers. Accommodations are allowed for students with disabilities, as are alternate assessments that include information similar to the standard forms.

Most schools provide accommodations. For example, last month I worked with two fifth-graders with LD who needed the accommodations of having a quiet room for test-taking and having the state test read out loud to them. The day before, the fifth-grade girl had tried to stab her mother and baby sister with a knife (she didn't succeed), so I made sure that all scissors and sharp implements were put away and that the I made the testing situation quiet, calm, and as conducive to good performance as possible. With my help, the girl was able to take the test calmly and without incident.

The No Child Left Behind Act also requires that schools must show adequate annual progress toward *all* students (including those with disabilities) being proficient in math and reading, or the schools will face penalties. Lastly, the No Child Left Behind Act mandates that teachers use scientifically based instruction in their classrooms.

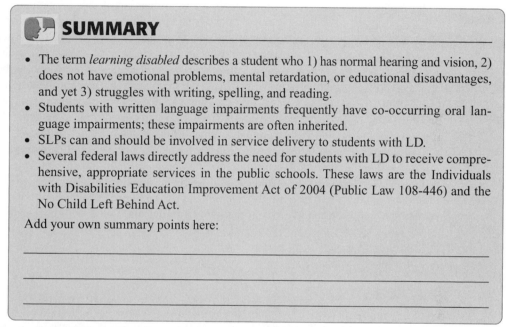

SUMMARY

- The term *learning disabled* describes a student who 1) has normal hearing and vision, 2) does not have emotional problems, mental retardation, or educational disadvantages, and yet 3) struggles with writing, spelling, and reading.
- Students with written language impairments frequently have co-occurring oral language impairments; these impairments are often inherited.
- SLPs can and should be involved in service delivery to students with LD.
- Several federal laws directly address the need for students with LD to receive comprehensive, appropriate services in the public schools. These laws are the Individuals with Disabilities Education Improvement Act of 2004 (Public Law 108-446) and the No Child Left Behind Act.

Add your own summary points here:

_____

_____

_____

ORAL COMMUNICATION PROBLEMS OF STUDENTS WITH LEARNING DISABILITIES

We said earlier that students with LD often have accompanying difficulties with oral language skills. These difficulties are seen most often in the areas of pragmatics skills, narrative skills, and semantic and grammatical skills.

Pragmatics Skills

Research has shown that, for the most part, students with LD may be less likely to find social acceptance with their peers due to poor pragmatics skills (Bender, 2004; Hallahan et al., 2005; Larson & McKinley, 1995). For example, students with LD may have difficulty with topic management or staying on the topic that other students are discussing (Seidenberg, 2002). They may also have difficulty being sensitive to the needs of their conversational partners (Kuder, 2003).

One manifestation of this is difficulty with conversational repair. For example, a listener may be confused by what the LD student is saying. A TD student would be able to repair the breakdown or explain something in a different and clearer way. A student with LD might offer a confusing explanation and have difficulty reformulating his message. In a reversed situation, students with LD are less likely to ask for clarification if they do not understand what someone else is saying.

Students with LD are often viewed as rude and insensitive because they have a hard time adjusting their language to accommodate the status of their conversational partner. They lack the ability to understand what kind of language is appropriate in various situations in order to function adequately in those situations. They might speak to the school principal in the same way they speak to their dog. Needless to say, this can cause true social and academic problems. A seven-year-old boy had a discussion with his parents about "playground language" versus "classroom language." His parents made it very clear that if he went to his classroom and repeated some of the things he heard on the playground, he could end up in the principal's office.

> Students with LD often have difficulty with pragmatics skills; these difficulties can especially cause problems during adolescence.

When students reach adolescence, difficulties with pragmatics skills can become a major problem. Brinton, Robinson, and Fujiki (2004, p. 283) state that "as children with language impairment grow into adolescence, they must navigate an increasingly complex social landscape." Adolescent conversations are fast paced, often removed from the here and now, and filled with innuendo, humor,

CASES TO CONSIDER

Tyrone L., an African American teenager with LD, came to our university clinic for assistance with his LD and also with his stuttering. We found out early in our conversations with him that Tyrone had been suspended from school a number of times. When we asked why, Tyrone shared that he was viewed as being "disrespectful and mouthy" to the teachers and principals at his school. As we worked more with Tyrone, we found that he consistently had difficulty changing the way he talked according to the listener's status. One of our therapy goals, then, was to help him learn to adjust his conversational tone and manner depending on who the listener was (e.g., a peer versus the school principal). What would you say to Tyrone? How would you help him understand the need for adjusting his conversational style according to the listener's status? What kinds of activities might you use to do this?

_____

_____

_____

and sarcasm. Adolescents greatly value perspective-taking in conversations with peers, and students with LD frequently have difficulty taking the listener's perspective.

Narrative Skills

In order to analyze students' spoken discourse skills, clinicians will often ask them to produce or listen to and answer questions about narratives. A narrative is a type of discourse that is often told in the past tense and concerns imagined or real memories of something that happened (McCabe & Bliss, 2003). In Chapter 7, we said that if preschoolers have problems with narratives, this can be predictive of an LI. As we discussed in Chapter 4, different cultures have different rules for narratives, and clinicians must take that into account.

For example, many Spanish-speaking children will deemphasize sequencing of events (McCabe & Bliss with Mahecha, 2003). In some Spanish American cultures, children will emphasize maintaining the flow of conversation among participants over telling a story-focused, monologic narrative (Meltzi, 2000). If clinicians compare students to their culturally and linguistically similar peers, they will have the best chance of accurately analyzing the appropriateness of a given CLD student's discourse skills.

In general, clinicians can be aware of the following signs of narrative difficulties that are typical of students with LD (Gillam & Carlile, 1997; Long, 2005; Thorardottir & Ellis Weismer, 2002; Wright & Newhoff, 2001):

1. In story retell, students with LD may have less knowledge of the world to help them interpret motivations and events in stories.
2. Students with LD have difficulty making inferences from stories; they may be able to recall simple facts verbatim, but they have trouble reasoning with the facts. These students may be more successful at making inferences about narratives they hear than about narratives that they read.
3. When students with LD retell stories, they reduce the amount of information that was in the original story. Often their spontaneous narratives are shorter and contain fewer complete episodes than those of TD students.

> Students with LD frequently have problematic narrative skills. SLPs must be careful to account for different cultural narrative styles.

4. Students with LD may appear to be egocentric and not take the needs and background of the audience into account. This may be due in part to inadequate discourse skills such as event sequencing and topic maintenance.
5. When LD students describe story characters, their descriptions may be shallow, with few references to internal states such as surprise, happiness, fear, or anger.

Semantic Skills

Current research suggests that students with LD have a generalized, underlying semantic deficit that results in two broad categories of problems: 1) word retrieval problems and 2) difficulties with word meanings (Hallahan et al., 2005; Long, 2005). When students with LD experience word retrieval problems, they know the word they want to use; they just can't think of the word at the moment they need it. You have probably experienced this yourself: a word was on the tip of your tongue, but you just couldn't think of it at the moment. It probably occurred to you the minute your conversational partner left! Research has suggested that LD students have word retrieval problems because they have learned words less completely than TD students, not because they have difficulty accessing these words (Kail & Leonard, 1986; McGregor & Windsor, 1996).

Students with LD may learn words less completely than TD students because they have underdeveloped lexical systems. Manifestations of underdeveloped lexical systems include poor metalinguistic skills and impoverished vocabularies. **Metalinguistic skills** include the ability to think and talk about language; these skills cut across both spoken and written language. For example, one four-year-old who had clearly had an excellent pre-school background talked about a "vowel-driven /r/." Another example of metalinguistic skill was given by the six-year-old who said, "Aunt Janice, do you want me to write your name in upper or lowercase letters?"

Students with LD may have impoverished vocabularies due in part to difficulties with multiple word meanings (Kuder, 2003). As we discussed in Chapter 1, the word *rock* can mean three or four different things (stone, type of music, motion made with a baby). Students with LD often can only think of one definition for a word such as *rock*. Students with LD also have difficulty with recognizing and using words that are structurally related (e.g., synonyms and antonyms).

When asked to define common words, students with LD may take longer and make more errors than TD peers (Wiig & Semel, 1975). Nippold (1999) showed that LD students also experienced problems with defining abstract nouns such as *friendship* and *burden*. As we will discuss later, vocabulary plays a very important role in reading, and having an impoverished vocabulary negatively impacts children's reading comprehension as well as their oral semantic skills (McGregor, 2004; Patterson & Pearson, 2004).

> Students with LD frequently have word retrieval problems. They may also have impoverished vocabularies.

One vocabulary problem for students with LD is the comprehension and use of nonliteral or abstract meanings (Kuder, 2003; Nippold, 1998). Research has shown that these students have more difficulty explaining sentences composed of idioms or metaphors than do their TD peers. For example, if you said, "What does this mean? *When it rains, it pours*," a student with LD might give you a literal response such as "whenever it rains, it rains really hard" rather than the correct abstract response that a TD peer might give.

Students with LD often do not understand humor, and this can cause difficulties with both the classroom curriculum and with peers. For example, my niece Jennifer, when she was eight years old, laughed and laughed at the following joke: "What does a ghost like on his sundae? Whipped scream!" A student with LD probably would not find that joke funny because she wouldn't understand it.

The lack of ability to understand nonliteral or abstract meanings can present a substantial hindrance to LD adolescents' relationships with their peers. For example, many adolescents today use the word "sweet" to mean "terrific" or "desirable." The LD adolescent might hear the word "sweet" and think of a food like candy. Older LD students are placed at a disadvantage when they misunderstand metaphors, puns, jokes, and sarcastic

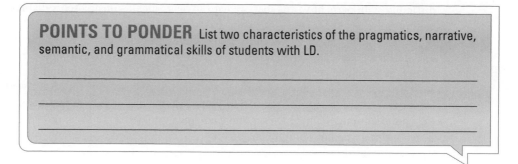

POINTS TO PONDER List two characteristics of the pragmatics, narrative, semantic, and grammatical skills of students with LD.

_____

_____

_____

remarks. As Larson and McKinley (1995, p. 73) state, "... their inadequate skills for rapid humorous verbal exchanges place older students with language disorders at a disadvantage when interacting with their peers."

SLPs must be careful when working with CLD students with LD because humor is very culturally based. CLD students may not understand humor because they come from a different cultural background, not because they have an LD. I mentioned earlier in the book that my family came to the United States from the Philippines to live permanently when I was seventeen years old. I remember sitting in freshman English in college while the whole class laughed at the professor's jokes. I was the only one not laughing, because I didn't understand the jokes—I had not grown up in the United States.

Grammatical Skills

With regard to grammatical skills, there appear to be two broad subgroups of LD students: 1) those who do not have grammatical problems and 2) those who do. With regard to the first group, recent research has suggested that students with LD with higher IQs may not have clinically significant grammatical problems (Scott & Windsor, 2000). However, many other students with LD do manifest difficulties with grammar in the areas of syntax and morphology.

Students with LD frequently have challenges with the syntactic and morphological aspects of spoken language. These challenges eventually affect written language also.

We will remember from Chapter 1 that syntax refers to the rules people use to put words together into sentences. With regard to syntax, some LD students may produce less syntactically complex sentences than same-age TD peers (Hallahan et al., 2005; Kuder, 2003; Scott & Windsor, 2000). They may also make more grammatical errors than TD peers. Comprehension of syntactically complex sentences is also problematic (Seidenberg, 2002). Many students with LD have trouble understanding sentences that use negation, that use the passive voice (e.g., The dog was petted by the little boy), and that use relative clauses (Kuder, 2003).

Morphological skills are frequently impaired in students with LD. We will recall that a morpheme is the smallest unit of meaning in language. Free morphemes (e.g., _bird, house, girl_) can stand alone while bound morphemes (e.g., past tense _-ed_, plural _-s_) cannot stand alone. Students with LD experience difficulty with parts of words that are hard to hear, such as unstressed syllables and word endings.

Thus, they may be slow acquiring morphological markers such as noun plurals, regular and irregular past-tense forms, comparatives and superlatives (bigg*er*, bigg*est*), and others. When their peers have advanced, children with LD may continue to make errors such as saying, "He runned yesterday" or "She gived it to me" (Rice & Wexler, 1996; Windsor, Scott, & Street, 2000). In the "grand scheme of things," morphological problems may not seem important. However, morphological problems are often reflected in LD students' writing; reading comprehension may also be impacted.

 SUMMARY

- Students with learning disabilities often have accompanying oral language deficits in the following skill areas: pragmatics, narratives, semantics, and grammar.
- Grammatical deficits include difficulties with receptive and expressive syntax and morphology.
- Students with LD may be slow acquiring morphological markers. This can eventually impact their reading and writing.

WRITTEN LANGUAGE PROBLEMS IN CHILDREN WITH LEARNING DISABILITIES

As we stated earlier, a hallmark of LD is difficulty with written language skills. We said that students with LD tend to have difficulty in several specific areas: reading, writing, and spelling. These are described below. (*Note*: We said earlier in this chapter that difficulties with reading, writing, and spelling tend to affect all academic areas; however, only reading, writing, and spelling are described here.)

Reading Disabilities (Dyslexia)

General Facts

As previously stated, most students with LD have difficulties with reading. Approximately 80 percent of students with LD have some deficits in reading comprehension or decoding (President's Commission on Excellence in Special Education, 2002). According to the NICHD (2000), approximately ten million students have problems learning to read; 10 to 15 percent of these drop out of high school; approximately 2 percent complete four-year college programs; approximately 50 percent of adolescents and young adults with criminal records have a history of reading problems, and 50 percent of youths with histories of substance abuse have reading problems. Clearly, reading problems are far ranging and quite expensive for our society. The reading characteristics of students with LD are listed in Table 8.2.

TABLE 8.2   Reading Characteristics of Students with Learning Disabilities

Poor Reading Habits

- Moves head jerkily from side to side
- May prefer to hold book within inches of face
- Shows tension while reading (e.g., fidgets, bites lips)
- Frequently loses place
- Shows insecurity by refusing to read or by crying

Comprehension Errors

- Difficulty recalling theme (e.g., can't give the main idea of the story)
- Difficulty recalling story sequence (e.g., can't explain order of events in the story)
- Difficulty recalling basic facts (e.g., can't answer questions directly from a passage)

Word Recognition Errors

- Slow, laborious reading
- Reversing words or letters (e.g., *ton* for *not*, *was* for *saw*)
- Transposing words or letters (e.g., *The man worked slowly* is read as *The man slowly worked*)
- Lack of attempting to read an unknown word by breaking it into familiar units
- Mispronouncing words (e.g., *hall* is read as *hill*)
- Substituting one word for another (e.g., *She went to the star* instead of *She went to the store*)
- Omitting a word (e.g., *She went to store* instead of *She went to the store*)

Other Characteristics

- Poor left-to-right orientation
- Possible difficulty with visual tracking skills

> Two main schools of thought on the causes of dyslexia involve 1) visual-perceptual/motor theories and 2) deficits related to phonological processing.

Many professionals use the term *dyslexia* to describe the specific problem of learning to read. A student with dyslexia is assumed to have normal-above average intelligence and no serious emotional or sensory disorders (Long, 2005; Nelson, 1998). Seidenberg (2002) emphasized the fact that dyslexia is not a unitary phenomenon, and a variety of causes underlie difficulties with reading. One cause may be difficulty with visual-perceptual/motor skills; this may be helped by an optical remedy. A second cause, which most experts today subscribe to, is difficulty with phonological processing. We shall look first into theories regarding visual-perceptual/motor skills in children with reading problems.

Visual-Perceptual/Motor Theories

With regard to visual-perceptual/motor theories, Bender (2004; pp. 9–10) summarizes these theories as follows:

> As the name implies, visual-perceptual/motor theorists were concerned with impaired visual perception and delayed motor development as possible causes of learning problems. This group of theorists believed that such visual-perceptual problems coupled with poor

fine motor control would result in learning deficits that were independent of intelligence. . . . From the late 1950s to the early 1970s, many public school classes for children with learning disabilities included various remediation exercises that were intended to correct these visual-perceptual problems. . . . Such exercises were assumed to improve visual perception and, therefore, reading. The assumption behind these training exercises suggested that if a teacher could remediate the visual-perceptual abilities, the improvement in design copying would result in improved reading scores for the children with learning disabilities. Of course, this assumption was highly questionable . . . and has been largely discredited (Moats & Lyon, 1993). Further evidence accumulated to indicate the futility of many of these early training programs. . . . In spite of these early failures, there is some recent evidence that reading disabilities . . . are associated with visual problems for some children (Eden, Stein, Wood, & Wood, 1995). Consequently, there are still many practitioners in the field who support the concept of some visual deficit as one potential cause of learning disabilities.

Thus, in sum, there may be a subgroup of students with LD who have visual-perceptual/motor problems that contribute to reading difficulty. A great deal of research is needed to verify this.

There have been some reports about an optical remedy for dyslexia. We have discussed the term *evidence-based practice* in this book, and thankfully, there is some preliminary research evidence to support this optical remedy (O'Connor, Sofo, Kendall, & Olsen, 1990; Whiting & Robinson, 1988). Beginning in 1983, a psychologist named Helen Irlen postulated that some students with reading problems might be overly sensitive to certain frequencies and wavelengths of the white light spectrum. These students were said to have *scotopic sensitivity syndrome*, a genetic condition where a person has cellular deficits in the portion of the brain that regulates low-contrast vision (Livingstone, Rosen, Drislane, & Galaburda, 1991; Robinson, Foreman, & Dear, 1996).

Scotopic sensitivity syndrome includes light sensitivity and problems with reading material on white high-gloss paper. People with scotopic sensitivity syndrome often manifest inefficient reading and a slow reading rate. They have writing problems such as trouble copying, unequal spacing of words and letters, writing uphill or downhill, and inconsistent spelling. Most have poor depth perception. Depth perception problems in those with scotopic sensitivity syndrome can cause clumsiness, difficulty judging distances, and difficulty catching balls (Irlen Institute, 2003).

> It is speculated that there may be a subgroup of people with dyslexia who have scotopic sensitivity syndrome that makes reading and writing difficult. This syndrome can be treated with colored spectacles and lenses.

Irlen began to treat students and adults with scotopic sensitivity syndrome by providing them with colored spectacles and lenses (Irlen, 2002). It was speculated that the colored lenses could help those people cope with their difficulties with low-contrast vision and allow their visual systems to function in a more normal manner. Irlen claimed that the lenses stabilized visual images on a page, thus making the perceptual component of reading easier. These special lenses had a highly beneficial effect for some people. Further research is needed to confirm the above-claimed findings and to inquire into whether all individuals with dyslexia have scotopic sensitivity, or whether this condition only affects a subgroup of dyslexic individuals (Long, 2005; Podell, 2004).

Deficits in Phonological Processing

Many experts today believe that for the vast majority of affected individuals, dyslexia may be a specific disorder of phonological processing (e.g., Cassar & Treiman, 2004; Ehri & Snowling, 2004; Goldsworthy, 2003; Lyon, 1996; Marshall, Snowling, & Bailey, 2001; Westby, 2004). Phonological processing is critical for literacy not only in English, but for other languages as well.

Cross-linguistic studies indicate that the interdependence of reading and phonological processing is most likely universal (Troia, 2004), and thus it is important to look at phonological processing in both monolingual and bilingual children. Three areas of phonological processing that have been studied in depth are 1) complex phonological production, 2) memory, and 3) phonological awareness.

Complex Phonological Production   In terms of phonological production, many students with LD are intelligible. However, even if they do not seem to have overt problems in producing their sounds, they often have difficulty producing complex words such as *aluminum, linoleum, statistics*. They also have difficulty repeating phonologically complex nonwords and difficulty repeating tongue-twisters (Goldsworthy, 2003). In addition, they may also have trouble saying phrases such as "Fly free in the Air Force" (Catts, 1986; Larrivee & Catts, 1999). Paul (2001) reminds us again that although a student may be intelligible, difficulties with literacy-related phonological processing can only be tapped by specially designed tasks such as imitation of complex sound sequences.

Memory Deficits   In Chapter 1, we looked at research that shows that students with specific language impairment have difficulties with memory. Students with LD also frequently have difficulty with short-term memory tasks (Gillam, Cowan, & Day, 1995; Goldsworthy, 2003; Owens, 2005; Seidenberg, 2002). For example, they have problems with repeating nonsense words (Larrivee & Catts, 1999; Snowling, 1996). As stated in previous chapters, the repetition of nonsense words holds promise for nonbiased assessment of CLD students because it rules out the factor of background knowledge and taps directly into language-learning ability (Dollaghan & Campbell, 1998; Laing & Kamhi, 2003; Meschyan & Hernandez, 2004; Montgomery, 1996).

Some researchers have believed that difficulty with short-term memory tasks in students with LD was limited only to verbal material (Snowling, 1996). However, other researchers today believe that there may be a subgroup of students with reading difficulties who have a deficit at the perceptual level that affects processing of both speech and nonspeech stimuli (Tallal, Merzenich, Miller, & Jenkins, 1998; Wright, Bowen, & Zecker, 2000). The auditory temporal deficit hypothesis posits that " . . . this deficit is specific to auditory temporal cues, affecting the perception of brief portions of the speech stimulus . . . that provide important cues for some phonemic contrasts . . . " (Breier et al., 2003). Paul (2001) states that more research is needed to confirm this hypothesis.

> Most experts today believe that dyslexia is related to deficits in phonological processing.

A related area of weakness for LD students is rapid automatic naming skills (Breier et al., 2003; Catts, 1991; Ehri & Snowling, 2004; Nelson, 1998; Seidenberg, 2002; Snowling, 2000). Rapid automatized naming is the ability to quickly name a small number of items (e.g., letters, colors, numbers, or objects). This has proven to be one of the best predictors of a student's printed word recognition (Goldsworthy, 2003). Professionals can assess rapid automatic naming skills by having a child quickly repeat a small number of items such as those listed above. They can also use tasks such as asking students to name the days of the week or months of the year as fast as possible.

Phonological Awareness We will remember that phonological awareness refers to the conscious knowledge that words in a given language are composed of various units of sound (Gillam & van Kleeck, 1996). Phonological awareness is the ability to consciously reflect upon and manipulate the sound component of language; the child needs to be able to analyze the structure of an utterance as distinct from its meaning (Gillon, 2004; Segers & Verhoeven, 2004). For example, many children know that the word *pancake* means something round that people eat for breakfast with butter and syrup. They would display phonological awareness if they were able to say that the word *pancake* has two syllables, begins with /p/, ends with a /k/ sound, and also has a /k/ sound in the middle.

Phonological awareness is strongly correlated with reading ability; it is a critical prereading skill (Justice & Kaderavek, 2004; Owens, 2005; Segers & Verhoeven, 2004). A number of researchers believe that difficulties in phonological awareness are central to students who have difficulty reading (Cassar & Treiman, 2004; Goldsworthy, 2003; Kuder, 2003, Nelson, 1998; O'Connor & Jenkins, 1999; Westby, 2004). The National Reading Panel (2000, pp. 2–11), after reviewing research on reading and phonological awareness, concluded that "phonological awareness measured at the beginning of kindergarten is one of the two best predictors of how well students will learn to read."

We talked earlier about the genetic component to LD/reading disabilities and language disabilities. Lyon (1996) discussed findings from research programs supported by the NICHD that have indicated that phonologically based reading disabilities are linked to neurobiological and genetic factors. Structural and functional neuroimaging studies indicate that poor phonological skills, which negatively impact reading development, are high related to aberrant neurophysiological processing.

There is mounting evidence from behavioral and molecular genetic studies that the phonological deficits observed in persons with reading disabilities are heritable. Longitudinal studies of genetic, neurobiological, and linguistic factors in reading disabilities provide

CONNECT & EXTEND

Phonological awareness and specific strategies for treating students with reading disabilities are described in detail in C. Goldsworthy (2003). *Developmental reading disabilities: A language based treatment approach* (2nd ed.). San Diego: Thomson/Delmar Learning.

POINTS TO PONDER Describe the two primary schools of thought about what causes reading problems in children.

strong evidence that reading disabilities are caused primarily by inherited deficits in phonological processing—specifically, phonological awareness (e.g., DeFries & Gillis, 1991; Stanovich & Siegel, 1994; Wood, Felton, Flowers, & Naylor, 1991).

It has been suggested that students who are slow to develop primary linguistic abilities (oral language abilities) during their preschool years may have some difficulty with higher-level skills like phonological awareness. Thus, as we said in Chapter 7, students who are slow in their oral language development during their preschool years can be considered at risk for written language problems later, even before they begin to fail in school (Ehri & Snowling, 2004).

Nelson (1998) points out that many students categorized as language delayed in preschool are recategorized in elementary school as LD. Researchers suggest that SLPs play an important role in helping identify students who are at risk for future reading problems (Apel, 2002; Catts, 1991; Goldsworthy, 2003; Larrivee & Catts, 1999). In order to identify at-risk students in preschool and kindergarten, SLPs can assess (among other things) phonological awareness as well as other literacy-related skills.

> Young children with oral language problems frequently evolve into older learners with written language problems. In order to identify at-risk young students, professionals can evaluate their phonological awareness skills.

Measures of phonological awareness such as the Comprehensive Test of Phonological Processing (CTOPP; Wagner, Torgesen, & Rashotte, 1999) can measure specific phonological awareness skills such as counting the number of syllables in words, the number of sounds in words, the number of words in a sentence, and others. However, clinicians must use caution in administering standardized tests of phonological awareness skills to CLD students.

For example, one study examined the performance of fifty-six low-income African American first graders on the Test of Phonological Awareness (TOPA; Torgesen & Bryant, 1994). Though the students' mean performance on a test of basic reading skills was within normal limits, their mean performance on the TOPA was "significantly below expected norms and negatively skewed" (p. 182). The authors stated that their findings suggested that the TOPA may not be a suitable assessment instrument for African American students, especially those who speak African American English. Interestingly, these same subjects performed significantly better on the CTOPP (Thomas-Tate, Washington, & Edwards, 2004).

Students who have been exposed at home to literacy experiences and reading-related media often have better phonological awareness skills than students who do not have this exposure (Foy & Mann, 2003). A problem for many CLD students is that they come from homes that may be rich in oral language exposure but that do not emphasize literacy-related activities. These students may need extra support in developing phonological awareness skills so that they do not fall behind in reading.

Writing Disabilities

Many students with LD have difficulty with writing. As Singer and Bashir (2004, p. 559) stated

> The demands of writing are staggering. It requires the coordination and accommodation of graphomotor and cognitive-linguistic abilities, as well as knowledge of social, rhetorical, and text production conventions. Writing is influenced by the writer's world knowledge, motivation, beliefs and attitudes. . . . For the individual with language learning disabilities, writing is an arduous process.

Students with LD may have trouble with the process of handwriting itself, and/or they may have difficulties with written expression. Let's consider the process of handwriting first. When students have trouble with handwriting (or **dysgraphia**), they write slowly and have difficulties with spacing. In addition, they often have poor letter formation, letters that are inconsistent in size, and letters that are crowded and cramped (Hallahan et al., 2005). When students write quite slowly, they are said to have difficulty with writing fluency.

Sometimes handwriting problems occur because the students do not have the developmental skills necessary for adequate writing. They may have fine-motor coordination and/or strength problems (Hardman et al., 2006). These problems may be amenable to intervention by a professional such as an occupational therapist, who can work with a student and his parents to do exercises that will help strengthen the student's coordination and strength.

Handwriting Without Tears, a commercially available program for students with handwriting problems, has been successfully used in various parts of the United States and Canada. Handwriting Without Tears is a simple, multisensory, "ball and stick" writing program that was created by an occupational therapist especially to help students with fine-motor problems (Olsen, 2003). Some schools in the district where I work use Handwriting Without Tears, and anecdotally, we find that it is especially helpful for kindergarteners who have not been exposed to writing or prewriting activities (such as coloring) in their home environments (many of the students I work with have not attended preschool).

> Writing problems in students with LD may be related to dysgraphia, poor written expression skills, or both.

Difficulties with written language expression may also characterize students with LD. LD students' difficulties in spoken language and reading comprehension often interact to create difficulties in written expression ability. Students with LD frequently have problems following information presented in narrative form and reproducing those narratives as we discussed earlier. All these oral language difficulties, added in with reading comprehension problems, impact written expression (Bender, 2004). These problems tend to become more pronounced as students get older. For example, in junior high and high school, students are required to express opinions or arguments in written form. Written expression can also be impacted by difficulties with spelling.

Spelling Disabilities

Students with LD are notoriously poor spellers. Spelling is a complex task that requires the child to integrate orthographic and phonological knowledge (Apel, Masterson, & Niessen, 2004; Kamhi & Hinton, 2000). Orthography is the formal name for the system of representing spoken language in a written form. For example, when we say the word *boat*, we usually pronounce it as [bout]. The orthographic representation is **boat**. We say the word women as [wImņ], yet the word is spelled **women**. The pronunciation and the written forms of these words are different. This presents difficulty for many students with LD, especially those who are English as a second language learners.

> Students with LD often have problems with spelling.

Many of these students come from language backgrounds (e.g., Spanish, German, Tagalog) where each phoneme corresponds with one grapheme. This is not the case in English. Hull (1981) states that there are 251 different spellings for the 44 sounds of English, and English has many irregularly spelled words. For example, the words *cough, rough, though, bough*, and *through* all end with the same letters but are pronounced differently (Hallahan et al., 2005). This can cause a great deal of confusion for students who are learning English as a second or third language.

In order to spell well, students have to be able to articulate the word correctly, recall the spoken pattern (the auditory sequence of the sounds or syllables), and recall correct visual letter sequences. They also have to remember the motor pattern for the word and execute the plan for the motor act (Hardman et al., 2006). Students with poor handwriting often have difficulty spelling because of two issues: legibility and speed. Errors in handwriting may make one word look like another word. Labored writing of letters may cause students to forget the word they were trying to spell or lose their place as they are spelling it (Hallahan et al., 2005).

Good phonological awareness skills are also critical to success in spelling (Cassar & Treiman, 2004; Clarke-Klein, 1994; Lewis et al., 2000; Moats & Lyon, 1993). Students with LD who lack phonological awareness skills have difficulty segmenting words and syllables into phonemes and their conventional, corresponding graphemes (Hallahan et al., 2005). It has been suggested that phonological awareness training that is tailored to a child's specific spelling difficulties may be effective in helping her to become a better speller (Bourassa & Treiman, 2001).

 SUMMARY

- Students with LD are frequently diagnosed with dyslexia, a specific reading disability. There are two major schools of thought about what causes dyslexia. One school of thought attributes it to visual-perceptual/motor problems, and another attributes it to phonological processing problems.
- Three areas of phonological processing that have been studied in depth with relation to dyslexia are 1) complex phonological production, 2) memory deficits, and 3) phonological awareness.
- Students with LD often have writing problems. These problems can be due to dysgraphia, written expression difficulties, or both.
- Spelling problems are also very common in students with LD. English spelling can be particularly confusing for students who are English Language Learners.

Add your own summary points here:

_____

_____

_____

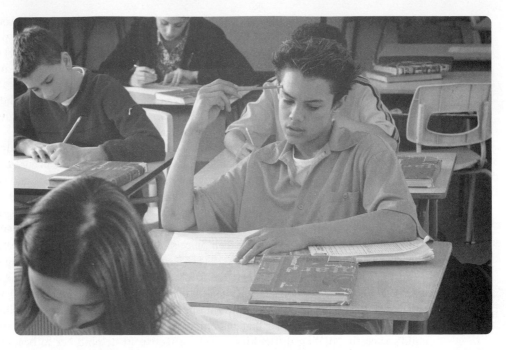

Speech-language pathologists need to provide intervention that addresses students' written as well as oral language difficulties.

ASSESSMENT OF STUDENTS WITH LEARNING DISABILITIES

Challenges in Nonbiased Assessment

Early identification of students with LD is critical, because as we shall discuss later, early intervention can prevent a host of academic difficulties later on. The purpose of assessment is twofold: 1) to discover if a student needs special education, and if so, 2) to determine the nature of the student's needs and ascertain what type of service delivery model will best meet those needs (Seidenberg, 2002). Assessments of students suspected as having LD must be made by multidisciplinary teams because the LD population is so heterogeneous.

In the school district where I work, this assessment is usually carried out by me or my SLP colleague, the resource specialist, and the psychologist. Our goal is to determine the student's social/emotional, cognitive, academic, and linguistic status. The psychologist will often use a formal intelligence test such as the Wechsler Intelligence Scale for Children:4 (WISC:4; Wechsler, 2003) while the resource specialist will evaluate the student's academic abilities using formal measures of academic skills. My SLP colleague and I will use formal tests to evaluate the student's oral language skills. (In the case of CLD students, we use primarily informal measures.)

A major concern in many public school districts is that some ethnic groups consistently achieve below the average for all students on standardized achievement tests. For example, many of these tests are biased against students who speak African American English (Thompson, Craig, & Washington, 2004). However, Woolfolk (2004) says that although there are consistent differences among ethnic groups on tests of cognitive abilities, most researchers agree that these differences can primarily be attributed to discrimination, cultural mismatches, or growing up in a low-income environment. Because many CLD students are from low-income homes, it is important to separate the effects of these two sets of influences on achievement in school and on performance on standardized tests. When we compare students from different racial and ethnic backgrounds who are all at the same socioeconomic level, the achievement levels are more comparable.

However, because of the bias inherent in standardized tests and the problems we have talked about with the existing discrepancy model, it is important to use informal measures with CLD students especially. Recall that in Chapter 3, we cited research that indicates that Basic Interpersonal Communication Skills, or BICS, take approximately 2 years for a second language learner to develop to a nativelike level under ideal conditions. We also said that Cognitive Academic Language Proficiency, or CALP, takes five to seven and even up to ten years to develop to a nativelike level.

There is a problem that I and many professionals nationwide encounter constantly. Many special-education teams believe that in order for a student to qualify as having an LD and thus be eligible for academic support, he must be assessed with formal measures and show a discrepancy as we have discussed. However, many formal measures (especially those that measure academic achievement in areas such as reading and spelling) are normed on monolingual, English-speaking students. CLD students who have not been exposed to English for five to ten years may do poorly on those measures, which really measure CALP, because they have not been exposed to English for a long enough time, not because they have genuine LD. Thus, "false positives" may occur where CLD students are wrongly identified as having learning disabilities and needing special education.

> It is especially challenging to assess CLD students for an LD because standardized assessment instruments, required by most districts, are biased against these students.

In addition, as we mentioned earlier, some children may not be provided with many opportunities for language learning because their caretakers don't read to them and they rarely observe writing and reading in their homes. They may have normal cognitive skills but just need a heightened exposure to literacy. Other students come from homes where there is a high degree of literacy but not in English, so school personnel may underestimate these students' linguistic competence. Others may have learned a dialect of English (e.g., Appalachian English, African American English) but never seen it in print. Teachers don't use this dialect, so these children may struggle (Hallahan et al., 2005; van Keulen et al., 1998). When school personnel are unaware of these variables, CLD students can be overidentified for special-education programs.

Unfortunately, there is also the potential for "false negatives." Ortiz (1997) pointed out that in some school districts, teachers are prohibited from referring students who speak English as a second language for a special-education assessment until they have been exposed to English for at least two years. While well-intentioned, these types of policies can have very negative effects and create long-standing problems for CLD students with genuine special-education needs.

What I often see happening (and not just in my own school district) is that special-education teams consisting of psychologists, resource specialists, and SLPs feel overwhelmed with the many referrals they get from teachers. Thus, they refuse to assess CLD students at all until they are in the upper elementary school grades. Some members of special-education teams are aware of the five to seven years a student needs to achieve CALP, and so they take a "hands-off" approach, knowing that their tests are biased and that students need time to develop CALP.

However, I have seen many younger students who I strongly suspected had LD and were unable to receive needed services because they were English Language Learners. This is a shame, because we have said that early identification and intervention are critical for students with LD. The "give them time" approach may cause some genuinely LD students to not receive needed services, as the case below illustrates.

Principles of Nonbiased Assessment

Principles of assessment for CLD students with potential LD can follow the ones discussed in Chapter 5. I will reemphasize here that in terms of their performance on formal and informal measures, CLD students must be compared to peers from similar cultural and linguistic backgrounds. There is no other nonbiased way to assess these students for the possible presence of LD. As we've emphasized, informal measures should especially

---

CASES TO CONSIDER

I assessed a Mexican, Spanish-speaking sixth-grader, Joel F., who was two months away from junior high school. Joel was born in Jalisco, Mexico, and came to California with his family at three years of age. Thus, he had all his elementary schooling in the United States. Joel was referred to me for "stuttering"; he didn't stutter. However, my assessment and examination of his school cumulative file revealed that in reading and writing, he was functioning at a first-grade level. His writing looked like that of most kindergarteners; he could only print and did not write in cursive at all. When I asked why Joel had never been assessed for a possible LD, the sixth-grade teacher shrugged and said that because Joel spoke Spanish as his primary language, no one had ever thought of that. I immediately referred Joel for a comprehensive evaluation involving the psychologist and resource specialist so that Joel could get much-needed support in junior high school, where he was bound to flounder without extra services. What should have happened in Joel's situation? What could school personnel have done differently?

_____

_____

_____

be used because of the lack of validity and reliability of formal measures which are usually standardized on White, monolingual English-speaking students (Bender, 2004; Brice, 2002; Duke, Pressley, & Hildren, 2004; Hearne, 2000; Roseberry-McKibbin et al., 2005). Informal measures can utilize principles of dynamic assessment discussed in Chapter 5.

> When assessing CLD students for possible learning disabilities, professionals can use informal measures such as criterion-referenced measures, curriculum-based assessment, and examination of students' school files.

The use of criterion-referenced measures is very relevant to CLD students with LD. Criterion-referenced testing measures of student achievement without reference to the levels of performance of other students within a group; this testing is individualized (Hearne, 2000). Professionals frequently use criterion-referenced testing to sample student progress toward curriculum goals.

Experts also recommend curriculum-based assessment based on a student's class work. This type of assessment is done once or twice a week. For example, the teacher might keep data on how long it takes a student to complete a writing assignment. The student's time can be charted on a daily basis, and the teacher can see the progress from day to day. A CLD student might be compared to other CLD students from a similar cultural and linguistic background; if she is seen

CASES TO CONSIDER

Quang N., a Vietnamese-speaking high school freshman, was struggling in school. He was getting Ds in Geometry and Geography, and had other academic difficulties as well. Quang was born in Texas and moved to California as a preschooler. He had gone from kindergarten through high school in my school district. The high school team was concerned about Quang, and wondered if he had a learning disability. However, they thought that his difficulties in high school might be due to the fact that Vietnamese was his primary language (although he told me he spoke mostly English now). The team asked me to assess him for the possible presence of a learning disability. When I examined Quang's school records, I found that every year since kindergarten, teachers had written comments such as "Quang struggles with learning the alphabet." "Quang works hard, but reading and writing are very difficult for him." "Quang is a sweet student who is substantially below average in spelling, reading, and writing."

Quang's records indicated that he had received special-education services since first grade. I found, in my assessment with Quang, that he could not spell basic words such as *chair, stomach, curtain*. His auditory memory was quite poor. He read slowly and hesitantly. Do you think that Quang might actually have had a learning disability, or that he was just experiencing difficulty because he was from a Vietnamese-speaking home? Explain your answer.

_____

_____

_____

to learn more slowly than her peers, it may be possible that she has an LD (Bender, 2004; Commission on Excellence in Special Education, 2001).

As discussed in Chapter 5, one strategy I have successfully used with older CLD students who are struggling in school is an examination of their school records. I use this in conjunction with other measures, of course, but I often find that a careful examination of students' school records can reveal consistent patterns that point to a possible LD. This is illustrated in the case of Quang N. on page 291.

 SUMMARY

- Assessment with CLD students is challenging because many standardized tests are biased against them. Unfortunately, this can lead to both over- and underidentification of CLD students with potential learning disabilities.
- A major challenge in assessing students who are English Language Learners is that it often takes them five to ten years to gain CALP skills that are commensurate with those of native English speakers. Thus, professionals often feel like they should take a "wait and see" policy with these students. This can prevent students with true learning disabilities from receiving much-needed early intervention.
- Professionals can use informal measures such as criterion-referenced testing, curriculum-based assessments, and inspection of school records to assess CLD students for potential learning disabilities.

INTERVENTION FOR SCHOOL-AGE CHILDREN AND ADOLESCENTS WITH LEARNING DISABILITIES

Service Delivery in the Public Schools

Public schools are legally obligated to provide appropriate intervention for all students with special-education needs, including students with LD. We talked earlier in this chapter about the discrepancy model for identifying students who qualify for services based on a diagnosis of LD. We said that hopefully, with the newly revised IDEA 2004, many school districts will stop using this model and instead provide a continuum of services to assist students who struggle in school. Specifically, the new IDEA targets *prevention* of reading problems by targeting students in earlier grades. I am so heartened to see this, because in my experience, many students with LD do not begin to receive services until they are in third or fourth grade and are experiencing a great deal of failure and frustration. Needless to say, their self-esteem has also suffered.

Students with LD may be served by SLPs. They are often served by resource specialists who have special training and expertise in written language as well as academic curriculum as a whole. Unfortunately, because resources in school districts are often scarce,

Services in public schools may be fragmented because of issues like territoriality and heavy caseload sizes.

CONNECT & EXTEND

A comprehensive text regarding building the literacy skills of students with written language problems is Ukrainetz, T.A. (Ed.) (2006). *Contextualized language intervention: Scaffolding PreK-12 literacy achievement.* Eau Claire, WI: Thinking Publications.

sometimes special-education teams will try to avoid "double dipping" by only giving a student services from one professional. In other words, special-education teams often will not provide services, for one student, from both the resource specialist and the SLP. In addition, SLPs are often afraid that if they serve students with written as well as oral language problems, they will double or triple their caseloads (Apel, 2002).

Even if both the resource specialist and the SLP serve the same children, issues of territoriality dictate that the SLP sees students for oral language disorders, and the resource specialist sees students for written language problems. In this situation, the student is taught isolated skills and services are often fragmented. It is critical for SLPs to be involved in providing intervention that addresses students' written as well as oral language problems (Duchan, 2004; Ukrainetz, 2006).

ASHA (2000) has taken a very strong stance on the importance of SLPs' involvement in serving students with written language problems because of the language bases of reading, writing, and spelling. However, many public school–based clinicians continue in the paradigm of serving students only in the area of oral language. Because I believe that it is best for LD students to receive integrated services, I have sometimes worked with students on written

CASES TO CONSIDER

I was seeing Rashina L. for speech-language services, and we were working on oral language. Rashina, a CLD fifth-grade student whose dominant language was English, could not even read basic safety signs. I decided that as part of my intervention for Rashina, who would be going to junior high school in a little over a year, I would teach her to read some basic safety signs. I thought that it would be good if she could read the words "Boys' Bathroom" and "Girls' Bathroom," for example. When I told the resource specialist I was doing this, he became angry at me for doing "his job." He told me that he had tried to teach Rashina to read, and it didn't work. He said she would "never learn to read those words." Fueled by this challenge, I worked with Rashina until she could read a list of about twenty safety words. That was one of the best victories of my career. But to this day, I will never forget the feeling of being told to "back off" on working with reading just because I was an SLP, not a resource specialist. What would you have done in my situation? Would you have worked with Rashina on reading safety signs, or would you have avoided this in order to not offend the resource specialist?

language skills. I have not always fared well with this as you will see from the case study of Rashina L on page 293.

Another consideration for SLPs who work in public schools is that federal law states that when possible, students must be served in the least restrictive environment (LRE) that appropriately meets their needs. This means that as much as possible, students with LD must be kept in classrooms and activities with their TD peers. This is accomplished to the extent possible depending on the student's level of need.

> SLPs can collaborate with classroom teachers to help students with LD improve their pragmatics skills in the general-education setting.

Reed and Spicer (2003) surveyed teachers regarding their opinions about the most important pragmatics skills for adolescents. The teachers ranked the following communication skills as the top five in importance: narrative skills, logical communication, clarification, perspective taking, and turn-taking. Reed and Spicer recommended that SLPs would do well to focus intervention on communication skills that are important in the classroom setting. This includes nonverbal as well as verbal skills (Turkstra, Ciccia, & Seaton, 2003).

We have referred several times to a study by Brice and Montgomery (1996), who examined the pragmatics skills of Latino adolescents in both general- and special-education settings. They found that even the adolescents in general-education classrooms had some difficulty acquiring mainstream pragmatic features, especially those related to affecting the listener's behavior through language. The TD Latino adolescents were not successful in this area. Brice and Montgomery concluded that SLPs and other professionals who work with both LD and TD CLD adolescents need to be aware that these students may need extra support in acquiring mainstream pragmatics skills that will help them succeed in the classroom setting. Students with LD who are CLD can also benefit from ideal listening conditions in the general-education classroom.

In Chapter 6, we discussed the fact that CLD students with and without language impairments can benefit from optimal listening conditions in classroom settings (Nelson, et al., 2005). Unfortunately, many classrooms have unfavorable listening conditions. These conditions include low-frequency, decontextualized information presented at a rapid rate with poor signal-to-noise ratios (Windsor & Kohnert, 2004). Thus, SLPs must work with classroom teachers in cases where CLD students also have LD. For these students, quiet classrooms with good signal-to-noise ratios are crucial. Recent research has shown that students with LD can also benefit from good listening conditions involving clear speech. Bradlow, Kraus, and Hayes (2003) showed, in their study, that students with LD especially benefited from hearing speech that was produced clearly, conversationally, and slowly.

> Students with LD also benefit from being in quiet classrooms where the teacher speaks slowly, clearly, and conversationally.

Professionals who work with LD students can try to be sure that they speak in quiet environments in a manner that is slow, conversational, and clear. Bradlow et al. concluded that (p. 94) "on the basis of the findings from the present study, we can conclude that a particularly effective means of enhancing speech perception under adverse listening conditions for students with and without learning disabilities is to modify the talker's speech production. . . . It is cost free, it requires no listener or talker training, and it is almost universally effective."

Specific Strategies for Teaching Students with Learning Disabilities

Basic Principles

SLPs, classroom teachers, and other professionals who work with students with LD can use many practical strategies. In Chapter 7, we discussed at length specific strategies for increasing phonological awareness in students, especially younger ones. Early intervention is crucial so that students with LD will fall behind as little as possible (Lyon, 1996; O'Connor & Bell, 2004). According to Cushen-White (2000), more than thirty-three years of NICHD-supported research has shown that for 90 percent to 95 percent of poor readers, prevention and early intervention programs that combine instruction in fluency development, phoneme awareness, phonics, and reading comprehension strategies, provided by well-trained teachers, can increase reading skills to average reading levels.

Providing Support for Written Language Skills

It is important to work on reading with all students with LD. According to Lyon (1996), students with extreme deficits in basic reading skills are much harder to remediate than students who have mild or moderate deficits. He states that it is not clear whether students in the most severe range can achieve grade- and age-approximate reading skills, even if they have normal intelligence and intensive intervention. Lyon reminds us that students with severe LD are likely to manifest an increased number of and severity of behavioral and social deficits; if these students have attention deficit hyperactivity disorder also, then the problem becomes even more complex.

While severe reading disorders are a major concern, even mild-moderate disorders can cause significant deficits in academic learning over time. When adolescents and young adults are not literacy proficient, there can be severe short- and long-term consequences. Low literacy achievement is correlated with underemployment, welfare dependency, crime, and a generally underprepared workforce (Ehren, Lenz, & Deshler, 2004; Sanger et al., 2004).

A difficult fact for most professionals who work with these students is that by the time they reach adolescence, they may be turned

Reading disorders cause a variety of problems, especially if these disorders are severe. Working with adolescents with reading disorders can be quite challenging, but professionals can implement a number of effective strategies to increase adolescents' motivation to read.

off to reading because it is so difficult for them. Professionals need to be especially proactive with adolescents with LD. Nippold, Duthie, and Larsen (2005) studied the free-time preferences and leisure activities of older children and adolescents. They found that the most popular free-time activities were watching TV or videos, listening to music/going to concerts, playing computer or video games, and playing sports. Reading was "moderately popular" (p. 93). Nippold et al. found that during the eleven- to fifteen-year age range, interest in pleasure reading declined. Boys were more likely than girls to report that they spent no time reading for pleasure.

According to Nippold et al. (2005), the amount of time spent reading predicts word knowledge; because word knowledge is so important to academic success, it is important for school-age children and adolescents to read a variety of materials. Reading a variety of materials is especially important in the vocabulary development of older students (McGregor, 2004). Nippold et al. stated that SLPs can work collaboratively with parents, teachers, and other professionals to encourage strong literacy habits in all students. They suggested that professionals can:

1. Encourage parents to read with their children at home and discuss what they have read.
2. Encourage parents to support the school library.
3. Explore with students their reasons for rejecting certain types of material and help them acquire reading materials that engage their interest.
4. Encourage students to visit the school library and take books home.
5. Provide blocks of class time each day (e.g., twenty-five minutes) for sustained silent reading where all students are required to read material of their choice.

> SLPs and others who work with students with LD need to create incentives for these students to read.

6. Organize book clubs at school; these clubs can have different themes such as Harry Potter and others.
7. Provide specific incentives such as prizes for reading. For older students especially, increasing their motivation to read is crucial (O'Connor & Bell, 2004).

There are many creative ways to provide incentives for students to read more. At my son's elementary school, the principal and librarian challenged the students to collectively read for more than a million minutes this last school year. All parents had to keep track of the number of minutes that they read with their children at home and turn in report sheets each month. Because the students succeeded and read for more than one million minutes, there was a special assembly at the end of the year where the school principal was dipped in goop and then covered with feathers. The students loved this, and many of us parents did too! It was interesting during the year to hear my son talk excitedly about reading more so he could "see Mr. Cook get all gooey and feathery." The opportunity to see the principal in this sorry state was definitely very motivating for my little boy to read more.

For students with reading problems, direct teaching of strategies and skills is especially important (Woolfolk, 2004). Paris (1991) suggests that students with reading comprehension problems be directly taught specific strategies that don't compete with decoding (a very hard skill for most of these students to master). For example, students can

Professionals can use a variety of strategies to motivate students to read. It is especially important to motivate older students who might be discouraged because reading has been so hard for them over the years.

examine the text before they read to identify the topic and think about what prior knowledge they have about the topic. They can pause at least at every paragraph to reread what they have read or paraphrase it. Many poor readers do not like to read because they feel inadequate; they believe that good readers can read something once and comprehend everything. Students with reading problems need to be reassured that strategies like pausing, rereading, and paraphrasing will be helpful to them and will not make them look "dumb."

Before reading, professionals should try to engage in prereading activities such as skimming the text, writing the title of the book and getting the students to predict what it will be about, developing questions about the story, and (if possible) telling the story in the students' primary language first. If students have "the big picture" before they try to decode the words in a story, they will frequently comprehend the story much better (Gibbons, 2002). If children look at the pictures in the story first, before reading, this can also help them to get the "big picture" before they begin to decode the words. Graves, Juel, and Graves (2001) suggest the following:

1. Set a purpose for reading.
2. Preteach key concepts and vocabulary.
3. Link students' background experiences and knowledge with the reading; relate the reading to students' lives.

CONNECT & EXTEND

Gibbons (2002) has written a very practical book entitled *Scaffolding language, scaffolding learning: Teaching second language learners in the mainstream classroom.* Portsmouth, NH: Heinemann. In this book, she describes excellent ideas that SLPs can share with classroom teachers to help CLD students be more successful in the regular classroom setting.

Many teachers of students with reading problems use the Neurological Impress Method (NIM). The NIM is a multisensory approach where the teacher sits beside the student and slightly behind her so as to speak clearly into the student's ear. The student is instructed to follow the reading passage in the book with her finger under each word as she reads it out loud. An adaptation of this is that the teacher can put his finger above each word while the student puts her finger under each word and they read the words aloud together. This utilizes the learner's kinesthetic, visual, and auditory senses together during reading (Hearne, 2000; Heckelman, 1978). I have successfully used this with some students who had great difficulty keeping their place during reading. The NIM helps students to not skip words or lose their place while reading.

Professionals can also use strategies to help students with LD improve their writing. In terms of writing, we have discussed the fact that many students with LD make grammatical errors. We said before that in terms of spoken language, when CLD students in the early stages of learning English make grammatical errors, it is important to not overtly correct these errors too often because this will discourage their use of English. The same principle applies to writing. We need to stress communication of meaning rather than grammar (Goldstein, 2000). In writing, it is recommended that students' ideas get communicated first, and then the focus moves to correct form or mechanics such as grammar and spelling (Ruiz, Rueda, Figueroa, & Boothroyd, 1995).

Some SLPs work on spelling skills with their students who have an LD. One straightforward procedure for helping LD students with spelling errors is as follows. Students can be tested daily on spelling words, and immediate feedback is given for errors. On the first day, students take a conventional spelling test and then write the error words five times, saying the letters aloud as they write them. The next day, the students take the spelling test again and are required to write the error words ten times while saying the letters out loud. Finally, the next day, students are required to retake the test and write the error words fifteen times, each time saying the letters out loud (Kearney & Drabman, 1993). Kearney and Drabman found that this procedure was very effective and speculated that the effectiveness might be related to the fact that the procedure is multisensory and that the students experienced both writing and saying the correct spellings on multiple occasions. They also pointed out that no special equipment is necessary to use this procedure.

> SLPs can use a variety of multisensory strategies to support students who have difficulty with spelling.

For students with LD who are learning English as a second language, word families can be most helpful in learning to spell. The SLP presents sound, word, and letter patterns to encourage the student to make a guess when she comes upon new words. The patterns can be presented orally, graphically, or both (Hearne, 2000). I have found that many of my English Language Learners with LD profit greatly from *seeing* as well as hearing new words. The following example illustrates the use of word families:

in   thin   grin   chin   tin   pin   win

Additional Considerations for CLD Students

CLD students are often learning English as a second or third language. Thus, they have two major challenges: 1) learning another language and 2) doing this with a system that has underlying problems characteristic of students with LD. Gibbons (2002) reminds us that children who are learning to read in a second language may need particular kinds of extra support. Some of this extra support can occur in the form of extra phonological awareness training.

Swanson, Hodson, and Schommer-Aikins (2005) conducted a study where they evaluated the effect of phonological awareness intervention, conducted in English, on reading development in adolescent poor readers. These poor readers spoke English as their second language and were predominantly bilingual. They spoke Spanish and African American English, as well as a number of Asian languages. The study was conducted in a primarily low-income, bilingual area and involved students who had a history of poor reading scores. The students (regardless of first language background) who received specific phonological awareness intervention (as compared to a group of students who did not receive this intervention) showed improvement in their ability to analyze the phonological construct of words. Swanson et al. (p. 343) concluded that

> The major clinical implication of this study is that literacy skills of junior high students with phonological awareness deficiencies, including individuals who are bilingual, can be enhanced. Direct, specific, systematic instruction in phonological awareness with applications to literacy . . . appears to be a means of removing a major obstacle to becoming literate.

Measurable gains were achieved in this study in only one semester . . . this line of research reveals the potential of late intervention for older students. . . . Students in middle and junior high schools may be able to remediate their literacy difficulties in time to benefit optimally from the educational years still ahead of them . . .

We can also support CLD students with LD by remembering that most children's books are written with the assumption that readers will already be fluent in the spoken language and will be familiar with the cultural aspects of the story. Gibbons encourages professionals to help English Language Learners to gain access to a culturally and linguistically diverse reading environment, a range of reading strategies, and a literacy program that aims to develop all the roles that effective readers take on.

It is also important to help these students focus on the *meaning* of what they read. As we said, sometimes students who struggle with reading are so focused on decoding that they comprehend little of what they read. Research has suggested that encouraging poor readers to focus on meaning helps increase their comprehension (Crowe, 2003). CLD students who speak English as a second language can profit from interactive book reading where adults engage them in discussions about what they have read (Kim & Hall, 2002). Reading comprehension in these students is also enhanced by supplemental, small-group tutoring in reading that focuses on both word-level and comprehension skills (Linan-Thompson, Vaughn, Hickman-Davis, & Kouzekanani, 2003).

> CLD students with learning disabilities have two major challenges: they must learn to be literate in a second language, and they also have intrinsic difficulties with written language.

Professionals can encourage families of CLD students with LD to use local libraries to encourage reading. This is especially helpful for CLD families where the parents do not speak English and/or do not have books in the home that are written in the student's primary language (Roseberry-McKibbin, 2008). I have talked previously about the fact that some libraries, such as the local one near us, have special programs like Reading with Delilah the Dog or Come in Your Pajamas Night (and be read to by local Rotarians). Many students who have difficulty reading enjoy these types of programs and will be encouraged to think of reading in a more positive light. Moore-Brown and Montgomery (2001) state that the read-aloud aspect of family literacy is especially relevant and appealing for CLD families.

There are many other ways to empower CLD students who are learning English as a second language in written form. Table 8.3 has some of these specific suggestions, some of which we have mentioned previously.

When we work with families of CLD students, we must be sensitive to the fact that they will have special challenges if they are low income. As we will discuss again in Chapter 10, poverty involves environmental risks such as inadequate nutrition and poor health care; thus, poverty places children at greater risk for LD and also affects how families are able to cope with a child with a disability. Severely strained psychological and financial resources may impact a family's ability to work with school personnel, and professionals must be aware of this (Haberman, 2005; Hallahan et al., 2005).

One way professionals can help these students is by recommending relevant computer programs. Some low-income families do own computers; if they don't, the students may be given extra time in the school's computer lab to take advantage of technology

TABLE 8.3   Encouraging Literacy Skills in CLD Students

- Have CLD students listen to books on tape
- Encourage CLD students to share their languages, cultural heritage, and even songs in their primary languages with the whole class
- Create a multicultural environment in the classroom
- Show interest in the students' primary language and culture; use maps of the world to locate countries of origin
- Provide opportunities for students to use English and their primary language in situations both inside and outside the classroom
- Help students find appropriate reading and learning materials for use in the home with family members
- Remember that some students come from homes where the parents are nonliterate; send home wordless books that can be looked at and discussed in the language of the home
- Use tutors or aides who speak students' primary languages to help classroom curriculum become more comprehensible. Student peer tutors can be very helpful.

resources for learning. Use of the Internet is becoming more common in today's schools. The Internet can be especially helpful for CLD students with LD because (Hearne, 2000)

- They can link with peers for collaboration and tutoring on schoolwork in both English and the primary language.
- They can access Web sites created especially for English Language Learners and/or students who have disabilities.
- They can access relevant Web sites in English and the primary language at home; if their parents are unable to help them with their English homework (as many of my parents can't), the students can obtain help from the Internet.
- The Internet provides parents with a way to link with the schools. This is especially helpful if the parents don't have transportation to the school.
- The Internet has thousands of free resources that can be quickly accessed. It provides a tool that allows students to delve into various subjects in ways that are not possible through any other source.

Two of my personal favorite free Web sites that encourage literacy are www.starfall.com (for younger children) and www.primarygames.com. Both of these Web sites uses music, animation, and voices to help students with phonological awareness skills, reading, and academics in general. For example, www.primarygames.com has games in math, science, and others. Computers may also be used for writing. Word processing programs can be most helpful for students with LD, especially those who are English Language Learners.

> Many CLD students with LD can benefit from using computer technology in learning.

Many students with LD are creative thinkers, but the mechanics of reading and handwriting are so difficult they become discouraged and don't want to write (Venkatagiri, 2002). Word processing programs can allow students to write, edit, and spell with ease. Today, a great deal of computer software can greatly enhance reading and writing for many students with LD.

For example, text-reading software lets the computer read text and highlight it either letter by letter or word by word. It can also provide spell checks (familiar to most readers) and definitions of terms. There are various types of writing templates for specific types of documents such as résumés, reports, and different types of outlines. Visual concept organization software provides graphic organizers for a student's words (Castellani & Jeffs, 2001). Bender (2004, p. 348) states that

> With this increasing emphasis on assistive technology in the schools, teachers must assure that all students—including those from ethnically diverse backgrounds or poorer students—have reading access to assistive technologies that will enhance their learning (Brown, Higgins & Hartley, 2001). For students with learning disabilities . . . assistive technology can be the difference between a successful school experience and an unsuccessful one. . . . Our students with learning disabilities deserve the very best instruction we can provide, and in many cases today, it will often involve assistive technology of one type or another.

 SUMMARY

- It is best for students with LD in the public school setting to receive integrated services. By law, they must receive these services in the least restricted environment.
- SLPs should work with general-education classroom teachers to promote LD students' success within the classroom setting. It is especially important to promote self-esteem and to make sure the classroom environment is ideal for listening.
- SLPs can work with students with LD to encourage reading; this is especially important with adolescents.
- It is also important to support students who have writing and spelling problems. Some practical methods can be used to do this.
- Special considerations for CLD students with LD include helping them to focus on meaning during reading and writing activities and working with families to promote literacy.
- Many CLD students with LD can benefit from using the computer both at home and at school to enhance learning in all domains.

Add your own summary points here:

_____

_____

_____

CHAPTER HIGHLIGHTS

- A student with a learning disability has normal hearing and vision, does not have significant emotional problems, mental retardation, or educational disadvantages, and yet struggles with reading, writing, and spelling.

- Oral and written language problems are related. They are often inherited. Young children who are identified with oral language problems early in life often are relabeled as LD during the school years. Federal laws mandate appropriate service delivery to students with LD in public schools.
- Students with LD may also have accompanying attention deficit hyperactivity disorder (ADHD). This is treated with medication, behavioral interventions, or both. Parents of children with ADHD may request a special plan that provides for appropriate classroom accommodations.
- Students with LD often have oral communication difficulties in the areas of pragmatics, narrative skills, semantics, and grammatical skills.
- Students with LD are frequently diagnosed with dyslexia. Two major theories about the cause of dyslexia are 1) visual-perceptual/motor theories and 2) phonological processing theories. According to phonological processing theories, dyslexic children have special difficulties in complex phonological production, memory (including rapid automatic naming), and phonological awareness.
- Writing problems in students with LD may include dysgraphia (difficulty with handwriting) and written expression skills. Students with LD frequently have difficulty with spelling also.
- Nonbiased assessment of students with LD is challenging, particularly when they come from CLD backgrounds. Traditional school districts use the discrepancy model, which is generally inappropriate for CLD students. SLPs can use informal measures with these students.
- It is ideal for students with LD to receive early intervention to prevent academic problems later. Ideally intervention services are integrated. Students must be served in the least restrictive environment that is appropriate for their needs. It is important for SLPs to collaborate with general-education classroom teachers.
- Support for written language problems for students with LD can include increasing motivation to read as well as providing assistance with writing and spelling.
- Special considerations for intervention with CLD students include being sensitive to family cultural and socioeconomic characteristics and encouraging literacy. The use of computer technology is especially promising for CLD students with LD.

Add your own chapter highlights here:

_____

_____

_____

STUDY AND REVIEW QUESTIONS

ESSAY

1. Describe the term *learning disability*. What are some characteristics of students with learning disabilities (LD)?

2. Describe the types of oral language problems that are typical of students with LD.

3. Let's say that you are working with an adolescent who has LD and is also from a CLD family who speaks Mandarin at home. What are some ways that you can help her to succeed in high school?

4. Why is it challenging to provide nonbiased assessment for CLD students with potential LD? What are some less-biased, informal ways that we can assess these students?

5. Describe the reading, writing, and spelling problems that typically characterize students with LD. What are some practical suggestions for helping students in these areas?

FILL-IN-THE-BLANK

6. Several federal laws impact provision of services to students with LD in the public schools. The _____ tries to minimize performance inequities between mainstream students and those who perform poorly; the _____ eliminates the need for a "significant discrepancy" in order to make a diagnosis of *learning disability*.

7. _____ skills include the ability to think and talk about language; these skills cut across both spoken and written language.

8. Some students with reading disabilities may have _____, a condition that is treated with colored lenses or glasses.

9. A student with _____ has difficulty with the actual process of handwriting; she frequently writes slowly and forms letters poorly.

10. The _____ for students with reading disabilities is a multisensory approach in which professionals sit beside and slightly behind the students and help students follow along with their finger under each word as they read.

MULTIPLE CHOICE

11. Which one of the following is *false?*
    a. There is a strong relationship between oral and written language impairment.
    b. Oral and written language impairments often co-occur in children and may be genetic.
    c. Students with written language impairments (students with LD) usually have a low IQ that impacts their ability to learn.
    d. SLPs should be involved in service delivery to students with LD.
    e. Early intervention is critical to prevent later problems in school.

12. A child with an LD who had difficulty repeating words such as *aluminum, linoleum,* or *statistics* and had difficulty repeating tongue-twisters would be said to have difficulty in
    a. Complex phonological production
    b. Memory
    c. Semantics
    d. Pragmatics
    e. Syntax

13. Remy S., a Filipino student, was diagnosed in a previous school district as having an LD. In the report, the SLP says that Remy especially has difficulty with conversational repair, adjusting his language to accommodate the status of his conversational partner, and staying on the topic that his peers are discussing. This indicates that Remy especially has difficulty with

    a. Semantics
    b. Pragmatics
    c. Narrative skills
    d. Syntactic skills
    e. Morphological skills

14. You have been asked to give a workshop to a group of parents who wish to understand the term *dyslexia*. You believe that dyslexia is due to deficits in phonological processing. Which of the following will you not tell the parents?

    a. Students with phonological processing problems are generally intelligible and do not have difficulty producing phonologically complex words such as *aluminum*.
    b. These students often have memory deficits.
    c. They also have phonological awareness problems.
    d. These students frequently have rapid naming problems.
    e. Phonological awareness is strongly correlated with reading ability.

15. You have been asked to provide support for Meuy, a seventh-grade Cambodian refugee student with an LD. The family speaks only Khmer at home, they are low income, and they have five children. Meuy enjoys computers but has great difficulty with reading and writing. Which of the following recommendations would be appropriate in this situation?

    i. The parents should purchase a computer for Meuy to use at home.
    ii. Meuy's teachers should permit her to use the computer lab at school as often as possible to complete her assignments.
    iii. Meuy's teachers should encourage her to utilize the school library as much as possible and take books home.
    iv. The resource specialist who works with Meuy in reading should not try to relate the reading to Meuy's life in Cambodia; this is America, and Meuy needs to blend in with American life and culture.
    v. When working with Meuy's writing, the resource specialist should pay careful attention to grammar, spelling, and punctuation; writing for meaning can come after these "basics" are mastered.
    a. All of the above
    b. i, ii, v
    c. ii, iii
    d. ii, iii, iv
    e. i, ii, iii, iv

See Answers to Chapter Study and Review Questions, page 465.

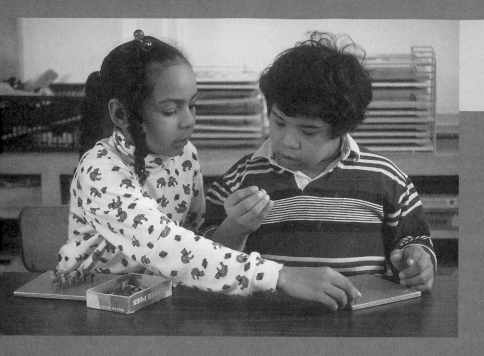

Language in Children with Developmental Disabilities

CASE STUDY

Donte stood out on the first day of kindergarten. The school where I work has navy and white uniforms, which we all wear, including me. Donte's uniform was dirty and rumpled. He would not look at the teacher and was very lackluster and unresponsive to her and his peers. As the weeks went by, Donte was not learning at the same pace as his peers. He continued to have little to no interaction with his teacher and peers and was clearly behind the other students in the class. Donte came from a culturally and linguistically diverse (CLD) home where English was spoken, so we knew that his difficulties could not be attributed to his having to learn English as a second language.

The other speech-language pathologist (SLP) at the school and I decided to place Donte into speech-language therapy. It took my colleague a whole year to teach Donte to label items and give their functions. For instance, she would hold up a ball and say, "Okay, Donte, tell me the name of this and what it does." After nine months of intensive work, Donte could finally do this. As the end of the year drew near, our team knew that there was no way Donte could be promoted to first grade. He still didn't know his alphabet and couldn't count from one to ten. He could not write his name. He continued to be very withdrawn in class and had no friends. Psychological testing eventually revealed that Donte had mental retardation.

We scheduled a meeting with Donte's mother to discuss a special day-class placement for him. In this placement, Donte would get more individual attention and structure as well as a slower pace of learning. Mrs. M. was late and full of apologies. Mrs. M. shared that she had five children; all of them had cognitive and linguistic challenges. The children's father (we were never sure if they were legally married at any point) was in Louisiana, and she was caring for the children alone. As the meeting progressed, it became quite clear to us all that Mrs. M. had mild mental retardation herself. At one point, I was verifying that Donte was five years old and shared that he had been telling us that he was six. She laughed and said, "Is he five? I've been telling him he was six!"

Clearly, it was necessary for us to use very simplified language and explain things several times. Because of Donte's mental retardation and extensive needs, my district spent a lot of money assessing him and placing him in one of the few available slots in a special day class at another school site. We did our best to help Mrs. M. understand that in first grade, a bus would come and pick up Donte each morning and take him to a special school (he walked to our school). She had to have him in the front yard, dressed and ready for school, by 8:15. She nodded, but we were not confident that she had understood. After the meeting, we realized that Mrs. M. might not even be able to have Donte in the front yard each morning at 8:15. That might be asking too much of her. However, we did hope that she would follow through so Donte could get the special class placement that he needed.

INTRODUCTION

Some children have language impairments that accompany developmental disabilities such as mental retardation, autism, or both. Mental retardation (MR) is a disability characterized by significant limitations in adaptive behavior and intellectual functioning. Mental retardation can be caused by a number of factors. These biological and social-environmental factors can bring about mental retardation singly or in combination. Children with MR have deficits in cognitive and linguistic skills. Down syndrome, a common form of MR, results from a chromosomal abnormality.

Some children are diagnosed with autism spectrum disorder (ASD). ASD can be but is not always accompanied by MR. Children with ASD display a variety of behavioral, cognitive, and linguistic characteristics that depend in part upon which subtype of ASD they have. There are five subtypes of ASD: autistic disorder, Rett disorder, childhood disintegrative disorder, Asperger syndrome, and pervasive developmental disorder not otherwise specified (PDD-NOS). It is believed that ASD is a neurologically based disorder and that there may be a genetic component .

Assessment and intervention for children with MR and/or ASD are usually conducted by multidisciplinary teams of professionals. Early intervention is considered critical for children with MR and/or ASD, and public school districts have taken on an increasingly prominent role in providing this early intervention. SLPs need to be especially sensitive when working with families of CLD children who have MR and/or ASD.

For cultural reasons, religious reasons, or both families may have an especially difficult time acknowledging that their child has MR and/or ASD. In these situations, SLPs must effectively utilize services of cultural mediators to support families as they deal with difficult diagnoses.

MENTAL RETARDATION: DEFINITION AND CAUSES

Definition and Classification

As many as three out of every 100 persons in the United States have mental retardation (MR). More than 614,000 children between the ages of six and twenty-one have some level of MR. One out of every ten children who needs special education services has MR (AAMR; American Association on Mental Retardation, 2002). The term **developmental delay** has also been used to describe these children. In this chapter, the term MR is used although it is important to acknowledge that in some circles, professionals use the term **developmental delay**.

The AAMR (2002) defined mental retardation as follows:

> Mental retardation is a disability characterized by significant limitations both in intellectual functioning and adaptive behavior as expressed in conceptual, social, and practical adaptive skills. This disability originates before the age of 18. . . . Mental retardation refers to a particular state of functioning that begins in childhood, has many dimensions, and is affected positively by individualized supports. . . . It includes the contexts and environment within which the person functions and interacts. . . . Mental retardation is thought to be present if an individual has an IQ test score of approximately 70 or below.

The AAMR stresses that limitations in present functioning have to be considered within the context of community environments typical of the person's age, peers, and culture.

Many educators are familiar with the classifications of MR as put forth by the AAMR (1992) as described in Table 9.1. Intelligence quotient, or IQ, is a ratio of mental age to chronological age. For example, if a child is six years old and his mental age is also six, he probably has an IQ of 100, which is average. It can be seen that most persons with MR have mild MR.

In 1992, the AAMR eliminated the above classification based on IQ. In an attempt to acknowledge the unique profiles of persons with MR, the AAMR recommended that children be evaluated on their functional abilities, including

- Physical and health status
- Intellectual and adaptive skills
- Emotional and psychological factors
- Environmental considerations

TABLE 9.1   Levels of Mental Retardation

IQ Range	Severity	% of MR	Characteristics
IQ of 50–69	Mild	89	Often have families; usually live and work independently in the community
IQ of 35–49	Moderate	6	Semi-independent; may live in community residences or with family; may work in supportive environments
IQ of 20–34	Severe	3.5	Can learn some self-care skills and may work in a supportive environment; may live with family or in a community residence
IQ below 20	Profound	1.5	Often have multiple handicaps; need constant supervision and care; may be able to learn basic life skills

Source: Adapted from Owens, 2004; American Association on Mental Retardation (1992, 2002)

Children with MR are a very diverse group. Some children have MR due to biological causes such as prenatal exposure to alcohol and drugs, or genetic syndromes such as Down syndrome and fragile X syndrome. Some children have MR due to social-environmental causes such as sensory deprivation (e.g., prolonged isolation) or an impoverished environment. Children with MR show a variety of communication problems, especially in the area of language. The severity of these problems exists in direct proportion to the severity of the retardation. Generally, children with MR show intellectual, social, and adaptive behaviors that are significantly below normal. Professionals who work with children with MR can develop a matrix to identify levels of support needed by individual children (see Table 9.2).

TABLE 9.2   Levels of Support

Intermittent Support = "as-needed" basis (e.g., a person doesn't need support all the time, just during certain times such as a medical crisis)
Limited Support = consistent, time-limited support
Extensive Support = regular, non-time-limited involvement (e.g., daily support at home)
Pervasive Support = high-intensity, constant support across environments (e.g., a constant companion around the clock)

Sources: Adapted from AAMR, 2002; Kuder, 2003; Woolfolk, 2004

Causes

As stated earlier, MR in children is caused by one of two things: biological or social-environmental factors. Of course, it is possible that a combination of these factors may contribute to MR in a child. Specific etiologies of MR in children are described as follows (AAMR, 2002):

Biological Factors

- Genetic and hereditary factors resulting in such syndromes as fragile X syndrome, Prader-Willi syndrome, Down syndrome, and cri du chat syndrome (for descriptions of these syndromes, see Roseberry-McKibbin & Hegde, 2006)
- Cranial abnormalities such as hydrocephaly (head enlargement due to an excessive collection of spinal fluids within the cranial vault) and microcephaly (extremely small head)
- Metabolic disorders such as Tay-Sachs disease
- Endocrine disorders, including hypothyroidism
- Prenatal factors such as mercury poisoning, lead poisoning, prenatal trauma, prematurity and low birth weight, maternal anoxia, maternal rubella, and maternal use of alcohol, drugs, or both during pregnancy
- Perinatal factors such as fetal anoxia and brain injury during the birth process (e.g., baby becomes stuck in the birth canal for an extended period of time)
- Postnatal factors (after birth) such as lead poisoning and postimmunization encephalitis
- Head trauma due to child abuse, gunshot wounds, or accidents such as car accidents

> MR can result from biological factors, social-environmental factors, or a combination of these.

Social-Environmental Factors

- Sensory deprivation (e.g., maternal deprivation or prolonged isolation)
- Impoverished environment (e.g., poor nutrition, exposure to lead, no books in home, few outside experiences)

I have found that children who have been in refugee camps have sometimes presented with MR. Their mothers had very inadequate nutrition during pregnancy, and the children have been malnourished all their lives after they were born. Many times they have had little schooling or cognitive-linguistic stimulation. This does tend to happen when people are fleeing for their lives.

In Chapter 4, we talked about internationally adopted children. Some of these children come from excellent environments in their home countries and do quite well. However, as we discussed, many come from orphanages where there was inadequate and very little stimulation. One researcher told me that when she visited a country in the former

USSR, she saw that in some orphanages, children spent three hours in the morning and three hours in the afternoon in a crib. A Ukrainian pastor I worked with said that in some Ukrainian orphanages, all the children had to eat was oatmeal with the occasional piece of candy. SLPs need to be especially aware of the possibility of MR in children who have spent extensive time in refugee campus or orphanages in their home countries.

CASES TO CONSIDER

A very bright student of mine at the university came to me and shared that her daughter's linguistic and cognitive skills had been deteriorating. Amy couldn't figure out what was wrong with her three-year-old Beth. Formerly a bright and precocious child, Beth was "going downhill" in Amy's words, and she was scared. To make a very long story short, the doctors finally identified that Beth had been exposed to high levels of lead in the low-income housing where Amy and her husband lived. What recommendations might you make to Amy regarding Beth's cognitive-linguistic skills and overall development in general?

_____

_____

_____

SUMMARY

- Mental retardation, also called developmental delay, originates before the age of eighteen. It is characterized by significant limitations in both adaptive behavior and intellectual functioning as expressed in conceptual, social, and practical adaptive skills.
- Mental retardation may range in severity from mild to profound. Individuals with mental retardation need varying levels of support, depending upon the extent of their needs.
- Mental retardation can be caused by biological factors, social-environmental factors, or a combination of these.

Add your own summary points here:

_____

_____

_____

COGNITIVE AND LINGUISTIC CHARACTERISTICS OF CHILDREN WITH MENTAL RETARDATION

The Relationship between Language and Cognition

Much has been written about the relationship between language and cognitive skills in people with MR. According to Kuder (2003), in children five years old and younger, there is a close relationship between language and cognitive development. In children six or seven years of age and older, there are specific language deficits that cannot be explained by age alone. Owens (2004) states that for approximately half the MR population, language comprehension and production levels are generally commensurate with cognitive levels. For the other half of the MR population, patterns vary; for example, some children have language production and comprehension skills that are below the level of cognition; others have commensurate language comprehension and cognition levels with lower production levels, and so forth.

Cognitive and Processing Characteristics

The first criterion in defining MR in a child is deficits in cognitive functioning. Usually, intelligence tests are used to measure cognitive functioning as we said before. Previously, experts thought that children with MR were "low across the board"; that they had equal deficiency in every aspect of cognitive functioning. Today, we know that this is not true. Each child has a unique profile where some cognitive skills are better than others. There are several areas that have been extensively researched with regard to cognitive functioning in MR children: attention, discrimination, memory, organization, and generalization (Hardman et al., 2006; Kuder, 2003; Owens, 2004; Paul, 2001).

> Children with MR usually have difficulty with attention, discrimination, memory, and organization

Children with MR can sustain attention as well as typically developing (TD) peers in many situations. Their problem is that they have difficulty selecting which stimuli to attend to (discrimination problems). This creates difficulty in learning, because MR children don't always attend to the important information in situations (Henry & Gudjonsson, 1999; Westling & Fox, 2000). In the intervention section of this chapter, recommendations are made for helping MR children in this area.

Children with MR have difficulty remembering information. Generally, long-term memory is better than short-term memory. Children with MR may forget new information seconds after they have heard it. There may be difficulties with storage of information as well as difficulties with associational strategies. In associational strategies, one symbol or word can aid recollection of another. For example, if you really want to remember the name of a woman you just met named Marsha Pickens, you might visualize her picking things out of a marsh. Many adults use associative strategies to help them remember names. Children with MR do not do this; they need to be explicitly taught.

Children with MR remember visual information better than they remember auditory information. They retain pictures better than letters or printed words. They remember non-linguistic auditory information (e.g., the music of the ice cream truck) better than linguistic auditory information (e.g., instructions for getting ready for bed).

Organization is hard for children with MR, especially with regard to categorizing information. In Chapter 1, we discussed this and gave the example of a file cabinet. When information comes in, TD children "file" it into a "mental drawer." For example, if a TD child hears "car, bike, boat, plane" she can file or categorize those as forms of transportation. Children with MR have difficulty with this. It is far more difficult to remember unrelated bits of information than to remember information that is categorized or "chunked."

Children with MR have a great deal of difficulty generalizing information that they learn (Beirne-Smith, Ittenbach, & Patton, 2002). So, for example, let's say that in a therapy session, you teach a child with MR to say "excuse me" if she needs to interrupt. She may be able to do this with 100 percent accuracy in the therapy room, but she will probably walk right out of the therapy room and interrupt others without remembering to say "excuse me" even once.

CASES TO CONSIDER

Donna L., a sixteen-year-old young lady from a White, monolingual English-speaking home, attended high school in the school district where I work. I was asked to come and assess Donna's speech and language, with particular attention to carryover of skills taught in speech-language therapy to Donna's daily environment. Upon examining Donna's file, I found that in early elementary school, she had been diagnosed with moderately severe mental retardation. Donna had attended special classes all through school and was in a self-contained special-education classroom at her high school campus.

In a long and acrimonious meeting with Mr. and Mrs. L., they stated that they were very angry at me for saying in my report that Donna had mental retardation. Apparently, Donna had accused one of the teachers in our school district of sexually molesting her. Without my knowledge, the teacher's attorney had subpoenaed my report and had used it in court to try and convince the jury that Donna did not have the mental capacity to make this type of accusation accurately.

I told Mr. and Mrs. L. that I felt very bad that my report had been used to discredit their daughter, and let them know that I thought Donna was a lovely, cheerful young woman who had been a pleasure to work with. I then talked with Mr. and Mrs. L. about the need for Donna to take what she was learning in speech-language therapy and generalize the information (e.g., curriculum vocabulary, vocabulary pertaining to activities of daily living) outside the therapy room. I asked them if they would be willing to work with her at home to help her generalize some of the vocabulary that the high school SLP was trying to teach her.

Mr. and Mrs. L. were angry that I asked them to work with Donna at home, and said that her progress was the school's job and that they did not have time to work with her.

How would you have handled their response? What would you tell them that might help motivate them to work with Donna in a home carryover program?

_____

_____

_____

Language Characteristics

Researchers have debated whether the language of children with MR is qualitatively or quantitatively different from that of TD children. Most researchers would agree that language of children with MR is quantitatively different; that is, these children develop language along the same lines as TD children, but more slowly. Below ten years of age, TD and MR children may demonstrate more quantitative language differences; language develops in a similar sequence, but MR children develop at a slower rate. After ten years of age, qualitative differences in the language skills of TD and MR children become more apparent (Owens, 2004). Children with more severe MR may manifest qualitatively different language behaviors such as **echolalia**, where they repeat verbatim what is said to them. Echolalia is not typical of any stage of the language development of TD children. We will now discuss phonological, morphological, syntactic, semantic, and pragmatic characteristics of children with MR.

> Some children with MR manifest echolalia, where they repeat verbatim what is said to them.

Phonological Characteristics

A thorough discussion of the phonological problems of children with MR is beyond the scope of this text; however, the reader is referred to previously cited sources for more information in this area (e.g., Bernthal & Bankson, 2004; Peña-Brooks & Hegde, 2000). Basically, children with MR frequently have consonant substitutions and distortions. Common characteristics include simplification of consonant clusters and especially final consonant deletion.

POINTS TO PONDER Describe the phonological, morphological, and syntactic characteristics of children with MR.

_____

_____

_____

Morphological and Syntactic Characteristics

Research suggests that children with MR develop morphemes in the same *sequence* as TD children, but at a slower *rate*. Commonly, children with MR omit bound morphemes such as plural -*s*, present progressive -*ing*, past tense -*ed*, and others. On a personal note, I have not had much success teaching bound morphemes to children with MR. I think that this is because bound morphemes are highly abstract. Imagine trying to teach possessive -*s* to a child who has difficulty remembering her own name and age.

Research suggests that initially, children with MR develop syntactic skills in the same sequence as TD children. However, there is probably a plateau. Children with MR tend to have simplified sentence structure with infrequent use of compound and complex sentences (defined in Chapter 1). When a child's mean length of utterance (MLU) in morphemes is less than 3.0, children with MR appear very similar to their TD peers in syntactic skills. Once MLU gets above 3.0, children with MR use shorter and less complex sentences than their mental-age peers. Children with MR learn grammatical morphemes in approximately the same sequence as their TD peers; however, they learn these morphemes more slowly.

> Children with MR may have telegraphic speech, where they leave function words out of sentences and only include content words.

Children with MR may have **telegraphic speech**, which we defined in previous chapters as speech where children leave function words out of sentences and only include content words. For example:

TD child: I want an ice cream cone, please.

Child with MR: Want ice cream cone.

Children with MR have difficulty with receptive syntactic abilities also; it is challenging for them to understand long and complex sentences. This may be related in part to their deficits in working memory (Facon, Facon-Bollengier, & Grubar, 2002).

Semantic Characteristics

As a general rule, children with MR are later to acquire their first words than TD children. The vocabularies of children with MR are smaller and more concrete than those of TD children. Abstract words present a great deal of difficulty for most children with MR, which has major implications for intervention as we shall see later. In addition, children with MR use many more nouns than verbs or adjectives. However, children with MR learn vocabulary more easily than syntax.

Pragmatic Characteristics

In Chapter 1, we discussed Fey's (1986) model of assertiveness and responsiveness. Children with MR have a variety of difficulties in these areas, depending on the cause and the extent of the MR. Some children may be physically aggressive, especially if they are frustrated or if they want something and don't have the linguistic ability to ask for it appropriately. I was working out at the gym one time, and a group of MR adults came in from a local community home. As I was sitting on a machine trying to bulk up my stringy muscles, one of the women came up and scratched me hard on the arm, breaking my skin. Clearly she wanted the machine I was using, and I had not noticed her wanting it. I quickly gave it to her.

In general, evidence seems to indicate that MR children have a tendency to be passive. They often do not initiate conversations. Topic maintenance is an area of difficulty for children with MR. They may not extend a conversational topic by adding new information; instead, they may just say "uh hum" (Kuder, 2003). In addition, these children have difficulty with conversational repair in terms of requesting clarification. For example, if a child with MR does not understand what someone is saying, she may not say, "I'm sorry—I don't understand. Could you tell me more?" Children with MR also frequently demonstrate **perseveration**, or excessive talking about a subject that has been previously addressed or is inappropriate.

Children with MR have more difficulty than TD children in judging the nonverbal emotions of their communication partners and may inadvertently offend them. I remember Melissa, a White, monolingual English-speaking sixth-grader with MR. Nicknamed "the roller derby queen," Melissa was an aggressive young woman who frequently got into fights on the playground, in part because she did not adequately judge the emotions and nonverbal cues of the other children. Part of my language intervention with her focused on helping her "read" other people's nonverbal cues and emotional states so that she could interact with them more successfully.

CASES TO CONSIDER

I was asked to evaluate a Vietnamese student named Van B. Van, the youngest of six children, was born in Vietnam. His mother was in her late 30s when he was born. Van's father was a first lieutenant of the old Saigon regime. According to the records that we were able to obtain from Saigon, Van had been a TD child up until the age of four, when he developed a very high fever and was hospitalized for ten days. According to Mr. B., "he became slow after that." Mr. B. shared that Van was "no longer able to do some of the things that he had once done." He described Van as "an eleven-year-old with the mind of a five-year-old."

The family had recently immigrated to California, where Van was put into school. Initially, he was defecating in his pants for the first week and had to be sent home. Van did not take care of his own hygiene; family members did this for him. Van was finally trained to take care of his own hygiene and was placed in a self-contained special-education classroom (where I first saw him). He reportedly wanted to interact with the other children, who all spoke English. Van spoke very little Vietnamese or English, and nonverbal IQ testing had shown that his skills were very low. When Van wanted to initiate interactions with the other children, he would spit, swear, hit, or pinch the children to get their attention. He had difficulty verbalizing even simple needs (e.g., that he needed food or to go to the bathroom).

What intervention goals might you have for Van? What would be your top priorities in language therapy with him?

_____

_____

_____

> The condition of Down syndrome results from trisomy 21, a chromosomal abnormality involving a third and extra copy of the twenty-first chromosome. People with Down syndrome exhibit problems in a number of cognitive and linguistic areas.

Children with Down Syndrome

The condition of **Down syndrome** results from trisomy 21, a chromosomal abnormality involving a third and extra copy of the twenty-first chromosome. People with Down syndrome experience mild to moderate retardation, intelligibility problems, oral motor problems, low muscle tone or hypotonia, brachycephaly (a face with a shortened front-to-back dimension), anomalies of the ear, and speech and language problems. Due to anomalies of the ear and upper respiratory tract, children with Down syndrome often have recurrent episodes of otitis media (middle ear infections), which further affect their language and phonological development. It is estimated that children with Down syndrome may have a fifty-two times greater incidence of infections than TD children due to a poorly functioning immune system.

Generally, the language development of children with Down syndrome follows the normal sequence; however, some atypical features may be present. These features are partially related to the aforementioned tendency toward otitis media as well as to craniofacial anomalies, which can severely impact intelligibility. Children with Down syndrome tend to have large tongues in relation to their oral cavities. I have found through the years that therapy to remediate articulatory-phonological disorders in children with Down syndrome is a real challenge. Progress may be minimal, and some SLPs turn to sign language or augmentative communication as illustrated in the case of Jessica R. below.

In terms of early vocabulary skills, comprehension does appear to be better than production, and this gap increases with age. Vocabulary comprehension skills keep pace with cognitive development, while expressive vocabulary skills do not. There is a similar situation with

CASES TO CONSIDER

Jessica R. was a first-grade girl with Down syndrome and accompanying cognitive-linguistic deficits. She was highly unintelligible, and I had difficulty getting her to even say simple CVC (consonant-vowel-consonant) words such as "mom" and "bed." Jessica was becoming quite frustrated in the classroom, where she would sometimes throw tantrums because of her difficulties in communicating. I recommended sign language as an adjunct to oral language. However, Jessica's mother, a doctor, was very opposed to this recommendation. What might you say to Jessica's mother if you had a chance to have a conversation with her? Would you agree with my recommendation that Jessica be taught sign language? Explain your answer.

_____

_____

_____

syntactic skills; production lags behind comprehension, and this gap increases with age. Research has verified that a hallmark of Down syndrome is expressive language skills that are depressed in comparison to comprehension skills (e.g., Chapman, Seung, Schwartz, & Kay-Raining Bird, 1998; Miles & Chapman, 2002). When expressive language is measured by MLU and the number of different words in conversational and narrative samples, children and adolescents with Down syndrome show greater impairment in expressive language than in nonverbal cognition and syntax comprehension (Boudreau & Chapman, 2000).

Professionals in the past often assumed that children with Down syndrome could not learn to read. However, it has been found that they can indeed learn to read, and their reading levels may be in advance of their cognitive and linguistic abilities. Some experts believe that children with Down syndrome learn to sight read whole words and do not necessarily use phonological awareness skills like TD children do (Paul, 2001).

Though experts have believed that Down syndrome children learn to read using minimal phonological awareness skills (if any), one study showed that phoneme segmentation (a phonological awareness skill) was positively associated with early oral reading skill in young children with Down syndrome. This suggests that young Down syndrome children's process of learning to read may be more qualitatively similar to that of TD children than was originally thought (Cupples & Iacono, 2000). However, results of a longitudinal study by Kay-Raining Bird et al. (2000) showed that over time, phonological awareness and word attack skills did not keep pace with word recognition skills. These researchers recommended that those who develop programs for children with Down syndrome use visual supports (to reduce demands on memory) as phonological awareness skills are taught.

Children with Down syndrome have poor verbal short-term memories. For example, if we ask a child with Down syndrome to "say these numbers: 5-9-2-4; (pause) now you say them," the child will have a great deal of difficulty (Jarrold, Baddeley, & Phillips, 2002). According to Laws & Bishop (2003), the working-memory difficulties of children with Down syndrome may be a significant predictor of language development in these children.

CONNECT & EXTEND

Language abilities of children with Down syndrome are described in Laws, G., & Bishop, D.V. M. (2003). A comparison of language abilities in adolescents with Down syndrome and children with specific language impairment. *Journal of Speech, Language, and Hearing Research*, 46, 1324–1339.

SUMMARY

- Children with MR have different profiles of cognitive-linguistic skills; patterns of language and cognitive deficits are unique to each child.
- Children with MR typically have difficulties with attention, memory, and organization. Generalizing learned information to other settings is a particular challenge.
- Children with MR often have phonological problems that lead to lack of intelligibility. They develop morphemes in the same sequence but at a slower rate than TD children. The syntax of children with MR tends to be simple and less complex than that of TD children.

(continued)

- Children with MR are later to acquire their first words than TD children. Their vocabularies are usually concrete because it is hard for them to grasp abstract words. In terms of pragmatics, these children tend to be passive in initiating interactions with others.
- Children with Down syndrome are often unintelligible. Research has shown that their expressive language skills are depressed in comparison to their comprehension skills.
- Children with Down syndrome have difficulty with reading and reading-related skills. This may be due in part to limited phonological awareness skills and problems with verbal short-term memory.

Add your own summary points here:

_____

_____

_____

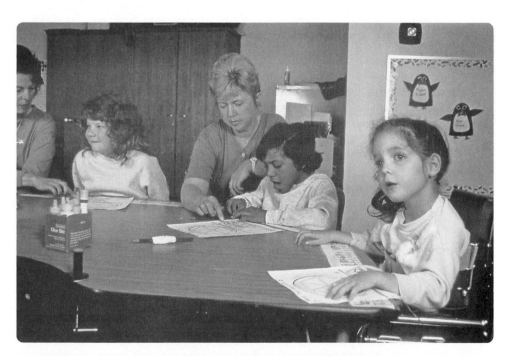

Because children with autism spectrum disorder and/or mental retardation frequently have difficulty discriminating what they need to pay attention to, those who work with them should highlight new or especially relevant information.

AUTISM SPECTRUM DISORDER: DEFINITION AND CAUSES

Definition

Pioneers in describing children with **autism spectrum disorder** (ASD) were Leo Kanner in 1943 and Hans Asperger in 1944. Leo Kanner worked in Baltimore, and Hans Asperger worked in Vienna, Austria. Both of these researchers believed that children with ASD had a fundamental biological disturbance from birth. They described a set of characteristics that was common to these children. They described, most of all, the overarching characteristic of disturbed social relationships.

Today, there are many estimates of the incidence and prevalence of ASD. It is very hard to estimate these parameters because of the differing subtypes of ASD (described below). I don't want to be flippant here; however, when I give workshops across the United States, usually audiences in every state from Washington to Georgia tell me that children with ASD are "coming out of the woodwork." There are experts who believe that today we do not have increasing numbers of children with ASD; we just have better means of identification (e.g., Frith, 2003). I must say that subjectively, from what I see in my own school district and in districts across the United States, I subscribe to the woodwork theory myself.

Fombonne (2003) summarized the data from large national surveys that indicated that in the United States today, there are approximately 425,000 children with ASD; 114,000 of these are younger than five years old. Fombonne stated that the available evidence indicates that recent rates for autism disorder and ASD (described below) are three to four times higher than they were thirty years ago. It is estimated that approximately one out of every 500 children has ASD.

> Autism spectrum disorder, also known as pervasive developmental disorder, involves a range of disabling behaviors that change and vary with development.

In previous decades, most professionals used the term **autism** to refer to a set of behaviors (described below) that occurred in children. Today, the term *ASD* is used to describe the profiles of a wide range of children who have impairments in their ability to initiate and sustain healthy, normal social relationships. The term *ASD* recognizes that autism is not a single condition; rather, it involves a range of disabling behaviors that change and vary with development (Schopler, 2001). The *Diagnostic and Statistical Manual*-IV-TR (DSM-IV-TR) of the American Psychiatric Association (2000) has systematized behaviors characterized by significant problems in communication and relationships under the category of **pervasive developmental disorder** (PDD). Today, PDD is more often referred to as ASD. There are five subtypes of PDD (or ASD):

- Autistic disorder (the more classic and severe form)
- Rett disorder
- Childhood disintegrative disorder
- Pervasive developmental disorder not otherwise specified (PDD-NOS)
- Asperger disorder

CONNECT & EXTEND

Full descriptions of each aspect of the autism spectrum disorder continuum are given by the National Institute of Mental Health (2004), available at www.nimh.nih.gov/publicat/autism.cfm.

Autistic disorder and Asperger disorder (also called Asperger syndrome) are the most commonly occurring types of ASD. If a child has symptoms of either of these disorders but does not meet the specific criteria for either, the diagnosis is called PDD-NOS. Childhood disintegrative disorder and Rett disorder are rarer and more severe.

To be diagnosed with any type of ASD, a child has to have developmental impairments in three areas: 1) verbal and nonverbal communication, 2) repertoire of activities and interests, and 3) reciprocal social interactions. Experts today believe that ASD can be diagnosed reliably by three years of age, and maybe even as early as eighteen months (National Institute of Mental Health, 2004). Sometimes children with ASD have accompanying conditions such as MR, seizures, or other conditions (Hogenboom, 2001). Interestingly, children with ASD—especially those with full-blown autistic disorder—are often described as being physically very beautiful (Frith, 2003).

One of the biggest changes in practice today is the recognition and treatment of children with Asperger syndrome (Klin & Volkmar, 1995). Asperger syndrome is generally thought of as milder than autism and it frequently is diagnosed much later. Children with Asperger syndrome have some unusual behaviors and social interaction problems, but they generally don't have impairments in other areas of language. Frith (2003, p. 11) states that

> People with Asperger syndrome are at the same time different from, and similar to, people with autism. The difference that is currently held key for the definition is that they show no language delay as children, nor delays in other aspects of their intellectual development. Yet at older ages they are not very different in their social impairments and obsessions from many of those who had such delays but were considered to have "high functioning" autism. . . . Their social communication impairments are especially evident in interaction with peers, and increase when expectations and demands increase with age. . . . Experts are divided as to whether Asperger syndrome and autism should be seen as different diagnostic categories. However, the consensus tends to favor the idea that both are variants of the same underlying developmental disorder, with autism being a more severe form, detectable at an earlier age.

Individuals with Asperger syndrome are often identifiable by their all-consuming interest in a particular topic. Researchers did a survey of parents of children with Asperger syndrome, and 100 percent of the parents indicated that their children had one or more special interests. The top five interests were 1) fads such as Pokémon, 2) video or computer games, 3) works of art, 4) movies, fictional books, or TV programs, and 5) computers (Blakemore-Brown, 2002).

Students with Asperger syndrome may have adultlike vocabularies and an all-consuming interest in a particular subject. They will talk incessantly about this interest, even if the listener does not want to hear more information.

There is a fine line between being very interested in a hobby and having an "Asperger-style" interest. Children with Asperger syndrome will conduct a monologue about their interests. They will not notice the other person trying to change the subject, looking disinterested, or even walking away. Listeners feel as if they are being lectured at rather than interacted with. They may feel that the child with Asperger syndrome is rude and self-centered (Blakemore-Brown, 2002). Children with Asperger syndrome often have a very impressive,

CONNECT & EXTEND

Asperger syndrome is described in depth by Mesibov, G.B., Shea, V., & Adams, L.W. (2001). *Understanding Asperger syndrome and high functioning autism.* New York: Kluwer Academic/Plenum Publishers.

adultlike vocabulary and an overly formal way of speaking (Bashe & Kirby, 2001). They are very different from those with frank autistic disorder (explained later), who are seen as mute and aloof.

Causes

One can very generally describe the cause of ASD as "neurologically based" (Mesibov et al., 2001). With the aid of modern technology such as computerized tomography (CT), positron emission tomography (PET), and magnetic resonance imaging (MRI), scientists have been able to study the functioning and structure of the brain in individuals

POINTS TO PONDER Describe characteristics of students with Asperger syndrome. What characteristics distinguish them from students with frank autistic disorder?

_____

_____

_____

CASES TO CONSIDER

Tommy B., a two-year-old boy from a Mexican family, was brought by his parents to the university clinic where I worked. Tommy's father, Dr. B., a pharmacist, shared with me that "Tommy seemed so normal up till a few months ago. Suddenly he didn't want hugs anymore, and he stopped talking. He was doing so well, and now he will hardly look at us or play with us. Something is wrong, and we don't know what it is." Dr. and Mrs. B. requested speech-language therapy, which we provided. My graduate students and I realized that Tommy had autism, but it was clear that Dr. and Mrs. B. were not prepared for this diagnosis. How would you handle this situation? What would you do to help Dr. and Mrs. B. recognize the fact that Tommy had autism? How might you be culturally sensitive in this situation?

_____

_____

_____

with ASD. MRI and postmortem studies have shown that many major brain structures are implicated in autism. These include the cerebral cortex, limbic system, brain stem, basal ganglia, and corpus callosum. Other research is focusing on the role of neurotransmitters such as epinephrine, dopamine, and serotonin. There is also increasing evidence that genetic factors play a large role in the causes of ASD (National Institute of Mental Health, 2004).

 SUMMARY

- Leo Kanner and Hans Asperger, two experts who lived and worked in the 1900s, described the characteristics of a group of children whose social relationships were particularly impaired.
- The term autism spectrum disorder (ASD) is used to describe children with particularly impaired social relationships. They may fall into one of five categories on the spectrum: classic autistic disorder, Rett disorder, childhood disintegrative disorder, pervasive developmental disorder not otherwise specified (PDD-NOS), and Asperger syndrome.
- Today, ASD is considered to be neurologically based. Genetic factors and differences in brain structure have also been implicated in ASD.

BEHAVIORAL, COGNITIVE, AND LINGUISTIC CHARACTERISTICS OF CHILDREN WITH AUTISM SPECTRUM DISORDER

> Some experts believe that children with ASD lack a theory of mind. They have difficulty understanding other people's behavior and taking other people's perspectives.

Theory of Mind

One hypothesis regarding cognitive and linguistic impairments in children with ASD states that these children lack a theory of mind (Frith, 2003). According to the **theory of mind** hypothesis, TD children have an understanding of the mental states of others. If this ability is impaired, children have problems understanding the behavior (including the communication behavior) of other people. They have difficulty taking others' perspectives.

Behavioral Characteristics

Children with autism exhibit certain characteristics very early in life, and these continue as they get older. Other times, children may appear to be developing in a typical fashion up till a certain point. Then, between twelve and thirty-six months of age, unusual behaviors become apparent (e.g., losing previously acquired social and language skills, rejecting other people), as in the case of Tommy B. This developmental regression occurs especially in regard to language and social skills (Hewetson, 2002). Behavioral characteristics of children with ASD may include the following in a variety of different combinations (depending on the child and the type of ASD he has) (Hardman et al., 2006; Roseberry-McKibbin & Hegde, 2006; Smith, Lovaas, & Lovaas, 2002):

- Lack of responsiveness to physical contact or affection (e.g., babies become rigid when picked up)
- Gaze aversion (avoidance of eye contact)
- Preference for objects rather than people
- Play behaviors such as excessive lining up of toys or other objects, strong attachment to one particular toy or object
- Doesn't smile
- At times seems to be hearing impaired
- Self-stimulation—e.g., rocking back and forth; flicking their hands in front of their faces; head banging (especially prevalent when the child wants to withdraw from the environment)
- Repetitive behaviors such as repeated flapping of the hands
- Sometimes repetitive behavior takes the form of an intense, persistent preoccupation; there is often a great interest in science topics, numbers, or symbols
- Possibly walking on their toes
- Resistance to change in routine or environment—even a minor deviation can cause an outburst (family often feels like they are "walking on eggshells")
- Tendency to "lose control," particularly in environments that feel strange or overwhelming; there may be temper tantrums
- Relatedly, children may perseverate on an item to be learned and have difficulty shifting to the next task
- Lower intelligence in children with "pure" autism; 75 percent of these children have IQs lower than 70
- Great difficulty understanding social cues and relating to others
- Sensory problems—e.g., great sensitivity to certain sounds, textures, tastes, and smells
- Approximately 10 to 15 percent of children with autism exhibit "splinter skills," or areas of ability where performance levels are quite high compared with other areas of functioning. For example, a child might have an excellent memory for numbers.

Some children with ASD have specific, strong, long-term memory skills. They are especially good at recalling factual information like dates, names, and numbers (Pring & Hermelin, 2002). The long-term memory skills of these students can equal those of their TD peers. Some readers may remember the movie *Rain Man* from some years ago. Dustin Hoffman, an adult with ASD, had incredible recall of numbers that could be very helpful in certain situations. The relatively strong long-term memory skills of some children with ASD can help them educationally.

Tiegerman-Farber (2002) states that as children with ASD get bigger, they can become physically uncontrollable and harder for parents and teachers to manage. This is illustrated in the case of Jerry (see page 324).

CASES TO CONSIDER

A friend of mine had two TD children, and then Jerry was born. Jerry was diagnosed with autism when he was two years old. My friend, his mother, put Jerry in special classes so that he could receive the education he needed. She and her husband kept Jerry living at home with them and his two siblings.

When Jerry was fifteen years old, he had a growth spurt and became quite tall and strong. He began to throw furniture, punch holes in walls, and be physically abusive to his mother and siblings. Jerry would slam my friend up against the wall and generally became out of control behavior-wise. My friend realized that she was no longer physically strong enough to control her son.

My friend and her husband decided that for Jerry's safety as well as their own and that of their two other children, they would place him in a comfortable, close-by group home that was run by competent, caring staff who were equipped to handle Jerry and others like him. Did my friend and her husband make the right decision? Should they have continued to try to have Jerry live with them? Explain.

_____

_____

_____

Phonological Characteristics

Research shows that children with ASD accompanied by MR often have phonological problems similar to those described in the previous section on mental retardation. Studies of the speech production of children with ASD without MR has shown that in those who develop spoken language, the course of development of phonological rules follows the same course as does that of TD children (Kuder, 2003; Owens, 2004). However, **suprasegmental features** may be deviant. Children with ASD may have disturbed prosody characterized by features such as flat intonation, a high-pitched voice, a "singsong" quality, inappropriate fluctuations in intensity, and others.

> Students with ASD often have deviant suprasegmental features; their voices may lack intonation and have a singsong quality.

Shriberg, Paul, McSweeny, Klin, Cohen, and Volkmar (2001) used standardized assessment instruments to study the speech and prosody (intonation)-voice profiles of thirty males with high-functioning autism or Asperger syndrome. They compared their findings to those that have been documented for typical speakers of comparable ages. The subjects ranged from ten to forty-nine years of age. Shriberg et al. found that the subjects in the high-functioning autism and Asperger syndrome groups had notable deficits in prosody; these subjects had distinctive differences in their loudness, pitch, stress, and resonance when compared with typical speakers.

Shriberg et al. suggested that SLPs screen speakers in the ten- to forty-nine-year-old age group for possible prosody-voice characteristics that might affect these speakers' vocational and social adjustment. If these characteristics are found, then clinicians can work in therapy to increase these clients' metalinguistic knowledge of appropriate suprasegmental targets. This can be followed by practice to apply this knowledge in practical situations where appropriate pragmatics skills are called for.

Morphological and Syntactic Characteristics

Children with ASD accompanied by MR will often have morphological and syntactic characteristics similar to those explained in the previous section. Children with autistic disorder are often delayed in acquisition of normal morphological and syntactic milestones. They may have specific difficulty with verb endings and pronouns. The sentences of children with ASD may be less complex than those of TD peers (Owens, 2004). However, children such as those with Asperger syndrome, who are higher functioning, often have sophisticated morphological and syntactic skills (Frith, 2003; Mesibov et al., 2001).

Some children with more severe autism will demonstrate **echolalia**—repeating back what was said to them. They may repeat words immediately, or even hours or days after hearing them. For example:

Clinician: Johnny, want to play with this car?
Johnny: Play with this car?

Not all children with ASD present with echolalia (Schuler & Fletcher, 2002). However, many will use "prefabricated" sentences; they have a specific deficit in creating novel sentences (Schuler & Fletcher, 2002). These children can be helped by visual, written cues as some of them do read fairly well. For many children with ASD, pragmatics and semantics skills are more adversely affected than those of language form (morphology and syntax).

Semantic Characteristics

The semantic development of children with ASD is extremely variable. As previously mentioned, some children demonstrate normal semantic development until they are eighteen to thirty-six months of age, and then they appear to "lose" the skills they gain. Other children remain mute throughout their lives. Some learn to use signs or augmentative/alternative devices such as communication boards. Some children have delayed language. Children whose ASD is accompanied by MR will usually have delays in their acquisition of vocabulary. Some children, especially those with Asperger syndrome, might have large and well-developed vocabularies that appear in almost startling contrast to their other language skills.

Children with ASD generally range from having poorly developed to very well-developed vocabularies; however, they may have difficulties using words appropriately in natural situations. They cannot always understand the appropriate use of words that they can define and spell (Iwanaga, Kawasaki, & Tsuchida, 2000). They may also have word-retrieval problems (Owens, 2004). When I worked with Brian, the thirteen-year-old with

Asperger syndrome whom I have discussed earlier in this book, I was impressed by his large and extensive vocabulary; at age thirteen, he had the vocabulary skills of a seventeen-year-old (as verified by standardized assessment). However, his other language skills were very low. For example, on a test of pragmatics skills, Brian performed five or six years below his age level.

Pragmatic Characteristics

The area of language most impacted in children with ASD is pragmatics, including deficits in discourse and limited uses of language (Condouris, Meyer, & Tager-Flusberg, 2003). Children with ASD have deficits in intentional communication. From early on (as early as one year of age), these children may demonstrate a lack of joint attentional behavior (described in Chapter 2) and may not respond to human voices. They may also avoid eye contact.

Children with ASD miss subtle social cues—they have difficulty interpreting what others are thinking. For example, if the mother of a TD six-year-old frowns and shakes her head in a social setting, he knows he'd better straighten up right now. But a child with ASD would not necessarily "read" these cues. In addition, as previously stated, children with ASD have difficulty seeing the world from another person's perspective.

When I talked with Brian's father after the assessment, his dad said he was "self-centered." I might not have quite used that term, but in a sense it's exactly right: the student with ASD has trouble putting himself in anyone else's shoes. Many times, the child with ASD will speak in a monologue, almost like the other person is not there. With Brian, he would frequently go off topic during the evaluation. I would have to keep getting him back on topic, and he generally ignored my attempts to do this and went right on talking as if I was not even in the room.

Sometimes students with ASD talk a lot with seemingly good vocabulary and sentence structure, but their communication is inappropriate to the situation (Westby & McKellar, 2000). They often have difficulty regulating their emotions. They may manifest "immature" behavior such as crying in class or having verbal outbursts that bewilder others.

> Some students with ASD talk a lot with seemingly good vocabulary and sentence structure, but their communication is inappropriate to the situation.

CONNECT & EXTEND

Language, Speech, and Hearing Services in Schools has an entire issue devoted to the discussion of children with ASD. See the July 2003 issue, volume 34, number 3.

Written Language Characteristics

Children whose ASD is accompanied by MR are generally delayed in reading, writing, and spelling. Children whose ASD is not accompanied by MR commonly manifest a condition called **hyperlexia**, where they have excellent word-recognition skills but little comprehension of what the words mean. They may read aloud flawlessly, but do not understand underlying meaning (Frith, 2003). Many children with ASD learn to read fluently; some individuals with Asperger syndrome who speak fluently prefer to use written language to communicate. They claim that it is easier to communicate in writing.

SUMMARY

- Children with ASD may exhibit a wide and varied range of behaviors. Language skills vary greatly depending upon whether the child's ASD is accompanied by mental retardation. However, the area most impacted in children with ASD is pragmatics.
- Some experts explain this by stating that these children lack a theory of mind, or the ability to understand the behavior of others or take others' perspectives.
- The suprasegmental features of ASD children's speech may be deviant. They may also demonstrate echolalia.
- Semantic skills of children with ASD vary widely, depending especially upon whether they have accompanying MR.
- Some children whose ASD is not accompanied by MR may manifest hyperlexia, where they have excellent word-recognition skills but little comprehension of what the words mean.

FOUNDATIONAL PRINCIPLES OF ASSESSMENT

Basic Principles

For children with MR and/or ASD, researchers have recommended that their language skills be evaluated in several primary ways: 1) parent interview and case history, 2) use of standardized language tests in structured settings, and 3) measurement and description of informal everyday conversational interactions. In combination, these methods are useful in obtaining a complete profile and description of the language skills of children with ASD and MR (Condouris et al., 2003; Hardman et al., 2006).

As with other populations of children whom we have discussed in this book, a comprehensive diagnostic evaluation for the child with suspected MR or ASD generally involves a team of professionals such as a psychiatrist, neurologist, SLP, and others. Because language is only one parameter of concern with these children, a comprehensive, multidisciplinary evaluation is always necessary. Usually this begins with a parent interview and gathering of a case history.

Parent Interview and Case History

Part of a comprehensive assessment is a parent interview and gathering a detailed case history.

In Chapter 5, we discussed the need for a case history. When we deal with families of children with ASD and MR, the gathering of a detailed case history is especially important (Schuler & Fletcher, 2002). But we must remember that in some cultures, as we have said before, personal questions are considered prying (e.g., the child's birth circumstances) (Sharifzadeh, 2004; Shipley & Roseberry-McKibbin, 2006).

It is best to have a cultural mediator who can help the family understand the need for the questions to be asked.

Specific Considerations in the Assessment of Children with ASD and/or MR

There are specific published instruments for use with children with ASD. Key items on these tests that help differentiate TD children from those with ASD include those that eval-uate pretend play. We will recall that children with ASD often do not play with toys in standard ways; they line them up, have difficulty generating play scripts that involve taking on the role of others, and do not engage in pretend play. They may manipulate a toy in uncon-ventional ways—for example, given a toy car, a child with ASD may bang it against a table instead of pretending to make it go somewhere (Westby & McKellar, 2000). Young children with ASD also have dif-ficulties with joint attention.

A discussion of specific tests for children with ASD is beyond the scope of this text; however, one very common one is mentioned here. The Childhood Autism Rating Scale (CARS; Van Bourgondien, Marcus, Schopler, 1992) is often used by professionals because it evaluates a number of parameters such as verbal communication, re-lationships to people, adaptation to change, body movements, and lis-tening response.

> **CONNECT & EXTEND**
>
> A summary of specific tests for children with ASD can be found in Tiegerman-Farber, E. (2002). Autism spectrum dis-orders: Learning to communi-cate. In D.K. Bernstein & E. Tiegerman-Farber, *Language and communica-tion disorders in children* (5th ed.) (pp. 520–564). Boston, MA: Allyn & Bacon.

As we have previously stated, in order for a diagnosis of MR to be made, frequently one or more IQ tests are given to a child. An IQ test is, ideally, a culture-free standardized test of general intelligence. There is a disproportionately higher percentage of mildly and moderately MR individuals among poor and minority populations. This can reflect the effects of poverty, but researchers also point out that middle-class professionals are more likely to classify CLD or low-income children as retarded (Hardman et al., 2006).

In Chapter 5, we discussed forms of possible bias that may be present when stan-dardized tests are used with CLD students. This is an especially important point here. American educational history is filled with examples of CLD students being overdiag-nosed with MR because professionals used IQ tests that were biased against them. In Chapters 3 and 5, I discussed Adam X., a Hmong-speaking high school student who was about to be placed into a self-contained special-education classroom on the basis of an IQ test given all in English. Adam's nonverbal or performance level was 30 points higher than his verbal level. No one saw anything amiss about this, and I felt so grateful to be in the right place at the right time to prevent him from being mislabeled and placed in a self-contained special-education classroom for all of his high school years.

> CLD students are dispro-portionately identified as needing special education. Professionals who admin-ister intelligence tests can modify these tests so that they are less biased toward CLD students.

The AAMR (2002) indicates that valid assessment considers cul-tural and linguistic diversity. To assess children with MR, we examine various developmental domains and age-appropriate achievement of milestones. It is important to remember that the age norms assigned to these various developmental domains primarily reflect White, middle-class child-rearing norms.

In Chapter 5, we discussed ways to modify standardized tests of language skills so they are less discriminatory against CLD students. Some of these suggestions are also applicable to IQ tests. Gopaul-McNicol and Armour-Thomas (2002) and van de Vijver (2000) make the following recommendations relative to modifying tests of intelligence:

- *Suspend time*. Many IQ tests have timed questions, which are very biased against CLD students. Allowing these students extra testing time helps to rule out cultural and linguistic variables that can lower their performance.

- *Allow students to codeswitch when necessary*. Children may perform better if they can respond to some questions in English and some in their primary language (Genesee et al., 2004). I have often found in my own assessment that counting answers in both the primary language and English yields the best profile of the student's skills, as we discussed in Chapter 5.

- *Give very detailed instructions with many examples*. We said this in Chapter 5—test tasks may be unfamiliar to students, and they often profit from having a number of examples and demonstrations of what they are supposed to do.

SLPs may also wish to use informal measures to evaluate the language skills of children with ASD and/or MR. Collecting spontaneous language samples in varied settings can be especially helpful with children with ASD, as their pragmatics problems usually stand out as being unusually deviant from the norm.

Frith (2003) points out that some children with ASD perform very well on standardized language tests. Frith differentiates between **school intelligence** and **world intelligence**. Children with ASD may appear to have high school/academic intelligence. They may have outstanding rote memory skills and have excellent reading and spelling ability as well as high capabilities in abstract math. However, because of their social impairments, their world intelligence (ability to relate to others) is compromised. Professionals must be aware that if only standardized tests are used with children with ASD—especially in the case of Asperger syndrome—the students may do quite well. It is only when professionals view these students in the "real world"—out among their peers—that true deficits can be seen.

POINTS TO PONDER Why is so important that professionals be extremely careful about administering standardized tests of intelligence to CLD students? How can these tests be modified so that they are more appropriate for these students?

_____

_____

_____

SUMMARY

- An evaluation of the language skills of any child with ASD and/or MR should begin with a detailed parent interview and case history.
- There are specific published assessment instruments for students with ASD; these particularly evaluate pretend play skills.
- Students with MR generally are assessed with measures of IQ. Great care must be taken here, because low-income and CLD students are often overidentified by these measures, which are usually administered by White middle-class professionals.
- Assessment of students with ASD and/or MR can be made more culturally and linguistically valid by modifying the tests that are administered.
- Informal assessment measures such as language samples can be quite helpful, especially with children with ASD whose performance on formal language tests is not representative of the way they interact in the "real world."

Add your own summary points here:

_____

_____

_____

FOUNDATIONAL PRINCIPLES OF TREATMENT

General Principles

Early intervention is critical for children with ASD and/or MR. Research indicates that for children with ASD, intervention provided before three years of age has a much greater impact than intervention provided after five years of age (Woods & Wetherby, 2003).

Sometimes medications are given to children with ASD and/or MR. If the child has severe tantrums, self-injurious behavior, aggression, or profound anxiety or depression, antidepressants may be given. Severe behavioral problems may be treated with antipsychotic medications. One in four persons with ASD has seizures, and these are treated with anticonvulsants. If a child has hyperactivity accompanying the MR or ASD, stimulant medications such as Ritalin may be prescribed as we will discuss in Chapter 10. These medications have been found to decrease hyperactivity and impulsivity in higher-functioning children with ASD.

Children with ASD and/or MR may have accompanying **sensory integration** problems. Sensory integration refers to the child's ability to organize, integrate, and use sensory information that she receives from the environment (Mauer, 1999). Children with sensory integration problems often benefit from receiving sensory-integration therapy

Some children with ASD and/or MR may have sensory-integration problems. They usually benefit from occupational therapy and small, structured classrooms.

from an occupational therapist. This therapy helps with modulating children's sensitivities and modifying their environments. A major goal is to diminish the student's sensory defensiveness while enhancing play, attachment, or language production (Huebner, 2001). Children with sensory-integration problems need to be in environments that are relatively calm, quiet, and not overly visually stimulating. Small, structured classrooms that are consistent and predictable work best.

For children up to three years of age, services are provided through an early-intervention system. As we discussed in Chapter 7, school staff work with the family to develop an Individualized Family Services Plan (IFSP) to describe the child's unique needs as well as the services she will receive to address those needs. When children are school-age, the staff and family will develop an Individualized Education Plan (IEP). Similar to the IFSP, the IEP describes the child's unique needs and the services that will be provided (at no cost) to address those needs.

When the child turns 14, the school district will begin transition planning. The **transition plan** is part of the IEP, and the goal of this is to figure out how to best help the child transition from the school into the community. The goal is to help the child to become as independent as possible. The student should take part in the planning when possible. After the student turns twenty-three years of age, the school district is no longer responsible for intervention. Some adults with MR and ASD may live independently; some live in foster homes or group homes where they are supervised in groups by professionals who help them with basic needs and activities of daily living. Table 9.3 shows the progression of special plans for students in public school settings.

In Chapter 6, we discussed the developmental/normative and the functional approaches to intervention. We said that many SLPs use a combination of these approaches. In my opinion, the functional approach is by far the most practical one to take when working

TABLE 9.3

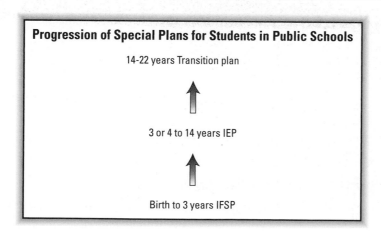

Progression of Special Plans for Students in Public Schools

14-22 years Transition plan

3 or 4 to 14 years IEP

Birth to 3 years IFSP

CASES TO CONSIDER

Marcos B. was born to immigrant parents from El Salvador who utilized welfare and did not have medical insurance. When Mrs. B. went into labor with Marcos, a doctor was called and told that he had to come and deliver the baby. He was at a party and had consumed some alcoholic beverages. He made some mistakes in Marcos's delivery, and Marcos was born with fetal anoxia (oxygen deprivation) and consequent substantial bilateral brain damage. Mr. and Mrs. B. were told that Marcos would never walk or talk. He was later diagnosed with profound mental retardation.

Mr. B. eventually left his wife and son, and it was around that time that I met Mrs. B. With my encouragement, she fiercely advocated for every possible service she could get for Marcos. Marcos was eventually able to walk, talk, and read. Some years later, I was called to perform a language assessment in Marcos' home. He was nearing eighteen years of age, and the school district needed to begin creating a transition plan for him.

I found out that Mrs. B. had demanded that Marcos be homeschooled for the last several years. He was quite depressed and had no friends. My assessment of Marcos's language skills revealed that he did have the ability to live semi-independently and work in a sheltered workshop arrangement under close supervision. However, Mrs. B. told me and the team that she had told Marcos that he ". . . could be anything he wanted—even a doctor." She hoped that maybe he would go to college and live totally independently.

How might you and the other members of the team help Mrs. B. to be more realistic about Marcos's skills and ability to live independently? What might you say and/or do to help her have a clearer picture of Marcos's potential?

_____

_____

_____

with students with ASD and/or MR. We can follow the norms on language development charts all we like; ultimately, however, these students need to function as effectively as possible in their daily environments. There are several specific intervention principles that we shall discuss in detail in the next section:

- using principles of behaviorism, including desired and appropriate reinforcers
- helping students generalize skills they learn during intervention
- utilizing practical techniques and strategies to increase overall language skills of students with ASD and/or MR

Utilizing Principles of Behaviorism

In Chapter 2, we discussed the behaviorist theory of language development. We said that one practical, clinical implication of this theory is that children learn language through stimulus, response, and reinforcement. Behavioral methods are believed by many experts to be highly effective with children with MR and/or ASD (Goldstein, 2002; Hardman et al., 2006; Prizant, 2004). Lovaas (1987) created a highly structured, behavioral approach for use with children with autism; this is described in detail a little later.

> Many experts believe that behavioral methods are highly effective for children with MR and/or ASD.

In Chapter 6, we discussed using the **mand-model** method as a potential intervention strategy. Let's return to that concept here. In the mand-model approach, the adult uses activities and objects that the student is using at the moment and initiates interaction. The clinician prompts a response by using a "mand" (command or request). This technique uses modeling as well as natural activities in the child's environment. An example follows:

The student is playing with a dollhouse.

Clinician: Tell me what you are doing.
Child: Doll.
Clinician: Say, "I have a doll."
Child: I have a doll.
Clinician: That's right, you have a doll who is going upstairs.

Highly structured behavioral methods are quite effective, but generalization of skills learned through these methods can be a challenge. I love the story told by a speaker at a conference I attended a few years ago. She and a colleague were targeting activities of daily living and had worked very hard with a group of MR adolescents to help them learn basic give-and-take scripts in a grocery store. They practiced and practiced in the therapy room and were finally ready to go forth into the real thing. All went well at the actual grocery store, but at the checkout counter, the bagger said, "So, are you all on a field trip?" One of the adolescents said, "Jesus Christ is the Son of God, and He loves you very much." So much for generalization! They had not practiced that one!

In Chapter 6, we discussed types of reinforcement that can be given to children during treatment sessions. We defined primary reinforcers as those with a biological basis— food and water, for example. We defined secondary reinforcers as those with a social, cultural basis—smiles, stickers, tokens, and charts, for example. Because children with ASD and/or MR can be very concrete, it is frequently more effective to give them primary reinforcers. In Chapter 6, I gave the example of Clint, a student with MR. Saying things like "Nice job, Clint! I'm proud of you!" was very ineffective. Words and phrases like "nice job" and "proud" mean little to a student who does not understand abstract language. However, M&Ms and sips of water were highly effective.

> Applied behavior analysis (ABA), created by Lovaas, involves intensive, one-on-one child-teacher interaction for 40 hours a week; the goal is to reinforce desirable behaviors and reduce undesirable ones.

Children with ASD frequently benefit from a program called applied behavior analysis (ABA) created by Lovaas (1987). This program involves intensive, one-on-one child-teacher interaction for 40 hours a week; the goal is to reinforce desirable behaviors and reduce undesirable ones. Mainly, the program builds on the child's interests, has a predictable schedule, actively engages the child's attention in highly structured activities, teaches tasks as a series of simple steps, and provides regular reinforcement (Marcus, Garfinkle, & Wolery, 2001; McEachin & Lovaas, 1993).

One premise of the ABA model is that initially, children with ASD don't benefit from larger-group learning environments until they have acquired basic skills in language, attention, compliance, and imitation. Once the child has mastered these skills, he can gradually go into a group setting. Some children go into regular large classroom settings alone; some need an aide with them (Ozonoff, Dawson, & McPartland, 2002). Increasingly, parents are being trained how to carry this out at home.

Tiegerman-Farber (2002) comments that ABA does work for some children with ASD; however, it is a methodology dictating *how* children are taught; it does not determine *what* they are taught. Increasingly, ABA is being viewed as one of many possible approaches that can be used successfully with children with ASD. The section on specific treatment strategies, introduced later, describes several other popular approaches that have succeeded with these children.

Generalization

We said earlier in this chapter that students with ASD and/or MR have difficulty generalizing what they learn to other contexts. You will recall that in Chapter 6, we said that ideally, in order to help children generalize what they learn in therapy, we need to vary the parameters of *settings, stimuli*, and *interlocutors*. This is even more important with children with ASD and/or MR. Because they are so concrete, they have much difficulty with generalization.

Let's take the example of teaching a child the word *shoes*. Instead of just drilling her with a picture of Reeboks, you might show pictures of Reeboks, loafers, high heels, children's shoes, adults' shoes, and others. Then, you might collect a variety of actual shoes to show her. Later, you might take a walk outside and point out all the kinds of shoes that people are wearing. Because you have varied the settings and stimuli, she will probably remember the word *shoes*. Again, generalization is a major issue for children with ASD and/or MR. They need to use skills and desired behaviors in a variety of settings, etc. (Marcus et al., 2001).

POINTS TO PONDER Describe the basic premise of behavioral approaches to intervention.

_____

_____

_____

CONNECT & EXTEND:

The relationship between phonological processing and intelligence is examined in a study by Conners, F.A., Carr, M.D., & Willis, S. (1998). Is the phonological loop responsible for intelligence-related difference in forward digit span? *American Journal on Mental Retardation, 103*, 1–11.

Written Language

Historically, many professionals did not expect that children with MR would learn to read and write. Part of the reason for this is that phonological ability is a key reading skill, and people believed that children with MR were so deficient in this area that learning to read was not possible (Kuder, 2003). However, Conners, Carr, and Willis (1998) found, in their study of children with MR, that phonological processing is not linked to intelligence and that phonological processing strategies may be successful in helping children with MR learn to read and write.

We said earlier that students with ASD may be able to learn to read and write, and that some high-functioning students with ASD may prefer writing to speaking. The written language abilities of students with ASD depend greatly on the type and severity of the ASD.

Practical Techniques and Strategies for Increasing Language Skills

Inclusion in General Education Classrooms

Practical techniques and strategies for increasing the language skills of children with ASD and/or MR have been categorized in different ways by various writers. I have not categorized various treatment approaches and techniques, explained below, because often, combinations of techniques work best. Also, the approaches used depend on such variables as the severity of the ASD, parents' preferences, and the background of the team who is implementing the intervention. However, one practical strategy that has been widely used to increase the language skills of students with ASD and/or MR is to include them in the general education classroom (Hardman et al., 2006).

> To the extent possible, children with ASD and/or MR should be included in supportive general education classrooms.

It is important for students with ASD and/or MR to be included in general education classrooms as much as possible. In previous chapters, we have discussed federal mandates in this regard. However, the general education classroom must be a safe, nurturing place where the child feels supported (Rees & Bellon, 2002). It may be hard for general education teachers to provide this type of environment in the classroom unless they have substantial support—for example, a full-time aide to work with the child. A friend of mine, whose son has severe autism, told me in frustration that "people worked so hard to provide special settings where my son's needs could really be met; now they're emphasizing inclusion!" Much has been written about the pros and cons of inclusion, but suffice it to say, it is a continuing and growing trend in the United States to place children with a range of disabilities in the regular education classroom.

Koegel, Koegel, Frea, and Green-Hopkins (2003) conducted a study of two students with ASD who were included in regular education classrooms. Both of them had low academic performance and many disruptive behaviors that interfered with the teaching. The researchers used a technique called "priming," where the students were exposed to school assignments before they were presented in class. Results of the study showed that priming was successful with both the five-year-old and the fifteen-year-old subject, who decreased their use of inappropriate classroom behaviors and increased the appropriateness of their academic responding. SLPs, other school personnel, and parents can be involved in priming.

Training Social Skills

Many things can be said about intervention for children with ASD and/or MR. However, researchers widely conclude that work on social skills (pragmatics) is a top priority in intervention. We will discuss this in detail here.

First, SLPs must evaluate the student's friendships and acceptance within his peer group. Students with ASD and/or MR usually need to be actively taught practical social skills. Social behavior is best taught in social settings with social skills groups that provide both the environment and the structure for this teaching.

These students need to be explicitly taught skills such as waiting, taking turns at being first, accepting when they don't win, working and playing quietly, and joining in a conversation or activity with other children in an appropriate manner. They also need to be directly taught how to take turns in conversation, take turns making decisions about what to play or do, read the emotions of others, introduce themselves, give compliments, share, and negotiate. Also, these children have to learn social problem-solving skills, such as how to handle teasing and being told "no," being left out, and others (Mesibov et al., 2001; Ozonoff et al., 2002).

I previously talked about a teenager I worked with who had attacked several adults and tried to burn his school down. I found out that he was teased a great deal by his peers; when this happened, he would react in great anger. Naturally, the teasing would escalate. I worked with this young man to help him learn to "shrug it off." I told him that when he was teased, he had to pretend that it didn't bother him even if it did. We role-played me being a peer who said nasty things like "Eric, you're stupid." He then had to respond, "So? No big deal," and walk away from me.

> Students with ASD and/or MR must be explicitly taught appropriate social skills—especially those skills that will help them to fit in with their peers.

Sometimes peers can be utilized to help students with ASD and/or MR to improve their pragmatics skills. However, SLPs must be careful how this is done. For example, in their research with school-age students with pervasive developmental delay (PDD), Thiemann and Goldstein (2004) showed that the PDD student's use of specific social initiation strategies did not improve through peer training alone. In other words, when peers were trained to help the PDD students improve in social initiation by saying things such as "start talking" and "say something nice" to get interactions going, this was not enough.

What was successful was combining peer training and written text instruction. The combination of working with peers and also having written cues was most successful in improving the initiation skills of students with PDD. So, for example, instead of a TD peer just saying "ask for something," the TD peer said "ask for something" and also held up a cue sheet where the same words were written. Other researchers have shown that children with ASD, especially if they are higher functioning, benefit from seeing written cues as an adjunct to auditory cues (Schuler & Fletcher, 2002).

Children with ASD especially need to learn to interpret the emotions of others. This can be taught through pictures, books, puppets, role plays, and interaction in outside settings. The Picture Exchange Communication System (PECS; Bondy & Frost, 1998) combines guidelines from alternative and augmentative communication and principles from applied behavior analysis; it was developed to help children with ASD develop a functional, self-initiating communication system. Unlike methods such as ABA, PECS does not direct the child to give an answer but rather begins with the child's observed interests and builds on them. Pictures are used to foster meaningful communication exchanges.

Training Attention and Listening Skills

Children with ASD and/or MR frequently have difficulty discriminating what they need to pay attention to, so we need to highlight new or relevant information. For example, if a new word is introduced, it could be written in a different color. If we introduce a new picture card, we might put a bright pink Post-it on the card (Marcus et al., 2001).

> Because children with ASD and/or MR have difficulty remembering what they hear, it is highly advantageous to use visual cues to help them learn new information.

Because children with ASD and/or MR have difficulty remembering what they hear, it is highly advantageous to use visual cues to help them learn new information. These children also need to learn rehearsal strategies so that they remember information. A specific program called Visualize and Verbalize trains children to create detailed mental pictures, or images, to assist with hearing (Bell, 1991). Children can be taught to visualize as an adjunct to listening; they might also be taught the strategy of **reauditorization**, where they repeat information aloud or silently a number of times.

Part of the attention and listening difficulties of students with ASD and/or MR involve categorization skills. I have found that it really helps to specifically teach these skills. For example, I might say to a child, "Okay, Janice, we are going to learn about zoo animals. I can think of lions, tigers, monkeys, and elephants. What zoo animals can you think of?" I also like to use a chart or whiteboard with pictures, with the category name as a heading and entries underneath. One fun thing to do is have Velcro attached to each picture so children can move the pictures easily. Some students with ASD and/or MR may remember pictures better than words, and I like to use visuals with both in order to facilitate memory of the printed word.

Students with Severe Deficits

It is important for all students with ASD and/or MR to keep targeting the development of language comprehension and especially language expression skills into adolescence (Chapman et al., 2000; Miles & Chapman, 2002). Training the family to carry over these skills into the home is critical (Taylor, 2003).

Experts recommend that for severely involved students with ASD and/or MR, functional communication training is best. In addition, some of these students may need alternative and augmentative communication (AAC) devices to supplement or replace their spoken communication skills. SLPs and other team members should be ready and willing to help students use these devices in both school and home settings (Bopp, Brown, & Mirenda, 2004; Johnston, Reichle, & Evans, 2004). More is said about these devices in Chapter 11.

Sometimes children with severe disabilities will act out in frustration because they do not know how to successfully and appropriately request and reject. These children can be taught these skills.

CONNECT & EXTEND

Strategies for SLPs who face challenges in using augmentative and alternative communication devices with beginning communicators with severe disabilities are found in Johnston, S.S., Reichle, J., & Evans, J. (2004). Supporting augmentative and alternative communication use by beginning communicators with severe disabilities. *American Journal of Speech-Language Pathology, 13(*1), 20–30.

In terms of specific language acts, researchers have suggested that students with severe disabilities specifically be taught how to make requests and rejections (Sigafoos, Drasgow, Reichle, O'Reilly, Green, & Tait, 2004). **Requesting** enables the speaker to gain access to activities, interactions, or objects. **Rejecting** allows the speaker to escape or avoid a situation that he does not want.

As we discussed in Chapter 2, rejecting appears very early in children's language development, and it is an important milestone. I gave the example of my son Mark, who when he was three years old and faced with the dreaded comb, said, "No thank you, please!" In another example, a child who has had enough to eat will say "no!" or "stop!" when she is full.

Children with severe disabilities sometimes act out in frustration; some of this is because they don't know how to request and reject in a socially acceptable manner. Children with ASD and/or MR frequently have difficulty asking for what they want, and temper tantrums are a common result. As Kumin (2002) says, protesting or rejecting empowers the child and helps to develop communicative intent. Clinicians who work with children with severe ASD and/or MR want to teach them how to request and reject things in as socially acceptable manner as possible. For example, if a child is offered a banana that he does not want, he can be taught to shake his head "no" or sign "no" rather than grabbing the banana and throwing it across the room.

One specific approach for more severely involved children with ASD is called **floortime** (Greenspan & Weider, 1998). This is a play-based technique that is nonstructured; the professional follows the child's lead. The main focus of floortime is to enhance the parent-child relationship and develop the child's affective experience. Floortime emphasizes engaging the child at the level where she is functioning socially and emotionally and building on this with the expectation that the child will develop improved cognitive, communication, and play skills (Marcus et al., 2001).

The **SCERTS** model (Prizant, 2004) is a specific, flexible, comprehensive, and integrated framework of specific goals and procedures for assessment and educational programming for children with ASD. The SCERTS model focuses on building a child's skills in several areas: social communication, transactional support, and emotional regulation. It is family centered and collaborative, and focuses on functional skills, communication, and socioemotional success in everyday routines of life.

Supports for Students with MR and/or ASD

The AAMR (2002) states that persons with MR need supports or the resources and individual strategies necessary to promote their development and well-being and optimize their potential. The supports approach recognizes that the needs and circumstances of a person with MR can change over time. (This can also be applied to children with ASD.) Supports can be provided by professionals, friends, family members, and agencies. Those who work with students with MR and/or ASD need to analyze the students' need for support in nine areas: home living, community living, human development, education, employment, health and safety, behavior, social skills, and protection and advocacy. Table 9.4 lists examples of supports areas and supports activities. SLPs can use this as a guide for creating functional intervention goals and objectives for students with MR and/or ASD.

Considerations for Working with CLD Students and Their Families

There is little research regarding CLD students with ASD and/or MR. However, there have been a few studies with CLD populations. A study comparing 330 Swedish children with Down syndrome with 336 TD Swedish children showed that vocabulary skills developed slightly ahead of pragmatics and grammar skills (Berglund, Eriksson, & Johansson, 2001). This is similar to findings of researchers who have worked with American children (Paul, 2001; Owens, 2002).

The authors recommended that early language stimulation programs for children with Down syndrome pay special attention to pragmatic and grammar skills. They stressed that early intervention for Swedish-speaking Down syndrome children was critical; this finding is supported by research on American English–speaking children, as we stated earlier. One might very cautiously extrapolate these findings to say that in children with Down syndrome from any CLD group, it is possible that vocabulary skills might be advanced compared to other language skills. More research is needed with children from a variety of cultural and linguistic backgrounds to confirm this speculation.

> Some CLD families may have difficulty accepting the fact that their child has ASD and/or MR because it can represent God's punishment and affect marriageability of siblings.

As we have previously discussed, some families—for cultural, or religious reasons, or both—may believe that a condition like ASD and/or MR is fate or the will of God. If the child has a syndrome associated with the MR, this is even more likely to be the case. Remember that for some families, a "defect" like this represents God's punishment. Parents may be very embarrassed, defensive, and even in denial about the extent of a child's problem. In some cultures, the marriageability of siblings may be affected (Santos & Chan, 2004).

If it becomes known that one child in a family has a condition such as ASD and/or MR, that child's siblings may not be able to find suitable marriage partners. Thus, parents may be unwilling to acknowledge the existence of the ASD and/or MR. It may be a genuine challenge to team with these parents to take active steps in intervention to help the child maximize her potential. Other families may want to use home or folk remedies to "cure" the disorder and may or may not believe in the value of treatment as recommended by US professionals.

Of course, the goal of any intervention—speech-language or otherwise—is to help the child with ASD and/or MR become as independent as possible. However, as we have discussed, in some cultures, "independence" may occur at ages later than those expected by US developmental norms. Families from some cultural groups feel very comfortable teaching their children to spoonfeed just before they enter kindergarten at five or six years of age; they do not feel the need to conform to the eighteen-month-old timeline on many US developmental checklists (Hanson, 2004). Many CLD families see no purpose in having a child drink from a cup before four or five years of age. There is also no pressure for children to dress independently if family members are around to help. In any plan

TABLE 9.4   Examples of Supports Areas and Supports Activities

Teaching and Education Activities

    Learning and using self-determination skills
    Interacting with teachers and fellow students
    Participating in decision-making
    Learning and using problem-solving strategies
    Using functional academics (e.g., counting change, reading signs)
    Using technology for learning

Human Development Activities

    Providing social and emotional developmental activities to foster trust, initiative, and autonomy
    Providing cognitive development opportunities such as reasoning logically about concrete events
    Providing physical development opportunities that include fine and gross motor activities

Home Living Activities

    Housekeeping and cleaning
    Preparing and eating food
    Using the restroom
    Taking care of clothes (e.g., doing laundry)
    Getting dressed
    Participating in leisure activities within the home
    Taking care of personal hygiene
    Operating home appliances

Community Living Activities

    Interacting with members of the community
    Using transportation
    Participating in leisure and recreation activities
    Going shopping and buying things
    Using public buildings and public settings such as the park or community pool

Employment Activities

    Completing work-related tasks with adequate quality and speed
    Learning and using specific job skills
    Interacting with coworkers and supervisors
    Changing job assignments
    Accessing and obtaining crisis assistance and intervention

Social Skills Activities

    Socializing within and outside the family
    Making and maintaining friendships
    Participating in recreation and leisure activities
    Communicating with others about personal needs
    Offering and receiving assistance
    Making appropriate sexual decisions
    Engaging in loving and intimate relationships

TABLE 9.4   Examples of Supports Areas and Supports Activities (*continued*)

Behavioral Activities

> Learning specific behaviors or skills (e.g., introducing oneself to a stranger)
> Maintaining socially acceptable behavior in public
> Controlling anger and aggression
> Making appropriate decisions
> Incorporating personal preferences into daily activities

Health and Safety Activities

> Communicating with health care providers
> Taking medication as directed
> Avoiding health and safety hazards
> Accessing and obtaining therapy services
> Accessing emergency services
> Maintaining physical health
> Maintaining a nutritious diet

Protection and Advocacy Activities

> Advocating for self and others
> Managing money and personal finances
> Exercising legal rights and responsibilities
> Protecting self from abuse and exploitation
> Belonging to self-advocacy and support organizations
> Using banks and handling checks

Source: Adapted from *American Association on Mental Retardation, 2002.*

for intervention, SLPs and other team members must take the family's cultural values into account, especially regarding timelines for independence (Valdivia, 2000).

Gronroos (2003) discusses recommendations for talking with CLD families who have a child with MR. Many of her suggestions are applicable to children with other types of issues also. First, Gronroos states that it is indeed ideal to have a cultural mediator present when parents first hear the news that their child has MR. However, she recommends that the district provide a cultural mediator rather than allow the parents to bring their own. This is because parents may not anticipate a diagnosis of MR, and having a family member or person from their community hear the diagnosis may be humiliating. Gronroos comments that the cultural mediator may dread giving the parents the news about the MR; the cultural mediator should be supported and encouraged in this type of situation.

Prelock, Beatson, Bitner, Broder, and Ducker (2003) discuss working with CLD families of children with ASD. They encourage SLPs to operate within a "strengths" perspective instead of a "cultural destructiveness" perspective. In the latter perspective, SLPs and other team members view cultural differences as a "pathology," and they may block the family and child's access to appropriate services. In the "strengths" perspective, the family's pain is acknowledged and the team works to facilitate a relationship of trust, believing that the family's strengths will be useful in providing solutions.

POINTS TO PONDER What are several important things to remember when we work with CLD children with ASD and/or MR and their families?

_____

_____

_____

A question I have heard many times is "Since children with ASD and/or MR have such severe language delays, shouldn't I just do therapy in English? Won't this be less confusing?" A related question is "Should I tell the parents to just speak to the child in one language instead of trying to raise the child in a bilingual environment?" This question was discussed in depth by Gutierrez-Clellen (1999) and was addressed at length by Genesee et al. (2004). These researchers stated that children with relatively low levels of intellectual ability are not differentially challenged in learning their first language as a consequence of being exposed to and learning a second language. In fact, children with challenges like MR can learn two languages successfully.

In one of the first studies of its kind, Kay-Raining Bird, Trudeau, Thordardottir, Sutton, and Thorpe (2005) compared the language abilities of children with Down syndrome who were being raised bilingually with those of three control groups matched on the developmental level: monolingual children with Down syndrome, monolingual TD children, and bilingual TD children. Kay-Raining Bird et al. found that there was no evidence that suggested a detrimental effect of bilingualism for the children with Down syndrome who were being raised bilingually. Their results suggested that children with Down syndrome can be successful in acquiring two languages, and they stated that there is no support for the recommendation that children with Down syndrome be restricted to input in just one language.

Anecdotally, when I conducted a workshop in Oregon last year, an audience member came up to me at a break and shared that she worked with children who had substantial intellectual deficits. She said that she had never had a problem with these children being exposed to and learning two languages. My conclusion is that both research and anecdotal evidence show that children with ASD and/or MR can and should be exposed to and learn two languages. These children do not have to be restricted to learning "just English."

 SUMMARY

- Early intervention is critical for children with ASD and/or MR. If they have severe behavior problems, medications may be helpful.
- For these students, public schools will make transition plans to help the students transition from the school to the community.

- For many children with ASD and/or MR, use of behaviorist principles can be extremely effective in increasing their language skills. They will need extra support in generalizing these language skills outside the therapy room.
- It is important for students with ASD and/or MR to be included in supportive general-education classrooms. A high priority in intervention for these students is to increase their pragmatics skills, especially relative to interacting with TD peers. These students also need training to increase their listening and attention skills.
- Students with severe deficits especially need functional communication training that may or may not involve the use of augmentative, alterative communication. They frequently need specific training in how to appropriately request and reject things.
- SLPs need to help provide supports for students with ASD and/or MR. In addition, SLPs may implement specific programs such as floortime or SCERTS.
- For various cultural and/or religious reasons, CLD families may find it especially difficult to hear a diagnosis of MR or ASD. Use of carefully selected cultural mediators can be very helpful here. Children can and should be exposed to two languages, even in the presence of a challenge such as ASD and/or MR.

Add your own summary points here:

_____

_____

_____

CHAPTER HIGHLIGHTS

- Mental retardation (MR) is a disability characterized by significant limitations in both intellectual functioning and adaptive behavior. MR can be caused by biological factors, social-environmental factors, or both.
- Children with MR have deficits in both cognitive and language skills. Some children with severe MR display echolalia, where they repeat verbatim what is said to them.
- Many children with MR have telegraphic speech, small vocabularies, and difficulty initiating interactions with others. Some may demonstrate perseveration, or excessive talking about a subject that has been previously addressed or is inappropriate.
- The condition of Down syndrome, a form of MR, results from a chromosomal abnormality involving a third and extra copy of the twenty-first chromosome. Children with Down syndrome generally show greater impairments in expressive language than in nonverbal cognition and syntax comprehension.
- Some children are diagnosed early in life with autism spectrum disorder (ASD). There are five subtypes of ASD: autistic disorder, Rett disorder, childhood disintegrative disorder, pervasive developmental disorder not otherwise specified (PDD-NOS), and Asperger syndrome. ASD is neurologically based, and there may be a genetic component.

- Children with ASD manifest a variety of behavioral characteristics depending on the subtype of ASD that they have. Many have phonological and suprasegmental problems as well as difficulties with semantics, pragmatics, and written language.
- When we assess the language skills of students with ASD and/or MR, we need to work as part of a multidisciplinary team. We must be sure to conduct a thorough parent interview and gather an extensive case history.
- There are published instruments available for assessing the language skills of children with ASD and/or MR. However, these instruments may be biased against low-income and CLD children, who tend to be disproportionately labeled as having MR especially. Tests can be appropriately adapted; also, informal measures and observations may be used.
- Early intervention is critical for children with ASD and/or MR. School districts have specific plans for children beginning at birth and ending at age twenty-three.
- It is often very helpful to use a behavioral approach in therapy. Primary reinforcers tend to work well. Generalization activities must be carefully planned and implemented.
- It is usually best for students with ASD and/or MR to be fully included in supportive, appropriate general-education classroom settings. These students must receive specific, extensive training in use of appropriate social skills. They also need training in listening and attention skills.
- Students with severe deficits may benefit from the use of augmentative, alternative communication. In addition, they can be specifically taught how to appropriately use specific language acts such as requesting and rejecting.
- The floortime and SCERTS models are several new comprehensive models for helping children with ASD increase their language skills.
- SLPs must be especially sensitive in working with families of CLD children with ASD and/or MR. For religious reasons, cultural reasons, or both, these families may have an especially difficult time acknowledging that their child has this type of disability. Appropriately selected cultural mediators can be very helpful.

Add your own chapter highlights here:

_____

_____

_____

STUDY AND REVIEW QUESTIONS

ESSAY

1. Describe the language, cognitive, and processing characteristics of children with MR. What are the clinical implications of these characteristics?
2. What does the term autism spectrum disorder mean? List the five types of ASD and briefly describe Asperger syndrome.
3. Discuss the problems that can occur when professionals administer standardized tests to CLD children to assess the possible presence of MR. How can these professionals adapt testing procedures to be more culturally sensitive?

4. Describe how we might apply the principles of behaviorism to intervention with children who have ASD and/or MR.

5. Discuss the necessity of training children who have ASD and/or MR to improve their social skills. Why is this so important? How do we accomplish this?

FILL-IN-THE-BLANK

6. Children with MR may exhibit_____, where they leave the function words out of sentences and only include content words.

7. Children with ASD and/or MR may demonstrate _____, or excessive talking about a subject that has been previously addressed or is inappropriate.

8. According to the_____ hypothesis, children with ASD have difficulty understanding the behavior of others; they have difficulty taking others' perspectives.

9. Children who have_____ have excellent word-recognition skills but don't understand what the words mean.

10. _____ refers to a child's ability to organize, integrate, and use sensory information that she receives from the environment.

MULTIPLE CHOICE

11. You are working in a public preschool where a three-year-old Middle Eastern child, Rajiv F., has been referred to the special-education team because his pediatrician suspects that Rajiv has autism. You and the other members of the special-education team carry out comprehensive testing with Rajiv, and all test results point to autism. You have worked closely with an interpreter who confirms that in Rajiv's first language, he demonstrates characteristics that are consistent with a profile of autism. You hear that Rajiv's pediatrician has already tried to tell his parents about the autism diagnosis, but his parents got quite angry and denied that their son had any problems at all. A meeting with the special-education team and Rajiv's parents is scheduled for the near future. Which of the following will probably be *appropriate* in this meeting?

   a. Be sure to have a cultural mediator from Rajiv's immediate community—the more familiar the family is with the cultural mediator, the better

   b. Be sensitive to the fact that early independence for Rajiv may not be high on the family's priority list, and be prepared to be flexible about recommendations for independence

   c. Remember that Rajiv's parents may be in denial; this is common, and team members should not negatively judge the parents for denying that Rajiv has autism

   d. b, c

   e. a, b, c

12. Casey P. is a six-year-old child with moderate MR. Casey's classroom teacher has asked you as an SLP for some specific suggestions that he can use in the classroom to help Casey work to her academic potential. Which of these recommendations would be inappropriate for you to make?

   a. Casey will need to be explicitly taught associative strategies to help her remember new words and concepts that she learns

b. It is ideal for the teacher to help Casey's parents learn how to carry over classroom lessons into the home, because generalization of lessons outside the classroom will be particularly challenging

c. Casey may demonstrate perseveration, and may also not be proficient in judging the nonverbal cues of others

d. Casey's speech may be telegraphic, and that is very common in children with MR

e. Casey will remember auditory information better than visual information, so he does not have to worry about having things like pictures around; just keep repeating new information, and Casey will eventually catch on

13. A parent comes to your private clinic concerned about her son Bradley. He is in third grade and does quite well in school academically. He is quite bright. However, he has no friends. Bradley is consumed by his interest in the computer game Dungeons and Dragons and will talk about it endlessly to anyone who will listen. Bradley's mother says that even when people begin to walk away out of boredom, Bradley will continue to talk about Dungeons and Dragons. Bradley's teacher thinks he is funny and has commented about his large vocabulary and about how he sounds like a "little adult." Based on this description, you might suspect that Bradley has

a. Childhood disintegrative disorder

b. Down syndrome

c. Asperger syndrome

d. Echolalia

e. Rett syndrome

14. One approach that has been successfully used with children with ASD is _____, which involves intensive one-on-one child-teacher interaction for 40 hours a week. The goal of this program is to reinforce desirable behaviors and reduce undesirable ones.

a. Lovaas' ABA program

b. Greenspan's floortime program

c. Prizant's SCERTS model

d. Mand-model reinforcement program

e. Generalization behaviorist program

15. One helpful skill that many children with ASD and/or MR can learn is _____, where they repeat information aloud or silently a number of times to help themselves remember what they heard.

a. Reauditorization

b. Picture Exchange Communication System

c. Requesting and rejecting

d. Mand-model

e. Expressive mnemonics

See Answers to Study and Review Questions, page 465.

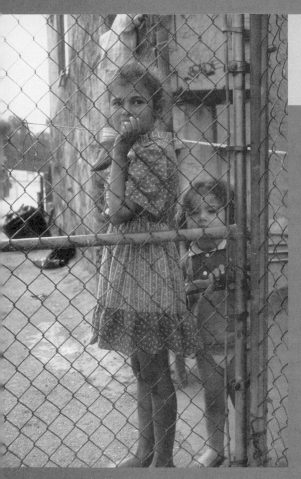

The Impact of Environmental Factors on Language Development

CASE STUDY

Harry was a ten-year-old culturally and linguistically diverse (CLD) student from a home where the family utilized Aid to Families with Dependent Children (welfare). I first met him when he was placed on my caseload in a south Sacramento school in a low-income area. Harry was in a special day class—a class specifically designated for children with language and learning disabilities. The teacher, Rose G., was quite young and inexperienced. Though she cared deeply for the children, the classroom could be appropriately described as "chaotic." When I went to pick up

Harry to bring him to speech-language therapy in the "Speech Room," he was often hiding under his desk. It would frequently take me five to ten minutes to get him to come with me and the other children for his twice-weekly small-group language intervention.

Harry's progress with me was quite minimal. I wanted to work with his family to teach them home carryover activities to promote his overall language and academic progress, as his language skills were closer to those of a six-year-old than a ten-year-old. I was advised that trying to work with the family was probably not going to be successful. I wanted to know why; I knew that if I could just involve his family in home activities, his prognosis for improvement would be much better.

I found out that Harry's family lived in a trailer. As I mentioned, they were on welfare. Harry's mother was not around; she had abused alcohol and drugs during her pregnancy with him and was no longer in the picture. As I understood it, the trailer where Harry's family lived was quite crowded, and basics such as food were scarce.

So I did my best with Harry during the therapy time we had together, trying to maximize his progress as best I could. I also worked with his classroom teacher to help him generalize the treatment targets I was addressing in small-group language intervention. One week, I noticed that Harry's behavior had taken a turn for the worse. He was extremely defiant toward me and would no longer make an effort in therapy. I talked with his teacher and found out that Harry was upset because his older sister had become pregnant. The baby's father? Harry's father. Harry's father had deliberately gotten his oldest daughter pregnant so that she would have a baby and they would be able to collect extra welfare money.

After this, I was transferred to another school site. I never did find out what happened to Harry. I hope he is not in jail; I hope that somehow, he "landed on his feet." He had major environmental issues to deal with, and for us at his school, it was quite challenging to deal with his issues and help him to learn and thrive despite those issues.

INTRODUCTION

In previous chapters, we have said that a child's developing language can be influenced by many variables. In this chapter, we discuss environmental factors that can interact with the child's intrinsic characteristics to contribute to a language impairment (LI).

Research consistently shows that regardless of cultural and linguistic background, children from low-income homes are vulnerable to a host of oral and written language problems that especially emerge when they begin elementary school. If children experience abuse and/or neglect, they frequently will manifest accompanying language problems. Children who are diagnosed with attention deficit hyperactivity disorder manifest their own unique language profiles. Children who are exposed to drugs and/or alcohol in utero have many special needs, including LI. For these and other populations of children described in this chapter, early intervention is crucial to future language, academic, and social outcomes.

Some children have the human immunodeficiency virus (HIV), or may have a full-blown case of AIDS (acquired immune deficiency syndrome). Speech-language pathologists (SLPs) work on multidisciplinary teams to meet the comprehensive social, medical, emotional, and communication needs of these children. Lastly, SLPs also work on multidisciplinary teams to support children with behavioral and emotional problems that may contribute to LI.

CHILDREN FROM LOW–SOCIOECONOMIC STATUS BACKGROUNDS

Background Information

When providing services to children from CLD backgrounds, SLPs have traditionally focused on ethnic background and the languages spoken in children's homes. While these factors are important, and we have talked a great deal about them in this book, professionals today are increasingly recognizing that socioeconomic status (SES) may be an even more important factor in understanding children's and families' behavior than ethnic or linguistic background (Roseberry-McKibbin, 2000). Woolfolk (2004, p. 157) states that

> Social class is a significant dimension of cultural differences, often overpowering other differences such as ethnicity or gender. For example, upper-class Anglo-European Americans, African Americans, and Hispanic Americans typically find that they have more in common with each other than they have with lower-class individuals from their own ethnic groups (Gollnick & Chinn, 1994).

I agree with the above statement and believe that SES issues often have a greater impact on children's and families' behavior and values than ethnic or linguistic factors. While these factors are important, understanding SES issues may be even more helpful to SLPs and other professionals who work with CLD students and their families. Thus, in this section, we will discuss special considerations to keep in mind in terms of providing appropriate and sensitive services to students and families from low-SES backgrounds. First, it is important to be aware of some basic background facts.

According to the US Bureau of the Census (2003), 17 percent of children under eighteen years of age live below poverty level The child poverty rate in the US is two to three times higher than that of most other major industrialized Western nations. Part of this is due to changes in family structure in past decades. In 1950, 22 percent of all householders were not married. In the year 2000, 48 percent of all householders were not married. In 1970, 40 percent of householders had children; in 2000, 24 percent of householders had children. Between 1990 and 2000, the number of families headed by single mothers increased by 25 percent to more than 7.5 million households (US Bureau of the Census, 2000).

Children in married-couple families are much less likely to experience poverty than children who live in homes headed by single mothers. In 1997, 49 percent of children in female-householder families lived in poverty compared to 10 percent of children in married-couple families. At all levels of educational attainment, median female wages in the United States are 30 to 50 percent lower than male wages at equal levels of educational attainment (US Bureau of the Census, 2000).

Homelessness is often a consequence of poverty (Morrison, 2003). Children who are homeless often have poor school attendance, and this can negatively impact their academic skills because

> Socioeconomic status may have a greater impact on a child's language development than linguistic or cultural background.

they are not consistently in the classroom. In addition, children who live in inner cities especially tend to attend schools that have fewer resources and poorer facilities than schools where middle- and upper-SES families reside.

Language and Behavioral Characteristics

There is no demonstrated causal relationship between LI and poverty. Some low-SES children come from homes where they receive good language stimulation. Others, however, show problems in language learning and development. Families who live in poverty often face conditions such as hunger, overcrowded and unclean housing, unsafe neighborhoods and schools, and limited access to health care (Park, Turnbull, & Turnbull, 2002) Research shows that while not directly causing LI, these variables in addition to low educational levels of caregivers are associated with lower language skills of children from low-SES homes (Hart & Risley, 1995; Roseberry-McKibbin & Brice, 1998).

Limited access to health care can impact language skills for a variety of reasons. Children who are often sick and don't get adequate medical care miss a great deal of school. This limits their academic and language exposure. If children do come to school when they are sick, they have difficulty concentrating and learning. I have worked with children who were sent to school with fevers of over 100 degrees. Needless to say, their caregivers were called to pick the children up.

Additionally, children who have limited access to health care may have untreated ear infections, which can negatively impact their language development. They may also be the product of a pregnancy where the mother was malnourished; this can impact the neural development of the fetus, and the child may be born with subsequent cognitive and linguistic deficits. Lastly, mothers who receive inadequate prenatal care tend to have babies who are premature and have low birth weight; these circumstances are associated with language and cognition problems (O'Hanlon & Roseberry-McKibbin, 2004; Robinson & Acevedo, 2001; Roseberry-McKibbin, 2000).

In terms of educational levels of caregivers, research has found that socioeconomic status is more critical to a child's language development than ethnic background, and the factor most highly related to socioeconomic status is the mother's educational level (Battle & Anderson, 1998; Dollaghan et al., 1999). As Hammer et al. (2004, p. 37) stated, "Research consistently demonstrates that higher maternal education fosters better outcomes for children."

Dollaghan et al. compared children's scores on different measures of language to maternal education in three categories: less than a high school graduate, a high school graduate, or a college graduate. Dollaghan and her colleagues found that maternal education correlated positively with children's mean length of utterance, the number of different words the children used, and the children's scores on a test of receptive vocabulary (their scores on this test increased significantly with the mother's increased education).

Research has documented a strong correlation between adults' education and their income levels. Long-term welfare dependency is strongly associated with low literacy levels and lack of a high school

> Low socioeconomic status is often accompanied by low educational levels of caregivers, especially mothers. Research shows that mothers with less education have children whose language skills are lower than children of mothers with more education.

diploma (Friedlander & Martinson, 1996). This can impact the language development of children from low-SES homes because some caregivers who have had limited educational opportunities may not provide adequate oral language stimulation for their children. They may not read to their children, and frequently do not have the money to purchase educational toys and supplies.

I have worked with low-SES kindergarteners who have never held a pencil or a crayon until they reached school. In one district where I worked as a twenty-three-year-old SLP right out of my master's degree program, I couldn't figure out why the children on my caseload never brought back their speech homework. I learned that most of them did not have paper, pencils, or crayons at home; in addition, some of their parents did not read. It was a shock to see the reality that many children did not have what I assumed were basics in every home.

In terms of oral language stimulation in low-SES homes, there is research to support the fact that low-SES parents provide less of this stimulation than middle- and upper-income parents (Hart & Risley, 1995; Smith, Landry, & Swank, 2000; Walker, Greenwood, Hart, & Carta, 1994). Smith et al. found that the amount of verbal stimulation provided to children, along with SES, significantly related to a child's verbal skills at five years of age. Children from low-SES homes who had received less verbal stimulation had lower verbal skills at five years of age than children from middle-SES homes who had received more verbal stimulation. Thus, low-SES children may be at risk for difficulties with oral language skills as they grow older. Woolfolk (2004, p. 160) gives the following, example, which contrasts the way a low-SES and a middle-SES mother might work with a child on a puzzle:

> *Low-SES mother:*   No, that piece goes here!
>
> *Middle-SES mother:*   What shape is that piece? Can you find a spot that is straight like the piece? Yes, that's straight, but look at the color. Does the color match? No—Look again for a straight, red piece. Yes—try that one. Good for you! You finished the corner.

You can see that the middle-SES child is benefiting from verbal elaboration, problem-solving opportunities, conceptual development, and encouragement to take initiative. The low-SES child is getting none of these opportunities. Over time, the difference between the two mothers' styles will dramatically impact how their children perform in school, where verbal elaboration, problem solving, and conceptual development are all highly valued.

Hart and Risley (1995) conducted longitudinal studies of families from various ethnic and SES backgrounds. There were three categories of SES: 1) welfare, 2) working class (blue collar), and 3) professional. The studies focused on the home environments of one- and two-year-old children, specifically looking at interactions and language stimulation within these homes. They concluded that SES made an overwhelming difference in how much talking went on in a family. The family factor most strongly associated with the amount of talking in the home was not ethnicity, but SES.

Hart and Risley extrapolated that in a 365-day year, children from professional families would have heard four million utterances, and children from welfare families

Low–socioeconomic status children are at risk for low oral and written language skills.

would have heard 250,000 utterances. Children from working-class or blue collar families fell in between. Hart and Risley stated that even by three years of age, the difference in the vocabulary knowledge between children from welfare and professional homes was so great that in order for the welfare children to gain a vocabulary equivalent to that of children from working-class homes, these welfare children would need to attend a preschool program for forty hours per week where they heard language at a level used in the homes of professional families. Thus, again, Hart and Risley showed that in terms of the amount of talking/language stimulation that went on in children's homes, ethnicity was not related; SES was.

There is research evidence that in addition to having depressed oral language skills, low-SES children may be at risk for difficulties in literacy and academic skills (Fazio et al., 1996; Qi & Kaiser, 2004). Research has shown that in many low-SES households, children are not read to as much as they are in households with a higher SES. This may be partially a function of lack of access to books. A number of variables contribute to depressed literacy skills in low-SES children. One is lack of money to purchase books. In a study of the number of books in the homes of various families, Bradley, Corwyn, Pipes-McAdoo, & Garcia-Coll (2001) found that across all ethnic groups, nonpoor children were much more likely to have ten or more developmentally appropriate books in their homes than their low-SES counterparts.

As we have said, low-SES mothers often have not had the benefit of education, which can affect the way they read to their children. Baker, Mackler, Sonnenschein, and Serpell (2001) found that a positive affective atmosphere during shared reading activities between mothers and children related positively to a child's reading activity in third grade. Better-educated mothers were found to generate more positive affective interactions during shared reading than less educated mothers.

Van Kleeck, Gillam, Hamilton, and Grath (1997) examined the type of language used by middle-class mothers and fathers when they were reading to their children. Van Kleeck et al. found that more than 60 percent of the language the parents used was at the level that their preschoolers had already mastered, and 40 percent was at a level that would challenge the children. Using lower-level language a greater percentage of the time gave the preschoolers a knowledge base from which to operate; language above their current abilities tested and challenged their language weaknesses. When parents read books to their children that the children had never heard before, there was an increased level of abstract language and also new vocabulary that stimulated language. Thus, middle-class parents appeared to consistently use language, during reading, that had many ideal characteristics for promoting their children's literate language skills.

Payne, Whitehurst, and Angell (1994) found a strong relationship between children's language and the literacy environment of their homes, especially with regard to the following parameters: frequency of parents reading to their children, number of picture books in the home, frequency that the child asked to be read to, frequency of visits to the library, and the child's age when shared reading began. Children with higher-level language skills were read to frequently, had begun reading with their parents very early, visited the library often, and had many picture books in their homes. Thus, like other studies, Payne et al.'s study showed that home literacy practices had a strong impact on children's language skills.

POINTS TO PONDER Describe how coming from a low-SES home can affect a child's language skills.

_____

_____

_____

There are other predictors of a child's reading ability that relate to SES. Dodd and Carr (2003) carried out a study in the United Kingdom in which they examined young children's letter-sound development at three levels: letter-sound recognition, letter-sound recall, and letter reproduction. They found that children from upper SES backgrounds had significantly higher scores on all three tasks than children from lower-SES backgrounds. They also found that children from lower-SES backgrounds had more difficulty with letter reproduction than letter-sound recall, while those from upper-SES families had similar scores on the same two tasks.

> In addition to being at risk for language delays, low-SES children may also be at risk for behavior problems.

Research has documented that low-SES children often have difficulty in other literacy areas, including phonological awareness and vocabulary (Justice & Ezell, 2001; Saint-Laurent & Giasson, 2001). Luster, Bates, Vandenbelt, & Peck Key (2000) showed in their study that the more a child was read to at a young age, the higher his scores on a standardized receptive vocabulary test. Sharif, Reiber, and Ozuah (2002) showed that the more young children were read to, the better their receptive vocabulary skills were as they developed.

An increasing amount of research shows that preschool children who grow up in low-SES homes are at increased risk for developing behavioral as well as language and academic difficulties later in life (Hester & Kaiser, 1998; Kaiser, Cai, Hancock, & Foster, 2002; Woolfolk, 2004). Low-SES children in Head Start have been shown to have higher-than-expected levels of externalizing behaviors and internalizing behavioral problems. Examples of externalizing behaviors include oppositional behaviors (e.g., running away, lying), physical aggression (e.g., biting and kicking) weak attention skills, hyperactivity, and impulsive behavior (Lochman & Szczepanski, 1999). Internalizing behaviors include problems of an introverted nature, such as worrying, social withdrawal, and depression.

Qi and Kaiser (2004) studied the language and social skills of sixty low-SES children enrolled in Head Start in Tennessee. They represented different ethnic backgrounds, and all spoke English as their dominant language. In one group, the children had typical language development. In the other group, the children had language delays. Qi and Kaiser found that children with language delays had poorer social skills and exhibited more problem behaviors on most but not all measures in comparison to the children whose language was developing normally. Qi and Kaiser suggested that children who are both low income

CONNECT & EXTEND

Language and behavioral skills of low–socioeconomic status CLD students were studied by Qi, C.H., & Kaiser, A.P. (2004). Problem behaviors of low-income children with language delays: An observation study. *Journal of Speech, Language, and Hearing Research, 47,* 595–609.

and LI are at risk for social and behavioral problems, and suggested that in intervention, clinicians might want to incorporate social-skills training that included conversational strategies for improved interactions with others.

O'Neill-Perozzi (2003) examined the language characteristics of twenty-five homeless mothers and their preschool children to ascertain whether or not there was a correlation between language deficits in mothers and language deficits in children. She found that 60 percent of the mothers had language deficits, and 69 percent of the children were identified as having language deficits. O'Neill-Perozzi also found that at the time of the study, 62 percent of the children were receiving no academic instruction and 60 percent of the mothers suffered from health problems, including depression. Maternal depression has been associated with lower quality of mother-child interactions, lower cognitive abilities in infancy, and more negative maternal views of children (Hammer et al., 2004).

Implications for Service Delivery

There is a strong relationship between SES and performance in school (Morrison, 2003; Woolfolk, 2004). High-SES students from all ethnic backgrounds have higher levels of achievement on tests and stay in school longer than low-SES students (McLoyd, 1998). Poverty during a child's preschool years appears to have the greatest impact; the longer the child lives in poverty, the greater the impact on her academic achievement. Even when we account for parents' educational levels, the chance that children will be placed in special education or retained in grades increases by 2 or 3 percent for every year they live in poverty (Sherman, 1994). Because low-SES children tend to struggle academically at a greater rate than children from homes where there are more financial resources, classroom teachers may refer these children to special education at a higher rate than they should (Morrison, 2003; Woolfolk, 2004). There are many problems with this.

One problem, for SLPs, is that many standardized tests of language skills are biased against low-SES students. (Roseberry-McKibbin, 2000, 2001b). Even if low-SES children are developing in a typical fashion, they may still be incorrectly identified as having LI and may be inappropriately placed into special education. We have previously mentioned a study by Fazio et al. (1996), who found that some low-SES children scored lower on cognitive and language tests than the normative sample, but this was not due to an underlying LI. Out of twelve children who scored lowest on tests of language in kindergarten, seven were later found to be typically developing (TD). Due to the effects of poverty, these children were incorrectly labeled as LI; as they became acculturated to the school environment, their language test scores improved.

Standardized language tests, especially those that measure language knowledge, may be biased against low-SES children.

In Chapter 5, we described a study by Campbell et al. (1997) that found that knowledge-based measures discriminated against CLD students. In an effort to ascertain if knowledge-based measures would discriminate against low-income children, Enos, Kline, Guillen-Green,

Weger, Roseberry-McKibbin, and O'Hanlon (2005) administered a commonly used knowledge-based measure of vocabulary to low-and mid-SES TD children in the Sacramento area of California. The purpose of the study was to ascertain whether there would be significant differences in the scores of the low- and middle-SES children on this measure.

Results indicated that there was a significant difference between the two groups' vocabulary test scores. The average percentile rank score for the low-SES subjects was 38; the average percentile rank for the middle-SES subjects was 51. Thus, there was a thirteen-point difference in the mean scores of the two groups when they only differed by the variable of SES. Enos et al. (2005) concluded that knowledge-based tests may indeed discriminate against TD low-SES children and recommended that processing-dependent measures be used to assess their language skills instead.

Most SLPs are middle-class, Anglo speakers of English. However, children who come to school from middle-SES backgrounds are decreasing in number and students who come from low-SES backgrounds are increasing in number. Middle-class SLPs and other professionals need to remember that schools operate from middle-class norms and follow the hidden rules of the middle class (Payne, 2003). There may be differences between the values of low-SES children and families and the middle-class professionals who provide assessment and treatment; two of these differences are described below (Payne, 2003).

First, mainstream middle-SES clinicians tend to be proactive, valuing planning for the future and setting goals. For example, these clinicians may recommend early intervention for a young child who is at risk for a language delay. However, the low-SES family's value might be that the present is the most important; decisions are made in the moment based on survival today. The future is uncertain and therefore not important. Thus, if the child is surviving as a three-year-old in the neighborhood, the family may not see the importance of planning for two years from now when the child enters kindergarten.

A second area of potential value conflicts between the middle-SES clinician and the low-income family. Most middle-SES clinicians believe that we all have choices and we can change or impact our future by making good choices now. But many low-SES families believe that there is little they can do to work against chance. Their current circumstances are their fate, and little to nothing can be done to change it. Thus, these families may not follow through with recommendations for home carryover programs or perhaps even bringing a child to an SLP for much-needed language intervention.

> When SLPs recommend language therapy, there may be a conflict between this recommendation and low–socioeconomic status families' values.

There are ways for SLPs and other professionals to reach out to families of low-SES children. First, caregivers from low-SES backgrounds who have children with communication disorders may need as much help as their children do. The caregivers may be unable to do homework, carryover activities, or other tasks without support from the entire team (Paul, 2001). If caregivers are struggling to put food on the table and pay rent, conducting language-stimulation activities or reading to their children may be low priorities. One thing that professionals can do to support caregivers like this is to conduct training through use of videos.

Payne (2003) stated that in many low-SES communities, caregivers cannot come to meetings or in-services because they don't have transportation. However, despite their poverty, many caregivers do own VCRs. Payne shared the story of a principal of a low-income school where 95 percent of the parents were on welfare. He and the teachers were success-fully able to reach these parents by providing information and instructions on fifteen-minute videotapes. SLPs who want to train caregivers in language-stimulation techniques might consider sending home short, simple videos that caregivers can watch repeatedly in their own homes.

A second practical thing that SLPs can do to support low-SES families is to have comprehensive, available lists of low-cost or free local health services for families and in-formation about transportation (Roseberry-McKibbin & Brice, 1998). There is a direct link between socioeconomic status and health-related problems (D'Andrea & Daniels, 2001). Many families with children with disabilities do not have health insur-ance that covers rehabilitation services.

> Low–socioeconomic status families often need support in a number of areas: health, transporta-tion, and others. Clinicians can have available lists of low-cost or free local services for these families.

Even if these services are available, families do not have trans-portation to the sites where services are provided. This can be a prob-lem in instances such as a child with many episodes of otitis media that affect hearing, language, and other aspects of communication (Gravel & Wallace, 2000). If that child cannot get to a service provider who can help her, the ear infections may continue unabated and have negative long-term consequences in terms of language de-velopment and other areas. Thus, again, SLPs need to be prepared to help low-SES families by providing suggestions for transportation to low-cost or free clinics where their health needs can be met.

When SLPs work with children and families who experience violence frequently, or who are surrounded by it daily, they may find an attitude of "why bother?" or "there's no hope" (Haberman, 1995). Haberman (1995, p. 71) states that

> Injuries, abuse, and even death are facts of daily life among children in poverty . . . profes-sionals frequently deal with students who are pregnant, on drugs, or in gangs, or who have dropped out and disappeared. All of these tragedies are deeply felt by professionals who have established close relationships with children and their families.

For families such as this, recommendations like reading books in the home or conducting language-stimulation activities might be met with resistance. Clinicians must be patient and nonjudgmental, perhaps obtaining the services of school personnel instead.

CASES TO CONSIDER

I remember Bobby R., a third-grader on my caseload in the schools. I was trying to work with his single mother to implement a language-stimulation program in the home, but she never responded to my notes or calls. Finally I found out from a colleague that sev-eral years before, she had seen Bobby's father kill a man and had called the police. The father was subsequently put in jail but was about to be released early and had vowed to find and kill his wife and children in revenge for the time he had spent in jail. Bobby and his family moved constantly in an attempt to hide from the father. What would you do in this situation? Would you continue to try working with Bobby's mother? What other resources might you use to help Bobby improve his language skills?

_____

_____

_____

In Chapter 7, we mentioned a study by La Paro et al. (2004) that examined 1,364 three-year-old children with LI. La Paro et al. found that when mothers experienced poverty, they were more likely to be depressed. Maternal depression impacted LI: at four-and-a-half years of age, the children whose mothers were less depressed tended to have LI that had resolved by this age. Children whose mothers were more depressed tended to have LI that had not resolved. Maternal sensitivity also contributed to the resolution of the children's LI (or lack thereof). La Paro et al. suggested that in therapy, it is very important to work closely with mothers of children with LI to optimize the child-caregiver relationship. They suggested that clinicians help mothers use more supportive interaction styles with their preschoolers who manifest LI.

SLPs may need to focus especially on increasing the phonological awareness and literacy skills of low-SES children with LI. Because research consistently shows that low-SES children have disadvantages in these areas, it is clear that they would be helped by intervention that increased skills in these areas. In a longitudinal study of the reading skills of low-income children, Chall, Jacobs, and Baldwin (1990) assessed children in grades two, four, and six and then followed up each group for two years. The most significant finding of the study was that low-SES children began to show deceleration of their reading skills in fourth grade. Skills in knowing word meanings or vocabulary were the first and strongest to decelerate. However, reading comprehension itself was not negatively impacted until sixth grade, when comprehension began to decline.

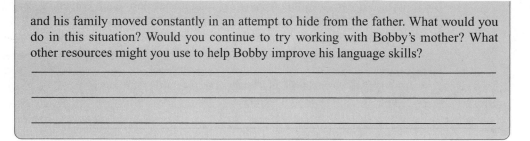

It is important to work closely with caregivers, particularly mothers of low–socioeconomic status children, to optimize the child-caregiver relationship and help mothers use more supportive interaction styles.

Chall et al. (1990) speculated that perhaps in fourth grade, the students were able to use context to compensate for their weakness in vocabulary skills. But when there were too many difficult words and reading material became more abstract, the students' comprehension decreased. Thus, Chall and her colleagues recommended that professionals who work with low-SES children focus on increasing their literacy skills, especially their vocabulary and reading comprehension skills. This is especially important as children stop learning to read and begin reading to learn (Chall & Jacobs, 2003).

Justice and Ezell (2001) examined the written language awareness skills of preschool children from low-SES homes. A battery of six measures was administered to assess skills in print awareness, word awareness, graphic awareness, and metalinguistic awareness.

TABLE 10.1   Written Language Awareness Attainments during the Preschool Period

By the time they are six years old, children should be able to

- display interest in reading and sharing books
- hold a book right side up
- identify the front and back of a book
- identify the top and bottom of a page
- look at and turn pages from left to right
- know that text runs from left to right
- identify where the title is on the cover of a book
- identify titles of favorite books
- distinguish between pictures and print on a page
- know where the story begins in a book
- identify letters that occur in their names
- print the first letter of their names
- recite the first ten letters of the alphabet
- point to the first letter in a word
- differentiate uppercase from lowercase letters
- use terms such as *letter, word, alphabet*
- point to words individually as they are read
- identify the space between two words
- respond to signs in the classroom
- recognize common environmental signs such as a stop sign
- recognize and read some signs in the environment (e.g., Boys, Girls [with regard to restrooms])
- ask for help to "read" signs in the environment

Adapted from Justice & Ezell, 2001; Goldsworthy, 2003; Hearne, 2000.

Analyses of the children's performance on the battery revealed that they had substantial knowledge gaps across all four dimensions of written language awareness.

Based on the findings of their study, Justice and Ezell recommended that SLPs and other professionals should implement early screening programs to identify children with difficulties in written language awareness before they begin kindergarten. These professionals should also work to stimulate early literacy skills. Some of these skills might include increasing the children's knowledge of the names of letters and improving their book-reading conventions.

Justice and Ezell recommended that professionals work to systematically increase children's participation in daily book-reading routines. In a separate study, Justice & Ezell (2002) found that intervention with low-SES preschool children that focused on increasing print awareness was successful in enhancing the children's overall performance in this area. Table 10.1 lists attainments in written language awareness that children should have mastered by age six years. Clinicians can use this list to guide them in assessment and intervention with low-SES children who may be at risk for reading problems.

It is critical to provide early intervention services to children who are at risk for difficulties in written language awareness skills.

Some low-SES caregivers may not be aware of the importance of talking with and stimulating the language of infants and young children

(Anastasiow, Hanes, & Hanes, 1982). SLPs can help these caregivers learn practical, inexpensive language-stimulation techniques like some of those we discussed in Chapters 6 and 7. For instance, as we discussed in Chapter 7, caregivers can be taught milieu techniques to support their children's language growth.

It is very important to help caregivers begin language stimulation as early in life as possible (Roseberry-McKibbin, 2001b). In a longitudinal study of children from various CLD backgrounds, it was found that those whose language enrichment began at four months of age had many long-term advantages over children whose language enrichment began at twelve months of age (Fowler, Ogston, Roberts-Fiati, & Swenson, 1995). Elsewhere in the book, we have mentioned other things that SLPs can do to support language development in children with LI; these things are applicable to low-SES children with LI.

First, we as SLPs can encourage caregivers to observe therapy and participate if they wish. Both caregivers and children can be encouraged to use the school and local community library as much as possible. If caregivers cannot work with their children for various reasons (e.g., substance abuse, illiteracy), peer tutors from the school might be assigned to spend extra time with the children (Roseberry-McKibbin, 2000, 2001b). At my school, many of the students are on welfare and are at risk for language and learning problems. We have free government-funded before- and after-school programs to support these children's academic skills, and tutors are provided. This is especially helpful for children whose parents don't speak English and thus can't help them with their homework.

Congress has provided a specific program to support low-SES children in public schools. Title 1 of the Elementary and Secondary Education Act provides funding for supplementary services in schools that have large numbers of low-SES children. SLPs might check to see if both their LI and non-LI low-SES children can participate in one or more Title 1 programs if the school site receives Title 1 funding. I have frequently referred low-SES children to Title 1 programs for extra language stimulation and academic support.

Weiner (2001) and Payne (2003) discuss the fact that for many low-SES children, school is somewhat of a culture shock. There is a mismatch between what the children are accustomed to in their home environment and what the school expects. Homes of low-SES families may be relatively unstructured, and it is a great transition for children to be in a kindergarten classroom, for example, when there is a slotted time for everything.

Accustomed to lack of structure, low-SES children may have difficulty adjusting to the regimentation of the school classroom. In my current part-time job in an elementary school in a low-income area, I work with many, many low-SES kindergarteners who come to school when they are still four years old. They have never been to preschool and struggle to adjust to the environment of the classroom. SLPs can help teachers and children by training the teachers to teach the children scripts, or routines that go on in the classroom. For example, the children can be taught about recess, lunch, circle time, and other parts of the kindergarten day.

CONNECT & EXTEND

Payne (2003) has written a practical book that helps professionals understand specific issues impacting children from low-SES backgrounds. The book is *A framework for understanding poverty.* Highlands, TX: aha! Process, Inc.

Professionals may have to help low-SES children adjust to the culture of school when these children enter kindergarten.

Kindergarten teachers should never assume that low-SES children have been to preschool. Instead, these teachers—in collaboration with SLPs—can help the children by explicitly teaching them how to behave appropriately in the classroom setting. For example, some children may not know that it is inappropriate to call out while the teacher is talking. Classroom/school language needs to be taught explicitly and without punitiveness to children who do not know the rules of school.

Additional Considerations for CLD Children

In the United States, the majority of low-SES children (about 65 percent) are White, because the total number of low-SES White families is greater than any other ethnic group. However, although the total number of low-SES African American and Hispanic American children is smaller than the number of low-SES White children, the percentages for the first two groups are higher. According to the US Bureau of the Census (2000), 22.1 percent of all African Americans and 21.2 percent of Hispanics live below the poverty level compared to 7.5 percent of the non-Hispanic White population. Residents of American Indian reservations have the highest poverty rate in the United States at 31 percent. In 2001, the unemployment rate for American Indians was 46 percent (Murphy, 2001).

In a review of research on literacy development of English Language Learners in the United States since the 1980s, Genesee and Riches (in press) found that SES was correlated with performance on a number of literacy measures. Specifically, Genesee and Riches found that students from low-SES backgrounds scored significantly lower than students from higher SES backgrounds. Genesee and Riches emphasized that, as we have said before, SES is not a causal factor within itself—however, it is associated with a variety of other factors that we have discussed (e.g., lower educational levels of caregivers).

Craig and Washington (2004b) discussed in detail the effects of poverty on the language and academic performance of African American students. They noted that African American children are more than three times as likely as their White peers to live in poverty and added that they are more likely than majority children to live in families in which the levels of parental education are low. Craig and Washington emphasized that poverty is one variable that is implicated in school reading failure for African American students. They went on to state that "although poverty and its covariables can have profound adverse effects on a child's well-being, recent research indicates that formal public preschool experience may mitigate some of these effects for literacy learning" (p. 234).

There is other research evidence to support the beneficial effects of early intervention programs on low-SES CLD children's cognitive development and academic skills (e.g., Barnett & Camilli, 2002; Halfon & McLearn, 2002; Li, 2003). Thus, we as SLPs can support the development and implementation of early intervention (before kindergarten) programs that will help all low-SES students, especially those from CLD backgrounds, to increase their chances of success in school.

In Chapter 4, we said that immigrants and refugees to the United States also experience a great deal of poverty. For most recent immigrants and refugees, their median income is approximately 58 percent of the income earned by US natives. The proportion of immigrant and refugee households that receive welfare benefits is 30 to 50 percent higher than that of native households (Center for Immigration Studies, 2001).

In Chapter 4, we mentioned migrant workers and some of the challenges they face. Because members of some CLD groups have migrant jobs (e.g., Mexicans in Texas), children from these families are at risk for poverty and academic difficulties. Forces that interrupt the continuity of children's schooling have a deleterious impact on general academic progress as well as relationships with teachers and peers (Nakagawa, Stafford, Fisher, & Matthews, 2002). Moving several times year creates much inconsistency in their schooling. They often have limited access to special-education services because they are never in one place long enough to be assessed and begin intervention (Hardman et al., 2006).

Migrant workers and their families are often socially and physically isolated from the larger community. Children may not always receive the language stimulation they need due to this isolation, in addition to the fact that hard physical labor makes their parents too tired to spend much time with them at the end of a day. For example, if parents who work in California's fields spend eight hours a day in 100-degree weather picking strawberries, they will have little energy left over for their children at night. In addition, many children in California's migrant families work alongside their parents in the fields and consequently are quite fatigued also. Each year in California for a long time, there was a large health fair (called Su Salud) in central California that provided free medical services for migrant workers and their families. Some of us who worked at Su Salud doing free speech and hearing screenings interacted with families who had not eaten for several days. It is challenging to recommend language-stimulation activities in the home to families who do not even have the basics of life.

> Immigrant/refugee and migrant families are particularly vulnerable to poverty and the problems that accompany poverty.

We have mentioned that lack of health insurance is a problem for many low-SES families. Lack of ability to access health insurance may be compounded by families' lack of English skills. In a survey of 254 migrant Hispanic families at Su Salud one year, Roseberry-McKibbin, Peña, Hall, & Smith-Stubblefield (1996) found that more than 90 percent of these families had no health insurance at all. SLPs must be particularly aware of health insurance needs in low-SES CLD families, and as previously stated, should have a list of affordable and accessible health care services to share with the families.

We have said before that some CLD parents' literacy skills may be limited. Because CLD children from low-SES backgrounds may be at additional risk of struggling in school (due to being unfamiliar with English and also being poor), we can encourage parents to share wordless books at home with their children. In this way, children can become familiar with at least some book conventions such as looking at pages from left to right, identifying the front and back of a book, holding a book right side up, and others.

It is very important, as we have said earlier in this book, to remember that immigrants and refugees from other countries may be low-SES in the United States, but that may have come from a lifestyle that was middle- or upper-SES in their countries of origin. Zuniga (2004, p. 205) reminds us that Hispanic Americans, for example

> . . . view class very similarly to others in the United States; for example, it is insulting to be called "low class" or to be assumed to be in a lower class group. Thus, it is critical that

interventionists understand the theme of class in all its complexity. Every family and parent needs to be addressed as an individual in terms of his or her particular reactions and perspectives on the disabilities or illnesses that affect his or her child.

In intervention, one thing that SLPs can do to support children with LI from low-SES families is to teach the them about basic safety. I have spent therapy time talking with eleven-year-olds about the dangers of smoking. I have dealt with gang members and discussed the dangers of drugs. I have spent much time in language therapy with my low-SES LI students teaching them to read and understand basic safety signs. This is especially important for low-SES language-impaired students from CLD backgrounds.

These students face the triple challenge of being low-SES, having a language impairment, and speaking English as their second or third language. I have found that it is difficult for these students to read and comprehend such signs as *No Trespassing, Don't Walk, Poison,* or *Danger.* One teenage CLD low-SES LI student, upon reading the warning label on the back of a household cleaner, said that he thought "flush your eyes upon contact" meant that he should stick his head in the toilet and flush it if the cleaner got in his eyes. Clearly, therapy time was spent clearing up this misconception.

Because many of my low-SES, CLD students with LI are left at home alone, I have also spent time helping them problem-solve what they would do if a stranger came to the door and/or tried to break into and enter their home. In Chapter 5, I mentioned a nine-year-old student, Sevon, who told me how his mother had taught him to point and shoot a gun. The loaded gun was kept beside the front door when she was at work, in case Sevon needed to use it. I have helped students such as Sevon understand how to call 911, circumstances in which they might need to call 911, and how to talk to 911 operators. I have been so surprised by how many of my low-SES, LI, CLD students do not know safety basics, and it has been very rewarding to teach them to understand these basics as part of language intervention.

> CLD students with LI from low–socioeconomic status backgrounds often benefit from learning basics of safety and self-care.

SUMMARY

- Socioeconomic status (SES) may have an even greater impact on children's language development than cultural and linguistic background.
- Research has consistently demonstrated that many low-SES caregivers tend to not have had the benefit of a higher education; maternal educational level is the greatest predictor of children's language skills. Higher maternal education fosters better outcomes for children.
- Low-SES children often have difficulties not only with oral language but with literacy and related skills such as phonological awareness. These children may also be at risk for behavioral problems.
- Low-SES children tend to be disproportionately referred to special education, where they are routinely given knowledge-based standardized tests that are biased against them.

> The use of processing-dependent measures is recommended for assessing the language skills of low-SES children.
> - SLPs and other professionals who work with low-SES children and their families must be prepared to provide or recommend comprehensive support (e.g., medical care, transportation).
> - Appropriate early-intervention programs can help low-SES children, especially those from CLD backgrounds, to be less at-risk for LI later on.

CHILDREN FROM BACKGROUNDS OF ABUSE AND/OR NEGLECT

Background Information

Nelson (1998) suggests that the terms *neglect* and *abuse* refer to a set of environmental conditions that may profoundly affect the development of children; they do not necessarily represent a clinical category. Recent research suggests that the prevalence of child neglect and abuse is approximately 12.2 cases per 1,000 children (US Department of Health and Human Services, 2003a). The highest rate of abuse is experienced by children in the birth to three-year-old age group. Both state and federal legislation have defined neglect and abuse of children. Each state is responsible for defining child abuse in conformity with the standards set by the Keeping Children and Families Safe Act of 2003 (P.L. 108-36). Most definitions include the following descriptions.

Neglect, the failure to provide for a child's basic needs, may be emotional, educational, or physical. Emotional neglect can involve exposure to domestic violence or inattention to a child's emotional needs. Research has found that children who are severely emotionally neglected may have cognitive problems, including difficulty with problem-solving skills and impulse control (Hildyard & Wolfe, 2002). Educational neglect can involve the caregivers' failure to attend to a child's general and/or special-education needs. Physical neglect can be characterized by lack of food, shelter, or medical care; it can also involve lack of appropriate supervision (e.g., leaving young children at home alone). Children who have been severely ignored and neglected may be apathetic and lethargic (Hardman et al., 2006). Parents may neglect their children for a variety of reasons; one of the major ones is a lack of financial resources.

Many low-SES parents neglect their children because they are literally unable to provide health care, food, clothing, or shelter for them. I used to work with a low-SES fourth-grade girl who we literally had to send home from school several times because her clothing was soiled from urine, and the smell was so bad that the classroom teacher and other children could not concentrate. Conducting language intervention with her in a small therapy room with no windows was particularly challenging. In winter, the girl had no sweater, and so some of us at the school brought sweaters from home for her to wear. Another low-SES boy I worked with at the same school had been referred for testing.

> Neglect, the failure to provide for a child's basic needs, may be emotional, educational, or physical.

As I was conducting the assessment, I could hear his stomach growling; he said he had not had breakfast. I obtained a snack for him so that he could focus and perform to the best of his capability during the assessment session.

Physical abuse is a physical injury that happens as a result of hitting a child with a hand, strap, or other object. The injury can also result from the child's being shaken, choked, beaten, or otherwise harmed. A child's injuries can range from mild (e.g., a bruise) to severe (e.g., a broken arm or head injury). Any injury to a child is considered physical abuse whether it happened on purpose or by accident (Gimpel & Holland, 2003). When my son Mark was four years old and in preschool, I had to take him to the hospital two days in a row for accidents that had happened at preschool (falling off the teeter-totter, stuffing a bead up his nose). The second day, the nurse looked at me quite intently and hinted that I might be abusing him. Thankfully, nothing more happened to him that week!

Emotional abuse is any pattern of behavior that impairs a child's sense of self-worth or emotional development. Examples of emotional abuse include constant rejection, threats, insults, and criticism as well as withholding guidance, love, or support (Caliber, 2003b). At the clinic in the university where I teach, one of my student clinicians worked with a nine-year-old girl with language impairment who appeared to have very low self-esteem. Upon talking with the girl's parents, my student discovered that they constantly told her she was fat, ugly, and would never get married. They were genuinely shocked when they were confronted with the fact that this was bad for their daughter's self-esteem. They said that they had no idea that their words were emotionally damaging her.

Sexual abuse includes sexual exploitation, assault, and incest. It involves any sexual activity that the child cannot or will not consent to. Girls are at greater risk than boys. Disabled children and youth are almost twice as likely as nondisabled children and youth to be sexually abused (US Department of Health and Human Services, 2003b). I worked with a sixth-grade girl who had a severe language impairment. After we all came back to school from Christmas break, Christina demonstrated selective mutism.

A medical examination of her vocal folds revealed no particular pathology, and all of us at the school were baffled by Christina's complete silence. Later, we found out that over the Christmas break, an uncle had moved into the home and had begun regularly sexually molesting this twelve-year-old girl. Although I am not aware of any research data along this line, it has been my personal clinical experience that selective mutism, where a

POINTS TO PONDER What are the differences between abuse and neglect? Describe.

_____

_____

_____

child does not speak for emotional reasons, often results from sexual abuse. The SLP confronting this type of situation must work closely with psychological and medical personnel; language intervention alone will usually be unsuccessful.

Children with special needs are especially at risk for neglect and/or abuse (NA) (Jaudes & Diamond, 1985; Knutson & Sullivan, 1993; Rossetti, 2001). Knutson and Sullivan suggest that mothers of infants with craniofacial anomalies may be less nurturing and attached to their infants than mothers of more physically attractive infants. Decreased attachment increases the chances of NA, and SLPs should be aware that infants who have craniofacial anomalies may be more at risk than more attractive babies.

Rossetti (2001) commented that an increased incidence of abuse is observed in families of children with a history of premature birth, low birth weight, and illness during infancy. Children with disabilities, including language impairments, put a great deal of stress on their caregivers. Without support, these caregivers may neglect and/or abuse the children. For example, some caregivers may shake their babies, resulting in "shaken baby syndrome," where the child experiences diffuse head injuries that can result in permanent cognitive, linguistic, and motor problems.

> Abuse generally takes one of three forms: physical, emotional, and/or sexual. Children with disabilities are especially vulnerable to abuse.

Child neglect and abuse occur at all socioeconomic levels and among all ethnic groups (US Department of Health and Human Services, 2003b). Thus, all professionals, including SLPs, must be aware of this and willing to address it appropriately. According to state law, educators and other professionals who work with children are mandated to report suspected NA to their administrators and/or appropriate child protection and law enforcement agencies (National Clearing House on Child Abuse and Neglect Information, 2003).

CASES TO CONSIDER

William C. was a sweet, eager-to-please eight-year old boy who transferred to my school with one of those infamous "thick files." He had been in speech-language therapy in his previous state due to speech and language delays, and so I immediately placed him onto my caseload. As I read through William's file, I found that his biological mother's rights to see him had been terminated. She had burned him and his siblings with cigarettes, and they were very neglected. William had constantly been hungry; his classroom aide at my school shared that at lunchtime in the cafeteria, William would "eat like there was no tomorrow." His father was apparently so obese that he was physically unable to drive a car; William took the bus to school. His language skills were similar to those of a five-year-old. In what areas of language do you think William might need extra stimulation? How might you obtain assistance in carryover/generalization activities?

_____

_____

_____

Although NA occurs at all socioeconomic levels, there is some evidence that there is a greater incidence among families who live in poverty (Trickett, Aber, Carlson, & Cicchetti, 1991). As we have said, families in poverty have multiple stressors and may be quite socially isolated (Hart & Risley, 1995). SLPs may need to help the child experiencing NA by joining with other professionals to help these families, particularly mothers, avail themselves of increased support and resources such as literacy programs, medical care, and treatment for any addictions.

Gimpel and Holland (2003) suggest that many children will not tell adults that they are being abused, particularly if they are being abused by their parents. I have worked with children who would not tell us at the school about abuse that we knew was occurring at home because they were afraid of being removed from their biological parents and put into foster homes. Thus, SLPs and other professionals who work with these children have to observe the children's behaviors to see if the behaviors suggest that abuse is occurring.

Children who have been physically abused tend to behave in a way that is destructive, oppositional, or aggressive. They may be verbally abusive, exhibit frequent tantrums and out-of-control behaviors, and show play themes that are often violent or destructive. Children who have been sexually abused may exhibit sexualized talk or behaviors, sexualized play themes, self-destructive behaviors, insecure attachments with their caregivers, and aggressiveness and hostility (Gimpel & Holland, 2003).

I worked with a five-year-old sexually abused kindergarten girl who, during the first session I attempted to spend with her, kicked me hard and repeatedly in the chest and stomach. Needless to say, this was a significant hindrance to working on her language skills. I got behind her and held her, eventually managing to turn her away from me so she was kicking and hitting outward. It turned out that I was unable to provide one-on-one intervention for her because of her aggressive and hostile behavior toward me, so I ended up collaborating with her classroom teacher to provide language-stimulation activities in the classroom.

Children who have undergone emotional abuse may manifest depression and lack of self-esteem. They may be overly seeking of others' approval, fear rejection, and have difficulty making decisions. They may also be verbally abusive, hostile, or aggressive to others (Gimpel & Holland, 2003).

> Children who have been abused may be destructive, aggressive, or depressed depending upon the type of abuse they have experienced.

Children who have been victims of NA may develop posttraumatic stress disorder. It has been estimated that approximately 50 percent of children who have been sexually abused will exhibit symptoms of posttraumatic stress disorder (Saywitz, Mannarino, Berliner, & Cohen, 2000). In these cases, children need specific intervention and support from qualified mental health professionals.

Language and Behavioral Characteristics

The effects of NA on a child's language development depend a great deal on the severity and extent of the NA. For example, a child who regularly undergoes severe emotional, physical, sexual abuse, or all three will have more severe language problems than the child who is neglected but not abused. It is difficult to make generalizations about the language of NA children because they are a very heterogeneous group, and there are many factors that impact these children's developing language. However, certain trends have emerged that have described the language skills of this population (Hildyard & Wolfe, 2002; Nelson, 1998).

Children who experience NA may have problems with expressive language especially (Roseberry-McKibbin & Hegde, 2006). Owens (2004) states that in general, NA children have lesser conversational skills than their peers and are less talkative. They are less likely than non-NA peers to volunteer information and discuss their feelings.

Among mother-child pairs where abuse has been identified, mothers have been observed to be less likely to engage in reciprocal interaction with their babies (Nelson, 1998). Research has shown that interactions between mothers and their NA infants do not provide the support for fostering effective communication or social skills; this can cause passivity, which leads to decreased initiative in interactions (Coster & Cicchetti, 1993). It The quality of the mother-child attachment is a more significant factor in language development than maltreatment and can exacerbate or moderate the effects of NA (Mosisset, Barnard, Greenberg, Booth, & Spicker, 1990).

Children who have been neglected and/or abused frequently show language delays.

Some mothers of NA children have been found to punish normal risk-taking and exploration that accompany a child's development (Nelson, 1998). Mothers who abuse their children may be more controlling, and thus they may ignore the child's initiations. This decreases the amount of verbal stimulation the child receives. Mothers who neglect their babies are unresponsive; therefore the babies' attempts at communication are not reinforced. In both these situations, the child's language development may be hampered (Owens, 2004).

It has also been found that in general, children who have been physically abused tend to be aggressive and noncompliant. Children who have been both neglected and physically abused experience more problems at school, including problems with adjustment and academic performance. Studies of language development have shown substantial correlations between language delay and maltreatment (Coster & Cicchetti, 1993; Nelson, 1998).

Research carried out in Minnesota in the Minnesota Mother-Child Project showed that physically neglected children had a significant decline in functioning during the early school years. They scored significantly lower on achievement tests than other children and had great difficulty coping with the demands of school. By second grade, all of them had been referred for special-education services (Egeland, 1991). They were also found to be uninvolved in learning and to have attention problems. Children who experienced emotional neglect during the first two years of their lives were found to perform substantially worse than their nonmaltreated counterparts on academic achievement testing in grades one, two, three, and six (Erickson & Egeland, 1996).

Eckenrode, Laird, and Doris (1993) found that neglect was associated with the lowest academic achievement levels in children. Other researchers found that although both physically neglected and physically abused children performed poorly on measures of academic skills, the academic deficits of the neglected children were more severe than those of the abused children. Both abused and neglected children differed from nonmaltreated children on standardized math tests, but neglected children performed significantly worse in reading and language.

Coster, Gersten, Beeghly, and Cicchetti (1989) studied the language development of maltreated thirty-one-month-olds as compared to that of a matched but lower-SES control group. More than 90 percent of the children in both groups were White. Coster et al. found that the maltreated children had a significantly shorter mean length of utterance than the control group, and they also had a more limited expressive (but not receptive) vocabulary during play sessions with their mothers. In addition, it was found that when compared with use of communication for instrumental purposes, a significantly smaller portion of the maltreated toddlers' communications was directed at exchanging information about their own feelings or activities. The maltreated toddlers made fewer decontextualized utterances (fewer references to events or people outside the immediate context). They engaged in shorter periods of continuous contingent discourse.

Coster et al. stated that overall, their findings suggested that the maltreated toddlers and their mothers had developed a communication style where language was used to get tasks accomplished, but it was used less frequently as a means of affective or social exchanges. Mothers who maltreated their children, compared with matched comparison mothers, focused more on controlling their children's behavior than on understanding their children's feelings, thoughts, or opinions.

> Children who have experienced neglect and/or abuse often experience substantial academic problems and are often referred for special education.

If this type of pattern persists across the child's life throughout the preschool years, it can restrict the child's ability to use language in several critical ways. First, the child may have reduced ability to sustain coherent dialogue and narrative, which is an important competence for social exchange with adults and peers. Second, the child may be restricted in her ability to use language to articulate her needs and feelings. Third, the child may have limited ability to use language to convey abstract concepts, which is a critical foundational skill for literacy.

In terms of social and behavioral problems, research has found that neglected children tend to be socially withdrawn and to avoid interacting with their peers. On the other hand, physically abused children tend to be more aggressive in terms of hitting, yelling, and engaging in destructive behaviors (Erickson & Egeland, 1996).

Implications for Service Delivery

An assessment of the NA child's language skills needs to be part of a broader interdisciplinary assessment of the child's overall development and of his family. Coster and Cicchetti (1993) suggest that assessment should go beyond examination of traditional aspects of language and include a thorough assessment of narrative and pragmatics skills. As discussed previously, research indicates that young maltreated children may have restricted ability to utilize language in connected discourse and to use a variety of language functions beyond strictly instrumental functions. In addition, maltreated children may have little experience in verbal methods of problem solving. They may have had limited experience in focusing on complex, lengthy communication exchanges and may find it hard to extract key ideas that are embedded in lengthy narratives.

When it is found that children are experiencing NA, they are generally asked to testify about this. SLPs may be called upon to assist in this process (Snyder, Nathanson, & Saywitz, 1993). Knutson and Sullivan (1993, p. 12) summarize some challenges for clinicians:

> Diagnostically, a valid interview cannot be conducted without a sound working knowledge of the child's language competence and performance. Without such knowledge, it is impossible

to discern specific meanings and abuse-related referents from the child's verbalizations. . . . . Children should not be asked questions about alleged abuse events that are beyond their developmental mastery. Many handicapped children, irrespective of age, will have difficulties recounting an experience and answering specific questions regarding that experience. . . . . Speech-language pathologists can help ensure that interviews are conducted at child's cognitive and linguistic developmental level.

Treatment of child NA is a complex process that needs to involve the entire family. Caregivers must be given information and support. Support could take many forms, including provision of food stamps, ways to deal with a child's crying, and others. As we said earlier, caregivers of children with special needs may be especially prone to abuse and/or neglect their children because they are under so much stress themselves.

SLPs who work with mothers of infants can teach the mothers to increase their responsiveness to their children's interactions, especially when the children are experiencing emotional challenges. Robinson and Acevedo found that when mothers increased their responsiveness to their babies during emotionally challenging times, the babies' emotional vitality increased. In addition, it was found that babies who scored as having high vitality scored higher than low-vitality babies on either the Preschool Language Scales-3 (Zimmerman, Steiner, & Pond, 1993) or the Mental Development Index of the Bayley Scales of Infant Development-II (Bayley, 1993). Thus, again, it is very helpful to support mothers in increasing their responsiveness to their babies.

> As with other populations of children, it is important for SLPs to help mothers of NA children to increase their responsiveness to their children's interactions.

Clinicians may need to facilitate "respite care," where the state or county provides a qualified service provider to come and care for the child so the caregivers can get a break. For example, if a child with autism does not sleep for three days straight, the caregivers will greatly profit by having a service provider come to care for the child for one or two days. Some caregivers have shared that when the service providers came to provide respite care, they went to motels and slept!

Children who have experienced NA often have a variety of problems, including language problems as we said earlier. These other problems can include regression in toileting habits, insomnia, eating disorders, ulcers, rage, and others (Hildyard & Wolfe, 2002).

Knutson and Sullivan (1993) state that in the case of LI children who have experienced NA, it may be especially important, in intervention, to increase these children's affective vocabulary or their ability to accurately describe their emotions. These children can also be encouraged to express their emotions. I remember Elinor, a second-grade girl with LI who had been placed in foster care due to NA in the home of her biological parents. Elinor had many anger issues, and as part of intervention, I taught her words to describe how she was feeling and also allowed her to talk about her anger in therapy. Although it is critical to make sure that children such as Elinor receive support from appropriate mental health professionals, SLPs can also be supportive as they carry out language intervention with children who have experienced NA.

A challenge for SLPs who provide intervention for NA children is that these children may try to behave violently toward the clinician (Coster & Cichetti, 1993). I gave a personal example of that earlier. Clinicians may need to enlist the help of others so that they can stay safe. I remember being asked to conduct a language assessment in the home of a teenage boy who had undergone NA (I have mentioned him in other chapters). He had attacked several adults at his school site and had tried to burn the school down. When I found out that my school district expected me to be at home alone with the boy during the evaluation, I asked that they ensure that at least one parent was on the premises. The mother ended up being there, and the assessment went well with no assaults on me. Again, clinicians need to do all they can to ensure their own safety and well-being.

Gimpel and Holland (2003) recommend that when professionals work with NA children, the therapy room needs to be perceived as a safe, warm, nurturing place with minimal distractions. Initially, the professional such as the SLP should remain child focused and nondirective. In the first session, the clinician needs to review the rules of the situation and discuss the purpose of therapy. For example, a clinician might tell a child something like (Gimpel & Holland, 2003, p. 154)

> My name is Kelly. I am someone children come and play with or talk to about things that are bothering them. Sometimes in here we will talk about things, sometimes we will play. You can play with whatever you want to in here. We will meet each week for about forty-five minutes. There are only three rules in here. The first rule is that you cannot hurt yourself, the second rule is that you cannot hurt me, and the third rule is that you cannot hurt the toys. . . . Everything that you do in here and talk about in here will stay between you and me. I won't tell anyone about it, unless you are going to hurt yourself or hurt someone else, or if someone else is hurting you. If one of those things is happening, I will have to tell someone to make sure that you are safe. We can talk about it if any of those things come up. Do you have any questions about what I just said?

Because this is a great deal for the child to take in during the first therapy session, the clinician may need to review the information in subsequent sessions.

Children who have experienced NA may need to spend a great deal of therapy time playing. Common toys that can be successfully used with these children include sand trays, puppets, dolls and dollhouses, animal figures, crayons/paints and paper, play food and dishes, and dress-up clothes. It can be very helpful if the clinician can observe and describe the child's actions as well as interpret the child's actions if appropriate. This nondirective approach helps the NA child feel much safer than direct questioning, which may be perceived as a further violation of the child's boundaries (Gimpel & Holland, 2003).

> Language therapy with NA children can often effectively utilize play in a relaxed, nonthreatening atmosphere.

Additional Considerations for CLD Children

It is important to remember that cultural factors can contribute to patterns of neglect and abuse (Fontes, 2005; Gimpel & Holland, 2003). For example, in some cultures, it is considered acceptable to use corporal punishment with children—including the use of belts, sticks, or other implements—when a child misbehaves. As Hardman et al. (2006, p. 499) state, when cultural values are contributing factors, this can indicate that the family " . . . is in need of information or assistance. When a family fails to use information and resources, and the child's needs continue to be unmet, then further intervention on the part of child welfare professionals may be required."

CASES TO CONSIDER

George V., a ten-year-old Vietnamese boy, was referred for language assessment by his classroom teacher. The teacher was especially concerned about George's written narrative skills. I looked through George's school records and saw that he had gotten excellent grades from kindergarten onward. There seemed to be no indicators that might predict LI. When I brought George to my office at the school to be tested, he began to cry. I was unable to accomplish any testing at all because he could not stop crying. Finally, he told me that his mother would beat him and his younger brother with household implements until the implements broke. He added that his bruises from a recent beating were fading nicely.

I went to Harold T., one of our school vice principals, who had past experience working for Child Protective Services. He and I arranged a meeting with George's parents; they both took time off from work to meet with us at the school. Harold explained to them that according to US law, their methods of discipline amounted to child abuse. Harold explained the consequences of this. Both parents were angry with Harold and me, but they understood and said that they would change their methods of discipline in the home. Given George's home situation and school history, do you think that he had a genuine LI or was primarily reacting to his home situation? Explain your answer.

_____

_____

_____

It is very important for CLD families especially to understand American laws regarding what constitutes child abuse. As SLPs, we are sometimes in positions where it is brought to our attention that a child is being disciplined at home in a way that does not conform to federal and state guidelines (Fontes, 2005). We are mandated to report child abuse to Child Protective Services, and I follow this practice myself. However, I have personally found that many CLD parents don't know that their discipline methods are illegal. In these cases, it can be effective for the SLP, working with appropriate colleagues such as school principals and social workers, to talk with families in a sensitive yet honest way to help them understand the consequences of continuing to use methods of discipline that are illegal in the United States. The case of George V. above illustrates this point.

SUMMARY

- The term *neglect* refers to failure to provide for a child's basic emotional, educational, or physical needs.
- Abuse can take three forms: emotional, physical, and sexual. Children who have been neglected and/or abused may manifest a variety of behavior problems.

(continued)

- NA children may have expressive language problems, academic difficulties, and over-all delays in linguistic and cognitive skills.
- Assessment and intervention for children who have experienced NA need to be comprehensive and multidisciplinary. Caregivers usually need a great deal of support.
- In some cultures, customary discipline practices are considered abusive by U.S. law. SLPs and other professionals need to help parents understand U.S. laws relating to discipline practices and help these parents understand what constitutes child abuse in the U.S.

CHILDREN WITH ATTENTION DEFICIT HYPERACTIVITY DISORDER

Background Information

In students with language problems, these problems often overlap with attention deficit hyperactivity disorder (ADHD), and researchers have been interested in the relationship between LI and ADHD (e.g., Breier, Fletcher, Foorman, Klaas, & Gray, 2003). There are three possible reasons for the overlap between LI and ADHD. First, the LI may precede

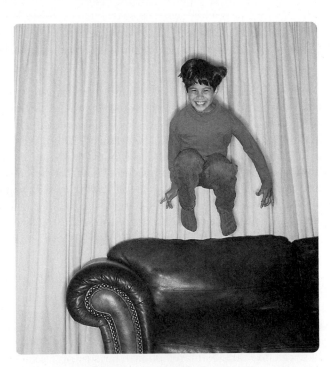

Students with ADHD often have difficulty remaining seated; they may move constantly and be fidgety.

and cause attention problems. Students who experience repeated failure may develop inattentive behaviors because they are frustrated.

Second, attention problems may precede the LI. A student who is not attending may fail to process important academic information and she may fall behind. Third, LI and attention problems may co-occur as separate conditions (Hallahan et al., 2005). The question of how many students with LI also have ADHD is unresolved. It is estimated that perhaps 10 percent of children with ADHD also have a LI, whereas 15 to 80 percent of children with LI also manifest ADHD (McKinney, Montague, & Hocutt, 1993).

In 1994, the American Psychiatric Association revised their classification system for describing different types of disorders. The DSM-IV (Diagnostic and Statistical Manual of Mental Disorders, fourth edition, American Psychiatric Association, 1994), describes several types of difficulties dealing with attention-related disorders in children. At this time, the term attention deficit hyperactivity disorder (ADHD) is considered the correct label for all disorders relating to attention.

In order to be diagnosed with ADHD, a student must manifest the characteristics in Table 10.2 no later than seven years of age. The symptoms must be seen in two or more settings (e.g., home and school) (Bender, 2004). Lastly, the attention problems must cause clinically significant impairment or distress in academic, social, or occupational functioning (American Psychiatric Association, 1994).

> A child may have one of three types of ADHD: primarily inattentive, primarily hyperactive, or a combination of the two.

Studies show that 3 to 5 percent of school-age children have been diagnosed with ADHD in the United States (National Institutes of Health, 1998). The most common subtype of ADHD is the combined type (50 to 75 percent of persons with ADHD). The second most common type is the inattentive type (20 to 30 percent), and the least common type is the hyperactive-impulsive type (less than 15 percent of the population) (Wilens, Biederman, & Spencer, 2002). Again, Table 10.2 describes these categories.

Language and Behavioral Characteristics

In Table 10.2, we have listed behavioral characteristics of children with ADHD. These children also have some distinguishing language characteristics that SLPs can be aware of as they work on teams to provide appropriate services for them.

Children with ADHD may manifest language and auditory processing problems (American Psychiatric Association, 2000; England, 1994; Long, 2005b; Roseberry-McKibbin & Hegde, 2006; Westby & Cutler, 1994). These problems especially include difficulties in pragmatics skills. For example, children with ADHD will often blurt out answers to questions before the questions have been completed. They often talk excessively and interrupt others. Children with ADHD often have difficulty with social entry; that is, they don't know how to successfully join a group or initiate ongoing interactions with others. These children also tend to be less talkative and responsive when others initiate interactions. Many children with ADHD manifest poor turn-taking skills. They may use non sequiturs during discourse.

TABLE 10.2   Behaviors of Students with ADHD

Primarily Inattentive ADHD

- loses books and work materials
- easily distracted
- ignores instructions; does not appear to listen
- short attention span
- poor attention to details; makes careless mistakes
- cannot finish homework in a timely manner
- has difficulty sustaining attention
- has difficulty with organization
- avoids or dislikes tasks requiring sustained mental effort
- is forgetful in daily activities

Hyperactive-Impulsive ADHD

- fidgety
- runs around the living room
- sits in unusual positions and moves constantly
- has difficulty remaining seated
- runs about or climbs excessively
- constantly talking
- impulsive and cannot wait for his/her turn; blurts out answers before questions have been completed
- interrupts or intrudes upon others

Combined ADHD

When children demonstrate the combined type of ADHD, any and all of the behavioral indicators reported above may be seen.

Source: Diagnostic and Statistical Manual, fourth edition (DSM-IV).

When they tell stories or describe things, children with ADHD frequently manifest false starts because they change their minds while structuring what they are going to say. They may use an excessive number of fillers and pauses because verbal expression occurs with minimal or no preplanning. It is difficult for these children to express themselves in a coherent, organized manner. Their disorganization and impulsivity of thought will often leave their listeners baffled.

Other language issues for children with ADHD include use of inappropriate register. For example, they may speak to the classroom teacher in the same way they would speak to the family dog. Clearly, as we discussed earlier, this lack of ability to appropriately shift register can get them into trouble! In addition, children with ADHD often do not accurately perceive their conversational partners' nonverbal cues.

> Language problems of students with ADHD include difficulties with pragmatics, auditory processing skills, and structuring expressive language appropriately.

POINTS TO PONDER List three behavioral and three language characteristics commonly found in children with ADHD.

_____

_____

_____

Implications for Service Delivery

There is no single test to diagnose ADHD; a comprehensive, multidisciplinary team evaluation is necessary to rule out other causes and determine the absence or presence of coexisting conditions. Professionals often use checklists for rating ADHD symptoms; these checklists are usually filled out by teachers and parents (people who are familiar with the child). Professionals who diagnose ADHD include psychologists, clinical social workers, neurologists, nurse practitioners, psychiatrists, and pediatricians.

ADHD tends to run in families, but it may also be related to other causal factors such as prenatal problems and low birth weight (CHADD; Children and Adults with Attention-Deficit/Hyperactivity Disorder, 2005). In addition, there has been research to indicate that the neurotransmitters dopamine and norepinephrine are out of balance in students with ADHD (Barkley, 2000; Solanto, 2002).

CONNECT & EXTEND

CHADD is a national organization that has been of help to many children, adolescents, and adults with ADHD. They can be accessed at www.chadd.org or www.help4adhd.org.

Treatment for ADHD is behavioral and/or medical (Bender, 2004). Medical treatment usually involves some form of medication such as a psychostimulants. Behavioral interventions are also an important component of managing ADHD. In school, classroom accommodations and behavioral interventions can be highly effective if used appropriately. For students with ADHD, early detection and intervention are critical to their success (CHADD, 2005).

Many, many strategies can successfully be used with students who have ADHD. These strategies can be used by SLPs, classroom teachers, and others who work with these students. Several are as follows (Barkley, 2000; Bender, 2004):

1. _Discuss with students what paying attention is_. Show them the advantages of finishing work more quickly and efficiently without being distracted. One mother I know had a first-grade son with ADHD who took one to one-and-a-half hours a night doing his homework. He became more efficient after she talked with him about the fact that if he focused and finished his homework in a timely fashion, he would have more time to play and watch TV. But if he took too long with his homework, there would be reduced playtime and no TV time at all.

2. _Keep external distractions to a minimum_. Make sure the classroom or homework environment at home is free from visual and/or auditory distractions such as people talking

nearby, a TV on, and others. Barkley (2000) talks about "beating the environment at its own game" by reducing environmental distractions as much as possible.

3. *Visually monitor a child's eye contact with the assigned task.* I remember observing a Romanian ten-year-old girl in her classroom; she had been referred for possible ADHD and LD issues. As I watched Estera trying to do her math worksheet, I counted thirty times that she looked up from her work within one minute. Adults need to make sure that students with ADHD literally keep their eyes on their work.

4. *Use special attention strategies.* For example, many students with ADHD like color. They can use colored highlighter pens, colored pencils, etc., to make work more arresting visually.

5. *Have a highly structured classroom.* Students with ADHD may not fare well in classrooms where students are constantly encouraged to make their own decisions. Because of their difficulties with organization, many students with ADHD benefit from a highly structured, very predictable schedule (Cooper, 1999).

6. *Give students with ADHD plenty of opportunities for physical movement.* Many public schools today ask students to sit still at their desks for an hour or more. This is usually very hard for students with ADHD. Frequent, small "movement breaks" as well as larger breaks (e.g., recess, lunch) can be of substantial benefit to students with ADHD.

7. *Provide speech-language therapy to address language and auditory processing problems that are related to the ADHD.* SLPs can especially help these children improve their social interaction skills. It is helpful to work on auditory processing as well as expressive organizational skills.

Treatment for attention deficit hyperactivity disorder can be medical, behavioral, or both. Parents may request a 504 plan to be implemented by the classroom teacher.

Parents of students with ADHD can encourage schools to adopt a *504 plan* to help meet the students' needs in the classroom. Section 504 refers to the section of the Rehabilitation Act of 1973 that guarantees certain rights to individuals with disabilities (including ADHD). This federal law states that no person ". . . shall, solely by reason of her or his disability, be excluded from the participation in, be denied the benefits of, or be subjected to discrimination under any program or activity receiving Federal financial assistance" (Sec. 504). A 504 plan can include elements of the list above that will help the student with ADHD succeed in the general-education classroom setting.

CASES TO CONSIDER

Two weeks ago a sixth-grader with attention deficit hyperactivity disorder (ADHD) was referred to me for speech-language testing. Nasir's family was from Syria and spoke Arabic in the home. English had become Nasir's dominant language, so I assessed him in English with a variety of formal and informal measures. I read in his very thick file that four years before, Nasir had been diagnosed in another city as having a central auditory processing disorder accompanied by ADHD. Nasir was given special-education support and placed on a psychostimulant medication to help him attend and focus better in the classroom. It worked, and teachers reported that when Nasir took his medication, there was a "big difference" in his performance. When I saw Nasir, he was no longer taking medication and performed poorly on many of the assessment tasks I gave him.

In a meeting with his mother later that day, my colleague and I asked her why Nasir was no longer taking his medication. Mrs. A. said that she was afraid of its potential side effects; she shared that the medication, though helpful to Nasir in school, was interfering with his sleep. She was also afraid the medication would inhibit Nasir's physical growth, and this dismayed her because he was already short for his age. Nevertheless, she was concerned about how he would perform in junior high school. My colleague and I said that when Nasir went to junior high school, we would send along my report, which was filled with comprehensive recommendations for the junior high school teachers to carry out in their classrooms. If you were the SLP in this situation, would you also try to persuade Mrs. A. to start readministering Nasir's ADHD medication? Why or why not? What would you do?

_____

_____

_____

Additional Considerations for CLD Children

It is critical to remember that various cultural groups define the construct of appropriate attention in different ways. Some cultural groups may have a greater tolerance than others for behaviors that are consistent with a mainstream definition of ADHD. Professionals must be careful not to overrefer children from such cultural groups. For example, research shows that African American boys are rated by teachers as having the most severe symptoms of ADHD, White girls as having the least severe symptoms, with African American girls and White boys being somewhere in the middle (Reid, Riccio, Kessler, DuPaul, Power, Anastopolous, Rogers-Adkinson, & Noll, 2000). Relatedly, research has also found that African American girls are 3.5 times more likely to screen positive for ADHD than White girls, and African American boys are 2.5 times more likely to screen positive for ADHD than White boys (Reid, Casat, Norton, Anastopoulos, & Temple, 2001).

> Professionals must be careful not to overidentify CLD students as having attention deficit hyperactivity disorder.

Researchers have found that rater bias might influence these findings. White teachers were more likely than African American teachers to rate African American students as having high levels of inattention and hyperactivity (Reid et al., 2001). Thus, professionals need to be careful to not be biased when they refer students for possible ADHD.

SUMMARY

- Students may have one of three subtypes of ADHD: primarily inattentive, primarily hyperactive-impulsive, or combined.
- ADHD is usually treated with medication, behavioral intervention, or both. Parents of students with ADHD can request a 504 plan, or a set of strategies implemented in the general-education classroom to give these students access to the curriculum.
- Language characteristics of students with ADHD often include difficulties with pragmatics skills and expressive language as well as auditory processing.
- It is critical for professionals to remember that various cultures may have more tolerance for behaviors that mainstream professionals might label as symptoms of ADHD. Professionals must not be biased when they refer CLD students for assessment and intervention for ADHD.

CHILDREN FROM BACKGROUNDS INVOLVING MATERNAL SUBSTANCE ABUSE

Background Information

Children with prenatal drug and/or alcohol exposure (PDAE) are a very heterogeneous group. Some have been exposed only to drugs, others only to alcohol. Many children are exposed to both, and so I am using the term PDAE very broadly with the realization that each child presents a unique and individual profile that must be considered by the SLP and other professionals who work with these children.

Paul (2001, p. 99) summarizes the heterogeneous nature of children with PDAE:

> . . . for those children who did show serious effects [of prenatal exposure to cocaine]. Cocaine was usually not the only risk to which they were exposed. Mothers who abused cocaine during pregnancy also tended to abuse other street drugs, as well as alcohol. Alcohol itself is known to be a serious teratogen and could cause many of the problems thought to be present in these babies, even without any other substance abuse. Further, mothers who abused cocaine and other drugs during pregnancy frequently continued to do so after the child was born. These mothers would not be available to their infants either for basic care or for social interaction. . . . We know that neglect during early development has a profoundly negative effect, particularly on language acquisition, for which the consequences are even more pronounced than those of outright abuse. . . . Finally mothers who abuse cocaine and other drugs tend to live in poverty. . . . A disorder of language development can rarely be fully accounted for by one direct, isolated causal condition. Language development is a complex psychological and interpersonal phenomenon and is almost always affected by a wide variety of biological and environmental factors.

Keeping these statements in mind, we will look at some of the effects of maternal substance abuse during pregnancy on the unborn child. We will start with fetal alcohol syndrome.

Fetal alcohol syndrome (FAS) involves damage to an unborn baby due to the mother's alcohol consumption during pregnancy. The child with fetal alcohol syndrome generally has mental retardation, a small brain, low birth weight, heart problems, and craniofacial abnormalities. In addition, the child may have delayed motor development, malformations of major organ systems, swallowing and feeding problems in infancy, and language problems (described later). The child who has fetal alcohol effects (FAE) has problems similar to those of a child with fetal alcohol syndrome, but to a lesser degree. Babies with fetal alcohol effects do not meet the diagnostic criteria for fetal alcohol syndrome. Fetal alcohol syndrome is the number-one cause of preventable mental retardation, and it is estimated that more than 50,000 infants with alcohol-related problems are born every year in the United States (National Organization on Fetal Alcohol Syndrome, 2000).

> The child with fetal alcohol syndrome generally has a number of medical problems accompanied by linguistic and cognitive deficits.

A mother's drug use during pregnancy has various effects on the baby. Drugs known to do the most serious damage are cocaine, morphine, heroin, and LSD (Hardman et al., 2006). In infancy and early childhood, children with PDAE may have feeding problems, sleep disturbances, and failure to thrive. They may have delays in motor milestones such as walking and may throw tantrums. They may be delayed in toilet training and be prone to otitis media (Sparks, 1993). Children with PDAE may have small head circumference; these children are at greater risk for chronic disabilities, but if their head growth catches up, this is a marker of a good prognosis for long-term development (Sparks, 2001).

During the school years, these children may have difficulty in school due to fine-motor difficulties, lack of inhibition, conduct problems, difficulty in understanding the consequences of their actions, poor judgment, and withdrawal and depression. Behavior problems in children with PDAE may include refusal to comply with simple commands and constant testing of limits (Sparks, 1993). A former student of mine worked with a three-year-old PDAE child who, upon hearing a polite request from her, said "No, -itch." Other behavior problems may include mood swings, aggressiveness, apathy, inability to modify their own behavior, and great difficulty with changes and transitions. Children with PDAE may also have decreased responsiveness to traditional forms of reinforcement such as praise and token rewards (Roseberry-McKibbin & Hegde, 2006).

Language and Behavioral Characteristics

Language and related problems are numerous in PDAE children. As we said earlier, the types of deficits children show are directly related to the pattern, type, and extent of drug and/or alcohol exposure during the pregnancy. Nevertheless, some tentative generalizations about the language skills of PDAE children may be made.

Some PDAE children may have good verbal facility, giving the impression of strong verbal skills, but may have difficulty with comprehension and receptive vocabulary. They may show poor abstract reasoning but perform well with concrete tasks. Word recognition may be easier than reading comprehension (Sparks, 1993; Streissguth, 1997).

A study by Rivers & Hedrick (1992) looked at the language characteristics of children prenatally exposed to cocaine. They found that the most striking behaviors of the children in the study were significant delays in receptive and expressive language skills. Even children who were considered to have normal mental abilities often exhibited subtle expressive and receptive language delays. Specifically, language-learning problems of drug-exposed children often include the following:

- fewer spontaneous vocalizations from infancy,
- lack of appropriate use of gestures and words to communicate needs
- decreased problem-solving skills
- word retrieval problems
- counting using a numerical system
- syntactic problems, especially disorganized sentences

PDAE children frequently have difficulties in the area of pragmatics. They have poor eye contact and may be poor at initiating social interaction. They may demonstrate indiscriminate attachment to new people. One PDAE girl I worked with in a mental hospital literally tried to block me from leaving her room after I had completed my assessment of her language skills. She constantly asked to sit on my lap throughout the entire evaluation. Her great affection for me was apparent the minute I walked through the door of her room, and the experience of evaluating her language was very memorable.

> Children with prenatal drug and/or alcohol exposure often have difficulties with pragmatics skills as well as attention and memory problems.

PDAE children frequently have difficulties in other areas such as decreased attention span, distractibility, hyperactivity, impulsivity, and difficulties with memory (Paul, 2001; Rivers & Hedrick, 1992; Sparks, 1993). In a study of cocaine-exposed children during the toddler period, Howard, Beckwith, Ridning, and Kropenske (1989) showed that in comparison to a control group with similar characteristics, the cocaine-exposed children (despite therapy) tended to throw toys or hit their toys without any provocation. They also found that the drug-exposed toddlers had fewer play sequences than the control group in a free play setting. The drug-exposed toddlers were more prone to temper tantrums, were less securely attached to their caregivers, and had more impulsive and less goal-directed behavior than the control group.

Implications for Service Delivery

Children prenatally exposed to alcohol and drugs may have language difficulties that are not easily detected by standardized language measures. Thus, such children may not readily receive services in public schools because they do not fit into a predetermined category such as learning disabled or mentally retarded. Informal assessment of these children's language skills in everyday settings may prove to be more helpful than the administration of formal, standardized measures.

PDAE children appear to benefit greatly from routine and structure. They also can profit greatly from early intervention and from programs designed to educate their caregivers. One relatively consistent characteristic of drug-exposed children is that they tend to not maintain treatment gains made in therapy sessions from one session to the next if the interval between sessions is too long (Rivers & Hedrick, 1992). Thus, it is important that therapy sessions be consistent and that caregivers regularly follow up treatment goals in the home.

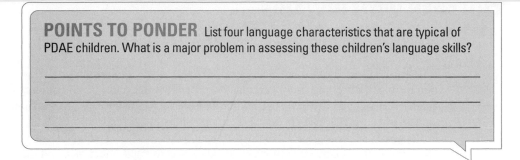

POINTS TO PONDER List four language characteristics that are typical of PDAE children. What is a major problem in assessing these children's language skills?

Additional Considerations for CLD Children

Alcoholism is prevalent in some CLD communities, and it is a serious problem in these communities because it often begins during the teen years. Alcoholism among women is a major issue; some women may not be aware that drinking during pregnancy can cause problems for their children. Drug use is more prevalent in urban than in suburban areas. This may be because residents of inner cities have greater access to drugs (Wallace, 1998).

Wallace (p. 318) states that "because a disproportionate number of minorities reside in urban America, it is likely that minority inner-city residents are more affected by the problem of substance abuse than the population at large." Thus, SLPs must remember that although substance abuse exists within every ethnic group and socioeconomic level of society, low-income CLD adults who live in inner cities may be more at risk than other members of the population.

 SUMMARY

- Children with prenatal drug and/or alcohol exposure (PDAE) make up a very heterogeneous group. They frequently manifest a number of behavioral, physical, emotional, linguistic, and cognitive problems.
- PDAE children may have language problems that are not easily detectable by standardized measures. Informal assessment of their language functioning in everyday settings is probably the optimal way to validly and reliably assess their language skills.
- In therapy, most PDAE children benefit from routine, structure, and predictability. Because they tend to have difficulty maintaining treatment gains between therapy sessions, it is critical that caregivers do carryover activities in the home to help maintain therapy gains.

CHILDREN WITH HIV/AIDS

Background Information

AIDS (acquired immunodeficiency syndrome) is the symptomatic clinical manifestation of impaired cellular immunity that is caused by infection with the human immunodeficiency virus type 1 (HIV-1). Children who have AIDS have the human immunodeficiency virus (HIV), which attacks certain white blood cells in the body, and/or the presence of antibodies to HIV in the tissues or blood as well as recurring bacterial diseases (Nickel, 2000). The purpose of white blood cells is to fight infections, and the body is defenseless without sufficient numbers and types of them.

In the United States, the average prevalence rate for cases of AIDS is 19.9 per 1,000 individuals. Approximately 8,600 children below age thirteen in the United States have been diagnosed with AIDS. Approximately 5,000 children or youth under fifteen years of age die in the United States each year due to AIDS (American Academy of Pediatrics, 2001). The incidence of pediatric HIV is highest in states where there are high percentages of low-SES Hispanic and African American women. Approximately 65 percent of children who have HIV are African American; 17 percent are Hispanic; 16 percent are White, and 2 percent are Asian-Pacific Islanders (Centers for Disease Control and Prevention, 2000).

Approximately 10 to 15 percent of infected children develop AIDS during their first months of life and die relatively quickly. Fifteen to 20 percent of infected children develop AIDS after the infancy period, and 65 to 75 percent of children who test HIV positive live and can thrive. Clearly, early diagnosis of infants with HIV is crucial because prophylactic treatment of opportunistic diseases as well as early antiviral therapy can have positive impacts on the child's prognosis over time (Jankelovich, 2001; Nehring, 2000).

> Early diagnosis of children with HIV is critical because early therapy can positively impact the children's prognosis.

HIV can be passed from one person to another through several methods. It can be passed by blood exchange through injection drug use, exchange of bodily fluids during sexual contact, blood transfusions, and breast milk (Nickel, 2000). HIV can also be transmitted from a mother to an unborn child. The virus crosses the placenta, infecting the fetus and damaging the unborn baby's immune system. When this happens, the child can have substantial intellectual deficits (Hardman et al., 2006). HIV is a major cause of preventable infectious mental retardation. Because the virus interrupts a baby's brain development in utero, the child may have extensive brain damage (National Association of School Psychologists, 2002).

Children who have AIDS move through a series of stages of the disease. The first is the exposure stage, or the period during which transmission of the HIV occurs. People may be infected with HIV but not yet exhibit the symptoms of AIDS. Children progress through various other stages of AIDS; about 50 percent of all individuals with HIV develop AIDS within ten years. In children, it can take between one and three years for AIDS to fully emerge. It is estimated that 80 percent of children who are infected by their mothers will develop full-blown symptoms of AIDS by the time they are two years old (National Association of School Psychologists, 2002). Approximately 33 percent of children who are exposed to HIV through any means remain free from AIDS until they are about thirteen years old (Nickel, 2000). Frequently, the most serious symptoms of AIDS don't appear until children enter school or begin adolescence (Hardman et al., 2006).

Many children who have AIDS don't gain weight appropriately and do not grow normally. They are slow to achieve key motor milestones such as crawling and walking. As HIV turns into AIDS, infected children get opportunistic infections that are life threatening. (Opportunistic infections are called that because they take the opportunity to cause illness in a person with a weakened immune system.) In addition, many children show signs of neurological damage associated with autism, cerebral palsy, seizure disorders, and mental retardation (National Institute of Allergy and Infectious Diseases, 2000).

> Children with AIDS have numerous physical problems, including neurological damage associated with various disorders.

At this time, there is no known cure for AIDS. However, there have been some medical breakthroughs. For example, research has found that retroviral medications can slow HIV's progression in children as they do in adults. In addition, it has been found that using the drug AZT with pregnant women can help in preventing the in-utero infection of babies (Davis-McFarland, 2002). Treatment for AIDS is usually provided by a multidisciplinary team composed of medical and educational professionals.

Language and Behavioral Characteristics

Because HIV manifests primarily in the central nervous system, children with HIV can have speech and language disabilities in addition to other problems (American Speech-Language-Hearing Association, 2004). They may have chronic otitis media with effusion, which impacts language development. Most research shows that HIV compromises the development and acquisition of communication milestones. As the children's medical condition worsens, they may have loss of the language milestones they have attained. A decline in language skills may precede or coincide with other losses in cognitive skills (Retzlaff, 1999).

> Children with HIV/AIDS may be diagnosed with mental retardation or learning disorders that require special education. Antiretroviral drugs can improve children's language skills and their life expectancy.

Approximately 25 percent of children with HIV/AIDS will be diagnosed with learning disorders or mental retardation and will need special education (Davis-McFarland, 2002). Unique manifestations in children with HIV include pragmatic language disorders and elective mutism. In addition, these children may have attention deficits, visual and auditory short-term memory problems, and academic difficulties. They may have severely withdrawn behavior and be labeled "autistic-like" (National Association of School Psychologists, 2002).

CONNECT & EXTEND

The communication problems of children with HIV/AIDS are detailed in Davis-McFarland, E. (2002). Pediatric HIV/AIDS—Issues and strategies for intervention. *The ASHA Leader, 7*, 10–21.

Some clinicians have found that with aggressive use of antiretroviral drugs, children's life expectancy improves and their language skills improve as well. Children make more rapid progress in therapy and are more likely to maintain the gains that they do make. However, it must be remembered that some of these drugs are ototoxic; they can compromise a child's hearing when used over long periods of time. Children must be regularly monitored by an audiologist to ensure that their hearing status remains stable (Davis-McFarland, 2002).

Implications for Service Delivery

Treatment for babies with AIDS can be challenging because they are so dependent and often, mothers who pass HIV on to their children can't provide proper care for their babies. These mothers often come from low-SES backgrounds where they have limited access to health care (Nehring, 2000). In addition, some of them are intravenous drug users and are not reliable caregivers (Hardman et al., 2006). Many infants and children with HIV/AIDS live in foster care, and it is important for clinicians to support these parents (Nehring, 2000; Pressman, 1992).

It can be quite challenging to treat adolescents with HIV and AIDS for several reasons. They might not comply with medical regimens, although it is important that they do this because missing a dosage of medication could place the student's health in serious danger. In addition, they may also experience depression and anxiety associated with their disease. These adolescents need instruction to help them and their families understand AIDS, communicate effectively with others, and make wise choices regarding their sexual behavior (National Institute of Allergy and Infectious Disease, 2000).

The law does not force students with AIDS or their parents to tell school personnel about their medical status. SLPs may be working with children with HIV/AIDS without even knowing it, and thus it is important to always use appropriate precautions. However, the information may be shared with a limited number of school personnel and should be kept strictly confidential. Students with AIDS are often fatigued, and this needs to be considered if adolescents with AIDS are on SLPs' caseloads.

> When SLPs work with children with HIV/AIDS, the focus should be on helping the children develop good oral-language and preliteracy skills.

While you as an SLP are not the key person to deal with the feelings of an adolescent with AIDS, it is possible that you might encounter one or more of these students on your clinical caseloads. It is important to be sensitive, a good listener, and to know good sources that you can refer them to for support. In addition, if the adolescent has a language impairment, it will be especially important to help him communicate clearly and directly with others regarding his situation. With adolescents, it is important to work on pragmatics skills, literacy skills, and academic skills (Davis-McFarland, 2002; Hardman et al., 2006).

According to Davis-McFarland (2002), there is little to no efficacy data on clinical intervention with children who have communication disorders related to HIV/AIDS. She recommends working directly with children and also with parents, commenting that many parents are highly motivated to help their children succeed. She states that with preschoolers, the focus of therapy should be on helping the child to develop good phonological, oral-language, and preliteracy skills. When children begin attending school, clinicians can focus on the communication skills necessary for academic success.

For children with HIV/AIDS who have severe communication problems, the use of augmentative and alternative communication (AAC) devices may be considered (Paul, 2001; Pressman, 1992). Pressman (1992) states that for children with full-blown AIDS who are terminally ill, in the final stages of life, eye-gaze communication may be encouraged because these children's ability to use AAC devices can change weekly or even every few days.

Additional Considerations for CLD Children

Members of CLD groups are disproportionately affected with AIDS (Morrison, 2003; Wallace, 1998). AIDS is a serious problem among CLD infants and children because the AIDS virus can be transmitted through the placenta (Wallace, 1998). SLPs and other professionals must be sensitive to the fact that, as we have said elsewhere in this book, members of some CLD groups feel that it is inappropriate to reveal private, personal information. This may be especially true in the case of HIV/AIDS, which can be accompanied by significant stigma (Hardman et al., 2006).

 SUMMARY

- Children with HIV/AIDS often have neurological damage and may get opportunistic infections that are life threatening.
- HIV compromises the acquisition and development of communication milestones. Approximately 25 percent of children with HIV/AIDS will be diagnosed with learning disorders or mental retardation and will need special education.
- Intervention should focus on increasing oral and written communication skills. For children who have severe communication problems, the use of augmentative, alternative communication devices may be considered.

CHILDREN WITH BEHAVIORAL AND EMOTIONAL PROBLEMS

Background Information

Researchers have historically focused on three distinct yet similar populations when reviewing the occurrence of language delays in children with emotional difficulties. These populations include 1) children labeled by the public schools as emotionally and behaviorally disordered who also display language disorders, 2) children with diagnosed psychiatric disorders who also have language disorders, and 3) children with LI who also display emotional and behavioral problems (Hardman et al., 2006). For purposes of this chapter, we will use the term "emotionally and behaviorally disordered" (E/BD) to describe these children.

Children with E/BD experience substantial difficulty in relating to peers and adults. The Council for Exceptional Children (CEC; 1991) has proposed a definition for E/BD:

> EBD refers to a condition in which behavioral or emotional responses of an individual in school are so different from his/her generally accepted, age-appropriate, ethnic, or cultural norms that they adversely affect educational performance in such areas as self-care, social relationships, personal adjustment, academic progress, classroom behavior, or work adjustment . . . [it persists] even with individualized interventions . . .

CASES TO CONSIDER

I was asked to evaluate the language skills of Jan S., a twelve-year-old girl who had tried to commit suicide but had failed. Jan swallowed a bottle of pills after a group of girls from her school followed her to the mall and tried to beat her up. There were major extenuating circumstances in her home that had contributed to severe emotional and behavioral problems. When I went to the mental hospital where Jan was staying, she was polite but would not look at me at all. She was deeply depressed. I did manage to evaluate her language skills fairly thoroughly and found that she was approximately two to three years behind norms in most areas of receptive and expressive language. I found out that Jan and her mother were going to be moving to a new area and a new school district. What types of recommendations might you make for Jan in terms of services that would support her linguistic, academic, and emotional growth?

> Over the past few years, SLPs have become increasingly aware of the co-occurrence of emotional and behavioral disorders and language impairments.

Paul (2001) suggests that there is somewhat of a "chicken and egg" situation with E/BD children: which comes first, the E/BD or the communication disorder? Does having LI, for example, create emotional and social problems that eventually become clinically significant? Or do children who originally have E/BD problems eventually develop language impairments because of the E/BD? We do not know the answers to these questions, and there is not enough research to allow us to establish causal relationships between E/BD and language impairments. However, numerous sources document their co-occurrence.

SLPs' awareness of the co-occurrence of language disabilities and challenging behaviors has increased over recent years (e.g., Fujiki, Spockman, Brinton, & Hall, 2004; Nungesser & Watkins, 2005; Woolfolk, 2004). Research over the last 20 years has suggested that 50 to 80 percent of children with LI have co-occurring emotional/behavioral disorders or psychiatric problems (Baltaxe, 2001; Hyter, Rogers-Adkinson, Self, Simmons, & Jantz, 2001). Additional research has indicated that these children have difficulties in all areas of language; however, pragmatic and expressive language difficulties have the potential to increase these children's risk of developing and maintaining behavioral and social-emotional problems and to affect educational success (Kuder, 2003; Prutting & Kirchner, 1983; Redmond, 2002).

Language and Behavioral Characteristics

We have said in previous chapters that children with LI are at risk for difficulty in social interactions because of pragmatics problems. This is especially true when they are dealing with peers (Brinton & Fujiki, 1999). We said that research shows that even as young as preschool, children with LI tend to be more rejected by their peers than children with TD language (Gertner, Rice, & Hadley, 1994; Rice et al., 1991).

It is possible that the pragmatics problems of children with LI are partially related to emotion regulation. Emotion regulation refers to a child's ability to control her emotions in various situations. Fujiki, Brinton, and Clarke (2002) conducted a study in which they looked at emotion regulation in children with LI. Fujiki et al. (p. 103) stated that "to borrow popular parlance, emotion regulation includes the need to both 'chill out' and 'psych up' emotions according to the child's social goals in specific contexts." For example, let's say a child is teased by peers and she becomes angry. A child with adequate emotion regulation might regulate her emotion of anger by reducing the intensity of her feelings through telling herself that those children need to "get a life" and then going to find some other friends to play with. A child who has difficulty with emotion regulation might become furious and talk angrily about the teasing for several days.

> Children with language impairments rate lower in emotion regulation than their peers; this is especially true for older boys.

Language skills are an important part of emotion regulation. Fujiki et al. (2002) gave the example of a child watching a scary movie who uses internal language to remind himself about things like "This isn't real. It's just a TV show. Maybe Dad will watch this with me. I'm going to be okay." A child with lower language skills would have more problems regulating her emotions in such situations than a child whose language skills were adequate.

Fujiki et al. found, in their study of LI children, that teachers rated LI children as substantially lower in emotion regulation than they did TD peers. Interestingly, inferential analyses showed among other things that older boys with LI appeared to have particular difficulty with emotion regulation; this was a concern because experience and maturity did not resolve the difficulties in emotion regulation for the children in this study.

An area of particular difficulty for the LI children was the ability to express if they were feeling fearful or afraid, angry or mad, or sad. Fujiki et al. recommended that clinicians and researchers more closely examine the relationship between emotion regulation and social competence in children with language impairment. One might speculate from this study that in intervention, children with LI be taught to identify and verbally express their emotions as well as learn to regulate them in order to facilitate social competence. More research needs to be done to see if this speculation is accurate.

Ruhl, Hughes, and Camarata (1992) gave a battery of language tests to a group of thirty children who had been labeled E/BD but were in general-education classes. The children had deficiencies in all language areas measured, but grammatical functioning stood out as an area of particular difficulty. The children tended to use simple sentences that only communicated one or two main ideas.

Implications for Service Delivery

Assessment of E/BD students can be difficult because their moods and behavior vary from day to day. For example, several days ago in my public school job, I was asked to assess the language of a kindergartener with E/BD. Another SLP had begun the assessment on a different day, and she asked me to help her as her schedule was very busy. When I went to pick Gary up, the class was having their pictures taken, and Gary was screaming and crying with fear because of the photography equipment. Thus, he met me at a very bad time. He clung to his full-time classroom aide and would not come with me. The aide walked him around outside to calm him down, and finally my colleague who had begun the testing finished the testing when Gary was calmer. You will probably agree that it was better for my colleague to assess Gary from beginning to end (instead of having me help her) because he was familiar with her and felt more comfortable. In addition, he had no negative associations with my colleague as he did with me (because I met him for the first time near the feared photography equipment).

In Chapter 5, we talked about the importance of test reliability. This is an especially relevant issue when we assess the communication skills of students with E/BD. They may or may not want to participate in testing depending upon the day, the circumstances, and their mood at the time as in the example above. In addition, some students with E/BD may perform adequately on formal language tests; however, they may have difficulty with communicative competence, or the ability to use their language skills in conversational contexts. Thus, it is often best to assess these students' communication in natural settings through such means as observations in different circumstances (e.g., classroom, playground, school cafeteria) (Kuder, 2003).

> Problems can occur when we try to use formal language tests with emotionally and behaviorally disordered students; it is often best to assess these students' functional communication in natural settings.

Earlier in the book I mentioned a teenage boy with E/BD who had attacked several adults and tried to set his school on fire. When I was asked to perform a comprehensive assessment of his pragmatics skills, I asked his parents if I could observe him several times, on different days, in the summer school setting he was participating in. I told them I wanted to observe his interactions with peers, since he appeared to have the most challenges in this area. His parents said absolutely not; they did not want me to "interfere" with their son's summer school. As previously mentioned, I assessed the boy in his home using informal and formal pragmatics measures.

He did very well alone with me in his home (with his mother upstairs), but I have always wished that his parents would have let me observe his peer interactions. The boy's behavior with me was courteous and appropriate, and to this day I greatly doubt that it was representative of his interactions with peers. In evaluating the language skills of children with E/BD, though it is ideal to conduct observations in their natural environments during peer interactions, this is not always possible; we have to do the best we can with what parents will permit us to do.

Kuder (2003) suggested that language intervention for children with LI and EB/D address three major categories: helping students improve peer interaction, become more effective communicators in the classroom, and learn and use vocabulary words to describe how they are feeling.

In intervention, it is very important to help the child become successful in using language with others in natural environments, especially peers (Hyter et al., 2001; Nungesser & Watkins, 2005). It has been recommended that when SLPs assess and treat children with LI and emotional/behavioral problems, they use a socioemotional perspective (Hummel & Prizant, 1993). The implication of this is that clinicians should target not only behavior and language skills, but also work on improving these children's emotional expression, self-concept, and relationship issues.

To this end, Hyter et al. (2001) conducted a study in which they worked with boys between eight and twelve years of age who attended a specialized educational facility for children with emotional/behavioral problems. The researchers administered several pretests measuring language and behavior along various dimensions, and then provided classroom intervention to improve communicative competence in four areas: describing objects, giving step-by-step directions, making judgments by stating personal opinions about inappropriate behavior, and negotiating for desired outcomes.

It was found that the subjects improved in their ability to describe objects to a naive listener and to provide sequenced directions. Subjects in the study improved in their ability (on a formal test) to express judgment and to consider and understand the listener. However, carryover of the latter skills to the classroom setting was limited. Hyter et al. suggested that perhaps the classroom intervention should have been supplemented by individual and small-group practice in monitored small-group settings in order to increase the students' confidence in and ability to carry over targeted pragmatics skills to the classroom setting. Hyter et al. suggested that SLPs be regularly involved in helping strengthen the pragmatics skills of students with emotional/behavioral problems.

> Research has shown that ideally SLPs work in the classrooms of emotionally and behaviorally disordered children, helping both the teachers and children with strategies for improved communication.

Based on their surveys of preschool teachers, Nungesser and Watkins (2005a) recommended that SLPs be involved in collaborative teams that help to train teachers to deal with challenging behaviors in the preschool classroom environment. In their study, they found that many preschool teachers did not necessarily acknowledge the role of language skills in children with challenging behaviors. Nungesser and Watkins recommended that SLPs work with both teachers and children in the preschool classroom environment, expanding these children's opportunities for academic and social success and advancement.

Nungesser and Watkins (2005a) recommended that in intervention, young children be taught communicative forms that function equivalently to the challenging behavior. For example, if a child wants to go to the bathroom, instead of having a tantrum or disrupting the class by running to the bathroom, she can be taught to say "I need the bathroom." Nungesser and Watkins particularly recommended that clinicians and teachers role model appropriate language alternatives.

In addition, they also recommended shadowing, where the adult (teacher or SLP) follows a child within the classroom during times such as free play to anticipate the potential occurrence of interactions and situations leading to challenging behaviors. The adult can provide communicative support to reduce the challenging behavior. For example, the adult might model "May I play with the dollhouse?" or point out appropriate behaviors displayed by other children ("Look, Jenna didn't grab the dollhouse; instead she said, 'May I play with the dollhouse?'")

Nungesser and Watkins (2005a), like other researchers, also recommended that clinicians teach children emotional language; that is, teach children to use labels to express how they are feeling. Clinicians and other adults can role-model this by saying things like "I feel happy. I feel happy because I just ate a nice snack" and smiling to convey accompanying facial expression. They can also use peers, as mentioned, as role models ("When Janey got mad at Suzy, she went off to play with Casey instead of yelling at Suzy.")

Other experts (e.g., Giddan, 1991; Paul, 2001) have also suggested that children with EB/D issues be taught vocabulary words that they can use to describe their emotional states. For example, instead of just using the words *mad, glad, sad*, the students can be taught words such as *worried, embarrassed, afraid*, and others that can capture the more subtle nuances of how they are feeling.

Paul (2001) listed some practical suggestions for incorporating socioemotional and behavioral aspects into language therapy. First, children can learn to use intentional communication to establish joint attention and to call attention to themselves. I would add here what is probably obvious: intentional communication in this context involves using appropriate verbal and nonverbal means that do not include biting, scratching, hitting, or other such behaviors. One Vietnamese ten-year-old boy I worked with was in a classroom for E/BD children. His problem was twofold: his English skills were very limited, and he had a number of cognitive-linguistic delays and emotional problems that greatly impacted his classroom performance. One of our number-one therapy goals was to help Chinh initiate verbally, not hit or bite to get attention.

Paul (2001) also recommended helping E/BD children learn acceptable means of expressing rejection and protest. You will recall that we discussed this in Chapter 9 in terms of children with developmental delays; these principles can apply here also. An example of this is that if a child wants to stop an activity, we can teach her to say, "I want to stop now" or "stop" rather than hitting others or crawling under the table. We can teach a child that if he does not want an item, he can say "no" rather than swatting it away.

Children can also be taught ways to communicate empathy to others. For example, the SLP can show the child a doll and say that the doll is scared because she had bad dreams. Then, the SLP can model how to comfort the doll. The child can then be asked to provide comfort to the doll. As an adjunct to this, I have found that when I am reading books with children, it can sometimes be effective to point to the expressions on the characters' faces and ask the children how they think the characters are feeling and why. Most children I have worked with feel comfortable with this activity, and it increases their ability to read and respond to others' feelings.

Children with emotional and behavioral disorders can be taught specific strategies to help them become more effective communicators. For example, self-regulation strategies can be quite helpful.

A final recommendation made by Paul (2001) is to teach children self-regulation strategies. For example, in the school where I work, we have a list on the whiteboard of our therapy room that has words like *stop, wait, look around you, think*. We find that many children with behavioral/emotional issues profit from this, especially if they are prone to impulsive behavior (which many are).

Additional Considerations for CLD Children

When working with CLD students who have LI and E/BD, it is extremely important to work with their families and also with cultural mediators to understand what behaviors are considered appropriate in the students' cultures. In the previous section, we just said that an important part of intervention is helping students learn how to express their feelings openly, especially through gaining the vocabulary to do this. However, we have also said that in some cultures, open expression of feelings is considered inappropriate (e.g., Chan & Lee, 2004; Fung & Roseberry-McKibbin, 1999; Roseberry-McKibbin, 2008).

In these cases, a cultural mediator can help parents to understand that although they may feel some discomfort with their child's open expressions of emotion, encouraging use of these expressions will probably help their child's behavior to improve. Parents from cultures that do not encourage open expressions of emotion often concurrently value good, respectful behavior in their children (Fung & Roseberry-McKibbin, 1999; Santos & Chan, 2004). Thus, SLPs and other professionals can emphasize that better behavior may be facilitated by allowing the child to more openly express how he is feeling. As always, parents love their children and want what is best for them. It is my personal clinical experience that even when CLD parents are asked to do or allow things that are uncomfortable for them, they will frequently agree to do or allow these things if they clearly see how they are in their child's best interest.

 SUMMARY

- In recent years, SLPs have been increasingly recognizing that there is a co-occurrence of language impairment (LI) and challenging behaviors in children.
- Students with LI, especially older boys, may have specific difficulties in the area of emotion regulation.
- In intervention, SLPs can help children effectively label and express their emotions. It is also important to work with classroom teachers to help students with LI and emotional and behavioral (E/BD) disorder integrate successfully into the classroom setting.
- Cultural mediators can be very useful when working with the families of CLD students with co-occurring LI and E/BD. Families can be taught how to help these students openly express their emotions.

CHAPTER HIGHLIGHTS

- Children from low–socioeconomic status (SES) backgrounds have a number of challenges such as limited access to health care, food, and other "basics" of life. In addition, many of them live with caregivers (especially mothers) who have not had the benefit of higher education. Research consistently shows that low maternal educational level is related to low oral and literate language skills.
- Some low-SES children develop behavior problems in addition to their language difficulties. Research suggests that children who are both low-SES and language impaired (LI) are at risk for social and behavioral problems.
- Standardized, knowledge-based assessment measures are often biased against LI, low-SES students; use of processing-dependent measures may be a better choice for these children. In terms of intervention, SLPs can support caregivers as well as provide

early-intervention programs to hopefully prevent future academic and language difficulties. This may be especially helpful for CLD children with LI from low-SES homes.

- Children may experience neglect and/or abuse in their homes. This can impact their language and behavioral skills. CLD parents may need to be educated about US laws regarding what discipline procedures constitute child abuse.

- In therapy, children who have experienced neglect and/or abuse may need to spend time playing in a nonthreatening, child-focused, nondirective atmosphere.

- Some children have attention deficit hyperactivity disorder (ADHD). Language problems manifested by these children may include difficulties with auditory processing, pragmatics skills, and overall expressive language skills.

- In addition to providing specific language intervention, SLPs can help develop 504 plans for these children to promote success in the classroom.

- Children with prenatal drug and/or alcohol exposure (PDAE) often have physical, emotional, cognitive, and linguistic problems.

- The language problems of these children are not always easily detected by standardized measures. Informal assessment of their functional use of language in natural settings is ideal. Therapy should be consistent and structured, with carryover activities to help children maintain gains between therapy sessions.

- Children with HIV/AIDS may have language delays, learning disabilities, or mental retardation. Intervention should focus on improving oral and written language skills.

- Children with HIV/AIDS who have severe communication problems may need to use augmentative, alternative communication devices.

- In recent years, SLPs have been increasingly recognizing the co-occurrence of LI and emotional/behavioral disorders (E/BD). Many of these students have difficulty with emotion regulation.

- Assessment of the language skills of E/BD students can be challenging because they may behave quite differently at different times. In intervention, it is important to help these students appropriately label and express their emotions in a nondisruptive manner.

STUDY AND REVIEW QUESTIONS

ESSAY

1. How does socioeconomic status (SES) affect the language skills of children? Describe.

2. Describe the language and behavioral characteristics of students who have experienced abuse and/or neglect (NA). How might we help these children improve their language skills?

3. What strategies can be used by SLPs and classroom teachers to support students with attention deficit hyperactivity disorder? Describe.

4. Some children have LIs that accompany exposure to drugs and/or alcohol in utero. What are two specific recommendations for optimizing intervention for these children?

5. Children with behavioral and emotional problems that accompany LI may be helped by focusing on certain specific skills in therapy. What are these skills?

FILL-IN-THE-BLANK

6. A program provided by Congress to support low-SES children in public schools is called _____.

7. The failure to provide for a child's basic educational, emotional, or physical needs is called _____.

8. A child who is fidgety, runs around, moves constantly, talks constantly, and has difficulty remaining seated may be said to have _____.

9. The number-one cause of preventable mental retardation is _____.

10. A condition that manifests primarily in the central nervous system and can cause speech and language disabilities as well as neurological problems is called _____.

MULTIPLE CHOICE

11. Which one of the following is *false?*

    a. If a child has HIV/AIDS, the family is legally mandated to disclose this condition to personnel who work with the child.
    b. Children with emotional and behavioral problems often have difficulties with emotion regulation.
    c. There is no demonstrated causal relationship between LI and poverty.
    d. Low-SES caregivers' lack of education is a major factor that affects their children's language development.
    e. Children with ADHD may especially have difficulty with pragmatics skills.

12. You are working in a school district that has a number of low-SES children from all ethnic backgrounds. At your school, the classroom teachers are referring many of these children to you because the teachers suspect that the children have LIs and need intervention. Which of the following things might be most appropriate for you to do in this situation?

    a. Tell the teachers that the referrals are inappropriate, and that these children can all be served through Title I programs.
    b. Work with both teachers and caregivers to help them learn additional methods of oral and literate language stimulation in the classroom and home.
    c. Use processing-dependent measures to assess these children's language skills because you know that knowledge-based measures tend to be biased against low-SES children.
    d. b, c
    e. a, b, c

13. Tilden F., a boy who has experienced both neglect and abuse, has been referred for testing by his classroom teacher. The teacher is concerned about Tilden's language

and behavioral skills and wants to know if Tilden needs language intervention. As you prepare to assess Tilden's language skills, you will of course keep in mind that each child will have an individual profile of linguistic strengths and weaknesses. However, based on available research, what might you suspect you will find when you conduct an assessment of Tilden's language skills?

a. Tilden will be reluctant to volunteer information and discuss his feelings.
b. Tilden might have a shorter mean length of utterance than his same-age peers.
c. Tilden might have limited ability to use language to convey abstract concepts.
d. a, b
e. a, b, c

14. Cathy N., a girl who has been diagnosed with ADHD, has moved into your school district with a 504 plan from her previous school district. Which one of the following would you NOT expect to find on her 504 plan?

a. Cathy will have plenty of opportunities for physical movement.
b. Cathy will be placed in a nonstructured classroom where she has plenty of freedom to make her own decisions.
c. Cathy will be placed in a classroom where external distractions are kept to a minimum.
d. Cathy will be allowed to use such learning aids as brightly colored highlighter pens and colored pencils.
e. Cathy's teacher will monitor her eye contact with assigned tasks.

15. Chinh B., a Southeast Asian first grader, has been diagnosed with LI accompanied by emotional and behavioral problems. His parents both work full time to support their family; they have six children. Chinh's parents want to help their son succeed in school and at home; however, they are busy and tired. They do not know how to help their child. You obtain the services of a cultural mediator to help Chinh's parents understand specific strategies to support their son. When you suggest that Chinh's parents allow him to fully express his emotions, they say that this is inappropriate in their culture. In this situation, what would be the *best* course of action for you to take?

a. Call Child Protective Services and report that Chinh's parents are being unsupportive.
b. Tell Chinh's parents in no uncertain terms that you think they are wrong; they must do things the way you recommend.
c. Utilize the support of the cultural mediator to help Chinh's parents understand that though they are uncomfortable with this recommendation, it will ultimately work for Chinh's greatest social, linguistic, and academic progress.
d. Tell Chinh's parents that the way they feel is okay, and they do not need to follow the suggestions that you have made.
e. None of the above.

See Answers to Study and Review Questions, page 465.

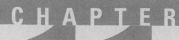

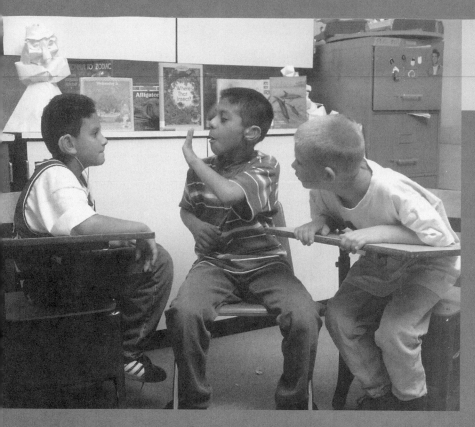

Language Impairment in Special Populations

It was going to be a tricky evaluation. James H., an eighteen-year-old culturally and linguistically diverse (CLD) high school senior, had vision and hearing impairments accompanying CHARGE syndrome. CHARGE is an acronym referring to *c*oloboma (eyeball fails to close), *c*ranial nerve involvement (which can lead to facial weakness and swallowing problems), *h*eart defects, *a*tresia of the choanae (blocking and narrowing of the passages from the back of the nose to the throat), *r*etardation of growth and development, *g*enital and urinary abnormalities, and *e*ar abnormalities with accompanying hearing loss.

I was called in to assess James's language skills because his mother fiercely disliked the speech-language pathologist (SLP) at the high school campus. I was told that Mrs. H. was thinking of taking our school district to court because she was so unhappy about the quality of speech-language services James was currently receiving. Because James was going to be graduating from high school in eight months, Mrs. H. and the school personnel were developing a transition plan for him. My evaluation was to be part of that transition plan, and my school district wanted very specific intervention recommendations that would be appropriate for James.

I called James's mother on the phone before the evaluation so that I could understand his history—especially his past and present medical circumstances. Mrs. H. said that her husband had died in the last year. After her husband's death, the doctors recommended that James have back surgery for scoliosis (curvature of the spine). When the surgeons began to operate, they discovered that there were blood vessels wrapped around James' spine. Continuing the surgery to repair the scoliosis would have caused James to bleed to death, so the surgeons had to stop operating and close James's back up without repairing the scoliosis. Mrs. H. also shared that James was blind in one eye, and his other eye was "drying up." Unless the "drying up" process could be stopped, James would lose all his vision in his better eye. James was hard of hearing but did not like to wear his hearing aids. Mrs. H. had a full-time job but had taken time off of work to be with her son during the back surgery. She was deeply worried about James and about what would happen to him after high school.

I thanked Mrs. H. for her willingness to talk with me and promised to do the most thorough assessment possible of James' language skills. When I went to pick James up in his classroom, he came to the testing room with an excellent attitude. I was so moved by his cheerfulness, cooperation, and willingness to work long and hard despite all his medical and physical challenges. Because of James' visual impairment, I did not use picture or written stimuli with him. I did make sure that James wore his hearing aids so that he could at least hear test stimuli. It was a real challenge to assess the language skills of a student who had difficulty with both vision and hearing! The challenge was compounded by James's lack of intelligibility. I could only understand about 50 percent of what he said.

To supplement my one-on-one evaluation of James's language skills, I interviewed personnel at his high school who were familiar with him. I also observed James in his classroom setting and walked around the high school campus with him several times. My observations and interviews revealed that James especially had difficulty with pragmatics skills. For example, on one of our walks, several students greeted James, but he did not look at them or reply. At one point, I asked another student named Jeremy to come over to James and talk with him. Jeremy asked James six or seven questions, which James answered appropriately. However, James did not ask Jeremy any questions about himself. Later the same day, as school was getting out, James's teacher said goodbye and told him to have a nice weekend. James kept walking and did not reply. I said "James, did you hear the teacher?" He said that he did and repeated back the teacher's exact words.

My recommendations for James were quite lengthy, as you can imagine. They focused on a number of areas, especially increasing his pragmatics skills. I requested that James participate in a peer-mediator program, where a peer would be assigned to spend time interacting with James each day. The peer would also be requested to facilitate James' communication with other TD students. The educational team took my recommendations into consideration as they designed a specific plan to help James transition into the community.

CHILDREN WITH HEARING IMPAIRMENTS

Introduction

In the United States, more than one million children are hearing impaired. More newborn babies are at risk for hearing impairment because advanced medical technology has enabled more high-risk, fragile, preterm infants to be saved. These babies are more vulnerable to hearing problems than are healthy, full-term infants (Tye-Murrary, 2004).

TABLE 11.1   Range and Categories of Hearing Loss with the Corresponding dB HL

Hearing Loss	Characteristics
Up to 15 dB	Normal hearing in children
16 to 40 dB	Mild hearing loss in children; difficulty hearing distant or faint speech; may be associated with language delay in children
41 to 55 dB	Moderate hearing loss; delayed speech and language acquisition; difficulty following conversation; difficulty producing certain sounds correctly
56 to 70 dB	Moderately severe hearing loss; can understand only shouted or amplified speech
71 to 90 dB	Severe hearing loss; difficulty understanding even amplified or loud speech; significant difficulty in learning and producing language
91+ dB	Profound hearing loss; typically described as deaf; hearing does not play a major role in learning, understanding, and producing speech and language

Note: Adapted from Hegde (2001a); Roseberry-McKibbin & Hegde (2006).

Hearing impairment can be very mild, creating few problems with communication. It can also be severe to profound, causing major communication problems. Table 11.1 shows the range of hearing loss in decibels hearing level (dB HL) and the corresponding categories. The term **hearing impaired** refers to the condition of being deaf or hard of hearing. The child who is **hard of hearing** has a loss between 16 and 75 dB; children who are hard of hearing acquire oral language and speech with variable proficiency. Children who are deaf are those who can't hear or understand conversational speech under normal circumstances. Their hearing loss is greater than 75 dB and in many cases is greater than 90 dB (Roseberry-McKibbin & Hegde, 2006).

The term **Deaf** with an uppercase **D** refers to deafness as a cultural identity, not as a disability (Helfer, 1998). We will discuss this in more depth later. In this chapter, I will use the term **hearing impaired** (HI) to describe children whose hearing difficulties are moderate to profound, whose hearing difficulties interfere with communication in their daily lives.

> The term hearing impaired refers to the condition of being deaf or hard of hearing. The term Deaf with an uppercase D refers to deafness as a cultural identity, not as a disability.

Congenital hearing loss, or hearing loss present at birth, has a greater impact on developing speech and language than a hearing loss developed later in life. Children with **prelingual deafness** become deaf before they acquire speech and language. Children with **postlingual deafness** have an HI that occurs after five years of age. Prognosis for the improvement of speech and language skills in HI children depends on several factors: 1) how early in life the child receives professional help; 2) the quality and scope of the services the child receives; 3) the extent to which parents and caregivers support HI children; and 4) the presence of other disabling conditions (e.g., brain damage, blindness).

An important consideration in the educational success of deaf and hearing-impaired children is the age at which the hearing loss is identified (Yoshinaga-Itano, 2003). The later a hearing loss is identified, the more disruptive it is to the process of language development. Children who have had even a little access to language demonstrate higher levels of linguistic achievement than children who have not had this exposure. One difficult factor is that when children are babies, it may not be obvious that they are deaf. Often, children are two years of age or more before their parents even realize that something is wrong and the children are identified (Schirmer, 2000). Thus, there is a great need for universal screening of babies to ascertain their ability to hear. Many states have made newborn infant hearing screening mandatory, although more work is needed to connect such identification with early intervention programs.

There are three kinds of hearing loss: **conductive, sensorineural,** and **mixed.** In conductive hearing loss, the efficiency with which the sound is conducted to the inner ear is diminished. In a pure conductive loss, the inner ear, acoustic nerve, and auditory centers of the brain are all working normally. Conductive hearing loss can be caused by abnormalities of the tympanic membrane (eardrum), the ossicular chain (middle ear bones), and other physical malformations. **Otitis media,** also known as middle ear effusion, is an infection of the middle ear that is often associated with Eustachian tube dysfunction and upper respiratory infections.

Children with otitis media frequently have fluid in the middle ear cavity. They do hear some sounds, but their hearing sensitivity is diminished. Otitis media usually creates a conductive hearing loss of 20 to 35 dB HL. Because otitis media generally occurs most often between birth and three years of age, it can have a dramatic and negative impact on a child's speech and language (Radziewicz & Antonellis, 2002). Conductive hearing loss often goes undetected in children, because in many physicians' offices and public schools, hearing screenings are conducted at 25 dB HL. It is very important for SLPs to be aware that a child can "pass" a hearing screening by the school nurse or pediatrician and still have an undetected conductive hearing loss.

CASES TO CONSIDER

Yesterday in my job in the public schools, I received a speech-language screening referral from a kindergarten teacher. Five-year-old Sharif F. was referred for "difficulty understanding instructions, expressing thoughts, articulating words clearly, and having difficulty repeating." When I screened Sharif on a one-on-one basis in my quiet speech room, I found that he was a bright, rather shy child who did an excellent job on the language screening measures I gave him in English. Baffled at the reason for the referral, I called Mrs. F. She said that her husband spoke English to Sharif and that she spoke exclusively Swedish to him at home. Sharif had never been to preschool. He had been in kindergarten for nine days at the time of the referral. Mrs. F. said that she was concerned about Sharif's hearing. She said that he had had a bad concussion when he was one-and-a-half years old, and that since then, she had noticed that he didn't respond readily when she called him. She thought that sometimes in noisy environments, he was reading her lips. The classroom teacher noticed also that Sharif, although well-behaved, spoke quite softly and somewhat unintelligibly and was often not responsive to directions in class. What do you think Sharif's problem might be? What courses of action would you take in this situation?

_____

_____

_____

The typical treatments for conductive hearing loss include antibiotics or pressure-equalizing tubes. These tiny tubes are inserted through the tympanic membrane and act as ventilators to the middle ear, draining the fluid out and thus restoring the child's hearing.

> There are three kinds of hearing loss: conductive, sensorineural, and mixed.

Differences in the incidence rate of otitis media have been found among various CLD groups (Eriks-Brophy & Ayukawa, 2000). African Americans have the lowest rate of otitis media; the highest rates are found among Native Americans, Alaskan Eskimos, and Aborigines. These differences in incidence rates may be related to differences in the function and structure of the Eustachian tube among various CLD groups (Scott, 2002).

In sensorineural hearing loss, the middle ear may conduct sound efficiently to the inner ear. However, damage to the acoustic nerve or to the hair cells of the cochlea may prevent the brain from receiving the neural impulses of sound. Sensorineural hearing loss is permanent; damaged hair cells in the cochlea and damage to the acoustic nerve are not reparable. Sensorineural hearing loss is not the same across all frequencies. Usually, the higher frequencies are more heavily impacted than the low frequencies. Children with severe to profound sensorineural hearing losses can experience major effects on their speech and language (Roseberry-McKibbin & Hegde, 2006).

A mixed hearing loss occurs when neither the middle nor the inner ear is functioning properly. A mixed loss is a combined conductive and sensorineural hearing loss. Mixed losses can be caused by two separate disorders in the same ear. For example, a child could have a sensorineural hearing loss and otitis media.

In terms of articulatory-phonological development, the speech of HI children may sound highly unintelligible even if they have received intervention. HI children tend to have difficulty with high-frequency sounds such as /s/ and /f/, and they have difficulty with other consonants as well as with vowels. In addition, HI children often have distinctive prosodic problems; they may have flat intonation, or their intonation may contain too much variety (Roseberry-McKibbin & Hegde, 2006). Young HI children who have received cochlear implants (described later) may sound more intelligible than those who have not received these implants, but research shows that they may still have noticeably impaired articulatory-phonological skills (Tobey, Greers, Brenner, Altuna, & Gabbert, 2003).

HI children often have difficulty acquiring semantic and syntactic skills. They may use a limited variety of sentence types and produce sentences of reduced length and complexity. They may also have problems comprehending and producing compound, complex,

POINTS TO PONDER Briefly describe the oral and written language skills that characterize a majority of children who have hearing impairments.

_____

_____

_____

and embedded sentences. They frequently show omission or inconsistent use of many morphemes, such as regular past tense *-ed*, third person singular *-s*, and so forth. Pragmatics skills may be impacted also. One area of pragmatics that may be especially challenging for HI children is repair of communication breakdowns.

> **CONNECT & EXTEND**
>
> A discussion of the repair strategies of hearing-impaired children is provided by Most, T. (2002). The use of repair strategies by children with and without hearing impairment. *Language, Speech, and Hearing Services in Schools, 33,* 112–123.

Most (2002) showed that the HI children in her study had difficulty in this area. When communication broke down, the HI children in her study most often repeated their statements. To a lesser extent, they used strategies such as revising their sentences and providing additional information. Most recommended that communication intervention programs for these children should explicitly introduce various repair strategies to facilitate HI children's successful interaction with others. For example, these children could be taught to use key words, simplifications of their utterances (if they are unintelligible), or expansions and additions (if they have good speech intelligibility). Most cautioned that the HI population is very heterogeneous, and repair strategies taught to HI children will depend upon a number of variables such as how intelligible their speech is to others.

For children with HI, reading and writing may be problematic. Although individual HI children have eventually achieved high levels of reading and writing, surveys of the reading abilities of older HI children and adults have suggested that their reading ability never got higher than a level commensurate with that of third-grade hearing children (Allen, 1986; LaSasso & Mobley, 1997; Radziewicz & Antonellis, 2002).

Many HI children have poor reading comprehension, and the writing of HI children may reflect oral language problems such as omission of grammatical morphemes and a limited variety of sentence types. The example below is one illustration of the types of writing difficulties that HI children tend to have into adolescence and adulthood. Figure 11.1 is an exact copy of an e-mail I received from Brent, a twenty-four-year old with HI whom I invited to guest lecture in one of my classes at the university. His wife, one of my students, was an audiology major in our program.

> Children with HI may have difficulties with both oral and written language.

Implications for Assessment and Intervention

Early Assessment and Intervention

We said earlier that early detection of hearing loss is critical. Various committees and health boards such as the Joint Committee on Accreditation of Health Organizations and the Department of Health and Human Services are encouraging all hospitals to provide newborn hearing screening programs. Audiologists are the key professionals who assess children's hearing and provide specific recommendations for intervention based on the child's exact nature and degree of hearing loss. Hopefully, this assessment and intervention begins when the child is a baby.

Speech and language development begin with a baby's earliest social exchanges between himself and his mother or other primary caregiver. The affective aspects of primary caregiver–infant interaction are critical to future language acquisition, and thus SLPs need

Hi DR. Celeste,

Wow, I would love to but Monday and Wednesday I work.

But I can be your class after 2 30 pm any days let me know. Yeah My Wife really work very hard To Become Audiology ya know. But let me know I

really really

want to share with your class.

But I hope to look forward to see you and meeting you smile thanks you for e-mail me. She very Smart and very out going and great question she has. She mostly asked me what it like, but ya know My Wife. She very

Special person to me. I do anything help you and

Help you and UR Classes too. Pls, let me know I really hope to come to UR class at after 2 30 pm.

Thanks

Brent

FIGURE 11.1   Writing Sample of a Young Adult with Hearing Impairment

to focus on programs that enhance and optimize primary caregiver–infant interaction. These programs educate parents about their crucial role in their HI child's development, and caregivers are taught a variety of strategies for stimulating the child's language skills and enhancing the environment so that it is optimal for the child's development.

As we discussed in Chapter 10, videotapes can be used to enhance primary caregiver–infant interactions. Parents can be trained to observe interactions that are successful and interactions that are not. In addition to helping parents work at home in an optimally facilitative manner with their HI children, SLPs can also facilitate aural rehabilitation programs for these children.

Basic Principles of Aural Rehabilitation

Aural rehabilitation is an educational and clinical program that is primarily implemented by audiologists, who may also work with SLPs and other team members such as *educators of the deaf* (special educators who teach American Sign Language as well as academic subjects to children with HI). It is designed to help those with HI achieve their full potential. Historically, professionals carrying out aural rehabilitation with HI children have focused intensive efforts on auditory training and speech-reading. Today, there is a greater focus on early identification and intervention, hearing-aid fitting and orientation, and optimizing the environment (Brackett, 2002; Martin & Clark, 2003; Schow & Nerbonne, 2002; Tye-Murray, 2004). Amplification is also emphasized.

> Aural rehabilitation is an educational and clinical program that is primarily implemented by audiologists who work with other team members.

Generally three types of amplification are used with HI children as part of an aural rehabilitation program: 1) hearing aids, 2) cochlear implants, and 3) auditory trainers. Advances in hearing-aid technology have greatly improved the quality of hearing aids. Digital hearing aids, which are commonly used today, provide a better **signal-to-noise ratio** than the older hearing aids. Signal-to-noise ratio refers to the difference in dB between the stimulus of interest and the competing background noise. State-of-the-art digital hearing aids are also programmable; they can be programmed to provide different types of amplification depending upon the settings (Gelfand, 2001).

By the year 2002, more than 7,000 American children had received **cochlear implants** (Ertmer, 2002). Cochlear implants are electronic devices. They are surgically placed into the cochlea and other parts of the ear, and they deliver sound directly to the acoustic nerve endings in the cochlea. Even if the child is profoundly deaf, there is often a large residual population of primary cochlear neural elements. A cochlear implant can take advantage of those residual elements. Where hearing aids deliver amplified sound into the ear canal, cochlear implants deliver electrical impulses, converted from sound, directly to the auditory nerve (Martin & Clark, 2003; Stach, 2003). Cochlear implants enhance children's speech-reading performance, give them better general sound awareness, and help them recognize environmental sounds (Gelfand, 2001).

Current US Food and Drug Administration (FDA)-approved guidelines specify that a child has to be at least twelve months of age or older to receive a cochlear implant (Cochlear Corporation, 2002). Ideally, with universal newborn screening programs, babies with HI will be identified shortly after they are born, fit with hearing aids, and will start receiving intervention in the first few months of life. If the baby has a profound hearing loss, gets the appropriate habilitative care, and doesn't make progress in developing auditory skills, then a cochlear implant may be recommended when the baby is twelve months old. Research shows that early access to sound, such as that provided by hearing aids or cochlear implants, has beneficial effects on the child's developing speech and language skills (Moeller, 2000; Teagle & Moore, 2002).

> Cochlear implants are electronic devices that are surgically placed into the cochlea and other parts of the ear, and they deliver sound directly to the acoustic nerve endings in the cochlea. Use of cochlear implants is somewhat controversial.

Studies show that under ideal conditions with some exceptions, children with cochlear implants may be able to achieve communication skills that are practically identical to those of children with normal hearing (Geers, Nicholas, & Sedey, 2003; Moog, 2002; Young & Killen, 2002). Recent research has shown that the earlier children receive cochlear implants, the higher their reading comprehension scores later (Connor & Swolan, 2004). Recent research has also shown that the most important characteristic that a child brings to the task of learning from a cochlear implant is good nonverbal intelligence (Geers, 2002).

The receipt of cochlear implants can be a determining factor in how quickly HI children are mainstreamed into general-education classrooms (Geers, Spehar, & Sedey, 2002). Children who receive cochlear implants are sometimes mainstreamed into general-education classrooms faster than HI children who do not receive cochlear implants (Niparko, Cheng, & Francis, 2000). Niparko et al. tracked use of support services and educational placements for thirty-five school-age children across their first four years of experience with their cochlear implants. Data for children with implants were compared to those of HI peers without implants. The primary finding of this research showed a positive correlation between the amount of implant experience and progress toward educational independence (for example, being included in a general-education classroom without extra support services).

Before they received their cochlear implants and for the first two years after the implants were placed, most of the children were in self-contained classrooms instead of general-education classrooms. In the third year of experience with the implants, there was a shift toward more mainstreaming or inclusion in general-education classrooms. By year four after implantation, 75 percent of the implanted children were enrolled in mainstream classrooms; most of them spent the entire school day in these classrooms. The children with cochlear implants who were in full-day general-education classrooms used about one-fourth of the support services (e.g., special education) that were received by the HI children who did not have implants.

Thus, the findings of this study suggest several things. First, the initial provision of intensive support services and special education provided a foundation for progress toward increasing independence. Second, there was a reduced need for special education programs for children with cochlear implants compared to HI peers without implants. The decreased reliance on special programs could save school districts many thousands of dollars over the years (Niparko et al., 2000). With the current federal law's emphasis on integrating special-education children into general-education classrooms (IDEA, 2004), it is very relevant that children wtih cochlear implants showed a significant ability to integrate into these classrooms faster than HI children without cochlear implants.

CONNECT & EXTEND

The July 2002 issue of *Language, Speech, and Hearing Services in Schools* contains a Clinical Forum devoted exclusively to the topic of cochlear implants.

There has been some criticism of cochlear implants (e.g., Crouch, 1997; Lane & Bahan, 1998). For example, cochlear implants do help to facilitate language development; however, as Bernstein Ratner (2005, p. 334) says, "Cochlear implantation has the potential to endanger Deaf culture and sign languages, which are rich, full-fledged linguistic systems, in much the same way that other cultures and languages have been endangered by social, political, and economic factors." Bagli (2002, p. 391) states that many members of the Deaf community are afraid of "cultural genocide," the gradual and eventual elimination of Deaf culture and language (sign). These members of the Deaf community are concerned that cochlear implants may eliminate the condition of deafness, which could lead to the total demise of Deaf language and culture. Their concerns are summarized by Pagliaro (2001, p. 174), who states that

> People who are Deaf . . . do not define themselves simply by their level of hearing loss . . . but rather by linguistic, social, and political aspects as well. They share a language (different from English) and a set of values, beliefs, and behaviors (different from hearing people) based on common experiences that bind them together and shape them as a people. . . . Their hearing loss is viewed not as a disability, but as a difference, similar to skin color. Nothing is "broken" nor needs to be "fixed." . . . Like other cultures throughout the world, Deaf culture is rich in history and tradition. Its people are a closeknit community. . . . Deaf culture is typically passed from generation to generation and from person to person. . . . Deaf people have long had to fight to preserve their language and traditions, and continue to do so.

In addition, many members of the Deaf community have questioned the ethics of making a decision for others who are too young to choose if they would like to reside solely in the Deaf community or try to interact in the hearing world (Helfer, 1998; Martin & Clark, 2003). Thus, though cochlear implants have been shown to greatly facilitate speech and language development, there is some controversy about their use. People who are uncomfortable with cochlear implants might be more comfortable with the implementation of auditory training.

> One key to the success of HI children in general-education classrooms is a favorable signal-to-noise ratio.

Auditory training is designed to teach an HI child to listen to amplified sounds, recognize their meanings, and discriminate sounds from each other. Sometimes the HI child uses a hearing aid; other times, she uses an **auditory trainer.** When auditory trainers are used, the child with HI wears headphones. The clinician's or the classroom teacher's speech is fed to an amplifier through a microphone, and the amplified sound is fed to the earphones and into the child's ear.

A widely used type of auditory trainer is the FM (frequency-modulated) auditory trainer, a wireless system that can be used in classrooms or even in individual therapy sessions. The teacher wears a microphone-transmitter, and the child wears an FM receiver that is either coupled to or built into a hearing aid. When the teacher speaks, his words transmit directly to the child's unit on a frequency-modulated radio carrier wave (Radziewicz & Antonellis, 2002). FM auditory trainers can be very helpful to children.

One thing that clinicians must consider is that extraneous or ambient noise in most school classrooms is approximately 60 dB. The **signal-to-noise ratio,** or the difference in dB between the stimulus of interest (the teacher's voice) and the competing background noise, is often negative; that is, the teacher's voice cannot be adequately heard due to the presence of background noise (Crandell, Smaldino, & Flexer, 2005). This negative signal-to-noise ratio is very detrimental to children with HI, and FM auditory trainers are quite beneficial in such situations. However, they can be expensive and may break down. School districts that use auditory trainers for HI children must be prepared to spend time and money in the purchase and maintenance of the trainers (P. Spears Lee, personal communication, June 24, 2005). The FM system should be checked regularly by an audiologist to ensure that the child is receiving an optimal signal.

Amplification for an entire classroom of children can be provided by a **sound-field amplification system.** The teacher wears a transmitter and microphone, and the speech signal is sent to speakers mounted on a desk, wall, or ceiling. All the children in the classroom can hear the teacher consistently at an enhanced level no matter where they are seated in the classroom. An HI child may need to wear a personal FM unit that is tuned to the same frequency as the sound-field unit (Lang, 2000).

Children who profit most from sound-field amplification systems are those with unilateral hearing loss, fluctuating hearing levels, and minimal hearing loss (Flexer, 1995). However, research has shown that background noise and reverberation interfere with speech perception of HI children in classrooms. If a classroom is noisy and reverberant, classroom devices are not beneficial to the speech perception of students who wear hearing aids. For HI students in this situation, the best listening benefits are provided by desktop sound-field systems or by personal FM auditory trainers.

Communication and Educational Approaches to Language Development for Hearing Impaired Children

As we have said, it is important to begin communication training as early as possible and also to involve the child's family. Some parents of HI children may choose to homeschool their children, and SLPs can help these parents with appropriate strategies for facilitating optimal learning in the home environment (Byrne, 2000). In school settings, SLPs who work with HI children should work closely with classroom teachers and educators of the deaf. The development of auditory skills must be integrated into the child's educational and speech-language programs.

There are three general approaches to the training of HI children: the **auditory/oral method,** the **manual approach,** and **total communication.** Proponents of the auditory/oral method (sometimes called aural/oral method) attempt to use amplification methods such as cochlear implants or hearing aids to tap into children's residual hearing. Children undergo intensive training in speech-reading and auditory training. It is expected that these children will eventually learn to speak clearly and fit into mainstream educational, social, and vocational settings.

The manual method is a means of nonverbal communication that involves finger-spelling and signing (Nicolosi et al., 2004). Proponents of the manual approach believe that early in life, HI children must be taught a comprehensive system of sign language. The sooner the child learns this system, the better. The sign language system is viewed as part of Deaf culture and is the standard means of communication in the community of people who are deaf. Thus, HI children learn not only a means of communication, but also a way of being integrated into the Deaf community and culture.

There are several types of sign language. A commonly used type is **American Sign Language,** or ASL. ASL is widely used in the United States and Canada. It is not considered a manual version of standard English but is viewed as a separate language. In ASL, signs are used to express concepts and ideas through complex hand and finger movements. Each sign expresses a different idea, and signs are made in quick succession much like spoken words are put into sentences. However, the syntax of ASL differs from the syntax of Mainstream American English. Children who use ASL write the way they speak. The prior example of the e-mail I received from Brent, who uses ASL, reflects some of these syntactic differences.

American Sign Language, widely used in North America, is viewed as a language separate from standard English.

CONNECT & EXTEND

The National Dissemination Center for Children with Disabilities has a detailed, informative Web site about services to children with severe impairments such as hearing loss and blindness. They can be contacted at www.nichcy.org.

In **total communication,** speech and signs are used simultaneously. Children with HI are taught both verbal and nonverbal means of communication; they are taught speech and language as well as a system of signs. There is no attempt to tap residual hearing through amplification. Some critics believe that it is unrealistic to expect children to follow signs, read lips, and sign simultaneously; however, despite this, total communication is a popular current teaching method for children with hearing losses in the profound-severe range (Martin & Clark, 2003; Tye-Murray, 2004; Woolfolk, 2004).

It is important for classroom teachers to make modifications for children with HI. The following strategies can be successfully used by classroom teachers to accommodate the needs of HI children (Lang, 2000; Pagliaro, 2001; Teagle & Moore, 2002):

1. The child should be seated where he can have full visual access to the teacher.

2. If the child needs to change seats for different activities in order to have this visual access, he should be accommodated.

3. The teacher's face should have full lighting with no shadows.

4. The teacher should only talk when she is facing the students. She should not talk when her back is turned and she is writing on the chalkboard, for example.

5. The child might profit from a peer "buddy" to assist him in understanding what the teacher is saying.

6. Visual aids should be used as much as possible to supplement what the teacher is saying. For example, when discussing math problems, the teacher can write them on the board or use an overhead projector with transparencies containing the math problems.

7. Teachers can pause at various points and ask the child to repeat instructions in order to verify that the information was heard and understood.

8. The child should be seated away from sources of noise such as telephones, pencil sharpeners, and open windows.

Additional Considerations for CLD Children and Their Families

According to the National Institute on Deafness and Other Communication Disorders (NIDCD, 1996), more than twenty-eight million individuals in the United States have a hearing disorder. Approximately 45.2 percent of deaf and hard of hearing children are from racial and ethnic minority groups. Of these, 20.4 percent are Hispanic, 17 percent are African American, 4.2 percent are Asian and Pacific Islander, 0.8 percent are American Indian, and the other 3 percent are multiethnic or "other" (Gallaudet Research Institute, 1998).

One thing that communication disorders professionals should remember regarding audiological assessment with CLD children is that in some cultures, it is considered inappropriate to touch the child's head (Scott, 2002). In these cases, professionals should carefully explain to the family the reason for assessment procedures such as putting on earphones.

Acceptance of a hearing loss can vary from culture to culture, and we have previously discussed some of the issues related to families' being told their child has a disability. It is important to be sensitive to some CLD families' reactions such as embarrassment, or the belief that God has given the family a deaf child as a cross they must bear (Nuru-Holm & Battle, 1998). Some families believe that a child with an HI reflects some fault on the part of one or both parents. Others believe that all children are gifts from God, and so they are perfect; parents should accept their children totally.

As an example of this, Aarts (2001) described her experiences providing audiology services in a private clinic in Saudi Arabia. In one particular instance, she (through an interpreter) told a mother that her baby was deaf. In Aarts' words (p. 34)

> The mother's reaction was swift and intense. She swung her chair over to the wall . . . and began wailing loudly. . . . My interpreter immediately started talking, very fast and very low. . . . Later [when the mother had left] and we had a few free minutes, I asked my interpreter what she had said to this mother. "Well," she said matter-of-factly, "I told her to stop

that crying, you know? By her crying she was questioning the will of Allah. I told her, 'your son has arms and legs and eyes, you should thank Allah for what he has given you, not wail about what he has not. . . .' " Arabic has no word for sadness.

It is possible that in cases such as this, parents may be reluctant to seek out intervention such as aural rehabilitation or a hearing aid. If they do, Scott (2002) recommends that communication disorders professionals consider the color of a hearing aid to be worn by a CLD child. Hearing aids will be more acceptable if they closely match children's skin tones.

Bagli (2002) discussed the African American deaf child, who must learn to deal with the prejudice associated with deafness and also with her ethnicity. Bagli pointed out that the deaf African American child in school usually has to deal with teachers who are neither African American nor deaf, and thus do not understand the child well. Bagli stated that "the deaf African American child must learn the rules of each culture, abide by them, and also develop his or her own values and self image" (p. 398).

Bagli pointed out that many deaf African American children come from single-parent homes headed by mothers who tend to be physical and firm in disciplining their children. In addition, in the home, toughness and self-sufficiency are valued. If school personnel such as teachers and SLPs behave differently than children expect of authority figures, especially when the children behave in ways that are unacceptable, the children may "run all over" school personnel (Bagli, 2002, p. 399).

Thus, it is recommended that when dealing with HI African American children, SLPs and other school personnel help these children to learn behaviors that are appropriate for home, and behaviors that are appropriate for school. Campbell (1993) talks about "home language" and "school language" for African American children. One can extend this distinction to "home behavior" and "school behavior." Students can be taught what kinds of behavior are appropriate for home and what kinds of behavior are appropriate for school. As Genesee et al. (2004) point out, CLD students must learn to become bicultural so that they will succeed in mainstream society as well as at home and in the neighborhood. This applies to CLD children with HI as well.

> Hearing-impaired children from some CLD homes may need to be taught that there is a set of behaviors that is appropriate at home and a set of behaviors that is appropriate at school.

Research with CLD children with HI has been conducted in Canada as well as in the United States. Eriks-Brophy and Ayukawa (2000) conducted a pilot study that investigated the potential benefits of sound-field amplification for Inuit first and second language learners. The study was conducted in Kangiqsualujjuaq, a village of approximately 650 Inuit in the Nunavik region of northern Quebec. The primary language in Nunavik is Inuttitut, and students are educated in this language from kindergarten through grade two by Inuit teachers. A transition takes place between Inuttitut and second language instruction in either French or English when children reach third grade. At this time, they are generally taught by non-Inuit teachers but they continue to have several classes a week in Inuttitut.

One challenge experienced by many Inuit children is a high prevalence of otitis media. Sometimes the hearing loss experienced due to otitis media presents such a challenge to Inuit children that they are fitted with hearing aids. However, having the children wear hearing aids consistently is problematic for several reasons (including replacement of broken hearing aids because of Nunavik's isolated geographic location). Consequently, many Inuit students with hearing losses do not receive consistent amplification in the classroom setting. This places them at risk for educational difficulties because of their reduced levels of hearing.

Accordingly, the purpose of this study was to investigate the usefulness of sound-field amplification in the classroom setting. Findings from the study indicated that in classrooms where FM systems were installed, students with and without hearing impairments showed significant improvement on a speech intelligibility task in noise. For some of the students who attended classrooms with FM systems, their overall scores in attending behavior improved significantly.

An analysis of teacher and student comments showed that the students in classrooms with FM systems learned new words more quickly. In addition, when FM systems were used, students participated more in discussions in the second language. Though there was only a small number of subjects in this pilot study, Eriks-Brophy and Ayukawa suggested that one might conjecture that sound amplification systems in classroom settings are beneficial to second language learners, especially those who are at increased risk for auditory difficulties.

FM systems (in this study) also benefited students with normal hearing and students with attentional or behavioral difficulties. More research on the efficacy of FM systems in classrooms with CLD students is needed; however, it is interesting to note that in this study, again, second language learners without HI benefited from the use of FM systems in the classroom.

Tur-Kaspa and Dromi (2001) conducted detailed analyses of spoken and written language samples of deaf eleven- to thirteen-year-old Hebrew-speaking children. The deaf children had significantly more grammatical deviations in their spoken and written language samples than matched typically hearing peers. These results are consistent with those reported about English-speaking HI children, and thus professionals may tentatively conclude that with CLD students who are deaf, it is important to know that these students may have written language difficulties that are clinically significant. More research with various CLD HI children is needed to support such a conclusion.

 SUMMARY

- Children can manifest various degrees of hearing impairment. Hearing impairment can be conductive, sensorineural, or a combination of these two.
- Children with hearing impairment can have both oral and written language challenges. Because of this, early detection of hearing impairment is critical.
- There are various approaches to the habilitation of children with hearing impairments. Devices such as hearing aids and cochlear implants can be used. There is some controversy surrounding the use of cochlear implants.
- Some children with hearing impairments undergo auditory training. In terms of communication approaches, professionals who work with hearing impaired (HI) children generally use the auditory/oral method, the manual approach, or total communication.

- Clinicians must be sensitive to the possible responses of CLD parents to a diagnosis of hearing impairment for their children. The limited research on CLD children with hearing impairments suggests that sound-field amplification systems can be useful in classroom settings for second language learners with and without hearing impairment. In addition, research suggests that CLD HI children may have clinically significant written language difficulties in their primary languages.

Add your own summary points here:

_____

_____

_____

CHILDREN WITH VISUAL IMPAIRMENTS

Introduction and Basic Principles

The rate at which visual impairments occur in individuals under eighteen years of age is 12.2 per 1,000. Severe visual impairments (totally or legally blind) occur at a rate of .06 per 1,000. In the educational context, children with visual impairments are described as follows. The term **partially sighted** indicates that the child has some type of vision problem that has resulted in a need for special education. Individuals with **low vision** have a severe visual impairment; they cannot read a newspaper at a normal viewing distance, even with the aid of contact lenses or eyeglasses (National Dissemination Center for Children with Disabilities, 2004).

Children with vision impairments can be described as partially sighted, blind, or having low vision.

These individuals may require the use of braille as well as adaptations in the size of print and lighting conditions. They use a combination of vision and other senses (e.g, hearing, touch) to learn. Individuals who are legally **blind** have less than 20/200 vision in their better eye or a very limited field of vision; they learn via braille or other nonvisual media. Some researchers have described the language development of children with visual impairments.

Children with visual impairments are a very heterogeneous group; however, some generalizations can be made about their language skills. Studies of the language development of blind children have found that its sequence and timing is similar to that of sighted children; however, there are some qualitative developmental differences.

Early semantic development differs for blind and sighted children in that they have different timelines for development of object permanence and they talk about different things. Andersen, Dunlea, and Kekelis (1984) found that visually impaired (VI) children in their study rarely used idiosyncratic forms of language or overextensions. Idiosyncratic words are words that children make up or create themselves. You will recall from Chapter 2 that *overextensions* refer to the child's extending a word beyond its conventional definition. Andersen et al. suggested that blind children were learning words, via imitation, as a whole; the blind children were not experimenting with words as sighted children would do. Andersen et al. concluded that blind children have less understanding of words as symbols and are slower than sighted children to form hypotheses about what words mean.

POINTS TO PONDER How do the language characteristics of blind children differ from those of sighted children? Describe.

_____

_____

_____

Bigelow (1987) studied the emergence of the first fifty words in three children who were blind from birth. She found that the growth and timing of blind children's first words was very similar to that of sighted children; also, the blind children generally talked about the same things that sighted children did. However, the specific referents named by blind children differed somewhat from those reported in research based on sighted children. The blind children tended to name referents that could be touched (e.g., *cat, mud*) or heard (*bird, piano*). Similar results were discovered by Sardegna and Otis (1991), who found that concepts and words that could be learned through other senses (e.g., *hot, cold, big*) were readily learned.

We previously defined language as a system of symbols used to represent concepts formed through exposure and experience (Bloom & Lahey, 1978). Blind children have been found to be slower to crawl and walk than sighted children, and thus frequently don't spontaneously explore their environment (Troster, Hecker, & Brambring, 1993). In addition, parents may be more protective of VI children and limit their chances to explore their environments. Thus, the children have less of a chance to explore their world than sighted children do, and so they do not gain the same quality and quantity of exposure and experience (National Dissemination Center for Children with Disabilities, 2004). This limited exposure and experience could contribute to delayed language and cognitive skills.

Bigelow (1990) studied the development of language and cognition in three young children with visual impairments. She found that in comparison to sighted children, blind children were slow to develop object permanence. We will recall that the development of object permanence is associated with the emergence of a child's first words.

It has also been found that blind children use imaginative play less frequently than sighted children and that they have some confusion with pronouns *I* and *you* (Erin, 1990; Nelson, 1998). For example, they call themselves "you" and call others "I" or "me." Blind children are often late to acquire vocabulary (Lahey, 1988).

> The language skills of blind children may show some differences with those of sighted children. This is partly because blind children have to use their other senses to learn language.

Researchers have found few differences between blind and sighted children with regard to syntax. Blind children's length of utterance has been found to be either similar to or slightly shorter than that of sighted children. Blind children use fewer sentence types than sighted children and tend to use a few sentence types repeatedly (Landau & Glietman, 1985; Erin, 1990). The syntactic development of blind children might be slow in the third year of life; however, by three years of age, blind children generally have age-appropriate mean length of utterance (Paul, 2001; Perez-Pereira & Conti-Ramsden, 1999).

Pragmatics skills of blind and sighted children show some subtle differences. One study reported that in comparison to sighted children, blind children raised their eyebrows inappropriately, smiled constantly and inappropriately, and nodded less frequently to signal understanding (Parke, Shallcross, & Anderson 1980). In addition, research has shown that blind children show less awareness of adapting their speech to the needs of the listener. Also, they tend to speak in a loud and strident voice—this may be the case because they are unaware of the distance between themselves and the listener (Erin, 1990; Freeman & Blockberger, 1987). In comparison to sighted peers, blind children initiate communication less often and have more trouble producing cohesive discourse and establishing and maintaining topics (Andersen, Dunlea, & Kekelis, 1993; Fraiberg, 1977). They have more trouble than their sighted peers in figuring out the purpose of language.

School-age VI children with severe visual problems may have difficulty in play situations, seek attention inappropriately, and ask a lot of irrelevant questions (Kekelis, 1992). In addition, the nonverbal aspects of language are difficult because, of course, the VI child cannot "read" others' body language. Children with visual impairments often send "mixed messages"; their nonverbal cues do not match what they are saying, and the listener may be left confused (Hardman et al., 2006). As Kuder (2003) states, there are some differences in the language development of blind and sighted children; however, "the good news is that these are factors that teachers and other education professionals can address in the classroom" (p. 175).

Implications for Assessment and Intervention

Assessment

When an SLP assesses the language skills of children with visual impairments, it is important to work with a vision specialist to adapt formal test materials so that they are appropriate for these children. Most standardized tests rely on visual stimuli and thus are inappropriate for these children. The SLP can make adaptations such as making the stimuli bigger and adjusting lighting for children who have some vision; however, when these adaptations are made, standardized scoring procedures cannot be used. It is probably more useful for the SLP to

When the language skills of a blind child are assessed, it is important for a vision specialist to be involved so that test materials can be appropriately adapted.

use informal assessment measures like some of those we described in Chapter 5. For example, the SLP can gather language samples, have parents fill out developmental questionnaires, and observe the child at play (Nelson, 1998).

Intervention

As we have said about other populations, early intervention is critical for children with visual impairments. It has been suggested that for VI children under three years of age, intervention might focus on consultation with parents so they can interact in ways that are appropriate and that facilitate cognitive-linguistic development (Hatton, McWilliam, & Winton, 2002; Paul, 2001). For example, when the children are babies, if parents approach silently, then the babies may become very still as they listen for the parents. A better alternative is for parents to talk softly to the babies as they approach, thus alerting the babies to their presence and encouraging cooing and smiling.

Some researchers have reported that parents of blind and sighted children interact differently with them. In infancy, much early communication is visual. You will recall that in Chapter 2, we talked about the development of mutual gaze and joint attention, which are achieved through the baby and caregiver watching each other's eye movements. Babies with visual impairments are not able to use these strategies, which are based on sight. Thus, blind children develop routines with their parents, but they do so ". . . through a more laborious auditory-tactile process" (Long, 2005b, p. 368).

When a child is attending auditorily (e.g., cocking her head or becoming still), it easy for the caregiver to not see it. Thus, mothers of VI children have been shown to use more directives and talk more (Perez-Pereira & Conti-Ramsden, 1999). They may also use body contact and touch to maintain their link to their child. Kekelis and Andersen (1984) found that parents of sighted children made more requests for information, while parents of blind children made more requests for action and gave more commands. In addition, the parents of blind children tended to label objects that their children interacted with (e.g., *Those are your ears*) while parents of sighted children gave richer descriptions, with more detail, about the objects. Thus, SLPs can work with parents to help them learn to give rich, detailed descriptions of things in the children's environments as well as help them learn to make more requests for information.

The parents of blind children can be taught how to provide appropriate language stimulation beginning in infancy.

In addition, Paul (2001) suggests that parents provide more variety in the topics that they discuss with their children; parents can talk about what is happening in the environment as well as talking about the child's own actions. Parents can also provide verbal signals as substitutes for nonverbal cues. For example, when they change or introduce materials, they can talk about what they are doing. Parents also need to be aware that if the child reacts negatively to being suddenly picked up or held, they should not be surprised. This is a response to being unexpectedly interrupted; it is not rejection. It is best for parents, as mentioned earlier, to speak gently to the child before they touch him in any way.

Early intervention and work with caregivers can have excellent results in terms of stimulating the language of VI children. VI children over three years of age, if they have language delays, may need direct services from an SLP. SLPs and other professionals who work with VI children can develop functional outcomes, or outcomes that promote the child's development while also making life easier for the child and his family. These functional outcomes can include (Hatton et al., 2002; McWilliam & Scott, 2001):

1. *Independence*—helping the child to function with as little assistance from others as possible. It is important to be aware of different cultures' views in this area. As we have said in other places in this book, some cultures do not value early independence in typically developing children the way that mainstream Anglo-Americans do. In some cultures, it is considered best to shield and protect the child with a disability and "do for" the child (Mokuau & Tau'ili'ili, 2004; Sharifzadeh, 2004; Zuniga, 2004).

2. *Engagement*—increasing the amount of time a child spends interacting with the environment in a contextually and developmentally appropriate manner. We previously referred to an article by van Kleeck (1994) where she discussed the possibility of using siblings in CLD families to assist in carryover of intervention goals because in some cultures, this is more culturally congruent than asking parents to engage in carryover activities.

3. *Social relationships*—helping the child develop trust, play and interact appropriately, get along with others, and form friendships.

Researchers have also made some specific suggestions for increasing the success of speech-language intervention for children with visual impairments (Freeman & Blockberger, 1987; Kekelis & Anderson, 1984; Kuder, 2003; Long, 2005b):

1. Help the child compensate for the visual impairment by using other sources of information (e.g., auditory and tactile sources).
2. Alter the behaviors that interfere with successful communication (e.g., using a voice that is inappropriately loud, smiling too much).
3. Help the child learn to vary his language for different communication situations.
4. Help the child learn to use pronouns accurately.
5. Keep the child informed about what people are doing around him.
6. When working with peer interaction in a play situation, introduce one peer at a time. Gradually increase the number of peers.
7. Work with the child's teacher in the general-education classroom to help optimize the classroom environment for the child and to help the teacher be aware of options that exist to support the child with a visual impairment.

Today, VI children in public schools may participate in one of a range of available options. First, many of these children (especially those with some residual, usable vision) may be accommodated in the regular-education classroom through the use of visual aids and specialized equipment. They might receive pull-out therapy from a vision specialist or participate in a part- or full-time self-contained special-education classroom. The student's placement into any of these options is based upon the extent to which the loss of vision affects her overall academic achievement (Hardman et al., 2006). No matter where the student is placed, a vision specialist should be involved in the educational process.

> Appropriate educational accommodations can be made to help visually impaired children succeed in general-education classrooms.

Materials are available to help VI children function in the school setting. These materials include software that converts printed material to braille or speech, large-print typewriters, personal organizers (such as BlackBerries) that have talking address books or appointment books, special calculators, three-dimensional maps, and others (National Dissemination Center for Children with Disabilities, 2004; Woolfolk, 2004). Teachers need to especially make sure that when VI students are asked to read print, the quality of the print is very good. Even if print is large, VI students will have difficulty if it is blurry.

The arrangement of the classroom and the speech-language therapy room are also important. Consistency is important, because VI students need to know where things are. If the teacher or SLP reorganizes the room, the VI student should be given a chance to learn the new layout. There should be plenty of space for the student to move around the room, and hazards such as trash cans in aisles or electrical cords that can be tripped over need to be carefully monitored (Friend & Bursuck, 2002).

 SUMMARY

- Children may have visual impairments that vary in severity. For children who are born blind, research has shown that they have language characteristics that differ somewhat from those of TD children.
- Assessment of the language skills of children with visual impairments needs to use procedures and materials that are modified to accommodate the children's needs. Informal assessment measures may be superior to formal assessment measures.
- SLPs can work with parents of visually impaired (VI) children beginning when the children are young infants. A major goal is to maximize communication opportunities and provide the most possible language stimulation early in life.
- SLPs can provide direct intervention for VI children with language problems. They can also work with classroom teachers to help optimize the child's classroom environment for learning.

Add your own summary points here:

_____

_____

_____

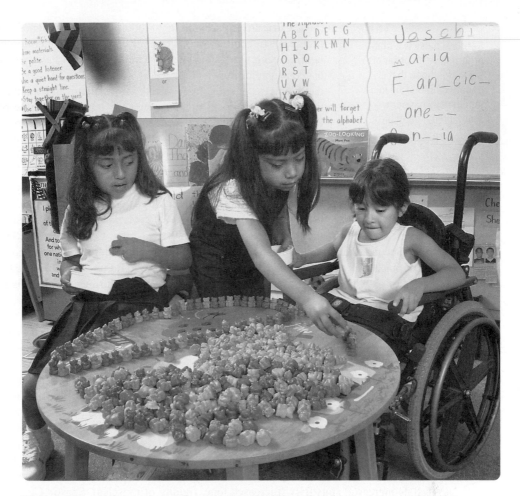

Students with special needs need as many opportunities as possible for active participation, communication, and interaction with typically developing peers.

CHILDREN WITH SEVERE/MULTIPLE DISABILITIES

Cerebral Palsy

Cerebral palsy (CP) is a disorder of early childhood. It is not a disease; it refers to a group of symptoms associated with brain injury in children. CP is not caused by problems in the nerves or muscles; rather, the central nervous system is affected, resulting in muscular incoordination and related problems. CP is a common childhood disability with an incidence rate of 2.5 per 1,000 children. It is estimated that approximately 764,000 adults and children in the United States manifest one or more symptoms of CP (Koman, Smith, & Shilt, 2004).

Cerebral palsy is a non-progressive disorder of early childhood that occurs due to brain injury that usually happens around the time of birth.

Currently, approximately 8,000 infants are diagnosed with CP each year. In addition, 1,200 to 1,500 preschool-age children are recognized each year as having CP (United Cerebral Palsy, 2001). Associated problems may include feeding difficulties, seizures, perceptual disturbances, hearing loss, visual impairment, and mental retardation. However, not all children with CP have all of these problems. Problems associated with CP can range from mild to severe.

CP is not progressive. However, secondary symptoms such as muscle spasticity can get better or worse (United Cerebral Palsy, 2001). CP generally occurs for one or more of the following reasons. First, there may be **prenatal brain injury** (injury to the brain while the baby is still in utero) due to maternal mumps, rubella, or other factors. Prenatal brain injury is responsible for congenital CP, which is present at birth but may not be detected right away. This type of CP is responsible for approximately 70 percent of the cases of CP in children (United Cerebral Palsy, 2001).

Second, there may be **perinatal brain injury,** or injury during the birth process. This is responsible for approximately 20 percent of the cases of CP. For example, if the baby is deprived of oxygen during the birth process, CP may result. A third cause of CP is **postnatal brain injury,** which can result from things like oxygen deprivation, infections, accidents, and diseases such as meningitis and scarlet fever. A friend of mine with CP is a twin. When he and his twin brother were born, they both were put on oxygen. My friend's oxygen machine was malfunctioning, and he got CP as a result. His twin brother, whose oxygen machine was functioning normally, ended up physically healthy and eventually very athletic.

Approximately 10 percent of children experience postnatal brain injury; they acquire CP after they are born. This can result from brain damage during the first few months or years of life. Brain damage can be caused by infections, such as bacterial meningitis, and by head injury. Head injury can occur through falls, car accidents, and child abuse (for example, when a baby is shaken or receives blows to the head).

Various types of CP have been described; most professionals categorize CP into three major types. Children with **spastic CP** manifest jerky, slow, stiff, and abrupt movements as well as increased **spasticity** (increased tone, rigidity of muscles). Spastic CP affects 70 to 80 percent of children with CP. Children with **ataxic CP** have an awkward gait, disturbed balance, and uncoordinated movements. This type of CP affects approximately 10 percent of individuals with CP. In **athetoid CP,** there are slow, writhing, involuntary movements. Athetoid CP affects approximately 20 percent of children with CP (United Cerebral Palsy, 2001). Some children have mixed CP, which involves more than one type of CP.

There are several types of cerebral palsy. Children can have paralysis of various parts of the body.

Children with CP can have paralysis of various parts of the body. If they have **hemiplegia,** only one side of the body (e.g., right or left) is paralyzed. If they have **paraplegia,** only the legs and lower trunk are paralyzed. In children with **monoplegia,** only one limb or a part thereof is paralyzed, while in children with **diplegia,** either both arms or both legs are paralyzed. Children who have **quadriplegia** have paralysis in both their arms and their legs (Roseberry-McKibbin & Hegde, 2006).

Because children with CP are such a heterogeneous group, there is no pattern of communication deficits that is always associated with them (Long, 2005b). Approximately 50 to 60 percent of children with CP have some degree of mental retardation, and the rest have normal intellectual capability (Haynes & Pindzola, 2004).

Some children with CP may have difficulties associated with mental retardation, visual impairment, hearing impairment, and others described in this book. Each child must be carefully and individually assessed so that SLPs and other professionals can determine his unique profile and combination of needs.

POINTS TO PONDER Describe the types of speech and language challenges that might characterize a child with cerebral palsy.

_____

_____

_____

One major consideration we have already discussed in this chapter is that children with physical problems such as visual impairment may be limited in exploring their environments. This applies to children with CP also. Even if they have normal vision, their motor impairments may prevent them from actively exploring their environments and thus learning about their worlds. Eventual communicative success for children with CP depends in large part upon their ability to compensate for their disability. For example, a child with CP who has normal hearing and vision might be able to learn about his world through books and storytelling instead of direct experiences.

A major problem for many children with CP is expressive language. They may be limited in using their hands to communicate through writing or sign language. They may be limited in their ability to speak by a disorder called **dysarthria,** which is produced by neuromuscular damage affecting voicing, breathing, and producing sounds. Children with dysarthria sound like they have slurred speech. The more upper-limb involvement a child has, the more likely he is to have dysarthria. Thus, a child with quadriplegic CP will be more likely to have dysarthria than a child with hemiplegic CP. Many children with CP may not develop expressive language skills that are commensurate with those of their same-age peers. However, they may develop high levels of language competence anyway (Long, 2005b).

When considering assessment and intervention for children with CP, it is important to remember that a multidisciplinary approach is greatly needed (Pellegrino, 2002). For example, SLPs often work with orthopedic surgeons, physical therapists, occupational therapists, ophthalmologists, vocational and rehabilitation specialists, and others to provide comprehensive services that meet the many needs of the child with CP (Bowe, 2000; Hardman et al., 2006). Recent developments in alternative and augmentative communication (discussed later in this chapter) have made a great impact on children and adults with CP.

It is crucial to implement early intervention for children with CP. Early signs of CP usually appear before children are eighteen months

Some children with cerebral palsy have dysarthria. They may use alternative and augmentative communication devices if they are severely unintelligible.

old; affected babies are usually slow to develop motor milestones such as sitting, crawling, and walking (United Cerebral Palsy, 2001). There are several central components to this intervention. One of those components is to assess and treat possible vision and hearing problems.

Another central component of any intervention program for a child with CP is proper positioning and handling. Because children with CP have problems with muscle tone, they can develop undesirable postures and movements that inhibit the development of skills. Usually, occupational and physical therapists will develop programs to help in positioning and handling; all professionals who work with the child, including SLPs, will be expected to assist with the program's implementation.

A major component of any intervention program for children with CP is to improve feeding and overall oral motor skills. There are specific feeding techniques and special exercises that can be implemented during infancy to help the baby reduce the interference of oral reflexes during chewing, biting, and swallowing. These techniques and exercises not only help the baby eat better, but they set the foundation for oral motor skills, which are critically related to speech.

When sensory and oral motor issues have been dealt with, then cognitive and linguistic development can be promoted through a home program of stimulation activities including social interaction (Long, 2005b). Elsewhere in this book, we have discussed activities that parents can do in the home to stimulate young children's language; many of those activities can be used by parents of children with CP.

> ### CONNECT & EXTEND
>
> United Cerebral Palsy is an organization dedicated to supporting persons with cerebral palsy and their families. They can be contacted at www.ucp.org.

> ### CASES TO CONSIDER
>
> Jarold S. was referred to me for an assessment of his language and articulation skills. He was a CLD fifteen-year-old high school student with severe cerebral palsy. His mother had abused alcohol throughout her pregnancy. Jarold was born two weeks after he was due. Due to difficulty during the birth process, he was deprived of oxygen for ten minutes. When Jarold was in preschool, his father shot and killed his mother; Mr. S. was put in prison. When I saw Jarold, he was living with his grandparents, who had devoted their lives to taking care of him. Jarold used an electric wheelchair and communicated through a device called a Dynavox. Intelligible speech was extremely hard for him; he drooled, had very poor oral-motor coordination, and could not even say basic words with three or four letters. However, I was called in to give a "second opinion" because Jarold's grandparents badly wanted him to speak clearly, not use his Dynavox. What might be the best way to handle this situation? How might you work with Jarold and his grandparents to foster realistic expectations and not frustrate Jarold by trying to force him to do something that he was incapable of?
>
> _____
>
> _____
>
> _____

Spina Bifida

Spina bifida is a birth defect involving an abnormal opening in the spinal column. Generally it originates in the early days of pregnancy before a woman even knows she is pregnant. The human nervous system develops initially from a small, specialized plate of cells along the embryo's back. Early in the development process, the edges of this plate begin to curl up toward each other, creating a neural tube. The neural tube is a narrow sheath that closes to form the embryo's spine and brain. As development progresses, the top of the tube becomes the brain and the rest of the tube becomes the spinal cord. Usually, this process is complete by the twenty-eighth day of pregnancy. Spina bifida is the most common neural tube defect in the United States, affecting between 1,500 and 2,000 babies each year (National Institute of Neurological Disorders and Stroke; NINDS, 2005).

> Spina bifida, a birth defect involving an abnormal opening in the spinal column, occurs during the early days of pregnancy and may be prevented if the expectant mother takes folic acid.

In a child with spina bifida, the neural tube fails to completely close; the reasons for this are not known. However, it is suspected that there may be a genetic component to spina bifida in at least some families. It is also possible that if the mother takes in harmful substances before, at the time of, or shortly after conception, spina bifida in the baby may result. **Teratogens** (poisonous agents) that may cause spinal malformations may include maternal high fever and high glucose levels. In addition, a maternal deficiency in folic acid has been strongly implicated in causing spina bifida. Pregnant women today are routinely advised to take folic acid supplements in order to prevent spina bifida in the developing fetus (NINDS, 2005).

Spina bifida often involves some paralysis of various parts of the body, depending upon where the opening in the spinal column is located. A child with spina bifida sometimes has accompanying intellectual impairment, but not always. Some children with spina bifida have little or no voluntary bowel or bladder control. However, as they get older, these children can be taught bladder and bowel management procedures.

Some students with spina bifida have hydrocephalus, a condition characterized by an excessive accumulation of cerebral spinal fluid within the brain. Surgery for hydrocephalus involves the inserting a small tube or shunt between the ventricles of the brain and connecting this tube to an absorption site in the abdomen. The excessive spinal fluid is diverted from the brain's ventricles to the peritoneum, a thin layer of tissue that lines the abdominal cavity.

CASES TO CONSIDER

I worked with a ten-year-old boy, Jamie, who had spina bifida. He was the seventh child of older Catholic parents, whose financial resources were stretched before he was born. Jamie's condition put the whole family into a crisis, and his parents were managing the best they could. At age ten, Jamie used crutches and wore diapers. He was very small for his age and had many emotional problems. One day I was seeing Jamie and two other boys for language therapy in a pull-out format at the school they attended. (The boys would leave

(continued)

their classroom and come to the speech room several times a week for a half an hour.) During this particular therapy session, Jamie became very frustrated, despite my best efforts, and he threw a pencil at me, which narrowly missed my eye. If you were in this situation, how would you handle it? Would you continue to provide therapy for Jamie in this format, or would you consider other possible ways of providing therapy for him? Explain your answer.

_____

_____

_____

School personnel can do a great deal to support the child with spina bifida. They can make sure that classrooms are laid out in such a way that students can move effectively around with crutches or wheelchairs. School personnel can also give these students support and privacy as they manage their toileting needs. For children who have shunts, it is important for school personnel to watch for signs of its malfunctioning. These signs can include headache, neck pain, irritability, reduced alertness, vomiting, and a decline in school performance (Hardman et al., 2006).

Most people with spina bifida have normal intelligence (NINDS, 2005). However, some children with spina bifida may have associated mental retardation or intellectual disabilities; speech and language problems result primarily from these (Long, 2005b). Language problems may also result from the children's lack of ability to explore their environments. Some children with more severe forms of spina bifida may have learning disabilities, including difficulty with math, reading comprehension, and paying attention. Early intervention is ideal for these children (NINDS, 2005).

Muscular Dystrophy

Muscular dystrophy is an inherited condition that involves progressive deterioration of muscle function. Some of the earliest signs of muscular dystrophy are difficulties with coordination and balance. As the child gets older, her muscles wither and weaken (Nicolosi et al., 2004). Affected muscles include those of the legs, hips, shoulders, and arms; children eventually lose their ability to walk and to use their arms and hands effectively. The muscles of the heart may also be impacted, and the child may experience consequent symptoms of heart failure.

> Muscular dystrophy is an inherited condition that involves progressive deterioration of muscle function. Duchenne muscular dystrophy is the most severe form.

The impact of muscular dystrophy depends on several variables: age of onset, heredity, the nature and physical location of onset, and how fast the condition progresses. Mothers who carry the gene for muscular dystrophy transmit the condition to their sons approximately 50 percent of the time. At least 40,000 people in the United States are affected by muscular dystrophy (Emery, 2000).

The most severe form of muscular dystrophy is Duchenne muscular dystrophy (DMD), which usually manifests between two and five years of age. One-third of the cases of DMD arise by mutation in families who have no history of the disease (Hardman et al., 2006). Boys are affected more often than girls. Often around age ten or thereafter, children with DMD use wheelchairs to move around.

Some children with DMD have deficits in their language skills, but research findings are inconsistent in terms of an exact profile of language problems in these children (Cotton, Vandouris, & Greenwood, 2001). Children with DMD often have dysarthria that worsens with time; the SLP's goal is to help the child compensate and be as intelligible as possible. The use of augmentative/alternative communication devices is frequently warranted.

As time goes by, children with DMD begin to lose respiratory function. In addition, they can't cough up secretions such as phlegm and may contract pneumonia as a result. DMD is terminal, and families and children often need much support to deal with this. Professionals should direct these children and families to specially designed programs that help them deal with the child's eventual death. Usually a child with DMD dies within ten to fifteen years after the first symptoms are noticed; this is often the result of acute respiratory infections (Muscular Dystrophy Campaign, 2004)

Muscular dystrophy is incurable. The goal of treatment is to help the child maintain independence as long as possible. Physical therapists are generally very involved with the child from early on and help her to function with various supportive devices (e.g., braces, walkers). Eventually, the child will probably need a wheelchair. The child may be given some type of medication to help counteract the effects of muscular dystrophy on the heart and to increase muscle strength. Professionals who are involved with the child will need to watch her carefully for any potential side effects of the medication (Hardman et al., 2006).

CASES TO CONSIDER

Yesterday in my job in the public schools, I was asked to assess the language skills of Stephen S., an eight-year-old boy with Duchenne muscular dystrophy. Stephen is currently in a foster home, and he transferred to our school district with a thick file from his prior school district. He is currently placed in a general-education second-grade classroom. In Stephen's previous district, he had been diagnosed with mental retardation, language problems, and microcephaly (small head/brain) in conjunction with the DMD. I had never seen Stephen before and attempted to give him a popular standardized test of language skills because in the public schools, we rely heavily on formal test scores. He achieved below the first percentile on the whole test, so I informally assessed functional language skills. Stephen could not tell me the days of the week, months of the year, date of birth, phone number, address, or his foster mother's name. He could not say the alphabet or count to twenty.

(continued)

You know that in ten to fourteen years, Stephen will probably die. He clearly is very delayed in his language skills. What language therapy goals might be appropriate for him? Should he continue in a general-education second-grade placement where he is now, or might there be a better alternative for him? Explain your answer.

_____

_____

_____

Spinal Cord Injury

Spinal cord injury occurs when the spinal cord is traumatized or severed. Trauma and severing of the spinal cord can result from a number of things: a sports injury, car accident, or extreme flexing or extension from a fall. In the United States, there are approximately 450,000 individuals with spinal cord injury. Each year, there are about 10,000 new cases (Spinal Cord Injury Resource Center, 2003).

The impact of spinal cord injury on a child depends on the nature and site of the injury. If the injury occurs in the lower back, paralysis only occurs in the lower extremities. If the injury occurs on the upper back or neck, the consequent effects are generally quite widespread (e.g., paralysis in a number of areas of the body). Many children with spinal cord injury have difficulties with bowel and bladder control. A child who sustains a spinal cord injury often has other bodily damage such as head injury and injury to the chest or neck.

> Children with spinal cord injury usually do not have speech-language problems unless they sustain a head injury along with the spinal cord injury.

When a child injures his spinal cord, immediate medical care is crucial. Once the child is stabilized and any accompanying medical conditions are treated, then he undergoes any necessary rehabilitation. For example, he might be taught to use braces, a headstick for typing, or some form of augmentative/alternative communication. Generally, the team who cares for the child with spinal cord injury is composed of an orthopedic specialist, occupational therapist, physical therapist, and others such as an SLP if necessary. A psychiatrist is often involved in the rehabilitation process, as the child and his family undergo a significant adjustment process in wake of the injury.

School personnel must be aware that some children with spinal cord injuries will not be able to feel pain or pressure in their lower extremities. Thus, skin breakdown and pressure sores may occur as a result of sitting for long periods of time. To prevent these problems from occurring, the child will need to be occasionally repositioned and moved. When a child with spinal cord injury reenters school, he may experience depression characterized by loss of appetite, reduced energy, irregular sleeping patterns, loss of interest in school activities, and avoidance of interaction with others (Hardman et al., 2006). SLPs may need to involve such a child in group therapy for social skills to help him readjust to interacting with peers post-accident. Most children with spinal cord injuries have no concomitant speech-language problems unless they sustain head injuries along with the spinal cord injuries.

SUMMARY

- Children with cerebral palsy have muscular incoordination and related problems due to damage to the central nervous system. This damage usually occurs before, during, or shortly after the birth process.
- It is common for children with cerebral palsy to have expressive language problems. If the children have accompanying mental retardation, receptive problems also occur.
- Children with spina bifida have a birth defect involving an abnormal opening in the spinal column. Most children with spina bifida have normal intelligence; however, some have associated mental retardation with its accompanying speech and language characteristics.
- Muscular dystrophy is an inherited, progressive condition that involves progressive deterioration of muscle function. Research has not yielded a "typical" profile of language skills for children with muscular dystrophy.
- Children with spinal cord injuries generally have normal speech and language skills. However, if they have accompanying head injuries, there will be associated speech, language, and cognition problems.

Add your own summary points here:

_____

_____

_____

AUGMENTATIVE AND ALTERNATIVE COMMUNICATION

Introduction and Basic Principles

Augmentative and alternative communication (AAC) methods supplement deficient oral communication skills or provide alternative means of communication for children with extremely limited oral communication skills. Increasingly, AAC is being used for children with receptive language problems as well. Children who are candidates for AAC usually have a condition such as autism, severe mental retardation, or a physical impairment such as cerebral palsy. In addition, AAC devices are increasingly being used with children who have behavior problems (Kuder, 2003; Nelson, 1998).

The child may use one of several forms of AAC: **gestural-unaided, gestural-assisted (aided),** or **neuro-assisted (aided)** (Roseberry-McKibbin & Hegde, 2006). In gestural (unaided) AAC, no external aids or instruments are used. Instead the child uses gestures and other patterned movements that may be accompanied by some speech. For example, the child might use **American Sign Language** (mentioned earlier) either alone

> There are several forms of augmentative and alternative communication: gestural (unaided), gestural-assisted (aided), or neuro-assisted (aided).

or with oral speech. Another type of sign language is **American Indian Hand Talk** (AMER-IND), a system developed by North American Indians. AMER-IND is not phonetic. Movements and gestures are used as pictorial representations of ideas and concepts. A third type of sign language is the **Left Hand Manual Alphabet,** which uses concrete gestures that approximate the printed letters of the alphabet. This is most appropriate for children with right-sided paralysis.

Other types of gestural (unaided) AAC include **eye-blink encoding** and **pantomime.** Eye-blink encoding is a simple system where the child learns to communicate messages by using a specific number of blinks. For example, one blink means *yes*; two blinks mean *no*. Eye-blink encoding is often used by children with paralysis. Pantomime uses the entire body or parts of the body to create gestures and dynamic movements. The child uses facial expressions, dramatizations of meanings, and **transparent messages.**

Transparent messages are those that can usually be understood by a communication partner who has no special training (Glennen & DeCoste, 1997). Balandin (2005, p. 387) states that transparency is the "ease of deciphering what a symbol means." For example, a child might cup her hand and bring it to her mouth in a drinking motion to indicate that she is thirsty. Conversely, the child might also use an **opaque** message, or one that is more difficult to decipher. For example, if the child waved both arms above her head to indicate that she was thirsty, this message would be opaque because it would be difficult for the average person to decipher. Clearly, transparent messages are the most desirable because they facilitate communication with a greater number of interlocutors, or conversational partners.

Children who use gestural (aided) AAC combine movements or gestures with an instrument or message-display device. Gestures are used for several purposes: 1) to scan or select messages displayed on a nonmechanical device such as a communication board or 2) to display messages on a mechanical device like a computer monitor. Usually mechanical devices involve sophisticated electronics and high technology. They are often run by computer software, and they generate speech or printed messages.

POINTS TO PONDER Describe the differences between mechanical and nonmechanical AAC devices.

_____

_____

_____

Nonmechanical devices do not use any electronic technology; there is no message storage, printed output, or speech output. One popular low-technology aided method of communication is called Picture Exchange Communication System (PECS). When using

PECS, the clinician initially teaches the child to exchange specific pictures to communicate with a partner. For example, to request a bowl of cereal, the child might hand his partner a picture of a bowl of cereal.

Neuro-assisted AAC is used with children who cannot use a manual switching device because they have limited hand mobility and profound motor impairments. Neuro-assisted AAC uses bioelectrical signals such as muscle-action potentials to activate and display messages on a computer monitor. The way this works is that the electrical activity of muscles, which is associated with their contraction, is used to activate switching mechanisms.

Electrodes, which are attached to the child's skin, pick up electrical discharges that are subsequently amplified so they can activate specific displays or special kinds of switches called *myoswitches*. When a switch or display is activated, the child receives feedback (e.g., onset of light or sound). Through biofeedback, the child learns to use muscle-action potentials for activating messages. Equipment for children who use neuro-assisted AAC is expensive, and maintenance of this equipment can be challenging for the average SLP, especially if she does not have ready access to an AAC technician.

> Children who use AAC devices may use dynamic displays, which allow them to select the exact vocabulary word they want.

Children who use AAC devices may send messages through **scanning** or **direct selection.** In scanning, the communication partner or mechanical device offers the child available messages. The messages are offered until the child indicates the one she wants to use to communicate. In direct selection, the child selects a message by pointing, touching a key pad, touching an item or object, pressing an electronic key, or other direct methods.

When AAC users want to communicate, they use **displays,** or devices or systems that show the message to their communication partner. For example, computer screens and communication boards are displays. **Dynamic displays** allow the child to navigate her way through layers of vocabulary (which is organized by category) until she arrives at the specific message she wants to convey. Categories of vocabulary available to the user can include *who, what, where, how*, and so forth. For example, symbols in the *who* category might include representations of teachers, classmates, and family members. Symbols in the *where* category might include symbols representing the playground, classroom, and home (Calculator, 2000).

Researchers caution that when working with young children, the appropriateness of AAC devices that use dynamic displays should be considered. In their study of three-year-old TD children who used dynamic displays to learn new vocabulary, Drager, Light, Carlson, D'Silva, Larsson, Pitkin, & Stopper (2004) concluded that after the first learning session, the subjects performed significantly better with AAC technologies in a contextual scene format than in a grid format. Drager et al. recommended that AAC technologies need to reflect appropriate developmental models for children, not just be based on conceptual models of adults without disabilities.

AAC users also use symbols to communicate. AAC symbols represent concepts. These symbols may be **iconic;** they look like the picture or object they represent. Put differently, a symbol's iconicity is defined as the degree to which a symbol is perceived to resemble the referent when the referent is known. For example, a hieroglyphic picture of a house is an iconic symbol that indicates the word *house*. The apple represented by Apple

Iconic symbols look like the picture or object they represent. Noniconic symbols are geometric, abstract, and arbitrary.

computer is also an iconic symbol. Symbols may also be **noniconic;** they are geometric, abstract, and arbitrary. They have to be specifically taught because they do not look like the object they represent. For example, chips and flexible plastic shapes are noniconic symbols.

When symbols are selected for an individual child to use with an AAC system, the team can ask several questions about these symbols (Reichle, 1991). First, how will the symbols be displayed? For example, a wallet, book, or board (electronic or nonelectronic) could be used. Second, what types of symbols should be used? This depends on the individual child. Third, how will the learner select the symbols? For example, will she use scanning, direct selection, or a combination of these methods? Fourth, how large should the symbols be? If the child has a visual impairment, the symbols will need to be larger.

Implications for Assessment and Intervention

Assessment

Fundamentally, when thinking about service delivery, it is important to remember that children who use AAC devices comprise a very heterogeneous population. Thus, in both assessment and intervention, a team approach is very important (DePaepe & Wood, 2001). Members of the team usually include an SLP, occupational therapist, physical therapist, social worker, psychologist, vocational counselor, nurse, teacher, and technical staff person.

SLPs provide assessment of and intervention for communication skills, and may coordinate the child's overall program because communication is so critical for children who use AAC devices (Moore-Brown & Montgomery, 2001). Occupational therapists help with the child's positioning and seating, while physical therapists provide support for the child's motor problems. Ideally, technical staff are available to assist with "troubleshooting" high-tech systems. As Moore-Brown and Montgomery (2001, p. 232) state, "The SLP is rarely qualified to be the repair person." AAC assessment has several goals. Balandin (2005, pp. 399–400) states that

> An AAC assessment involves more than assessing a child's current level of communication and suggesting a communication aid. . . . The goal of AAC assessment is not only to identify a system that will be functional for a child but also to select one that will allow the child to develop language skills and meet future communication needs. . . . It is also important to remember that assessment is only a part of any AAC intervention. Providing a suitable communication system does not, in itself, ensure that a child will use it or will communicate more effectively. . . . training the child in the use of the system coupled with training of communication partners is important.

We will say more about training communication partners a little later.

In conducting an assessment with a child who needs an AAC device, it is possible to use standardized tests and modify them appropriately to fit the individual child's needs. However, as we said earlier in this chapter, when adaptations are made, standardized scores cannot be used. Standardized tests are not ideal with children who use AAC devices

(Ianoco & Cupples, 2004). It is best to use a combination of in-depth interviewing with the child's communication partners as well as observation of the child attempting to communicate in a variety of settings with a variety of communication partners (Sigafoos, Woodyatt, Keen, Tait, Tucker, Roberts-Pennell, & Pittendreigh, 2000).

> A comprehensive assessment of a child who will be using an AAC device includes the assessment of motor, perceptual, and sensory skills. This is usually done by occupational and physical therapists.

It is important to gather a detailed case history. Research has shown that interviewing people who are familiar with a child (e.g., parents and teachers) can yield valuable information about the child's language use in a variety of settings (Sigafoos et al., 2000). Calculator (2000) recommends the portfolio method for children in public school settings. In the portfolio method of assessment, the SLP interviews the classroom teacher and reviews the child's classroom portfolio. In Chapter 5, we said that a portfolio contains examples of a child's ongoing work samples.

The child's motor, perceptual, and sensory skills must be assessed. The physical therapist and occupational therapist can evaluate things such as ways of optimizing the child's posture, positioning for use of the AAC device, and types of switches that can be used to help the child activate the AAC system. The occupational therapist and physical therapist can also provide information about the child's ability to use signs and gestures. Does the child have the motor skills to use signs and gestures? If not, then clearly signs and gestures should not be taught as methods of communication (Calculator, 2000).

In terms of perceptual skills, the occupational therapist needs to assess how to organize and present symbols on the AAC device so that the child can easily perceive and access them. The occupational and physical therapist can also give input about the number of items on a display, the size of the items, and the spacing that needs to be between the items so that they will be most optimally perceived. Sensory skills such as vision and hearing must also be assessed. Students with cerebral palsy often have accompanying vision problems, and this needs to be considered in terms of what type of device is used. Hearing problems can impact the child's ability to send and receive messages. Hearing and vision must be thoroughly assessed before any type of device is selected (Calculator, 2000).

It is also important to assess the child's behavior, especially her motivation to communicate (Calculator, 1998; Paul, 2001). Sometimes a child who is frustrated about her ability to communicate will scream, cry, have tantrums, abuse herself, be aggressive, and exhibit other disruptive behaviors. In my school district, we worked with one ten-year-old boy with severe cerebral palsy who would literally lie on the floor and cry all day. It was a challenge to create an AAC system to meet his needs and reduce his frustration. Calculator (2000) states that probably the best way to reduce a child's behavior problems is to help him communicate, not to use behavioral programs like we discussed in Chapter 6.

When the child has undergone a comprehensive assessment, it will be necessary for her to have follow-up assessments also. The purpose of these follow-up assessments is to ensure that the AAC device is still appropriate for the child's needs. In addition, because technology evolves so rapidly, it is important for the assessment team to ensure that the child has the most currently available, appropriate equipment to help her communicate as successfully as possible.

> An AAC device is intended to supplement talking, not replace it.

Intervention

As we said earlier, an AAC device is not intended to replace talking. Rather, the AAC system is a set of strategies, techniques, and tools added to the child's communication possibilities. An AAC device can actually facilitate a child's speech production. For example, children who use AAC devices are often passive; they do not often initiate interaction, and thus have fewer chances to practice language than their TD peers (Kuder, 2003). If these children can use their AAC devices to initiate and maintain interactions, their language skills will have many more chances to develop and flourish.

When an AAC device is developed for a student, the following learner characteristics should be considered (Mirenda & Ianoco, 1990):

1. *Sensory-perceptual*: What are the learner's vision and hearing skills like?

2. *Cognitive/linguistic*: What types of symbols are most likely to be successful with this learner given her cognitive/linguistic skills?

3. *Mobility*: Evaluators need to assess the student's ability to walk and her overall mobility.

4. *Communication*: How does the student currently communicate? Does she have any speech at all? Does she use gestures or other nonverbal means of communication?

5. *Manipulation:* The student's fine-motor skills need to be considered. Can she use a gestural communication system such as sign language? If she is going to use a high-tech device, will it need to be adapted to her fine-motor needs?

For children with physical disabilities, it is important that they are able to use their AAC devices comfortably and without getting too tired. These children need to be trained in how to use their systems to promote successful interaction with others (Balandin, 2005). In addition, it is important to assure that these systems are portable. The child needs to be able to use the system with relative ease. If a system is bulky and hard to take around in various settings, it will be of limited use to the child.

As part of intervention, SLPs help children learn to use AAC devices in a variety of settings outside the therapy room. These settings include the school, home, and various places in the community (Glennen & DeCoste, 1997). Successful language intervention for children who use AAC devices needs to include natural-speaking partners in natural environments. Natural-speaking partners must be trained regarding the use of AAC and how to best facilitate the child's language development. It is ideal for peers to be trained to interact appropriately with the child who uses an AAC device, because this can increase the child's language skills.

When children who use AAC devices have chances to talk about real situations with conversational partners in real settings, they have a greater chance of generalizing their skills (Calculator, 1988). As Johnston, Reichle, and Evans (2004, p. 23) stated, "An effective augmentative communication system requires a commitment from all social partners, including family members, professional staff, and peers."

When AAC devices or systems are being designed, the interactional styles and preferences of the child's communication partners must be considered. Often, these communication partners are TD peers.

Johnston et al. (2004) added that when designing an AAC system, it is important to consider the interactional styles and preferences of the child's communication partners as well as those of the child himself. It must be remembered that communicating through an AAC device can be slow and frustrating, requiring patience on the part of the listener as well as the AAC user (Bedrosian, Hoag, & McCoy, 2003). Many times, the listener is a TD peer.

There has been research examining the reactions of TD peers to children who use AAC devices. Beck and Fritz-Verticchio (2003) described a school-based intervention designed to increase the positive attitudes of TD peers toward children who used AAC devices. One group of TD peers was given information about AAC. The other group was given both information and opportunities to role-play being a nonspeaking person. The results of the study showed that there was a greater positive effect for the group of TD peers who had been given both information and role-play experience. This was particularly true of boys and older children. Beck and Fritz-Verticchio suggested that in order to help TD peers have more positive attitudes toward and interactions with children who use AAC devices, SLPs might use a combination of information provision, role-playing, and explicit instruction regarding how to communicate with the child who uses an AAC device.

We must remember to focus on the most critical skills for the student: participation, interaction, and communication. The student who uses an AAC device is probably accustomed to having decisions made *for* him. Others have usually anticipated his wants and needs (Calculator, 2000). It is important to help the student be an active initiator and interactor during communication exchanges.

It is critical for the child's AAC system to contain vocabulary that is relevant to her daily environments (e.g., home, school). Communication boards can be designed with overlay that can be changed for various activities and functions. For example, one overlay might contain pictures of a classroom; another overlay might contain pictures that pertain to the home environment. Most electronic AAC devices can be reprogrammed and the overlay changed to meet the child's communication needs in different situations. However, it is important to consider how easy or difficult it might be for the device to be reprogrammed and changed (Kuder, 2003). Clinicians should be careful to not have the communication be solely focused on the present. The child needs a way to communicate about the past and future also (Paul, 2001).

Students who use AAC devices may have difficulty in the area of literacy, especially if these students have severe impairments (Paul, 2001; Fallon, Light, McNaughton, Drager, & Hammer, 2004; Ianoco & Cupples, 2004). Based on their research with five severely impaired students who used AAC devices, Fallon et al. suggested that daily reading instruction (as opposed to two or three times a week) is recommended for students who are beginning readers. Fallon et al. also suggested that the subjects in their study might have benefited more from the reading program if phonological awareness skills had been firmly established first. They recommended that literacy intervention target phonological awareness skills as a foundation for reading.

> Reading may be especially difficult for students who use AAC devices. These students may benefit from receiving foundational instruction in phonological awareness as well as daily reading instruction.

For children in the public schools, SLPs must remember that the Individuals with Disabilities Education Act (IDEA, 2004) mandates that if these children need AAC devices, the school district has to provide them. AAC devices can be purchased by the district or by the family. Devices can also be leased or borrowed. If an AAC device is found to be medically necessary for the student, Medicaid or an insurance company might purchase the equipment. However AAC devices are obtained, school districts must procure them in a timely manner. The school makes AAC decisions based on what is most educationally beneficial for the student (Moore-Brown & Montgomery, 2001).

The SLP in the public-school setting often has many children to see each week, and time can be quite limited. Calculator (2000) suggests that the SLP might best serve the child with an AAC device by using her time in a consultative role to help others engage students in meaningful activities during the day. For example, the SLP might provide instruction and support to the classroom teacher to help him integrate the child into daily curriculum activities. The SLP might also work with the classroom aide to instruct her in specific ways to make the curriculum more accessible to the child. In addition, the SLP can go into the classroom and model, for the teacher and children, how to communicate effectively with the child using the AAC device.

Steps can be taken to integrate children who use AAC devices into regular classroom settings. First, educational priorities need to be established collaboratively with parents and other team members. Second, as we have said, assessment and intervention need to take place in the child's natural environmental settings where she spends most of her time. Third, functional, practical skills should be taught throughout the day and not restricted to a specific time slot. Lastly, the effectiveness of intervention needs to be evaluated in regard to its impact on the child's performance in natural settings.

Calculator (2000) lists some practical suggestions to foster optimal interactions with students who use AAC devices in natural settings, especially the school setting:

1. Find ways of incorporating the device into lessons. For example, students can create worksheets for science using Boardmaker (Myer-Johnson Co., P.O. Box 1579, Solana Beach, CA 92075-7579). Boardmaker software allows users to select from thousands of line drawings to customize displays; there may be words accompanying these displays, or no words may be used.

2. As needed, modify and replace vocabulary on the AAC system so that it corresponds with school activities and the curriculum. For example, the child will need a different set of vocabulary symbols for lunch in the cafeteria and for social studies in the classroom.

3. Model total communication when appropriate. For example, instead of just talking, use gestures, objects, and other methods. Convey the notion that all methods of communication are acceptable and valued.

4. Do not bombard the child with questions. Comments will help to create more stimulating and interesting interactions.

It is necessary for professionals to help children who use AAC devices to integrate successfully into the school setting.

5. If the child has deficits in comprehension, it may be necessary to restrict conversation to here-and-now topics that correspond with predictable routines in the child's life.

6. Encourage and reinforce all the child's attempts to communicate.

7. When the child is communicating, be sure to understand how the child would like you to verbalize. For example, some children who use nonelectronic devices want to construct the entire message before the conversational partner verbalizes it. Other children prefer for the communication partner to verbalize the message one symbol at a time as it is being constructed.

8. Be sure to give the child enough time to respond. Some children may take a minute or more to reply, and the conversational partner needs to be patient.

Additional Considerations for CLD Children and Their Families

It is projected that by the year 2020, the largest non–European American population of AAC consumers in the United States (460,000) will be within the Hispanic community (Soto et al., 1997). When working with CLD children who need AAC and their families, it is extremely important to be sensitive to whether or not the family wants the child to use AAC (Huer & Parette, 2003). We have said that some families may believe that a disability is fate or God's will, and that intervention is not appropriate. For these families, probably the introduction of an AAC device is insensitive and inappropriate. However, the family should always be made aware of their options and given choices about whether to use AAC devices or not (Parette, Huer, & Wyatt, 2003).

Some families, if they have immigrated from rural areas in developing countries, may be overwhelmed and intimidated by AAC devices—especially high-technology ones. If a family has lived most of their lives in a rural area with no cars or electricity, the idea of using a high-tech device can be very uncomfortable because it is totally outside their experience. It is possible that with the help of a cultural mediator, the SLP can help the family become comfortable enough with the AAC device to use it in helping the child to successfully communicate. But SLPs must also be prepared to accommodate the family by introducing a low-tech device that they are more comfortable with. Even if an AAC device is very expensive and high-tech, it won't be helpful if the family can't or won't help the child use it!

In one of the few studies to examine the use of AAC devices with CLD children, Huer, Parette, and Saenz (2001) obtained information from focus groups consisting of family members of children with disabilities. These family members provided information for identifying and understanding issues impacting AAC practices within a Mexican American community. Seven family members participated in the focus groups; these family members ranged from twenty-nine to fifty-three years of age, and the average age was forty. The families all spoke Spanish and were Mexican

American; several had lived in Mexico. Collectively, the participants of the focus groups represented the families of four children (three girls and one boy) who were between nine and ten years of age. Three of the children were in wheelchairs; one was ambulatory with assistance. Two of the children used Alpha Talkers (a form of augmentative communication utilizing a keyboard with pictures for communication). The four children had communication boards and knew sign language; their verbalizations were quite limited.

When the transcripts from the focus groups were subjected to a content analysis, several general themes emerged. First, all seven focus-group participants expressed deep gratitude toward the group leaders and toward SLPs for helping their children. Participants' attitudes toward professionals were very positive. Second, five out of seven parents frequently referred to the difficulty they experienced with having a child with special needs. References were made to the lack of support available in Mexico for children with multiple needs. A third finding from this study was that there was a recurring theme of having families of children work together—there was extensive family involvement. As Huer et al. stated, "These families emphasized their commitment to caring for their family member to the extent that they nurtured and advocated dependence on the family" (p. 203). In addition, group participants often mentioned working together with professionals.

> When working with CLD families of children who use AAC devices, it is important to remember that many of them emphasize extensive family involvement.

One interesting finding from this study is that the Mexican American families interviewed preferred that their children use sign language or speech over assistive technology. There were family concerns about the cost of equipment, and some family members felt uncomfortable with the responsibility of using expensive equipment. They did not want to feel liable should this equipment malfunction or break down. Huer et al. also conjectured that perhaps the AAC devices recommended for the children were not useful in the homes because they were programmed in English for use at school.

POINTS TO PONDER Describe two considerations that SLPs need to keep in mind when working with CLD families of children who need AAC devices.

_____

_____

_____

Huer et al. (2001) recommended that SLPs who work with CLD families keep several facts in mind. First, the families in this study liked to talk and tell stories; SLPs should be prepared to take time to listen and not rush families. Second, as we discussed earlier in this book, the results of this study agree with the fact that within the Hispanic community, the most valued institution is the family. SLPs should be prepared to select therapy strategies that focus on family involvement.

> Families need training so they can feel comfortable using AAC devices.

CONNECT & EXTEND

An informative resource for those who work with CLD children who use AAC devices is Huer, M.B., & Parette, H.P. (2003). Issues in family interventions: Working with parents cross-culturally. In S. von Tetzchner and M.H. Jensen (Eds.), *Perspectives on theory and practice in augmentative and alternative communication.* (pp. 154–167). Toronto, Ontario: International Society for Augmentative and Alternative Communication.

In addition, an interesting finding in this study was that when families were asked to "Tell me about your child," most of the parents described their children's personal grooming skills (e.g., that a child could go to the bathroom and brush his teeth). In therapy, it is important for the SLP to ascertain parents' priorities; for some Hispanic parents from Mexican backgrounds, priorities may include self-care/personal grooming skills such as described by the parents in this study.

Lastly, Huer et al. (2001) found that all the families wished for devices that would speak in Spanish. They also wanted more training in how to operate their children's AAC devices. Possibly, although there are few AAC devices programmed in various languages, SLPs might utilize the services of cultural mediators to help families at least become comfortable with the devices and be able to understand how to operate them.

As Huer et al. (2001) stated, it is important not to make generalizations based on one study involving a small number of participants. Nevertheless, this study provides an interesting foundation for SLPs who work with CLD children who use AAC devices and their families. The study also highlights the importance of spending time with family members of these children to ascertain their circumstances as well as possible strategies for improving service delivery to the children.

 SUMMARY

- Some children use augmentative and alternative communication (AAC) devices to supplement oral communication skills. AAC devices generally fall into one of three categories: gestural-unaided, gestural-assisted, and neuro-assisted.
- The child who uses AAC can send transparent (easy to read) or opaque (hard to read) messages. She can use symbols that are iconic (look like the picture or object they represent) or noniconic (geometric, abstract, and arbitrary).
- A thorough AAC assessment will involve gathering a detailed case history, observing the child in various communication settings, and evaluating motor, perceptual, and sensory skills. The child's behavior, language skills, and motivation to communicate must also be assessed.

(continued)

- Intervention for children who use AAC devices involves, among other things, making sure the device is appropriate and updated and facilitating communication with TD peers in various naturalistic settings.
- CLD families from rural areas may feel intimidated by high-technology AAC devices. Some families would like devices that use their primary language. SLPs, using cultural mediators, need to spend time with families ascertaining their needs, comfort levels, and goals for their children who will be using the devices.

Add your own summary points here:

_____

_____

_____

CHAPTER HIGHLIGHTS

- Children with hearing impairment can be categorized as deaf or hard of hearing. A hearing loss can be conductive, sensorineural, or both. Children with hearing impairments frequently have accompanying problems with oral and written language skills.
- Early detection of a hearing loss is critical. Habilitation for children with hearing impairments can include the use of hearing aids or cochlear implants. Auditory training can also be used.
- Three general approaches to communication training for hearing-impaired (HI) children are the auditory/oral method, the manual approach, and total communication. It is important for classroom teachers to make necessary modifications for HI children. Clinicians may need to account for special circumstances surrounding CLD children with hearing impairments.
- Children can have varying degrees of visual impairment. The language of blind children has been shown to differ in some ways from the language of sighted children.
- Because of the language differences, SLPs should work with the parents of blind children from the infant period onward, providing ideas for appropriate language stimulation.
- Direct language intervention for children with visual impairments focuses especially on helping these children communicate appropriately in social settings. SLPs can also help classroom teachers made modifications to optimize the classroom environment for learning.

- Children with cerebral palsy have nonprogressive central nervous system damage. They may have more problems with expressive than with receptive language. A key factor associated with language development in children with cerebral palsy is whether or not these children have accompanying mental retardation.
- The presence of language impairments accompanying mental retardation is also a factor to consider with children who have spina bifida. Children with spina bifida who do not have mental retardation generally have normal language skills.
- Research has not yielded a specific profile of the language skills of children with muscular dystrophy. However, these children may become unintelligible as the muscular dystrophy worsens; in these cases, they may benefit from the use of augmentative and alternative communication devices.
- Children with spinal cord injury usually have normal language skills. If the spinal cord injury is accompanied by head injury, however, usually language and cognitive problems will result.
- Alternative and augmentative communication (AAC) is used to supplement deficient oral language communication skills in children. There are various types of AAC devices and forms of communication. Some can be regarded as "high technology"; others can be regarded as "low technology."
- Assessment and intervention for children who need AAC is carried out by a multidisciplinary team. Critical members of this team include occupational therapists, physical therapists, and technical staff people who are trained in maintenance and repair of AAC equipment.
- Language intervention for children who use AAC is often focused on helping these children interact successfully in naturalistic environments, especially with peers. Peers and other conversation partners must be trained to interact successfully with children who use AAC.
- CLD families may have a variety of reactions to AAC. Their choices and preferences should always be honored. The SLP, using the services of a cultural mediator, needs to spend enough time with these families to ensure that they can help their children use AAC successfully.

STUDY AND REVIEW QUESTIONS

ESSAY

1. Discuss the use of cochlear implants with hearing-impaired children. What are the benefits of cochlear implants? What might be some of the drawbacks?

2. Describe how an SLP might work with the parents of a blind baby to provide optimal language stimulation for the baby.

3. What types of problems might a child with cerebral palsy have relative to language development? What can be done to support this child?

4. List and briefly describe several key components of intervention for a child who uses an augmentative and alternative communication (AAC) device.

5. What issues may come up when working with CLD families whose children need AAC devices? How can we be sensitive to these families?

FILL-IN-THE-BLANK

6. An infection of the middle ear that is often associated with Eustachian tube dysfunction and upper respiratory infections is called _____.

7. A child with _____ cerebral palsy manifests jerky, slow, stiff and abrupt movements along with increased tone and rigidity of muscles.

8. A severe form of muscular dystrophy is called _____ muscular dystrophy. Usually children with this type of muscular dystrophy die ten to fifteen years after the first symptoms are noticed.

9. In AAC, a(n) _____ message is one that is more difficult for the communication partner to decipher.

10. Hearing-impaired children who use both speech and signs simultaneously can be said to use _____.

MULTIPLE CHOICE

11. The head of the private practice where you work tells you that tomorrow, you will be assessing the language skills of a nine-year-old boy with a severe hearing impairment. He wears his hearing aids sporadically and uses American Sign Language most of the time. What types of language problems might you expect to find?
    a. Difficulty repairing communication breakdowns
    b. Written language that closely mirrors Standard American English
    c. Inconsistent use of morphemes such as past tense -*ed* and plural -*s*
    d. a, c
    e. a, b, c

12. In the private practice where you work, a mother calls and tells you that she just found out that her two-month-old son Benjie is blind. The mother wants to consult with you and see what recommendations you have for her for helping Benjie to develop language as normally as possible. Which one of the following recommendations would **not** be appropriate to give this mother?
    a. Be sure to restrict Benjie's movements around the premises when he begins to crawl; he needs to be kept safe, and his physical exploration of his environment must be limited.
    b. When she approaches Benjie, she should make soft noises such as gently calling his name or cooing to let him know that she is coming; she should make these sounds before she picks him up.

    c. When playing or interacting with Benjie, she should provide rich and detailed descriptions of what is happening in his environment.

    d. When she changes activities, she can talk about what she is doing to cue Benjie that the activity is changing.

    e. It would be good if she could monitor herself to make sure that she does not overuse directives with Benjie as he grows older and more mobile.

13. You become aware of a girl named Tara who has cerebral palsy. She has been diagnosed with *ataxic cerebral palsy,* which means that she

    a. Has increased tone and rigidity of her muscles

    b. Has slow, writhing involuntary movements

    c. Walks with an awkward gait and disturbed balance and has uncoordinated movements

    d. a, b

    e. b, c

14. Which of the following are important to remember when working with children who have spina bifida?

    a. They may or may not have language problems accompanying intellectual impairments.

    b. If they do have language problems, the language problems may be related in part to their lack of ability to physically explore their environments.

    c. If these children have shunts due to hydrocephalus, school personnel should watch for possible malfunctioning of the shunts; this malfunctioning can produce reduced alertness, vomiting, and head and neck pain.

    d. b, c

    e. a, b, c

15. Lupita S. is a low-income four-year-old Mexican American preschooler who has cerebral palsy. She needs to use an AAC device. You have been informed by other personnel at Lupita's preschool that her parents "won't listen to advice" and are "totally close minded" about the possibility of an AAC device for Lupita. However, when you see Lupita's parents come to pick her up at the end of the day, they seem very loving, affectionate, and caring toward her. You find out that they speak a minimal amount of English. School personnel have not found a Spanish-speaking interpreter to help them discuss the possibility of an AAC device for Lupita because they are very busy. All communication has taken place in English when Lupita's parents have come to pick her up at the end of the day. In this situation, the best thing for you to do would be to

    a. Not interfere; clearly, Lupita's parents have spoken and they are not at all interested in an AAC device for their daughter

    b. Find a Spanish-speaking cultural mediator and, together, conduct a home visit where you and the mediator spend time talking with Lupita's parents and trying to understand why they seem disinterested in an AAC device for her

    c. Ask Lupita's parents if you can meet with them; when you do, bring some brochures about the usefulness of AAC devices and recommend that they find out more about these devices on the Internet

    d. Meet with Lupita's parents and a Spanish-speaking cultural mediator who has been instructed to try to persuade them to use a specific AAC device with their daughter

    e. Meet with Lupita's parents and the preschool director; in this meeting, tell them that they are neglecting their daughter's needs if they refuse to use an AAC device with her

See Answers to Study and Review Questions, page 465.

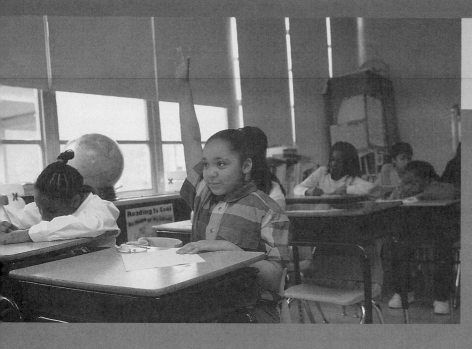

School Language and Classroom Programs for Children with Language Impairments: Collaborating with Parents and School Personnel

Alejandro E. Brice and Roanne G. Brice

CASE STUDY

Marisa J. was from a Mexican family who lived near the school. In kindergarten, her teacher (who spoke both Spanish and English) noticed that Marisa was very shy and seemed somewhat delayed, even in her Spanish skills. But the teacher knew that Marisa's parents worked hard in low-paying jobs and had four children; they did not have a lot of time, money, or energy to provide extra language stimulation for Marisa and her siblings. Also, Marisa had never been to preschool.

The school team met, and it was decided that Marisa would be provided with extra support in the classroom. A special-education professional who spoke Spanish came in each day to work

439

with Marisa in math and reading. The special-education professional also worked collaboratively with the kindergarten teacher, and together they taught some lessons to the whole kindergarten class. The special-education professional particularly modeled techniques for increasing the children's listening comprehension and for increasing their verbal interaction skills.

By the end of kindergarten, Marisa was doing very well. She had learned some English but had also maintained her Spanish skills because she had extra support in that area. Marisa was talking a lot more and had several good friends. Her parents reported that at home, Marisa talked more too; they proudly said that she had become quite interested in reading books.

INTRODUCTION

In this book, we have talked about the language needs of students with varying kinds of disabilities. We know that no matter what type of disability a student has, she has the right to a free and appropriate education that will support her language skills. This includes both special and general education. The nature of special-education services for students with disabilities has changed over the past decade. At the center of this change has been access to the general-education curriculum via the inclusion movement.

The Council for Exceptional Children (CEC; 1993) in a policy statement declared that ". . . CEC believes children, youth, and young adults with disabilities should be served whenever possible in general-education classrooms in inclusive settings" (p. 1). Inclusion involves services in the general-education classroom with the educational supports provided to ensure student learning and success. One of the tenets of the inclusion movement has been the "zero rejection" philosophy. This philosophy states that no student is deemed to be too disabled or that a disability classification is deemed too severe for the student not to be included in general-education classrooms.

The National Association of State Boards of Education (1992) suggested that mainstreaming and labeling students have been ineffective strategies for children receiving special-education services. Kauffman (1989) also stated that all students are more alike than different: The (handicapped-nonhandicapped) and exceptional-nonexceptional distinctions are not useful for educational purposes. Stainback and Stainback (1996; 1987; 1984) have stated that such labeling is very detrimental to the education of students with disabilities.

> Students with special-education needs are to be served in the least restrictive environment. Students who are included in the general-education classroom need to be provided with educational supports.

Other educators have focused on the need to maximize the education of all students (Braaten & Mennes, 1992; Braaten, Kauffman, Braaten, Polsgrove, & Nelson, 1988; Kauffman, 1989; McGregor & Vogelsberg, 1998; Stainback & Stainback, 1996; Stainback, Stainback, Stefanich, & Alper, 1996). It is apparent that many school districts have implemented changes toward an inclusion and/or collaborative model. Services using the pull-out model have diminished and instead more districts have been using resource rooms and self-contained classrooms. Figure 12.1 shows a typical hierarchy of services for students with special needs.

LEVEL 1

Regular general-education classroom — classroom teacher ideally implements strategies to help student access the curriculum

LEVEL 2

Regular-education classroom with collaboration/consultation between teacher and special educator such as an SLP, resource specialist, psychologist, or some combination thereof

LEVEL 3

Regular-education classroom with DIS (designed instruction and services). Usually this involves pull-out services, where the student leaves the classroom and spends a half hour to one hour in a separate room with a professional such as a resource specialist; usually students are seen in small groups

LEVEL 4

Participation in campus learning center where the student spends part of the day in the regular classroom and part of the day in a separate room receiving speech-language therapy, resource assistance, or both

LEVEL 5

Student spends all her time in a special-education classroom taught by a teacher with special credentials

LEVEL 6

Special separate public school where large numbers of students with certain types of disorders are grouped together

LEVEL 7

Nonpublic-school setting within the community (e.g., group home for students with severe autism)

FIGURE 12.1

Inclusive services for students are provided in the context of the general-education classroom as the least restrictive environment (LRE). Inclusion also attempts to minimize the use of separate curriculums for students with speech disorders, language disorders, or learning disabilities. Since 1990, the focus of the inclusion debate has changed from *whether* inclusion should be the major delivery model to *how* inclusion and access to the general-education curriculum can best be accomplished (for a further discussion of these issues the reader is referred to the work of Stainback & Stainback, 1996). Inclusion and collaboration with general-education classrooms can be summarized as including the following critical features: (a) the inclusive classroom setting is an integrated setting in which all children learn together; (b) the inclusive classroom setting does not unduly label or identify students as special-needs learners; (c) the inclusive classroom maximizes educational benefit; and (d) the inclusive classroom minimizes the need for a separate curriculum and facilitates access to the general-education curriculum.

The separation of general education from speech-language programs or special education has led to certain inequities in education. As a result, some students have not had access to the mainstream or core curriculum. A solution to this dilemma is for schools to provide special education or speech and language instruction in the classroom. This requires collaborative efforts between the special-education teacher and/or speech-language pathologist (SLP) and the general-education classroom teacher. This rationale is based on four aspects: (a) the classroom is the most natural context for the use of language; (b) carryover and generalization is more likely to occur if instruction/therapy occurs in the classroom; (c) more children will benefit from special education or SLP services in the classroom; and (d) success of instruction or therapy will be measured in skills that enhance academic and classroom success.

> Speech-language and special programs have been separated from general education; a solution for this is to provide special education or speech and language instruction in the classroom.

Educational Reform

In January of 2002, the most recent educational reform legislation was enacted when President George W. Bush signed into law the *No Child Left Behind Act (NCLB) of 2001.* The US Department of Education (2002) stated that

> . . . since the *Nation At Risk* report was issued nearly 20 years ago, there has been vigorous national debate over how to improve our nation's schools and our children's achievement.

POINTS TO PONDER Why is it important for special-education students to be fully included in general classroom settings?

Out of these years of debate, a general consensus has emerged that schools and districts work best when they have greater control and flexibility, when scientifically proven teaching methods are employed, and when schools are held accountable for results. These are the guiding ideas behind the NCLB Act (p. x).

The new reauthorization specifies four key principles: (a) stronger accountability for students' education performance; (b) greater flexibility for states, school districts, and schools in the use of federal funds; (c) more choices for parents of children from disadvantaged backgrounds; and (d) an emphasis on teaching methods that are scientifically based and have been demonstrated to be effective. The US Department of Education (2002) stated that in order to assure educational accountability the "data will be disaggregated for students by poverty levels, race, ethnicities, disabilities, and limited English proficiencies [i.e., those students who are English language learning] to ensure that no child—regardless of his or her background—is left behind" (p. x).

> The No Child Left Behind Act, enacted in 2002, has increased emphasis on greater accountability of schools, increased emphasis on reading, enhancing teacher quality, and teaching English to English language learning (ELL) students.

In addition, the NCLB Act increases emphasis on reading, enhancing teacher quality, and teaching English to English language learning (ELL) students. The US Department of Education (2002) stated that "the goal of the program is for *all* [emphasis added] children to read at or above grade level by the end of third grade (p. 13)." The NCLB Act has increased the accountability requirements for the academic and reading achievements of all students, including data on specified student groups from major racial and ethnic backgrounds (e.g., Hispanic), students with English learning needs, and students with disabilities. One means of providing accountability of student performance is for SLPs and special-education teachers to provide instructional services in classrooms. This inclusion of services will require collaboration, co-teaching, and at times consultation with general-education classroom teachers.

CONNECT & EXTEND

Detailed information about No Child Left Behind is available at http://www.ed.gov/nclb.

Program Types

The most common models for inclusion of speech, language, and special-education instruction to students have consisted of **collaboration** (working with the teacher in the classroom), **co-teaching** (sharing the responsibility for planning and teaching lessons), and **consultation** (instructing the teacher on instructional strategies for children with special needs). Typically, instruction, speech and language services, and special-education services have been provided in resource rooms, in an itinerant fashion (e.g., pull-out model), or as a consultative model.

> Collaboration is a form of working together and co-teaching with other school professionals.

For some special-education services, **resource rooms** may be the least restrictive environment where students are removed from their general-education classrooms for a portion of the school day. The amount of time that a student spends in the resource room is dependent upon the student's particular needs as specified by their Individualized Education Plan (IEP). Usually the resource room is a room on the school campus that is specifically designated for students with language impairments and academic deficits stemming from these impairments. In the resource room, the students work with a resource specialist and sometimes other professionals to improve language and academic skills.

The **itinerant model** is used for certain categories that require less contact and less specific classroom instruction. The itinerant SLP typically pulls students from their instructional classrooms to work on specific speech (e.g., articulation, fluency, voice), language (e.g., oral language, emergent literacy, and related reading skills), or hearing-related objectives (e.g., auditory processing disorder).

Collaboration is defined here as a form of working together and co-teaching with other school professionals (Idol, Nevin, & Paolucci-Whitcomb, 2000). Collaboration is also defined as providing instruction in the classroom or inclusively. Collaboration may involve the SLP in the resource room, the special-education teacher in the general-education classroom, or the SLP in the general-education classroom.

> In the itinerant model of service delivery, children are pulled out of their classrooms to work on specific skills.

SUMMARY

- The nature of special-education services for students with disabilities has changed over the past decade. One of the greatest changes is providing these students access to the general-education curriculum via the inclusion movement.
- Inclusive services for students with special-education needs are provided in the context of the general-education classroom as the least restrictive environment.
- The No Child Left Behind Act of 2002 mandated a number of changes in education. A major change was to ensure that school districts would be held accountable for all children's progress, especially those from low-income and English as a second language backgrounds.
- Collaboration involves SLPs' working together and co-teaching with other professionals. In the itinerant model, children are pulled from their classrooms to work on specific skills.

Add your own summary points here:

_____

_____

_____

COLLABORATION VERSUS CONSULTATION

Definitions

No one takes an expert role under the collaborative model; i.e., knowledge and responsibilities are shared. The collaborative focus is to facilitate instruction for the special needs students. One type of collaboration is to provide instruction for these students in the

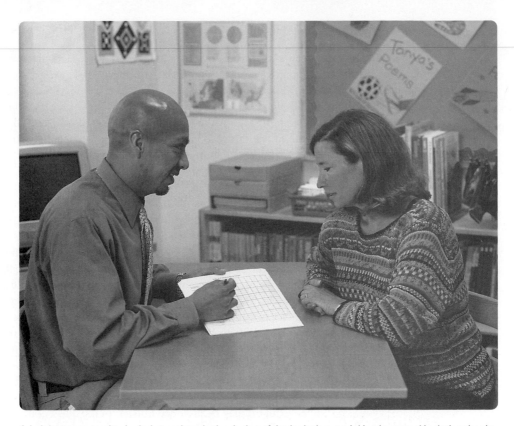

Administrators need to include teachers in the design of the inclusion model implemented in their schools.

general-education classroom. This model uses an inclusion framework for service delivery where all professionals come together as experts in their own fields. The role of a collaborator is to be a facilitator and team member. Collaboration is a cooperative effort focusing on problem solving; e.g., how to best teach the student with disabilities. Intervention and implementation of teaching efforts should follow problem-solving models (Idol, Nevin, & Paolucci-Whitcomb, 2000). Collaboration is direct service delivery as the SLP or special-education teacher is in direct contact with the students. Collaboration needs to be distinguished from consultation. A brief description of consultation follows.

Consultation is defined as the sharing of expertise with others. The recipient (i.e., general-education classroom teacher) perceives that there is a problem and that someone else's expertise (i.e., the SLP) is needed. It should be noted that being an expert does not mean that the information to be shared is presented in an authoritative manner. Consultation is voluntary in that the recipient does not have to implement the suggestions. Consultation can be thought of as

> Consultation refers to sharing one's expertise with others who then work directly with children. For example, an SLP might consult with a classroom teacher, giving recommendations for modifying the curriculum to meet certain children's language needs.

indirect service delivery since the consultant (SLP or special-education teacher) does not directly teach or work with the special needs students.

The degree of involvement taken by consultants may vary with the flow of assistance and information existing along a continuum of services. However, resistance to change is likely to occur. Maintaining familiar roles and familiar service-delivery models can become obstacles to implementation. Other obstacles include time, space and resource allocations and training and support of the key persons involved (i.e., the SLP, special-education teacher, general-education teacher, students, family members and other school personnel). A discussion of various collaborative models follows.

Models of Collaboration

Several service-delivery models are recommended when directly providing speech-language services or special-education services (American Speech-Language-Hearing Association, 1999; Borsch & Oaks, 1993; Westby, 2006): (a) **co-teaching** or **classroom-based team teaching,** wherein the classroom teacher and the SLP or special educator share the responsibility for planning/teaching the lesson, monitoring progress, and making decisions regarding any needed modifications; (b) **classroom-based complementary teaching** wherein the classroom teacher is responsible for teaching the lesson and the special educator or SLP focuses on specific skills or instructional strategies; (c) **supportive teaching** wherein the SLP or special educator incorporates teaching supplemental instructional information related to the curriculum either in the general-education classroom or in a pull-out setting; (d) **pull-out resource management** wherein the SLP collaborates with the classroom; teacher and observes in the classroom; however, instructional support may be provided outside of the classroom; and (e) **self-contained programs** wherein the special educator or SLP is the classroom teacher responsible for both academic/curriculum instruction and speech-language or special-education instruction.

> Speech-language or special-education services can be directly provided through several different service-delivery models.

The first example of collaborative teaching illustrated here consists of **supportive alternate teaching** (Montgomery, 1993). The SLP and special-education teacher alternate in assisting the general classroom teacher. The SLP or special educator may also assist the teacher by outlining lectures on the chalkboard, underlining main points, spelling out new vocabulary, sequencing main ideas, and in general providing strategies for learning. Individualized Education Plan (IEP) goals and objectives may be written for instruction to occur in the general-education classroom to reflect such skills as sequencing, literacy and written language, attainment of main ideas, and categorization. Other examples may include reading fluency and comprehension activities.

> One type of supportive collaboration is the three-week pull-out one week in class alternation sequence.

Another supportive collaborative example consists of a **"three-week pull-out one week in class"** alternation sequence (Montgomery, 1993). In essence, the SLP or special-education teacher provides instruction or services using the pull-out model for three weeks. During the fourth week the SLP or special-education teacher observes the classroom lesson. The special-education teacher or SLP answers questions, assists cooperative learning groups, and/or conducts language

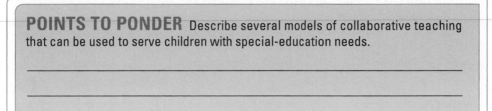

POINTS TO PONDER Describe several models of collaborative teaching that can be used to serve children with special-education needs.

_____

_____

_____

enrichment activities and emergent literacy activities (e.g., assists with phonemic aware-ness, phonics skills, vocabulary, or reading fluency).

An example of a literacy activity may include the following: (a) the SLP or special-education teacher meets with the regular classroom teacher and determines which core reading books are being used that year; (b) the general-education teacher and special-education teacher or SLP share the weekly lesson goals of teaching phonemic awareness and phonics; (c) the SLP or special-education teacher can assist the teacher on those days or conduct the lessons for those days. Lessons may include initial sound identification, final sound identification, and letter identification of one- and two-syllable short words. Students are encouraged to practice good listening habits, discrimination skills, and auditory memory skills. Refer to Table 12.1 for an overview of the different instructional models.

Becoming a collaborative teacher requires that certain steps or procedures be followed in order to ensure cooperation from others. Specifically, the SLP or special-education teacher must obtain the class schedules for each student that she or he wishes to teach in the general-education classroom. The SLP or special-education teacher should then observe those classrooms to find out what the expected classrooms demands are for language (speaking, reading, and writing) and communication.

The SLP or special-education teacher must possess good communication skills. Critical communication and interaction skills include effective listening, appropriate questioning, acceptance and respect of others, and an ability to maintain focus (Vaughn, Bos, & Schumm, 2003). Effective listening requires that the special-education teacher or SLP be able to understand the main concepts in conversation and communicative exchanges. In addition, he or she should allow opportunities for messages to be clearly conveyed and understood (e.g., not hurrying the speaker).

Appropriate use of questions involves knowing when to ask open-ended questions (i.e., questions that require a full range of responses) versus closed questions (i.e., questions that require a minimal answer). Crucial to effective communication is the acceptance of others and the ability to show respect for other teachers and professionals. In sum, the special-education teacher or SLP must be able to maintain a focus to the task of collaboration in the classroom. Schools and classrooms are busy learning environments, and it takes determination to stay focused.

CONNECT & EXTEND

More specific suggestions on communication between professionals are given by Vaughn, S., Bos, C.S., & Schumm, J.S. (2003). _Teaching exceptional, diverse, and at-risk students in the general education classroom_ (3rd ed.). Boston: Allyn & Bacon.

TABLE 12.1   Types of Instructional Models Employed by SLPs and Special-Education Teachers

Environment	SLP or Special-Education Teacher Role	Model
1. General-education classroom	Working with the teacher in the classroom	Collaboration or inclusion
2. General education classroom	Assisting the general-education classroom teacher	Collaboration with supportive teaching
3. General-education classroom	Sharing the responsibility of planning and teaching lessons	Co-teaching
4. Separate classroom	Instruction in another classroom for a portion of the day	Resource room
5. Separate classroom	Academic instruction and specialized instruction (e.g., speech-language or special education) is provided by the SLP or special educator	Self-contained classroom
6. Therapy room	Instructional support is provided outside the classroom	Pull-out or itinerant model
7. Outside the classroom	Information is provided to the general-education classroom teacher. No direct instruction is provided in the general-education classroom, separate classroom, or therapy room	Consultation

> Successful collaboration with classroom teachers requires the SLP or special-education teacher to have good communication skills. These skills include respect for and acceptance of the teachers.

Some other stumbling blocks for collaboration include the fact that all school professionals need to redefine their own roles and perceptions regarding the role of collaboration. The special-education teacher or SLP needs to realize that change involves struggles in role expectations and role release. Therefore, the SLP or special-education teacher will need to take active steps to initiate, choose, and maintain a collaborative program.

Becoming a "team player" is not always an easy transition for either the special-education teacher or SLP. Reviewing the characteristics of successful collaboration will facilitate the transition toward collaborative teaching: (a) teams share common goals; (b) all members contribute equally; (c) leadership is distributed equally; and (d) responsibility for implementing team decisions is shared. The following six steps toward role release or role transition should also facilitate a move toward collaboration.

1. Role extension (information sharing). When new information becomes available then everyone examines how the information can be applied to the needs of the students and making the general education curriculum accessible.

2. Role enrichment. Each professional adds to her knowledge base information gained from another discipline. Examples include examining curriculum materials, attending grade-level meetings, conferencing with teachers, and observing in the classrooms.

3. Role expansion. The SLP or special-education teacher uses new information from other disciplines to better serve the children. The special-education teacher or SLP examines communication in the classroom as a whole, and also communication at school as a whole.

4. Role exchange. SLPs, special-education teachers, and classroom teachers exchange roles. For example, the SLP or special-education teacher assumes the responsibility of teaching content lessons in the general education classroom.

5. Role release. The special-education teacher or SLP allows another professional to take his or her responsibility. It means letting go and trusting the other professional (e.g., the classroom teacher).

6. Role support. Each professional knows that the others bring specific knowledge and skills, and support is given to all members of the collaborative team.

> In optimal collaborative teaching, teams share common goals, all members contribute equally, and responsibility for implementing team decisions is shared.

In sum, successful collaboration includes conviction and commitment of those involved. Components of successful collaboration include the knowledge that administrative support is crucial for success to occur. In addition, responsibility must be shared and parents must be included in the teaching of their children. Martin, Donovan and Senne (2003) stressed the relationship of collaboration and respect for teachers and parents. When this occurs, then the child benefits. Communication with parents can be accomplished with parent-teacher conferences and via regular communication with parents and caregivers (e.g., communicating through the student's daily/weekly planners). Two case studies are presented next to illustrate how best practices and instructional strategies may be implemented with parents, classroom teachers, and other school professionals.

Instructional Strategies for Use with Miguel

What follows are successful strategies that the teacher and paraprofessional implemented in the general-education classroom. These strategies are not time consuming and can be implemented by all educators. In essence, they can be thought of as "good teaching" practices. These teaching practices are informal due to student needs. However, as student needs increase because of disability or other educational issues, then co-teaching planning becomes a much more structured process.

1. Teaching should have a foundation in real learning or learning that is based on contextualization (Figueroa & Ruiz, 1997), or authentic examples. Figueroa and Ruiz stated that reading, writing, listening, and speaking defines 90 percent of special-education programs. Their advice is to let Spanish speakers take risks in English.

CASES TO CONSIDER

Miguel (not his real name) is a bilingual Spanish-English student enrolled in second grade. Spanish is the language of the home. He receives English as a second language (ESL) instruction for reading and some mathematics (in a pull-out type of model for ESL). He receives the rest of his instruction, for the majority of the day, in the general classroom where he has a paraprofessional for mathematics help. He is seated near an English-proficient, Spanish-speaking schoolmate. He is also seated at the front of the classroom near the teacher. Miguel does not present with any language disorders or learning disabilities. Hence, any language or learning difficulties that Miguel experiences are solely attributable to his learning English as a second language. He has been listening to and speaking English for approximately two years. However, information from his experiences in the general classroom shall be reported here.

The general classroom consists of fourteen students. Four students including Miguel are bilingual Spanish-English. Miguel is seated in a cluster of four desks at the front of the room. Desks are arranged so that the students in that cluster face each other. Lessons are conducted in approximately one-hour blocks (e.g., reading for one hour, mathematics for one hour). It may be inferred that Miguel's greatest hurdle in learning is understanding and following directions (e.g., teacher commands) and completing assignments. Note the typical language listening demands placed upon Miguel and how he will need to decipher the key pieces of information to complete the task.

> *Teacher:* "Okay, if you have a book please put it away. And then take out your English book and turn to page 30. Page 30. Remember your English book is the one with the red cover. And you do need a pencil out, but you're not going to need it right away. Start on problems one through ten. Then do problems twenty to thirty. Afterwards we will have our milk break."

Such exchanges are the norm within the general classroom, which proceeds at a fast pace of instruction and which necessitates fast processing abilities. Not only was Miguel able to keep up with the fast pace of instruction, he was also able to learn English as both content and the medium of instruction and he was able to perform well in this classroom and achieve high marks. Can you think of any other classroom modifications that might have been helpful for Miguel? Describe.

_____

_____

_____

2. Teaching should incorporate instances where all students are included in lessons. In one exchange between the teacher and Miguel, he responded to a teacher question about the main topic of "cars" in a short story that was read to the class. Although Miguel's answer and comment were not completely on-task and related, the teacher allowed

Miguel's example from a real situation to be brought into the classroom. She in essence allowed for real language to be contextualized in the lesson. In addition, she acknowledged his response and allowed him to practice his English skills within the lesson. She also acknowledged his response as being acceptable. Miguel, for the most part, comprehended the question, formulated a response, and used his English to participate in the lesson.

> Good teaching practices include using authentic examples and incorporating instances where all students are included in lessons.

3. The teacher in this classroom allowed for longer wait response times from Miguel. While the expected and recommended wait time is from five to seven seconds, the teacher allowed up to 40 seconds for Miguel to respond to higher-level questions in order to accommodate his second language processing needs. In addition, he was given extra time to complete classroom assignments. It should be noted that expectations of his performance were not diminished; he was provided some modifications in order to learn.

4. Miguel was paired with a bilingual, Spanish-English peer, who had higher English skills and could assist him when needed. This assistance was encouraged with Miguel being allowed to look upon the other student's work when following instructions for completing a task. The teacher also circulated around the entire classroom, assisting all students with individual needs. The paraprofessional spent approximately 90 percent of her time with Miguel in explaining and rewording instructions so that he would understand the tasks or content being taught orally.

5. The teacher and paraprofessional used several overt language strategies such as reiterating information and checking for vocabulary understanding. These served to reinforce language comprehension, maintain on-task behaviors, and learn English as a content subject.

6. The general classroom teacher met frequently with the ESL teacher to discuss Miguel's progress and his inclusion in the general-education classroom. These meetings were informal (i.e., when the need arose and for five minutes or less). Although a formalized co-teaching plan had not been set, an informal one did exist. As importantly, the teachers and paraprofessionals were all communicating. The school encouraged an atmosphere of communication. This was evidenced by two facts: all classrooms doors were open, and teachers frequently approached and entered each other's classrooms at any time to request assistance or communicate any pertinent information.

> One variable in Miguel's favor was that his teachers communicated frequently, feeling free to approach and assist each other.

The strategies employed by the general-education teacher and paraprofessional included the following: (a) making learning authentic based on contextualizing lessons and including all students in lessons; (b) allowing for longer wait times; (c) pairing Miguel with a more English-proficient student; (d) using overt strategies of reiterating key words and continuous monitoring for understanding; and (e) meeting with other teachers to discuss individual student needs.

What is notable about these interventions is that all teachers may incorporate these teaching strategies. In addition, these strategies have been found to be successful, yet may

CASES TO CONSIDER

An example of the inclusive environment as a restrictive model can be seen in the following example. The student, whom we will call John (not his real name), was sitting in the back of the classroom with a paraprofessional beside him. It was the beginning of the school day. The general-education teacher was at the front of classroom and after some general classroom activities told the students that it was "time for reading." All of the students, except John, got their reading materials and moved to a designated area on a rug for reading instruction. During classroom reading instruction, John remained in the back of the room working with his paraprofessional. During reading time, John traced his hand on a piece of paper with the assistance of the paraprofessional. Next came math period. The general classroom teacher gave instructions for the students to get out their materials, and the teacher provided instruction. John, however, remained in the back of the room working with his paraprofessional for this additional hour. During this class, John again traced his hand on a piece of paper. John remained in the back of the classroom for the majority of the school day doing activities that were disengaged from those completed by his peers.

Everyone involved in this example was extremely pleased with how the co-teaching model was working in this school (with the possible exception of John's parents). The general-education teacher was pleased because he was given a paraprofessional to work with John in the back of the room, and John was not a particular burden for instruction. The special educator was pleased because John was included with his peers in the general-education setting, and a paraprofessional had been assigned to work with him. The principal was pleased because her school was at the "cutting edge," and all students with disabilities were fully included in the general classroom. It appeared that the paraprofessional had received no training specific to John's needs, but she was pleased with the inclusion model because she was helping John to be "fully included." In addition, she was receiving much reinforcement from the staff for her one-to-one work with John.

During reading and math John was to trace his hand on a piece of paper. This method of co-teaching is an example of an excellent educational concept taking on a life of its own and becoming more important than the education of the student for whom the concept was developed. In this example, we would guess that little or no pretraining was done with teachers regarding methods, materials, or strategies to make co-teaching successful prior to the implementation of the model.

The results are tragically obvious. In this case, collaboration was a more restrictive environment than many of the educational alternatives. It was, in fact, a segregated setting in which the methods and materials of instruction identified the student as too disabled to participate in activities even closely related to those of his nondisabled peers. Why was John not participating in reading or prereading activities during the reading hour? Why was John not participating in mathematics-related activities at an appropriate level during the same time period as his peers? He was certainly capable of learning at the same level of his peers with instructional modifications. Had the instructional team sat down to design a plan to include John with his peers in appropriate or similar activities to the maximum extent possible, or was, in fact, the act of placing of John within the walls of the general-education classroom the criterion for "full inclusion"?

_____

_____

_____

not be implemented with a change in teacher perspective. This is illustrated in the second case presentation where inclusion did not work.

Instructional Strategies for Use with John

It is suggested that this tragic example of ineffective collaborative practices could have been avoided with the use of some simple yet more formal strategies.

1. Placement of any student in a collaborative learning environment should occur only after the educational team, including the general-education classroom teacher, SLP, special-education teacher, paraprofessional assigned to work with the student, and parent(s) have had the opportunity to sit down and design a co-teaching plan that addresses the needs of the student. The collaborative plan should (a) specifically designate the level of co-teaching on a scale from physical inclusion to full academic participation with peers; (b) identify the amount of support from other education professionals, including paraprofessionals, that will be needed to maximize the opportunity of the student to be successful in the inclusive setting; (c) provide for specific training needs of the paraprofessional staff assigned to the student to guarantee quality instruction as well as continuity of instruction across academic settings, and (d) identify who will provide what instruction and during what period of the school day. Specificity in developing this inclusion plan will minimize future disagreements as to who is responsible, who is accountable, what the instruction will be during a specific class period, as well as where the instruction will take place within the classroom.

> Successful collaboration takes careful preplanning and training for all involved with the student.

2. The team must decide what training is needed for the co-teachers to successfully implement the instructional plan. Regardless of who is providing direct instruction for a period of the school day, that person must be provided the skills to implement that portion of the inclusion plan.

When teachers and other school professionals are not provided the skills to implement inclusion successfully, one should anticipate frustration and resentment by teachers and staff toward the inclusion model as well as possible frustration and resentment toward the included student. In environments where training is not provided to meet the needs of students included in the general-education classroom, one should expect that inclusion will be less successful than would be the case with appropriate preparation.

3. Successful collaboration requires formal and informal communication for teams to meet and discuss the progress of students in the inclusive environment. The student's co-teaching plan must be monitored for midcourse corrections in order to remain meaningful.

4. Any educational innovation such as collaborative co-teaching will require that administrators allow for and build into the educational schedule a point in time for teachers and paraprofessionals to meet, discuss, plan, and modify instruction. Collaboration will not occur without the planned intervention of the educational team. Planning takes time, effort, and commitment.

Strategies for Collaboration with Classroom Teachers: Enhancing Listening and Attention Skills

As early as 1960 it was reported by Griffin and Hannah that children spend as much as one-half or more of their time listening to teachers talking. Children move from being incessant talkers to being passive learners in classroom settings beginning as early as kindergarten (Cazden, 1998; McDevitt & Oreskovich, 1993). The pattern of situations where children ask few questions in elementary school settings has been noted by various researchers (Cazden, 2001; Cazden, 1998; Dillon, 1982; Good, Slavings, Harrel, & Emerson, 1987). You will recall that in Chapter 2, we discussed the importance of young children's having a solid foundation in auditory-oral skills, or listening and speaking skills. We said that most schools assume that young children have this solid foundation. However, some children do not.

The estimate of students having to spend their day listening to teachers talking increases dramatically for high school students who may spend up to 90 percent of their school time listening. It has been noted that school discourse places great demands upon listening comprehension, i.e., the ability to understand language (Nelson, 1991). This becomes even more of an issue as age and grade level increase. Therefore, it is essential that the special-education teacher or SLP be able to teach effective listening and auditory processing skills to students with disabilities.

> In most schools, students spend much of their day listening. The amount of time spent listening in school increases greatly as students enter high school.

Nelson (1991) stated that "communication in the classroom relies more on the meaning being expressed within teachers' spoken words or the written words of textual material" (p. 80). Nelson (1991) further stated that

> In addition to language use, the content of language events occurring in classrooms differs widely depending on grade level. Whereas in the earlier grades greater emphasis is placed on learning to read and write and perform basic mathematical computations, in the later grades much of teacher talk centers on topics of substance in the content areas of science, geography, social studies, and literature (p. 82).

POINTS TO PONDER Why is it so important for children to have good listening skills? How can we help them to improve their listening skills?

_____

_____

_____

However, it has been said that **listening skills** are the most neglected area of the language curriculum (Donahue, 1997). Researchers have stated that listening comprehension in schools is very rarely the focus of instruction (Cazden, 2001; Wolvin & Coakley, 1988). Listening plays an important role in the education of students and children as they are expected to listen for a significant amount of time during their school day. Furthermore, Cazden (2001) stated that students' listening comprehension abilities greatly influence their later academic success. However, Cazden stated that instruction in communication most often and typically focuses on reading and writing. The language domains of speaking and listening are assumed to develop without any directive and planned instruction. Consequently, some students will need specific instruction in listening and auditory comprehension. The following strategies are for use in the general-education classroom during content instruction focusing on **enhancing listening comprehension and interaction:**

1. Give instructions during quiet times to enhance auditory comprehension (Brice, Roseberry-McKibbin, & Kayser, 1997).

2. Encourage students to ask questions. Roseberry-McKibbin (2008) suggests that teachers avoid rhetorical, ambiguous, and run-on questions, as they do not encourage dialogue and classroom discourse. In addition, multiple questions are difficult to process for students with auditory comprehension difficulties, and bilingual students needing additional processing time. Questions using vague language (e.g., the teacher or SLP says, "Are there any questions?" or "Is that clear?") may not be understood by students with a different cultural background. Students from some cultural groups may feel that it is rude to indicate that they did not comprehend and, thus, show signs of teacher disrespect by asking for clarification (Roseberry-McKibbin, 2008).

3. Review the previous day's material. Students need advanced organizers and longer lead statements (one or two sentences) as to what is to be taught during a lesson (Brice, Mastin, & Perkins, 1997). Students may also need to hear statements restated and/or summarized from what has been said.

4. Break lessons down into shorter components and scaffold lessons (Brice et al., 1997; Roseberry-McKibbin, 2001). In answering

CONNECT & EXTEND

Detailed information about language use in the classroom is available in Cazden, C.B. (2001). _Classroom discourse: The language of teaching and learning_ (2nd ed.). Portsmouth, NH: Heinemann.

> Because students spend so much of their time listening, general-education teachers should use strategies to support listening comprehension and interaction.

questions, keep in mind that Bloom's (1957) (Knowledge, Comprehension, Application, Analysis, Synthesis, Evaluation) hierarchy should be applied to the different levels of responding that promote higher-level thinking skills. Montgomery (1993) has adapted this taxonomy from least to most difficult:

    i. **Nonverbal responses (Knowledge).** "Show me the picture of the rainforest."

    ii. **Yes/no questions (Comprehension).** "Did Ellen find the painted box?"

    iii. **Embedded in the question (Comprehension).** A closed choice set. "Is this a frog or a toad?"

    iv. **One-word answer (Knowledge).** Also known as a factual question. "What was under the umbrella?"

    v. **Lists (Application).** "Name three animals in Asia."

    vi. **Elicit information (Comprehension).** "What happened to the parrot's home?"

    vii. **Analysis.** "Why is this soup so spicy?"

    viii. **Synthesis.** "What does this picture book have that all books have?"

    ix. **Evaluation.** "Why is this form of plant life so important?"

    5. Relate the information to the student's previous knowledge (Figueroa & Ruiz, 1997). Students retain more in memory when the information is tied to personal experiences (Gathercole & Baddeley, 1993).

Collaborative Instruction

Teachers should implement strategies to enhance attention skills. It has already been noted that school discourse and classroom instruction place great emphases upon listening skills.

> Teachers need to implement strategies to enhance students' attention skills. This will maximize students' listening abilities.

Student seating can be a means to resolve and maximize listening abilities and also minimize auditory and/or visual distractions. The student should be seated in a quiet section of the classroom, i.e., away from noise and possible distractions such as high-traffic areas, open windows, pencil sharpeners, air conditioners, heaters, telephones, the overhead, etc.

Classroom organization strategies for special needs learners, e.g., ELL students and monolingual or bilingual students with language impairments (LIs), may also include use of advance organizers, lead statements, or preparatory sets; that is, the use of language to start lessons (Brice et al., 1997). Children with LI as well as English Language Learner students will need more elaborate lead statements and explanations to be able to follow the teacher's directions, rather than a single sentence. In assessing the student's comprehension, ask for a brief summary of what was said. In addition, ask the student's opinion of the material. The special-education teacher or SLP may use clarification requests to assure comprehension; for example, "Can you tell me what you mean by that?" The following suggestions to make input more comprehensible to students are given: (a) slow down the rate of verbal delivery,

Administrators are responsible for making sure teachers are properly trained in methods, strategies, and materials for collaboration and consultation.

Successful collaboration requires commitment on the part of administrators to allow time to meet and plan as well as time for training.

(b) pause frequently to allow more comprehension time, (c) use shorter sentences and phrases, (d) use fewer multisyllabic words, (e) avoid excessive use of slang or idiomatic speech (e.g., "she really put her foot in her mouth"), and (f) emphasize key words through increased volume and slightly exaggerated rising intonations or variations in pitch.

Strategies for Collaboration with Administrators

Before schools can implement a model of collaboration and consultation, school professionals must be prepared with methods, materials, and strategies for use of these methods. Too often, schools implement co-teaching of students with disabilities without providing teachers with the proper training and support to include students successfully. Collaboration is much more than placement; it must be a planned philosophy of instruction. Administrators have much responsibility to ensure that inclusion will work in their school through proper training of teachers. In many cases, teachers do not feel as if they have been involved in the design of the inclusion model implemented in their schools.

In a study of 211 members of the Minnesota Council for Exceptional Children (MCEC), Brice and Miller (1996) found that 49 percent of special educators and 33 percent of general educators stated that they were "not very involved" or "not involved at all" in the development of the inclusion model in place within their school. Further, Brice and Miller (1996) found that 61 percent of special-education teachers and 47 percent of general-education teachers rated themselves as "not involved" or "not very involved" in the implementation of collaboration services in their school. In order for inclusion to be truly successful in meeting the needs of all students, schools need to plan and prepare teachers for successful implementation. Administrators should ensure that all educators have been provided with the tools to be successful, and teachers must be strongly encouraged to implement the model of inclusion.

As a team, the decision must be made as to what training is needed for the school professionals to successfully implement the collaborative plan. Brice and Miller (1996) found that too few teachers had been provided any training in methods, materials, or strategies for inclusion prior to implementation of the inclusion model. Specifically, these authors found that 29 percent of educators received very little training (one to five hours) and 11 percent of educators received no training or in-service (zero hours) prior to the implementation of their school's inclusion model. Thus, 40 percent of all educators in the study by Brice and Miller (1996) received "very little" or "no" training or in-service.

Successful collaboration requires formal and informal training and opportunities for the teams to meet and discuss the progress of the students in the inclusive environment. The students' inclusion

POINTS TO PONDER Why might students with language impairments have low self-esteem?

_____

_____

_____

plan must be monitored for midcourse corrections in order to remain meaningful. Any educational innovation such as collaboration will require that administrators allow for and build into the educational schedule a point in time for teachers and paraprofessionals to meet, discuss, plan, and modify instruction. Inclusion will not occur without the planned intervention of the educational team. Planning takes time, effort and commitment.

Strategies for Collaboration with Classroom Teachers: Enhancing Students' Self-Esteem

It is important to help students with special needs to communicate successfully with teachers and peers in the classroom setting and vice versa (Westby, 2006). SLPs can work with teachers to facilitate peer interactions within the classroom (Falk-Ross, 2002). Because many students with special needs have difficulties relating to peers (as we have discussed before), teachers may need to "go the extra mile" to promote successful interactions with peers (Beilinson & Olswang, 2003). This is especially true with adolescents (Brinton et al., 2004; Sanger, Moore-Brown, Montgomery, & Hellerich, 2004). Successful classroom interactions help to increase students' self-esteem.

CONNECT & EXTEND

Research regarding the self-esteem of students with language impairments was conducted by Jerome, A.C., Fujiki, M., Brinton, B., & James, S.L. (2002). Self-esteem in children with specific language impairment. *Journal of Speech, Language, and Hearing Research, 45,* 700–714.

A study by Jerome, Fujiki, Brinton, and James (2002) showed that while younger children with language impairments did not differ significantly in their self-esteem from typically developing (TD) peers, older students had lower self-esteem than their TD peers. The older students perceived themselves more negatively in social acceptance, behavioral conduct, and scholastic competence. Sometimes older students who become frustrated act out in violent ways, and this is an increasing problem in our society (Sanger et al., 2004). It is important for professionals who work with these students to help them feel as confident and successful as possible, especially in the classroom. SLPs can collaborate with classroom teachers to help implement strategies for increasing students' self-esteem. Table 12.2 provides specific suggestions for how this might be done. These suggestions can also be applied to the speech-language therapy setting.

TABLE 12.2   Enhancing Self-Esteem for Students with Special Needs in Classroom Settings

Create a climate of trust in the classroom
Examples:

1. Always follow through with fair consequences when students violate rules.
2. Don't make students stay in at recess as a punishment; most students with special needs greatly need the "break time" from class.
3. Avoid unnecessary comparisons between students; highlight students' strengths. For example, the poor reader might be an excellent artist.

Help students recognize and express their feelings
Examples:

1. Provide a vocabulary of emotions beyond "mad, sad, glad." Help students learn terms like "frustrated," "annoyed," "excited," and others that are more specific and descriptive.
2. Be clear and descriptive of your own emotions. For example, one teacher told her students that she felt tired and grouchy because she had slept poorly the night before. She provided a model of describing her emotions without being unkind to the students because of her bad night's sleep.
3. Encourage students to journal about their own feelings, and protect the privacy of these writings.

Help students recognize emotions in others
Examples:

1. For young children, say something like "Look at Jose's face. How do you think he feels when you tell him that you don't want to play with him anymore?"
2. For older students, use readings, videos, and role plays to help them accurately identify emotions in others.

Provide strategies for coping with emotions
Examples:

1. Discuss and practice alternatives such as stopping and thinking about how the other person feels, seeking help, and using anger management strategies such as self-talk or leaving the scene. Many students will understand the concept of "giving myself a time-out to cool down."
2. Model strategies for students. Talk about how you handle anxiety, anger, disappointment, and other emotions. For example, one SLP talks to students about how she exercises as a way to manage stress and the emotions that accompany stress.

Help students recognize cultural differences in the expression of emotion
Examples:

1. Have students write about or discuss how they show emotions in their family.
2. If students have immigrated from another country to the United States, have them share ways that they express various emotions in their country in contrast with those ways emotion is expressed in the United States.
3. Teach students to "check it out"—ask other people how they are feeling.

Adapted with permission from Woolfolk, A. (2004). *Educational psychology* (9th ed.). Boston: Allyn & Bacon.

SUMMARY

- Collaboration occurs when the SLP or special-education teacher has direct contact with the students. Consultation occurs when the SLP or special-education teacher shares his expertise with the teacher but does not directly serve the student.
- When directly providing speech-language or special-education services to students, there are several types of service delivery models: classroom-based team teaching, classroom-based complementary teaching, supportive teaching, pull-out resource management, and self-contained programs.
- All professionals involved in collaboration need to be "team players" who share common goals and responsibilities. Good communication is essential.
- Teachers can implement specific strategies to help students listen and pay attention so they can get the most out of the curriculum. Teachers and SLPs can also help students increase their self-esteem.
- Administrators are responsible for providing training, instruction, and time for team members to meet and collaborate to best serve the needs of all students.

Add your own summary points here:

_____

_____

_____

CONCLUSIONS

In order for collaboration or consultation to become successful, it will require planning and preparation, appropriate communication, and training of teachers, administrators, and educational staff. Brice, Miller, and Brice (in press) have identified five instructional strategies that will facilitate co-teaching and collaboration among SLPs, special-education teachers, and general education teachers. These strategies emphasize **planning** and **communication**:

1. **Plan** lessons and establish what expected learning outcomes should result from the lessons. Outline what adaptations may be needed for children learning English and students with disabilities. Engage in teaching and demonstrating learning strategies that the students may incorporate. Teachers should incorporate lessons beyond use of workbooks. These skills will increase a student's ability to start lessons, comprehend lessons, ask questions, speak out loud, give informative responses, and end lessons.

2. **Plan** lessons jointly with other teachers so that continuity of information may occur across classrooms. Key terms and concepts should be reinforced in both classrooms to

enhance vocabulary and concept acquisition. As a consequence students will be better able to seek clarification due to the unity of lessons across the two classrooms.

3. Plan lessons that allow students to be successful and allow for opportunities to use language in purposeful dialogue, e.g., to accomplish a small group assignment, speak out loud, provide information, ask questions, or to engage and turn-take in other classroom discourse events.

> If professionals plan and communicate appropriately, collaboration will be successful.

4. Establish a routine of **communicating with students.** Engage in turn-taking and exchanging ideas. Incorporate pauses and listen to the students. Communicate frequently with students in one-to-one exchanges. Involve all students in whole-classroom and small-group activities. This will facilitate answering and responding, heuristic, and informational exchanges.

5. Establish a pattern of **communicating with other teachers.** This should be formalized for discussing lessons, students, and educational outcomes. Specific times and days should be set for these co-teacher conferences. Planning will facilitate an easier transition for the students as they move from the ESL classroom to the general-education classroom.

In addition, a significant commitment by the administration to support the collaborative classroom will be necessary. Collaboration will not be successful if implemented in a haphazard manner. If students are to receive the best services according to practices under IDEA or No Child Left Behind, then the students with special needs must receive the most appropriate education in the least restrictive environment. It is anticipated that teachers feel positive about special needs children, that educators become involved in how services are to be delivered, and that SLPs and teachers receive adequate preparation. If this is accomplished, then education to students with disabilities will be provided in a least restrictive environment. It is anticipated that all educators will rise to the opportunities of truly collaborative classrooms.

CHAPTER HIGHLIGHTS

- Over the past decade, the nature of special education has changed in that there is an increased emphasis on giving special-education students access to the general-education curriculum. This is happening through the inclusion movement.
- Inclusion for special-education students involves placing those students in the least restrictive environment.
- The No Child Left Behind Act of 2002 specified four key principles: (1) stronger accountability for students' education performance; (2) greater flexibility for states, school districts, and schools in the use of federal funds; (3) more choices for parents of children from disadvantaged backgrounds; and (4) an emphasis on teaching methods that are scientifically based and have been demonstrated to be effective.
- The most common models of inclusion of speech, language, and special-education instruction to students have consisted of collaboration, co-teaching, and consultation.

- Collaboration is defined as working together and co-teaching with other professionals, providing direct services to students. Consultation means sharing one's expertise with someone else so that person can provide direct and appropriate services to students.
- Various models of collaboration include co-teaching, classroom-based complementary teaching, supportive teaching, pull-out resource management, and self-contained programs.
- Successful collaboration depends heavily upon good communication between professionals, appropriate training, and being given time to collaborate.
- Administrative support is extremely critical to this process. Administrators must provide time and training for general and special educators in order for collaboration to truly work.
- Teachers can be trained to use specific strategies to enhance students' listening comprehension, interaction, attention, and self-esteem.

Add your own chapter highlights here:

_____

_____

_____

STUDY AND REVIEW QUESTIONS

ESSAY

1. What are the key specifications of No Child Left Behind? Describe.

2. Compare and contrast collaboration and consultation. How do they differ from one another?

3. List and briefly describe four things classroom teachers can do to help increase students' listening comprehension and interaction skills.

4. List and briefly describe three things classroom teachers can do to help increase students' self-esteem.

5. What is the role of the administrator in collaboration? Why is the administrator's role so important?

FILL-IN-THE-BLANK

6. The _____ model of service delivery is used for certain categories that require the professional to have less contact with a student and provide less specific classroom instruction.

7. When the special educator or SLP is the classroom teacher, this is a(n) _____ program.

8. When the special education teacher or SLP allows another professional to take one's responsibility, this is called _____.

9. Some experts believe that _____ skills are the most neglected area of the language curriculum.

10. An adaptation of Bloom's hierarchy of skills lists these skills from the least to the most difficult. If a teacher asks a child, "Why is this soup so spicy?" this would be an example of _____.

MULTIPLE CHOICE

11. Trang N., a Laotian student with a language impairment, is fully included in the sixth-grade general-education classroom. His teacher tells you that his self-esteem is quite low and that she is concerned about him. Which of the following would *not* be an appropriate strategy for her to implement to increase Trang's self-esteem?

   a. Tell him that he must only say positive things; he may not talk about his emotions if they are negative because this will just make him feel worse.
   b. Make him stay in at recess as a "time-out" if he violates classroom rules.
   c. Model how she deals with her own emotions, even negative ones.
   d. a, b
   e. a, b, c

12. You work at a public high school where the teachers have been told they need to collaborate with the SLP and other special educators to fully include students with disabilities in their classrooms. These teachers have been accustomed to students with disabilities being served through an itinerant model where they were pulled out of class. Now the teachers are being told that they are responsible for meeting the students' needs inside the classroom. In the teachers' lounge, you hear that most of them are very unhappy at being asked to implement this collaborative model. How can you help them have a positive attitude toward collaboration and work with you without resenting you?

   a. Make sure the principal is not involved; this would only make the teachers feel more resentful.
   b. Obtain class schedules for each special-education student that you wish to teach in the general-education classroom, then go and observe those classrooms to see what the curriculum demands are.
   c. When communicating with the teachers, be careful to ask primarily closed-ended questions, as this will save time and help them to feel like you are being efficient.
   d. b, c
   e. a, b, c

13. Successful strategies for helping English Language Learners and special-education children succeed in the general classroom include

   a. Allowing longer wait response times (e.g., giving these students more time to answer questions)

   b. Having all professionals involved with these students design co-teaching plans that address the needs of these students
   c. Encouraging students to ask questions
   d. b, c
   e. a, b, c

14. You are collaborating with a classroom teacher and are sharing with him how to promote higher level thinking skills in his students. One of the things that you will tell him is that higher-level questions involve

   a. Nonverbal responses and yes/no questions
   b. Yes/no questions and comprehension questions
   c. Analysis, synthesis, and evaluation questions
   d. Comprehension and synthesis questions
   e. One-word answer (factual) questions and yes/no questions

15. Successful collaboration with administrators involves

   a. Making sure that administrators involve the teachers in the design of the inclusion model implemented in their schools
   b. Making sure that administrators strongly encourage teachers to implement the inclusion model
   c. Telling administrators not to worry about having to provide extra time for teachers to collaborate; this can be done during the weekly staff meeting
   d. a, b
   e. a, b, c

See Answers to Study and Review Questions, page 465.

Answers to Chapter Study and Review Questions

Chapter 1
6. morpheme, allomorph
7. compound, complex
8. kernel sentence, phrase, base
9. narrative
10. telegraphic
11. D
12. D
13. C
14. E
15. A

Chapter 2
6. Language
7. Noam Chomsky, Language Acquisition Device
8. Echoics
9. behaviorist, stimulation, response, reinforcement
10. Lev Vygotsky, function, structure
11. A
12. C
13. D
14. E
15. B

Chapter 3
6. Acculturation
7. Transfer/Interference
8. codeswitching
9. subtractive bilingualism
10. monolingual norm assumption/ limited capacity hypothesis
11. D
12. C
13. A
14. D
15. B

Chapter 4
6. cultural pluralism
7. Situational
8. acculturated
9. call-and-response
10. Culture
11. D
12. C
13. A
14. E
15. B

Chapter 5
6. Static
7. format, situational
8. Interjudge
9. Screening
10. concurrent
11. B
12. B
13. A
14. D
15. C

Chapter 6
6. satiation
7. parallel
8. mand-model (or elicited imitation)
9. receptive
10. fixed
11. B
12. C
13. E
14. D
15. A

Chapter 7
6. cultural mediator
7. Language Development Survey
8. direct intervention
9. phonological awareness
10. Public Law 99-457
11. D
12. C
13. A
14. B
15. A

Chapter 8
6. No Child Left Behind Act; Individuals with Disabilities Education Improvement Act of 2004 (Public Law 108-446).
7. metalinguistic
8. scotopic sensitivity syndrome
9. dysgraphia
10. Neurological Impress Method
11. C
12. A
13. B
14. A
15. C

Chapter 9
6. telegraphic speech
7. perseveration
8. theory of mind
9. hyperlexia
10. Sensory integration
11. D
12. E
13. C
14. A
15. A

Chapter 10
6. Title I of the Elementary and Secondary Education Act
7. neglect
8. hyperactive-impulsive ADHD
9. fetal alcohol syndrome
10. HIV (or AIDS)
11. A
12. D
13. E
14. B
15. C

Chapter 11
6. otitis media
7. spastic
8. Duchenne
9. opaque
10. total communication
11. D
12. A
13. C
14. E
15. B

Chapter 12
6. itinerant
7. self-contained
8. role release
9. listening
10. analysis
11. D
12. B
13. E
14. C
15. D

References

Aarts, N.L. (2001). Audiology overseas: A Saudi experience. *Hearsay: Journal of the Ohio Speech-Language-Hearing Association, 14,* 28–39.

Allen, T. (1986). Patterns of academic achievement among hearing impaired students. In A. Schildroth & M. Karchmer (Eds.), *Deaf children in America.* Austin, TX: Pro-Ed.

Alt, M., Plante, E., & Creusere, M. (2004). Semantic features in fast-mapping: Performance of preschoolers with specific language impairment versus preschoolers with normal language. *Journal of Speech, Language, and Hearing Research, 47,* 407–420.

American Academy of Pediatrics (2001). Adolescents and human immunodeficiency virus infection: The role of the pediatrician in prevention and intervention. *Pediatrics, 107,* 1–5.

American Association on Mental Retardation (1992). *Mental retardation: Definition, classification, and systems of support* (9th ed.). Washington, DC: Author.

American Association on Mental Retardation (2002). *Definition of mental retardation and fact sheet: FAQs about mental retardation.* Retrieved July 10, 2004, from www.aamr.org.

American Psychiatric Association (1994). *Diagnostic and statistical manual of mental disorders* (4th ed.). Washington, DC: Author.

American Psychiatric Association (2000). *Diagnostic and statistical manual of mental disorders: DSM-IV-TR* (4th ed., text revision). Washington, DC: Author.

The ASHA Committee on Language, Speech, and Hearing Services in the Schools (April, 1980). Definitions for communicative disorders and differences. *ASHA, 22,* pp. 317–318.

American Speech-Language-Hearing Association (2000). *Roles and responsibilities of speech-language pathologists with respect to reading and writing in children and adolescents: Guidelines and technical report.* Rockville, MD: ASHA.

American Speech-Language-Hearing Association (2004). *Special populations: Pediatric HIV/AIDS—2004 edition.* Retrieved 7/28/05 from www.asha.org/members/research/reports/hiv_aids

American Speech-Language-Hearing Association (2005). Introduction to evidence-based practice: What it is (and what it isn't). Retrieved 6/4/05 from www.asha.org/members/ebp/default.

Anastasiow, N.J., Hanes, M.L., & Hanes, M. (1982). *Language and reading strategies for poverty children.* Baltimore, MD: University Park Press.

Andersen, E., Dunlea, A., & Kekelis, L. (1984). Blind children's language: Resolving some differences. *Journal of Child Language, 11,* 645–664.

Andersen, E., Dunlea, A., & Kekelis, L. (1993). The impact of input: Language acquisition in the visually impaired. *First Language, 13,* 23–50.

Anderson, K.L. (2004). Speech perception benefits of FM and infared devices to children with hearing aids in a typical classroom. *Language, Speech, and Hearing Services in Schools, 35,* 169–184.

Anderson, R.T. (1999). Impact of first language loss on grammar in a bilingual child. *Communication Disorders Quarterly, 21,* 4–16.

Anderson, R.T. (2004). First language loss in Spanish-speaking children: Patterns of loss and implications for clinical practice. In B.A. Goldstein (Ed.), *Bilingual language development and disorders in Spanish-English speakers* (pp. 187–212). Baltimore, MD: Paul H. Brookes Publishing Co.

Apel, K. (2002). Serving students with spoken and written language challenges: It's in the cards. *The ASHA Leader, 7,* 6–7.

Apel, K., Masterson, J.J., & Niessen, N.L. (2004). Spelling assessment frameworks. In C.A. Stone, E.R. Silliman, B.J. Ehren, & K. Apel (Eds.). *Handbook of language and literacy: Development and disorders* (pp. 644–660). New York: The Guilford Press.

Aram, D.M., & Nation, J. (1980). Preschool language disorders and subsequent language and academic difficulties. *Journal of Communication Disorders, 13,* 159–170.

Aram, D.M., Ekelman, B., & Nation, J.E. (1984). Preschoolers with language disorders: 10 years later. *Journal of Speech and Hearing Research, 27,* 232–244.

Atkin, R., Bray, R., Davison, M., Herzberger, S., Humphreys, L., & Selzer, U. (1977). Cross-lagged panel analysis of sixteen cognitive measures at four grade levels. *Child Development, 48,* 944–952.

Bagli, A. (2002). Multicultural aspects of deafness. In D.E. Battle (Ed.), *Communication disorders in multicultural populations* (3rd ed.) (pp. 361–414). Woburn, MA: Butterworth-Heinemann.

Baker, C. (2000). *A parents' and teachers' guide to bilingualism* (2nd ed.). London: Anness Publishing.

Baker, L., Mackler, K., Sonnenschein, S., & Serpell, R. (2001). Parents' interactions with their first-grade children during storybook reading and relations with subsequent home reading activity and reading achievement. *Journal of School Psychology, 39*, 415–438.

Balandin, S. (2005). Language impairment and augmentative and alternative communication (AAC). In V.A. Reed, *An introduction to children with language disorders* (3rd ed.) (pp. 384–403). Boston: Allyn & Bacon.

Baltaxe, C. (2001). Emotional, behavioral, and other psychiatric disorders of childhood associated with communication disorders. In T. Layton, E. Crais, and L. Watson (Eds.), *Handbook of early language impairment in children: Nature* (pp. 63–125). Albany, NY: Delmar Publishers.

Barkley, R.A. (2000). *Taking charge of ADHD: The complete, authoritative guide for parents* (rev. ed.). NY: Guildford Press.

Barnett, W.S., & Camilli, G. (2002). Compensatory preschool education, cognitive development, and "race." In J.M. Fish (Ed.), *Race and intelligence: Separating science from myth* (pp. 369–406). Mahwah, NJ: Lawrence Erlbaum.

Bashe, P.R., & Kirby, B.L. (2001). *The Oasis guide to Asperger syndrome: Advice, support, insights, and inspiration*. New York: Crown Publishers.

Battle, D.E. (2002). Language development and disorders in culturally and linguistically diverse children. In D.K. Bernstein and E. Tiegermann-Farber, *Language and communication disorders in children* (5th ed.) (pp. 354–386). Boston: Allyn & Bacon.

Battle, D.E., & Anderson, N. (1998). Culturally diverse families and the development of language. In D.E. Battle (Ed.), *Communication disorders in multicultural populations* (2nd ed.) (pp. 213–246). Newton, MA: Butterworth-Heinemann.

Bauman-Waengler, J. (2004). *Articulatory and phonological disorders: A clinical focus* (3rd ed.). Boston: Allyn & Bacon.

Bayley, N. (1993). *Bayley Scales of Infant Mental Development—Revised (ed. 2)*. New York: Psychological Corporation.

Beck, A., & Fritz-Verticchio, H. (2003). The influence of information and role-playing experiences on children's attitudes toward peers who use AAC. *American Journal of Speech-Language Pathology, 12*, 51–60.

Bedore, L.M. (2004). Morphosyntactic development. In B.A. Goldstein (Ed.), *Bilingual language development and disorders in Spanish-English speakers* (pp. 163–186). Baltimore, MD: Paul H. Brookes Publishing Co.

Bedore, L.M., & Leonard, L.B. (2001). Grammatical morphology deficits in Spanish-speaking children with specific language impairment. *Journal of Speech, Language, and Hearing Research, 44(*4), 905–924.

Bedore, L.M., Peña, E.D., Garcia, M., & Cortez, C. (2005). Conceptual versus monolingual scoring: When does it make a difference? *Language, Speech, and Hearing Services in Schools, 36*, 188–200.

Bedrosian, J.L., Hoag, L.A., & McCoy, K.F. (2003). Relevance and speed of message delivery trade-offs in augmentative and alternative communication. *Journal of Speech, Language, and Hearing Research, 46*, 800–817.

Beilinson, J.S., & Olswang, L.B. (2003). Facilitating peer-group entry in kindergarteners with impairments in social communication. *Language, Speech, and Hearing Services in Schools, 34*, 154–166.

Beirne-Smith, M., Ittenbach, R.F., & Patton, J.R. (2002). *Mental retardation* (6th ed.). Upper Saddle River, NJ: Merrill.

Bell, N. (1991). *Visualizing and verbalizing for language comprehension and thinking*. Paso Robles, CA: Academy of Reading Publications.

Bender, W.N. (2004*). Learning disabilities: Characteristics, identification, and teaching strategies* (5th ed.). Boston: Allyn & Bacon.

Bennett, C.I. (2003). *Comprehensive multicultural education: Theory and practice* (4th ed.). Boston: Allyn & Bacon.

Berglund, E., Eriksson, M., & Johansson, I. (2001). Parental reports of spoken language skills in children with Down syndrome. *Journal of Speech, Language, and Hearing Research, 44*, 179–191.

Bernstein, D.K. (2002). The nature of language and its disorders. In D.K. Bernstein & E. Tiegerman-Farber, *Language and communication disorders in children* (5th ed.) (pp. 2–26). Boston: Allyn & Bacon.

Bernstein, D.K., & Tiegerman-Farber, E. (2002). *Language and communication disorders in children* (5th ed.). Boston: Allyn & Bacon.

Bernstein, D.K., & Levey, S. (2002). Language development: A review. In D.K. Bernstein & E. Tiegerman-Farber, *Language and communication disorders in children* (5th ed.) (pp. 27–94). Boston: Allyn & Bacon.

Bernstein Ratner, N. (2005). Atypical language development. In J.B. Gleason (Ed.), *The development of language* (6th ed.), pp. 324–395. Boston: Allyn & Bacon.

Bernthal, J., & Bankson, N. (2004). *Articulation and phonological disorders* (5th ed.). Boston: Allyn & Bacon.

Berko Gleason, J. (2005). *The development of language* (6th ed.). Needham Heights, MA: Allyn & Bacon.

Betancourt, H., & Lopez, S.R. (1993). The study of culture, ethnicity, and race in American psychology. *American Psychologist, 48*, 629–637.

Beverly, B.L., & Williams, C.C. (2004). Present tense *be* use in young children with specific language impairment: Less is more. *Journal of Speech, Language, and Hearing Research, 47*, 944–956.

Bhatia, T.K., & Ritchie, W.C. (1999). The bilingual child: Some issues and perspectives. In W.C. Ritchie & T.K. Bhatia (Eds.), *Handbook of child language acquisition* (pp. 569–646). San Diego: Academic Press.

Bialystok, E. (1997). Effects of bilingualism and biliteracy on children's emerging concepts of print. *Developmental Psychology, 33*, 429–440.

Bialystok, E. (2001). *Bilingualism in development: Language, literacy, and cognition*. New York: Cambridge University Press.

Bigelow, A. (1987). Early words of blind children. *Journal of Child Language, 11*, 645–664.

Bigelow, A. (1990). Relationship between the development of language and thought in young blind children. *Journal of Visual Impairment and Blindness, 84*, 414–419.

Bishop, D.V.M., & Adams, C. (1990). A prospective study of the relationship between specific language impairment, phonological disorder, and reading retardation. *Journal of Child Psychology and Psychiatry, 31*, 1027–1050.

Bishop, D.V. M., & Edmundson, A. (1987). Language-impaired four year olds: Distinguishing transient from persistent impairment. *Journal of Speech and Hearing Disorders, 52*, 155–173.

Bishop, D.V. M., Price, T.S., Dale, P.S., & Plomin, R. (2004). Outcomes of early language delay: II. Etiology of transient and persistent language difficulties. *Journal of Speech, Language, and Hearing Research, 46*, 561–575.

Blachman, B.A. (1991). Early intervention for children's reading problems: Clinical applications of the research in phonological awareness. *Topics in Language Disorders, 12*, 51–65.

Blakemore-Brown, L. (2002). *Reweaving the autistic tapestry: Autism, Asperger syndrome, and ADHD*. London: Jessica Kingsley Publishers.

Bliss, L.S. (2002). *Discourse impairments: Assessment and intervention applications*. Boston, MA: Allyn & Bacon.

Bliss, L.S., McCabe, K., & Mahecha, N. (2001). Analyses of narratives from Spanish-speaking bilingual children. *Contemporary Issues in Communication Sciences and Disorders, 28*, 733–739.

Bloom, B. (1957). *Taxonomy of educational objectives: The classification of educational goals by a committee of college and university examiners*. New York, NY: McKay.

Bloom, L., & Lahey, M. (1978). *Language development and disorders*. New York: Macmillan.

Bohannon, J.N., & Bonvillian, J.D. (2005). Theoretical approaches to language acquisition. In J. Berko Gleason, *The development of language* (6th ed.) (pp. 230–291). Boston: Allyn & Bacon.

Bondy, A.S., & Frost, L.A. (1998). The picture exchange communication system. *Seminars in Speech and Language, 19*, 373–388.

Bopp, K.D., Brown, K.E., & Mirenda, P. (2004). Speech-language pathologists' roles in the delivery of positive behavior support for individuals with developmental disabilities. *American Journal of Speech-Language Pathology, 13*, 5–19.

Boudreau, D. (2005). Use of a parent questionnaire in emergent and early literacy assessment of preschool children. *Language, Speech, and Hearing Services in Schools, 36*, 33–47.

Boudreau, D.M., & Chapman, R.S. (2000). The relationship between event representation and linguistic skill in narratives and adolescents with Down syndrome. *Journal of Speech, Language, and Hearing Research, 43*, 1146–1159.

Bourassa, D.C., & Treiman, R. (2001). Spelling development and disability: The importance of linguistic factors. *Language, Speech, and Hearing Services in Schools, 32*, 172–181.

Bowe, F. (2000). *Physical, sensory, and health disabilities*. Upper Saddle River, NJ: Merrill.

Braaten, B., & Mennes, D. (1992). A model of collaborative service for middle school students. *Preventing School Failure, 36*, 10–15.

Braaten, S., Kauffman, J.M., Braaten, B., Polsgrove, L., & Nelson, C.M. (1988). The regular education initiative: Patent medicine for behavioral disorders. *Exceptional Children, 55*, 21–27.

Brackett, D. (2002). Management options for children with hearing loss. In J. Katz (Ed.), *Handbook of clinical audiology* (5th ed.) (pp. 758–766). Baltimore, MD: Lippincott Williams and Wilkins.

Bradley, R.H., Corwyn, R.F., Pipes-McAdoo, H., & Garcia-Coll, C. (2001). The home environments of children in the United States Part I: Variations by age, ethnicity, and poverty status. *Child Development, 72*, 1844–1867.

Bradlow, A.R., Kraus, N., & Hayes, E. (2003). Speaking clearly for children with learning disabilities: Sentence perception in noise. *Journal of Speech, Language, and Hearing Research, 46*, 80–97.

Brady, N.C. (2004). Introduction to the clinical form on communication interventions for individuals with severe disabilities. *American Journal of Speech-Language Pathology, 13*, 3–4.

Breier, J. I., Fletcher, J.M., Foorman, B.R., Klaas, P., & Gray, L.C. (2003). Auditory temporal processing in children with specific reading disability with and without attention deficit/hyperactivity disorder. *Journal of Speech, Language, and Hearing Research, 46*, 31–42.

Brice, A. (2002). *The Hispanic child: Speech, language, culture, and education.* Boston: Allyn & Bacon.

Brice, A., & Anderson, R. (1999). Code mixing in a young bilingual child. *Communication Disorders Quarterly, 21,* 17–22.

Brice, A., & Brice, R. (2007) (Eds.). *Language development: Monolingual and bilingual acquisition.* Old Tappan, NJ: Merrill/Prentice Hall.

Brice, A., Mastin, M., & Perkins, C. (1997b). English, Spanish, and code switching use in the ESL classroom: An ethnographic study. *Journal of Children's Communication Development, 19,* 11–20.

Brice, A., Miller, K., & Brice, R.G. (submitted). A case study of two classrooms: Implications for speech-language pathologists and special education teachers. *Communication Disorders Quarterly.*

Brice, A., & Miller, R.J. (1996, March). Minnesota council for exceptional children inclusion survey. *MCEC Newsletter, 8,* 7.

Brice, A., & Montgomery, J. (1996). Adolescent pragmatic skills: A comparison of Latino students in English as a second language and speech and language programs. *Language, Speech, and Hearing Services in Schools, 27,* 68–81.

Brice, A., & Perkins, C. (1997). What is required for transition from the ESL classroom to the general education classroom? A case study of two classrooms. *Journal of Children's Communication Development, 19,* 13–22.

Brice, A., & Roseberry-McKibbin, C. (1999). A case example of a bilingual evaluation: A tutorial. *Florida Journal of Communication Disorders, 19,* 25–31.

Brice, A., Roseberry-McKibbin, C., & Kayser, H. (1997, November). *Special language needs of linguistically and culturally diverse students.* Paper presented at the annual convention of the American Speech-Language-Hearing Association, Boston, MA.

Brinton, B., & Fujiki, M. (1999). Social interactional behaviors of children with specific language impairment. *Topics in Language Disorders, 19,* 49–69.

Brinton, B., & Fujiki, M. (2004). Social and affective factors in children with language impairment: Implications for literacy learning. In C.A. Stone, E.R. Silliman, B.J. Ehren, & K. Apel (Eds.), *Handbook of language and literacy: Development and disorders* (pp. 130–153). New York: The Guilford Press.

Brinton, B., Robinson, L.A., & Fujiki, M. (2004). Description of a program for social language intervention: "If you can have a conversation, you can have a relationship." *Language, Speech, and Hearing Services in Schools, 35,* 283–290.

Brown, L.B. (2002). *Reweaving the autistic tapestry: Autism, Asperger syndrome and ADHD.* London: Jessica Kingsley Publishers, Ltd.

Brown, R. (1973). *A first language: early stages.* Cambridge, MA: Harvard University.

Brown, M.R., Higgins, K., & Hartley, K. (2001). Teachers and technology equity. *Teaching Exceptional Children, 33,* 32–49.

Bruner, J. (1968). *Processes of cognitive growth: Infancy (Vol. III, Heinz Werner Lecture Series).* Worcester, MA: Clark University Press.

Bryne, M.R. (2000). Parent-professional collaboration to promote spoken language in a child with a severe to profound hearing loss. *Communication Disorders Quarterly 21,* 210–223.

Calculator, S.N. (2000). Augmentative and alternative communication. In E.P. Dodge (Ed.), *The survival guide for school-based speech-language pathologists* (pp. 345–366). San Diego: Singular/Thomson Learning.

Camarota, S.A. (2003). Immigration in a time of recession: An examination of trends since 2000. Retrieved July 23, 2004, from www.cis.org/articles/2003/back16003.html.

Campbell, L.R. (1993). Maintaining the integrity of home linguistic varieties: Black English Vernacular. *American Journal of Speech-Language Pathology, 2,* 85–86.

Campbell, T., Dollaghan, C., Needleman, H., & Janosky, J. (1997). Reducing bias in language assessment: Processing-dependent measures. *Journal of Speech, Language, and Hearing Research, 40,* 519–525.

Cassar, M., & Treiman, R. (2004). Developmental variations in spelling: Comparing typical and poor spellers. In C.A. Stone, E.R. Silliman, B.J. Ehren, & K. Apel (Eds.). *Handbook of language and literacy: Development and disorders* (pp. 627–643). New York: The Guilford Press.

Castellani, J., & Jeffs, T. (2001). Emerging reading and writing strategies using technology. *Teaching Exceptional Children, 33,* 60–67.

Catts, H. (1986). Speech production/phonological deficits in reading disordered children. *Journal of Learning Disabilities, 19,* 504–508.

Catts, H.W. (1991). Early identification of reading disabilities. *Topics in Language Disorders, 12*(1), 1–16.

Catts, H.W. (1993). The relationship between speech-language impairments and reading disabilities. *Journal of Speech and Hearing Research, 36,* 948–958.

Catts, H.W., Fey, M.E., Tomblin, J.B., & Zhang, X. (2002). Longitudinal investigation of reading outcomes in children with language impairment. *Journal of Speech, Language, and Hearing Research, 45,* 1142–1157.

Catts, H.W., & Kamhi, A.G. (1999). *Language and reading disabilities.* Boston: Allyn & Bacon.

Cazden, C.B. (1998). *Two meanings of discourse.* (ERIC Document Reproduction Service No. ED 420198).

Cazden, C.B. (2001). *Classroom discourse: The language of teaching and learning* (2nd ed.). Portsmouth, NH: Heinemann.

Centers for Disease Control and Prevention (2000, August). Pediatric AIDS cases by exposure category and race/ethnicity, reported through December, 2000. *HIV/AIDS Surveillance Report, 12*(2).

Center for Immigration Studies (2001). Available at www.cis.org/articles/2001/back101.html.

Chall, J.S., & Jacobs, V.A. (2003). Research round-up: Poor children's fourth grade slump. *American Educator,* Spring 2003. Retrieved 12/3/04 from www.aft.org/pubs-reports/american_educator/spring2003/chall.html

Chall, J.S., Jacobs, V.A., & Baldwin, L.E. (1990). *The reading crisis: Why poor children fall behind.* Cambridge, MA: Harvard University Press.

Champion, T., & Mainess, K. (2003). Typical and disordered narration in African American children. In McCabe, A., & Bliss, L.S., *Patterns of narrative discourse: A multicultural, lifespan approach* (pp. 55–70).

Chan, S., & Lee, E. (2004). Families with Asian roots. In E.W. Lynch and M.J. Hanson (Eds.), *Developing cross-cultural competence: A guide for working with young children and their families* (pp. 219–298). Baltimore, MD: Paul H. Brookes Publishing Co.

Chao, R. (1995). Chinese and European American cultural models of the self reflected in mothers' childrearing beliefs. *Ethos, 23,* 328–354.

Chapman, R.S., Seung, H.-K., Schwartz, S.E., & Kay-Raining Bird, E. (1998). Language skills of children and adolescents with Down syndrome: II. Production deficits. *Journal of Speech, Language, and Hearing Research, 41,* 861–873.

Chapman, R.S., Seung, H.-K., Schwartz, S.E., & Kay-Raining Bird, E. (2000). Predicting language production in children and adolescents with Down syndrome: The role of comprehension. *Journal of Speech, Language, and Hearing Research, 43,* 340–350.

Chasnoff, I.J., & Griffith, I.N. (1989). Cocaine, pregnancy, and the neonate. *Women and Health, 15,* 23–25.

Cheng, L.L. (1991). *Assessing Asian language performance* (2nd ed.). Oceanside, CA: Academic Communication Associates.

Cheng, L.L. (2002). Asian and Pacific American cultures. In D.E. Battle (Ed.), *Communication disorders in multicultural populations* (3rd ed.) (pp. 71–112). Woburn, MA: Butterworth-Heinemann.

Children and Adults with Attention-Deficit/Hyperactivity Disorder (CHADD, 2005). *The disorder named AD/HD—CHADD Fact Sheet #1.* Retrieved June 13, 2005, from www.chadd.org.

Chomsky, N. (1981). *Lectures on government and binding.* Dordrecht, The Netherlands: Foris.

Chomksy, N. (1982). *Some concepts and consequences of the theory of government and binding.* Cambridge, MA: MIT Press.

Clark-Klein, S.M. (1994). Expressive phonological deficiencies: Impact on spelling development. *Topics in Language Disorders, 14,* 40–55.

Cochlear Corporation (2002). *Package insert for Nucleus 24 Contour* [Brochure]. Sydney, Australia: Author.

Cognitive Concepts (1997–2003). *Earobics: Sound foundations for reading and spelling.* Evanston, IL: Cognitive Concepts.

Coles-White, D. (2004). Negative concord in child African American English: Implications for specific language impairment. *Journal of Speech, Language, and Hearing Research, 47,* 212–222.

Coleman, T. (2000). *Clinical management of communication disorders in culturally diverse children.* Boston: Allyn & Bacon.

Collier, V.P. (1987). Age and rate of acquisition of second language for academic purposes. *TESOL Quarterly, 21,* 617–641.

Coltrane, B. (2003). Working with young English language learners: Some considerations. *ERIC Digest, 5/03,* 1–5. Available at www.cal.org/ericcll/digest/0301coltrane.html

Commission on Excellence in Special Education (2001). Revitalizing special education for children and their families. Available from www.ed.gov/inits/commissionsboards/whspecialeducation

Condouris, K., Meyer, E., & Tager-Flusberg, H. (2003). The relationship between standardized measures of language and measures of spontaneous speech in children with autism. *American Journal of Speech-Language Pathology and Audiology, 12,* 349–358.

Conners, F.A., Carr, M.D., & Willis, S. (1998). Is the phonological loop responsible for intelligence-related differences in forward digit span? *American Journal on Mental Retardation, 103,* 1–11.

Connor, C.M., & Zwolan, T.A. (2004). Examining multiple sources of influence on the reading comprehension skills of children who use cochlear implants. *Journal of Speech, Language, and Hearing Research, 47,* 509–526.

Conti-Ramsden, G. (2003). Processing and linguistic markers in young children with specific language impairment (SLI). *Journal of Speech, Language, and Hearing Research, 46*(5), 1029–1037.

Conti-Ramsden, G., & Botting, N. (2004). Social difficulties and victimization in children with SLI at 11 years of age. *Journal of Speech, Language, and Hearing Research, 47*(1), 145–162.

Conti-Ramsden, G., Simkin, Z., & Pickels, A. (2006). Estimating familial loading in SLI: A comparison of direct assessment versus parental interview. *Journal of Speech, Language, and Hearing Research, 49,* 88–101.

Cooper, P. (1999). ADHD and effective learning: Principles and practical approaches. In P. Cooper & K. Bilton (Eds.), *ADHD: Research, practice, and opinion* (pp. 138–157). London: Whurr Publishers.

Coster, W., & Ciacchetti, D. (1993). Research on the communicative development of maltreated children: Clinical implications. *Topics in Language Disorders, 13*, 25–28.

Coster, W.J., Gersten, M.S., Beeghly, M., & Cicchetti, D. (1989). Communicative functioning in maltreated toddlers. *Developmental Psychology, 25*, 1020–1029.

Cotton, S., Voudouris, N.J., & Greenwood, K.M. (2001). Intelligence and Duchenne muscular dystrophy: Full-scale, verbal, and performance intelligence quotients. *Developmental Medicine and Child Neurology, 43*, 497–501.

Council for Exceptional Children (1991). *Report of the CEC advocacy and governmental relations committee regarding the new proposed U.S. federal definition of serious emotional disturbance.* Reston, VA: Author.

Council for Exceptional Children (1993). CEC policy on inclusive schools and community settings. *Supplement to Teaching Exceptional Children, 25*, 1.

Craig, H.K., & Washington, J.A. (2002). Oral language expectations for African American preschoolers and kindergarteners. *American Journal of Speech-Language Pathology, 11*, 59–70.

Craig, H.K., & Washington, J. (2004a). Grade-related changes in the production of African American English. *Journal of Speech, Language, and Hearing Research, 47*, 450–463.

Craig, H.K., & Washington, J. (2004b). Language variation and literacy learning. In C.A. Stone, E.R. Silliman, B.J. Ehren, & K. Apel (Eds.), *Handbook of language and literacy: Development and disorders* (pp. 228–243). New York: The Guilford Press.

Craig, H.K., Thompson, C.A., Washington, J.A., & Potter, S.L. (2004). Performance of elementary-grade African American students on the Gray Oral Reading Tests. *American Journal of Speech-Language Pathology, 13*, 141–154.

Craig, H.K., Washington, J.A., & Thomson-Porter, C. (1998). Average C-unit lengths in the discourse of African American children from low-income, urban homes. *Journal of Speech-Language-Hearing Research, 41*, 433–444.

Crandell, C.C., Smaldino, J.J., & Flexer, C. (2005). *Sound field amplification: Applications to speech perception and classroom acoustics* (2nd ed.). Clifton Park, NY: Delmar Learning.

Creaghead, N. (1994). Collaborative intervention. In N. Creaghead & D. Ripich (Eds.). *School discourse problems* (2nd ed.), (pp. 373–386). San Diego, CA: Singular Publishing.

Crouch, R. (1997). Letting the deaf be deaf: Reconsidering the use of cochlear implants in prelingually deaf children. *Hastings Center Reports, 27*, 14–21.

Crowe, L.K. (2003). Comparison of two reading feedback strategies in improving the oral and written language performance of children with language-learning disabilities. *American Journal of Speech-Language Pathology, 12*, 16–27.

Crowley, C.J. (2003). *Diagnosing communication disorders in culturally and linguistically diverse students. ERIC Digest E650.* Arlington, VA: ERIC Clearinghouse on Disabilities and Gifted Education.

Crowley, C.J. (2004). The ethics of assessment with culturally and linguistically diverse populations. *The ASHA Leader, 9*, 6–7.

Cummins, J. (1984). *Bilingualism and special education: Issues in assessment and pedagogy.* San Diego, CA: College Hill Press.

Cummins, J. (1992). The role of primary language development in promoting educational success for language minority students. In C. Leyba (Ed.), *Schooling and language minority students: A theoretical framework* (pp. 3–50). California State University, Los Angeles: Los Angeles, CA.

Cummins, J. (2000). *Language, power, and pedagogy: Bilingual children in the cross-fire.* Clevedon, England: Multilingual Matters.

Cummins, J. (2002). Foreword. In P. Gibbons, *Scaffolding language, scaffolding learning: Teaching second language learners in the mainstream classroom.* Portsmouth, NH: Heinemann.

Cupples, L., & Ianoco, T. (2000). Phonological awareness and oral reading skill in children with Down syndrome. *Journal of Speech, Language, and Hearing Research, 43*, 595–608.

Currenton, S.M., & Justice, L.M. (2004). African American and Caucasian preschoolers' use of decontextualized language: Literate language features in oral narratives. *Language, Speech, and Hearing Services in Schools, 35*, 240–253.

Cushen-White, N. (2000). The Slingerland multisensory structured language approach. *The International Dyslexia Association Northern California Branch Winter Newsletter,* 4–6.

Dale, P.S., Price, T.S., Bishop, D.V.M., & Plomin, R. (2003). Outcomes of early language delay: I. Predicting persistent and transient language difficulties at 3 and 4 years. *Journal of Speech, Language, and Hearing Research, 46*, 544–560.

Damico, J., & Damico, S. (1993). Language and social skills from a diversity perspective: Considerations for the speech-language pathologist. *Language, Speech, and Hearing Services in Schools, 24*, 236–243.

D'Andrea, M., and Daniels, J. (2001). *Respectful counseling.* Pacific Grove: Brooks/Cole.

Davern, L. (1996). Listening to parents of children with disabilities. *Educational Leadership, 4*, 61–63.

Davis-McFarland, E. (2002). Pediatric HIV/AIDS—Issues and strategies for intervention. *The ASHA Leader, 7*(4), 10–20.

de Rivera, C., Girolametto, L., Greenberg, J., & Weitzman, E. (2005). Children's responses to educators' questions in day care play groups. *American Journal of Speech-Language Pathology, 14*, 14–26.

DeFries, J.C., & Gillis, J.J. (1991). Etiology of reading deficits in learning disabilities: Quantitative genetic analyses. In J.E. Obrzut & G.W. Hynd (Eds.), *Neuropsychological foundations of learning disabilities: A handbook of issues, methods, and practice* (pp. 29–48). San Diego: Academic Press.

DeGroot, A.M.B., & Kroll, J.F. (1997). *Tutorials in bilingualism: Psycholinguistic perspectives.* Mahwah, NJ: Lawrence Erlbaum.

DePaepe, P.A., & Wood, L.A. (2001). Collaborative practice related to augmentative and alternative communication: Current personnel preparation programs. *Communication Disorders Quarterly, 22*, 77–86.

Deevy, P., & Leonard, L.B. (2004). The comprehension of wh-questions in children with specific language impairment. *Journal of Speech, Language, and Hearing Research, 47*, 802–815.

Delgado, C., Mundy, P., Crowson, M., Markus, J., Yale, M., & Schwartz, H. (2002). Responding to joint attention and language development: A comparison of target locations. *Journal of Speech, Language, and Hearing Research, 45*, 715–719.

Dickinson, D., & McCabe, A. (1991). The acquisition and development of language: A social interactionist account of language and literacy development. In J.F. Kavanagh (Ed.), *The language continuum: From infancy to literacy* (pp. 1–40). Parkton, MD: York Press.

Dickinson, D.K., McCabe, A., & Clark-Chiarelli, N. (2004). Preschool-based intervention of reading disability: Realities versus possibilities. In C.A. Stone, E.R. Silliman, B.J. Ehren, & K. Apel (Eds.). *Handbook of language and literacy: Development and disorders* (pp. 209–227). New York: The Guilford Press.

Diehl, S.F. (2003). Prologue: Autism spectrum disorder: The context of speech-language pathologist intervention. *Language, Speech, and Hearing Services in Schools, 34*, 177–179.

Dillon, J.T. (1982). The multidisciplinary study of questions. *Journal of Educational Psychology, 74*, 147–165.

Dodd, B., & Carr, A. (2003). Young children's letter-sound knowledge. *Language, Speech, and Hearing Services in Schools, 34*, 128–137.

Dollaghan, C. (2004). Taxometric analyses of specific language impairment in 3- and 4-year-old children. *Journal of Speech, Language, and Hearing Research, 47*, 464–475.

Dollaghan, C.A., & Campbell, T.F. (1998). Nonword repetition and child language impairment. *Journal of Speech, Language, and Hearing Research, 41*, 1136–1146.

Dollaghan, C.A., Campbell, T.F., Paradise, J.L., Feldman, H.M., Janosky, J.E., Pitcairn, D.N., & Kurs-Lasky, M. (1999). Maternal education and measures of early speech and language. *Journal of Speech, Language, and Hearing Research, 42*, 1432–1443.

Donahue, M.L. (1997). Beliefs about listening in students with learning disabilities: Is the speaker always right? *Topics in Language Disorders, 17*, 41–61.

Dore, J. (1975). Holophrase, speech acts, and language universals. *Journal of Child Language, 2*, 21–40.

Drager, K.D.R., Light, J.C., Carlson, R., D'Silva, K., Larsson, B., Pitkin, L., & Stopper, G. (2004). Learning of dynamic display AAC technologies by typically-developing 3-year-olds: Effect of different layouts and menu approaches. *Journal of Speech, Language, and Hearing Research, 47*, 1133–1148.

Drew, C.J., & Hardman, M.L. (2004). *Mental retardation: A lifespan approach to people with intellectual disabilities* (8th ed.). Columbus, OH: Merrill.

Duchan, J.F. (2004). *Frame work in language and literacy: How theory informs practice.* New York: Guilford Publishing, Inc.

Duke, N.K., Pressley, M., & Hilden, K. (2004). Difficulties with reading comprehension. In C.A. Stone, E.R. Silliman, B.J. Ehren, & K. Apel (Eds.). *Handbook of language and literacy: Development and disorders* (pp. 501–520). New York: The Guilford Press.

Dunn, L.M., & Dunn, L. (1997). *Peabody Picture Vocabulary Test-3.* Circle Pines, MN: American Guidance Service.

Eadie, P.A., Fey, M.E., Douglas, J.M., & Parsons, C.L. (2002). Profiles of grammatical morphology and sentence imitation in children with specific language impairment and Down Syndrome. *Journal of Speech, Language, and Hearing Research, 45*, 720–732.

Eckenrode, J., Laird, M., & Doris, J. (1993). School performance and disciplinary problems among abused and neglected children. *Developmental Psychology, 29*, 53–62.

Eden, G.F., Stein, J.F., Wood, M.H., & Wood, F.B. (1995). Verbal and visual problems in reading disability. *Journal of Learning Disabilities, 28*, 272–290.

Egeland, B. (1991). A longitudinal study of high risk families: Issues and findings. In R. Starr & D.A. Wolfe (Eds.), *The effects of child abuse and neglect* (pp. 33–56). New York: Guilford Press.

Ehren, B.J., Lenz, B.K., & Deshler, D.D. (2004). In C.A. Stone, E.R. Silliman, B.J. Ehren, & K. Apel (Eds.). *Handbook of language and literacy: Development and disorders* (pp. 681–70). New York: The Guilford Press.

Ehri, L.C., & Snowling, M.J. (2004). Developmental variation in word recognition. In C.A. Stone, E.R. Silliman, B.J. Ehren, & K. Apel (Eds.). *Handbook of language and literacy: Development and disorders* (pp. 433–460). New York: The Guilford Press.

Ellis Weismer, S., & Evans, J. (2002). The role of processing limitations in early identification of specific language impairment. *Topics in Language Disorders, 22(3),* 15–29.

The Elementary and Secondary Education Act of 1965 Title, I. Improving the Academic Achievement of the Disadvantaged. (20 U.S.C. 6301 et seq.).

Ellis Weismer, S., Plante, E., Jones, J., & Tomblin, J.B. (2005). A functional magnetic resonance imaging investigation of verbal working memory in adolescents with specific language impairment. *Journal of Speech, Language, and Hearing Research, 48,* 405–425.

Emery, A.E.H. (2000). *Muscular dystrophy: The facts (2nd ed.)*. New York: Oxford Press.

England, C.A. (1994). Assessing students with attention deficit hyperactivity disorder: Student interactions within social context. *California Speech and Hearing Association, 20,* 4–6.

Enos, L., Kline, L., Guillen-Green, S., Weger, L., Roseberry-McKibbin, C., & O'Hanlon, L. (2005, April). *The influence of poverty and maternal education on children's language.* Paper presented at the annual meeting of the California Speech-Language-Hearing Association, Santa Clara, CA.

Erickson, M.F., & Egeland, B. (1996). Child neglect. In J. Briere, L. Berliner, J.A. Bulkley, C. Jenny, & T. Reid (Eds.), *The APSAC handbook on child maltreatment* (pp. 4–20). Thousand Oaks, CA: Sage Publications.

Eriks-Brophy, A., & Ayukawa, H. (2000). The benefits of sound field amplification in classrooms of Inuit students of Nunavik: A pilot project. *Language, Speech, and Hearing Services in Schools, 31,* 324–335.

Erin, J. (1990). Language samples from visually impaired four- and five-year olds. *Journal of Childhood Communication Disorders, 13,* 181–191.

Ertmer, D. (2002). Challenges in optimizing oral communication skills in children with cochlear implants: Prologue to a clinical forum. *Language, Speech, and Hearing Services in Schools, 33,* 149–152.

Ervin, M. (2001). SLI: What we know and why it matters. *The ASHA Leader, 6*(12), 4–31.

Eyer, J.A., Leonard, L.B., Bedore, L.M., McGregor, K.K., Anderson, B., & Viescas, R. (2002). Fast mapping of verbs by children with specific language impairment. *Clinical Linguistics and Phonetics, 16,* 59–77.

Ezell, H.K., & Justice, L.M. (2000). Increasing the print focus of adult-child shared book reading through observational learning. *American Journal of Speech-Language Pathology, 9,* 36–47.

Facon, B., Facon-Bollengier, T., & Grubar, J.C. (2002). Chronological age, receptive vocabulary, and syntax comprehension in children and adolescents with mental retardation. *American Journal on Mental Retardation, 107,* 91–98.

Fadiman, A. (1997). *The spirit catches you and you fall down: A Hmong child, her American doctors, and the collision of two cultures.* New York: Farrar, Straus, and Giroux.

Falk-Ross, F.C. (2002). *Classroom-based language and literacy intervention: A programs and case-study approach.* Boston: Allyn & Bacon.

Fallon, K.A., Light, J.C., & Paige, T.K. (2001). Enhancing vocabulary selection for preschoolers who require augmentative and alternative communication (AAC). *American Journal of Speech-Language Pathology, 10,* 81–94.

Fallon, K.A., Light, J., McNaughton, D., Drager, K., & Hammer, C. (2004). The effects of direct instruction on the single-word reading skills of children who require augmentative and alternative communication. *Journal of Speech, Language, and Hearing Research, 47,* 1424–1439.

Fazio, B.B. (1996). Serial memory in children with specific language impairment: Examining specific content areas for assessment and intervention. *Topics in Language Disorders, 17,* 58–71.

Fazio, B.B., Naremore, R.C., & Connell, P. (1996). Tracking children from poverty at risk for specific language impairment: A 3-year longitudinal study. *Journal of Speech and Hearing Research, 39,* 611–624.

Fenson, L., Dale, P., Reznick, S., Thal, D., Bates, E., Hartung, J. et al. (1992). *The MacArthur Communicative Development Inventories: User's guide and technical manual.* San Diego, CA: Singular Publishing Group.

Fey, M.E., Windsor, J., & Warren, S.F. (1995). *Language intervention: Preschool through elementary years.* Volume 5, Communication and Language Intervention Series. Baltimore, MD: Paul H. Brookes Publishing Co.

Fey, M.E. (1986). *Language intervention in young children.* Boston: Little, Brown and Company.

Fey, M.E., Long, S.H., & Finestack, L.H. (2003). Ten principles of grammar facilitation For children with specific language impairment. *American Journal of Speech-Language Pathology, 12,* 3–15.

Fiestas, C.E., & Peña, E.D. (2004). Narrative discourse in bilingual children: Language and task effects. *Language, Speech, and Hearing Services in Schools, 35,* 155–168.

Figueroa, R.A., & Ruiz, N.T. (1997, January). *The optimal learning environment*. Paper presented at the Council for Exceptional Children Symposium on Culturally and Linguistically Diverse Exceptional Learners, New Orleans, LA.

Flax, J.F., Realpe-Bonilla, T., Hirsch, L.S., Brustowicz, L.M., Bartlett, C., & Tallal, P. (2003). Specific language impairment in families: Evidence for co-occurrence with reading impairments. *Journal of Speech, Language, and Hearing Research, 46*(3), 530–543.

Fletcher, P., Leonard, L.B., Stokes, S.F., & Wong, A. M.-Y. (2005). The expression of aspect in Cantonese-speaking children with specific language impairment. *Journal of Speech, Language, and Hearing Research, 48*, 621–624.

Flexer, C. (1995). Classroom amplification systems. In R.J. Roeser & M.P. Downs (Eds.), *Auditory disorders in school children*. New York: Thieme Medical Publishers, Inc.

Fombonne, E. (2003). *Autism statistics: The prevalence of autism*. Retrieved July 12, 2004, from www.autisticsociety.org.

Fontes. L.A. (2005). *Child abuse and culture*. New York: Guilford Publications, Inc.

Fowler, W. (1995). *Talking from infancy: How to nurture and cultivate early language development*. Cambridge, MA: Center for Early Learning and Child Care.

Fowler, W., Ogston, K., Roberts-Fiati, G., & Swenson, A. (1995). Patterns of giftedness and high competence in high school students educationally enriched during infancy: Variation across educational and racial/ethnic backgrounds. *Gifted and Talented International, 10*, 31–36.

Foy, J.G., & Mann, V. (2003). Home literacy environment and phonological awareness in preschool children *Differential effects for rhyme and phoneme awareness. Applied Psycholinguistics, 24*, 59–88.

Ford, J.A., & Milosky, L.M. (2003). Inferring emotional reactions in social situations: Differences in children with language impairment. *Journal of Speech, Language, and Hearing Research, 46*(1), 21–30.

Foy, G., & Mann, V. (2003). Home literacy environment and phonological awareness in preschool children: Differential effects for rhyme and phoneme awareness. *Applied Psycholinguistics, 24*, 59–88.

Fraiberg, S. (1977). *Insights from the blind: Comparative studies of blind and sighted infants*. New York: Basic Books.

Freeman, R., & Blockberger, S. (1987). Language development and sensory disorder: Visual and hearing impairments. In W. Yule and M. Rutter (Eds.), *Language development and disorders* (pp. 234–247). Philadelphia: J.B. Lippincott.

Friedlander, D., & Martinson, K. (1996). Effects of mandatory basic education for adult AFDC recipients. *Educational Evaluation and Policy Analysis, 13*, 327–337.

Friend, M., & Bursuck, W. (2002). Including students with special education needs (3rd ed.). Boston: Allyn and Bacon.

Frith, U. (2003). *Autism: Exploring the enigma* (2nd ed.). United Kingdom: Oxford.

Fritjers, J.C., Barron, R.W., & Brunello, M. (2000). Direct and mediated influences of home literacy and literacy interest on pre-readers' oral vocabulary and written language skill. *Journal of Educational Psychology, 92*, 466–477.

Fujiki, M., Brinton, B., & Clarke, D. (2002). Emotion regulation in children with specific language impairment. *Language, Speech, and Hearing Services in Schools, 33*, 102–111.

Fujiki, M., Brinton, B., Isaacson, T., & Summers, C. (2001). Social behaviors of children with language impairment on the playground: A pilot study. *Language, Speech, and Hearing Services in Schools, 32*, 101–113.

Fujiki, M., Spackman, M.P., Brinton, B., & Hall, B. (2004). The relationship of language and emotion regulation skills to reticence in children with specific language impairment. *Journal of Speech, Language, and Hearing Research, 47*, 637–646.

Fung, F., & Roseberry-McKibbin, C. (1999). Service delivery considerations in working with clients from Cantonese-speaking backgrounds. *American Journal of Speech-Language Pathology, 8*, 309–318.

Gabriels, R.L., & Hill, D. E. (Eds.) (2002). *Autism—from research to individualized practice*. London: Jessica Kingsley Publishers.

Garcia, G.E. (1999). Bilingual children's reading: An overview of recent research. *ERIC/CLL News Bulletin, Fall/Winter 1999*. Available at www.cal.org/ericcll/News/199909/main.html

Garcia, G.E., Jimenez, R.T., & Pearson, P.D. (1998). Metacognition, childhood bilingualism, and reading. In D.J. Hacker, J. Dunlosky, & A.C. Graesser (Eds.), *Metacognition in educational theory and practice* (pp. 193–219). Mahwah, NJ: Erlbaum.

Garcia, B., Mendez Perez, A., & Ortiz, A.A. (2000). Mexican American mothers' beliefs about disabilities: Implications for early childhood intervention. *Remedial and Special Education, 21*, 90–102.

Garnett, K. (1986). Telling tales: Narratives and learning-disabled children. *Topics in Language Disorders, 6*, 44–56.

Gallaudet Research Institute (1998). *Regional and national summary report of data from 1998–1999. Annual Survey of Deaf and Hard-of-Hearing Children and Youth*. Washington, DC: Gallaudet University.

Gathercole, S.E., & Baddeley, A.D. (1993). *Working memory and language*. Erlbaum Associates: Hillsdale, NJ.

Geers, A. (2002). Factors affecting the development of speech, language, and literacy in children with early cochlear implantation. *Language, Speech, and Hearing Services in Schools, 33*, 172–183.

Geers, A., & Moog, J. (1987). Predicting spoken language acquisition of profoundly hearing-impaired children. *Journal of Speech and Hearing Disorders, 52*, 84–94.

Geers, A,. Nicholas, J., & Sedey, A. (2003). Language skills of children with early cochlear implantation. *Ear and Hearing, 24*, 46S–58S.

Geers, A., Spehar, B., & Sedey, A. (2002). Use of speech by children from Total Communication programs who wear cochlear implants. *American Journal of Speech-Language Pathology, 11*, 50–58.

Gelfand, S.A. (2001). *Essentials of audiology* (2nd ed.). New York: Thieme Medical Publishers.

Genesee, F., Paradis, J., & Crago, M.B. (2004). *Dual language development and disorders: A handbook on bilingualism and second language learners*. Baltimore, MD: Brookes Publishing Co.

Genesee, F., & Riches, C. (in press). Literacy development: Instructional issues. In F. Genesee, K. Lindholm-Leary, W. Saunders, & D. Christian, *Educating English language learners: A synthesis of research evidence*. Washington, DC: Center for Applied Linguistics.

Gertner, B.L., Rice, M.L., & Hadley, P.A. (1994). Influence of communicative competence on peer preferences in a preschool classroom. *Journal of Speech and Hearing Research, 37*, 913–923.

Gibbons, P. (2002). *Scaffolding language, scaffolding learning: Teaching second language learners in the mainstream classroom*. Portsmouth, NH: Heinemann.

Giddan, J.J. (1991). School children with emotional problems and communication deficits: Implications for speech-language pathologists. *Language, Speech, and Hearing Services in Schools, 22*, 291–295.

Gilger, J.W., & Wise, S.E. (2004). Genetic correlates of language and literacy impairments. In C.A. Stone, E.R. Silliman, B.J. Ehren, & K. Apel (Eds.), *Handbook of language and literacy: Development and disorders* (pp. 25–48). New York: The Guilford Press.

Gillam, R.B. (1998) (Ed.). *Memory and language impairment in children and adults: New perspectives*. Gaithersburg, MD: Aspen.

Gillam, R.B. (1999). Computer-assisted lnauge intervention using Fast ForWord: Theoretical and empirical considerations for clinical decision-making. *Language, Speech, and Hearing Services in Schools, 30*, 363–370.

Gillam, R.B., & Carlile, R.M. (1997). Oral reading and story retelling of students with specific language impairment. *Language, Speech, and Hearing Services in Schools, 28*, 30–42.

Gillam, R.B., Cowan, N., & Day, L. (1995). Sequential memory in children with and without specific language impairment. *Journal of Speech and Hearing Research, 38*, 393–402.

Gillam, R.B., & Ukraintez, T.A. (2006). Language intervention through literature-based units. In T.A. Ukrainetz (Ed.), *Contextualizing language intervention: Scaffolding PreK-12 literacy achievement* (pp. 59–94). Eau Claire, WI: Thinking Publications.

Gillam, R.B., & van Kleeck, A. (1996). Phonological awareness training and short-term working memory: Clinical implications. *Topics in Language Disorders, 17*, 72–81.

Gillon, G.T. (2000). The efficacy of phonological awareness intervention for children with spoken language impairment. *Language, Speech, and Hearing Services in Schools, 31*, 126–141.

Gillon, G.T. (2004). *Phonological awareness: From research to practice*. New York: Guilford Publications, Inc.

Gimpel, G.A., & Holland, M.L. (2003). *Emotional and behavioral problems of young children*. New York: The Guilford Press.

Girolametto, L., Weitzman, E., & Greenberg, J. (2003). Training day care staff to facilitate children's language. *American Journal of Speech-Language Pathology, 12*, 299–311.

Girolametto, L., Weitzman, E., & Greenberg, J. (2004). The effects of verbal support strategies on small-group peer interactions. *Language, Speech, and Hearing Services in Schools, 35*, 254–268.

Girolametto, L., Wiig, M., Smyth, R., Weitzman, E., & Pearce, P.S. (2001). Children with a history of expressive vocabulary delay: Outcomes at 5 years of age. *American Journal of Speech-Language Pathology, 10*, 358–369.

Glennen, S.L. (2002). Language development and delay in internationally adopted infants and toddlers: A review. *American Journal of Speech-Language Pathology, 11*, 333–339.

Glennen, S.L., & DeCoste, D.C. (Eds.) (1997). *Handbook of augmentative and alternative communication*. San Diego: Singular Publishing Group.

Glennen, S.L., & Masters, M.G. (2002). Typical and atypical language development in infants and toddlers adopted from Eastern Europe. *American Journal of Speech-Language Pathology, 11*, 417–433.

Goldstein, B.A. (2000). *Cultural and linguistic diversity resource guide for speech-language pathologists*. San Diego: Singular/Thomson Learning.

Goldstein, B.A. (Ed.) (2004). Bilingual language development and disorders: Introduction and overview. In B.A. Goldstein (Ed.), *Bilingual language development and disorders in Spanish-English speakers* (pp. 3–20). Baltimore, MD: Paul H. Brookes Publishing Co.

Goldstein, H. (2002). Communication intervention for children with autism: A review of treatment efficacy. *Journal of Autism and Developmental Disorders, 32*, 373–396.

Goldsworthy, C.L. (2001). *Sourcebook of phonological awareness activities: Volume II children's core literature.* San Diego: Singular/Thomson Learning.

Goldsworthy, C.L. (2003). *Developmental reading disabilities: A language based treatment approach* (2nd ed.). Clifton Park, NY: Thomson/Delmar Learning.

Gollnick, D.A., & Chinn, P.C. (1994). *Multicultural education in a pluralistic society* (4th ed.). New York: Merrill.

Gollnick, D.M., & Chinn, P.C. (2002). *Multicultural education in a pluralistic society* (6th ed.). Columbus, OH: Merrill.

GoPaul-McNichol, S., & Armour-Thomas, E. (2002). *Assessment and culture: Psychological tests with minority populations.* San Diego: Academic Press.

Good, T.L., Savings, R.L., Harel, K.H., & Emerson, H. (1987). Student passivity: A study of question asking in K-12 classrooms. *Sociology of Education, 60,* 181–199.

Gorbet, F. (1979). To err is human: Error analysis and child language acquisition. *English Language Teacher, 34,* 22–28.

Gravel, J.S., & Wallace, I.F. (2000). Effects of otitis media with effusion on hearing in the first 3 years of life. *Journal of Speech, Language, and Hearing Research, 42*(3): 631–644.

Graves, M.F., Juel, C., & Graves, B.B. (2001). *Teaching reading in the 21st century* (2nd ed.). Boston: Allyn & Bacon.

Gray, S. (2003). Word-learning by preschoolers with specific language impairment: What predicts success? *Journal of Speech, Language, and Hearing Research, 46*(1), 56–67.

Gray, S. (2004). Word learning by preschoolers with specific language impairment: Predictors and poor learners. *Journal of Speech, Language, and Hearing Research, 47,* 1117–1132.

Greenhalgh, K.S., & Strong, C.J. (2001). Literate language features in spoken narratives of children with typical language and children with language impairments. *Language, Speech, and Hearing Services in Schools, 32,* 114–125.

Greenspan, S.L., & Weider, S. (1998). *The child with special needs.* Reading, MA: Addison-Wesley.

Griffin, K., & Hannah, L. (1960). A study of results of an extremely short instructional unit in listening. *Journal of Communication, 10,* 135–139.

Grimes, B. (2003). *Ethnologue: Languages of the world* (web version). Retrieved July 11, 2004, from www.ethnologue.com/web/asp.

Gronroos, N. (2003). *Cultural considerations in discussing mental retardation.* National Mental Health and Education Center, retrieved 7/14/03 from www.naspcenter.org/teachers/culture_conferencing.html

Guiterrez-Clellen, V.F. (1999). Language choices in intervention with bilingual children. *American Journal of Speech-Language Pathology, 8,* 291–302.

Gutierrez-Clellen, V.F. (2004). Narrative development and disorders in bilingual children. In B.A. Goldstein (Ed.), *Bilingual language development and disorders in Spanish-English speakers* (pp. 235–258). Baltimore, MD: Paul H. Brookes Publishing Co.

Gutierrez-Clellen, V.F., Calderon, J., & Ellis Weismer, S. (2004). Verbal working memory in bilingual children. *Journal of Speech, Language, and Hearing Research, 47,* 863–877.

Gutierrez-Clellen, V.F., & Peña, E. (2001). Dynamic assessment of diverse children: A tutorial. *Language, Speech, and Hearing Services in Schools, 32,* 212–224.

Gutierrez-Clellen, V.F., & Quinn, R. (1993). Assessing narratives of children from diverse cultural/linguistic groups. *Language, Speech, and Hearing Services in Schools, 24,* 2–9.

Gutierrez-Clellen, V.F., Restrepo, M.A., Bedore, L., Peña, E., & Anderson, R. (2000). Language sample analysis in Spanish-speaking children: Methodological considerations. *Language, Speech, and Hearing Services in Schools, 31,* 88–98.

Haberman, M. (1995). *Star teachers of children in poverty.* Bloomington, IN: Kappa Delta Pi.

Haberman, M. (2005). *Star teachers: The ideology and best practice of effective teachers of diverse children and youth in poverty.* Houston, TX: The Haberman Educational Foundation.

Hadley, P.A., Simmerman, A., Long, M., & Luna, M. (2000). Facilitating language development for inner city children: Experimental evaluation of a collaborative, classroom-based intervention. *Language, Speech, and Hearing Services in Schools, 31,* 280–295.

Halfon, N., & McLearn, K.T. (2002). Families with children under 3: What we know and implications for results and policy. In N. Halfon and K.T. McLearn (Eds.), *Child rearing in America: Challenges facing parents with young children* (pp. 367–412).

Hallahan, D.P., Lloyd, J.W., Kauffman, J.M., Weiss, M.P., & Martinez, E.A. (2005). *Learning disabilities: Foundations, characteristics, and effective teaching* (3rd ed.). Boston: Allyn & Bacon.

Halliday, M. (1975). *Learning how to mean: Explorations in the development of language.* London: Edward Arnold.

Hammer, C.S., Miccio, A.W., & Wagstaff, D. (2003). Home literacy experiences and their relationship to bilingual preschoolers' developing English literacy abilities: An initial investigation. *Language, Speech, and Hearing Services in Schools, 34,* 20–30.

Hammer, C.S., Miccio, A.W., & Rodriguez, B.L. (2004). Bilingual language acquisition and the child socialization process. In B.A. Goldstein (Ed.), *Bilingual language development and disorders in Spanish-English speakers* (pp. 21–52). Baltimore, MD: Paul H. Brookes Publishing Co.

Hammer, C.S., & Weiss, A. (1999). Guiding language development: How African American mothers and their infants structure play interactions. *Journal of Speech, Language, and Hearing Research, 42*, 1219–1233.

Hammer, C.S., & Weiss, A. (2000). African American mothers' views of their infants; language development and language-learning environment. *American Journal of Speech-Language Pathology, 9*, 126–140.

Hanson, M.J. (2004a). Ethnic, cultural, and language diversity in service settings. In E.W. Lynch and M.J. Hanson (Eds.), *Developing cross-cultural competence: A guide for working with young children and their families* (pp. 1–2). Baltimore, MD: Paul H. Brookes Publishing Co.

Hanson, M.J. (2004b). Families with Anglo-European roots. In E.W. Lynch and M.J. Hanson (Eds.), *Developing cross-cultural competence: A guide for working with young children and their families* (pp. 81–108). Baltimore, MD: Paul H. Brookes Publishing Company.

Hardman, M.L., Drew, C.J., & Egan, M.W. (2006). *Human exceptionality: Society, school, and family* (8th ed.). Boston: Allyn & Bacon.

Harris, G. (1985). Considerations in assessing English language performance of Native American children. *Topics in Language Disorders, 5*, 42–52.

Harris, M.D., & Reichle, J. (2004). The impact of aided language stimulation on symbol comprehension and production in children with moderate cognitive disabilities. *American Journal of Speech-Language Pathology, 13*, 155–167.

Hart, B., & Risley, T.R. (1995). Meaningful differences in the everyday experiences of young American children. Baltimore, MD: Paul H. Brookes Publishing Co.

Hatton, D.D., McWilliam, R.A., & Winton, P.J. (2002). *Infants and toddlers witch visual impairments: Suggestions for early interventionists*. Arlington, VA: The Eric Clearinghouse on Disabilities and Gifted Education. Retrieved July 9, 2005, from ericec.org.

Haynes, W.O., & Pindzola, R.H. (2004). *Diagnosis and evaluation in speech pathology* (6th ed.). Boston: Allyn & Bacon.

Hearne, J.D. (2000). *Teaching second language learners with learning disabilities: Strategies for effective practice*. Oceanside, CA: Academic Communication Associates.

Heckelman, R.G. (1978). *Using the neurological impress reading technique: Solutions to reading problems*. Novato, CA: Academic Therapy Publications.

Hegde, M.N. (2001a). *Introduction to communication disorders* (3rd ed.). Austin, TX: Pro-Ed.

Hegde, M.N. (2001b). *PocketGuide to treatment in speech-language pathology* (2nd ed.). San Diego: Singular/Thomson Learning.

Hegde, M.N. (2001c). *PocketGuide to assessment in speech-language pathology* (2nd ed.). San Diego: Singular/Thomson Learning.

Heilmann, J., Ellis Weismer, S., Evans, J., & Hollar, C. (2005). Utility of the MacArthur-Bates Communicative Development Inventory in identifying language abilities of late-talking and typically developing toddlers. *American Journal of Speech-Language Pathology, 14*, 40–51.

Helfer, K.S. (1998). In C.M. Seymour & E.H. Nober (Eds.), *Introduction to communication disorders: A multicultural approach* (pp. 277–305). Newton, MA: Butterworth-Heinemann.

Hemphill, L., Uccelli, P., Winner, K., Chang, C., & Bellinger, D. (2002). Narrative discourse in young children with histories of early corrective heart surgery. *Journal of Speech, Language, and Hearing Research, 45*, 318–331.

Henry, L.A., & Gudjonsson, G.G. (1999). Eyewitness memory and suggestibility in children with mental retardation. *American Journal of Mental Retardation, 104*, 491–508.

Hester, P., & Kaiser, A.P. (1998). Early intervention for the prevention of conduct disorder: Research issues in early identification, implementation, and interpretation of treatment outcome. *Behavioral Disorders, 24*, 57–65.

Hewetson, A. (2002). *The stolen child: Aspects of autism and Asperger syndrome*. Westport, CT: Bergin & Garvey.

Hildyard, K.L., & Wolfe, D.A. (2002). Child neglect: developmental issues and concerns. *Child Abuse and Neglect, 26*, 679–695.

Hoag, L.A., Bedrosian, J.L., McCoy, K.F., & Johnson, D.E. (2004). Trade-offs between informativeness and speed of message delivery in augmentative and alternative communication. *Journal of Speech, Language, and Hearing Research, 47*, 1270–1285.

Hoffman, L.M., & Gillam, R. (2004). Verbal and spatial information processing constraints in Children with specific language impairment. *Journal of Speech, Language, and Hearing Research, 47*, 114–125.

Hogenboom, M. (2001). *Living with genetic syndromes associated with intellectual disability.* London: Jessica Kingsley Publishers Ltd.

Holliday, P.A.C. (2001). Demand may exceed supply in future job market. *The ASHA Leader, 6,* 18.

Houwer, A.D. (1999). Two or more languages in early childhood: Some general points and practical recommendations. *ERIC Digest, July 1999.* Available at www.cal.org/ericcl/digest/earlychild.html

Howard, J., Beckwith, L., Rodning, C., & Kropenske, V. (1989). The development of young children from substance-abusing parents: Insights from seven years of intervention research. *Zero to Three, 9,* 8–12.

Huebner, R.A. (Ed.) (2001). *Autism: A sensorimotor approach to management.* Gaithersburg, MD: Aspen Publishers.

Huer, M.B., & Parette, H.P. (2003). Issues in family interventions: Working with parents cross-culturally. In S. von Tetzchner and M.H. Jensen (Eds.), *Perspectives on theory and practice in augmentative and alternative communication* (pp. 154–167). Toronto, Ontario: International Society for Augmentative and Alternative Communication.

Huer, M.B., & Saenz, T.I. (2003). Challenges and strategies for conducting survey and focus group research with culturally diverse groups. *American Journal of Speech-Language Pathology, 12,* 209–220.

Huer, M.B., Parette, H.P., & Saenz, T.I. (2001). Conversations with Mexican Americans regarding children with disabilities and augmentative and alternative communication devices. *Communication Disorders Quarterly, 22,* 197–206.

Hugdahl, K., Gundersen, H., Brekke, C., Thomsen, T., Rimol, L.M., Ersland, L., & Niemi, J. (2004). fMRI brain activation in a Finnish family with specific language impairment compared with a normal control group. *Journal of Speech, Language, and Hearing Research, 47,* 162–172.

Hulit, L.M., & Howard, M.R. (2002). *Born to talk: An introduction to speech and language development* (3rd ed.). Boston: Allyn & Bacon.

Hull, M.A. (1981). *Phonics for the teacher of reading: Programmed for self-instruction* (3rd ed.). Columbus, OH: Merrill.

Hummel, L.J., & Prizant, B.M. (1993). A socioemotional perspective for understanding social difficulties of school-age children with language disorders. *Language, Speech, and Hearing Services in Schools, 24,* 216–224.

Hwa-Froelich, D., Hodson, B., & Edwards (2002). Characteristics of Vietnamese phonology. *American Journal of Speech-Language Pathology, 11,* 264–273.

Hwa-Froelich, D., & Westby, C. (2003). Frameworks of education: Perspectives of Southeast Asian parents and Head Start Staff. *Language, Speech, and Hearing Services in Schools, 34,* 299–319.

Hwa-Froelich, D., & Matsuo, H. (2005). Vietnamese children and language-based processing tasks. *Language, Speech, and Hearing Services in Schools, 36,* 230–243.

Hyter, Y.D., Rogers-Adkinson, D.L., Self, T.L., Simmons, B.F., & Jantz, J. (2001). Pragmatic language intervention for children with language and emotional/behavioral disorders. *Communication Disorders Quarterly, 23,* 4–16.

Hyun, J.K., & Fowler, S.A. (1995). Respect, cultural sensitivity, and communication: Promoting participation by Asian families in the individualized family service plan. *Teaching Exceptional Children, 28,* 25–28.

Ianoco, T., & Cupples, L. (2004). Assessment of phonemic awareness and work reading skills of people with complex communication needs. *Journal of Speech, Language, and Hearing Research, 47,* 437–449.

Idol, L., Nevin, A., & Paolucci-Whitcomb, P. (2000). *Collaborative consultation* (3rd ed.). Austin, TX: Pro-Ed.

Individuals with Disabilities Education Act Amendments of 1997 [U.S. Code of Federal Regulations 303.12(4)(b)(2)].

Individuals with Disabilities Education Improvement Act of 2004 (IDEA; 2004). *Public Law 108-446, 108th Congress.* Retrieved on June 14, 2005, from www.copyright.gov/legislation/al108-446.html

Irlen, H. (2002). *Reading by the colors: Overcoming dyslexia and other reading disabilities through the Irlen method.* New York: Berkley Publishing Group.

Irlen Institute (2003). Irlen syndrome/scotopic sensitivity: A piece of the puzzle for reading problems. *Learning difficulties, AD/HD, dyslexia, headaches and other physical symptoms through the use of colour.* Retrieved June 12, 2005, from www.irlen.com/sss_main.htm

Isaacs, G.J. (1996). Persistence of non-standard dialect in school-age children. *Journal of Speech and Hearing Research, 39,* 434–441.

Iwanaga, R., Kawasaki, C., & Tsuchida, R. (2000). Brief report: Comparison of sensory-motor and cognitive function between autism and Asperger syndrome in preschool children. *Journal of Autism and Developmental Disorders, 30,* 169–174.

Jackson, S.C., & Roberts, J.E. (2001). Complex syntax production of African American preschoolers. *Journal of Speech, Language, and Hearing Research, 44,* 1083–1096.

Jackson-Maldonado, D. (2004). Verbal morphology and vocabulary in monolinguals and emergent bilinguals. In B.A. Goldstein (Ed.), *Bilingual language development and disorders in Spanish-English speakers* (pp. 131–162). Baltimore, MD: Paul H. Brookes Publishing Co.

Jackson-Maldonado, D., Bates, E., & Thal, D. (1992). *Fundacion MacArthur: Inventario del desarrollo de habilidades comunicativas.* San Diego, CA: San Diego State University.

Jacob, N. (2004). Families with South Asian roots. In E.W. Lynch and M.J. Hanson (Eds.), *Developing cross-cultural competence: A guide for working with young children and their families* (pp. 415–440). Baltimore, MD: Paul H. Brookes Publishing Co.

Jacobs, E.L., & Coufal, K.L. (2001). A computerized screening instrument of language learnability. *Communication Disorders Quarterly, 22*, 67–75.

Jankelovich, S. (2001, February). *Serious bacterial infections in children with HIV*. HIV InSite Knowledge Base Chapter. Retrieved May 24, 2003, from hivinsite.ucsf.edu/InSite.jsp?page=kb-05&doc=kb-05-01-01-01

Jarrold, C., Baddeley, A.D., & Phillips, C.E. (2002). Verbal short-term memory in Down syndrome: A problem of memory, audition, or speech? *Journal of Speech, Language, and Hearing Research, 45*, 531–544.

Jaudes, P.I., & Diamond, L.J. (1985). The handicapped child and child abuse. *Child Abuse and Neglect, 9*, 341–347.

Jerome, A.C., Fujiki, M., Brinton, B., & James, S.L. (2002). Self-esteem in children with specific language impairment. *Journal of Speech, Language, and Hearing Research, 45*, 700–714.

Jia, G. (2003). The acquisition of the English plural morpheme by native Mandarin Chinese-speaking children. *Journal of Speech, Language, and Hearing Research, 46*, 1297–1323.

Joe, J.R., & Malach, R.S. (2004). Families with American Indian roots. In E.W. Lynch and M.J. Hanson (Eds.), *Developing cross-cultural competence: A guide for working with young children and their families* (pp. 109–149). Baltimore, MD: Paul H. Brookes Publishing Co.

Johnson, B.A. (1996). *Language disorders in children: An introductory clinical perspective.* Albany, NY: Delmar Publishers.

Johnson, C.J., Beitchman, J.H., Young, A., Escobar, M., Atkinson, L., Wilson, B., et al. (1999). Fourteen-year followup of children with and without speech/language impairments: Speech/language stability and outcome. *Journal of Speech, Language, and Hearing Research, 42*, 744–760.

Johnson, V.E. (2005). Comprehension of third person singular /s/ in AAE-speaking children. *Language, Speech, and Hearing Services in Schools, 36*, 116–124.

Johnston, J., & Wong, M.-Y. (2002). Cultural differences in beliefs and practices concerning talk to children. *Journal of Speech, Language, and Hearing Research, 45*, 916–926.

Johnston, S.S., Reichle, J., & Evans, J. (2004). Supporting augmentative and alternative communication use by beginning communicators with severe disabilities. *American Journal of Speech-Language Pathology, 13*, 20–30.

Justice, L.M., & Ezell, H.K. (2000). Enhancing children's print and word awareness through home-based parent intervention. *American Journal of Speech-Language Pathology, 9*, 257–269.

Justice, L.M., & Ezell, H.K. (2001). Written language awareness in preschool children from low-income households: A descriptive analysis. *Communication Disorders Quarterly, 22*, 123–134.

Justice, L.M., & Ezell, H.K. (2002). Use of storybook reading to increase print awareness in at-risk children. *American Journal of Speech-Language Pathology, 11*, 17–29.

Justice, L.M., & Ezell, H.K. (2004). Print referencing: An emergent literacy enhancement strategy and its clinical applications. *American Journal of Speech-Language Pathology, 35*, 185–193.

Justice, L.M., Invernizzi, M.A., & Meier, J.D. (2002). Designing and implementing an early literacy screening protocol: Suggestions for the speech-language pathologist. *Language, Speech, and Hearing Services in Schools, 38*, 84–101.

Justice, L.M., & Kaderavek, J.N. (2004). Embedded-explicit emergent literacy intervention I: Background and description of approach. *Language, Speech, and Hearing Services in Schools, 35*, 201–211.

Justice, L.M., Chow, S-M., Capellini, C., Flanigan, K., & Colton, S. (2003). Emergent literacy intervention for vulnerable preschoolers: Relative effects of two approaches. *American Journal of Speech-Language Pathology, 12*, 320–332.

Justice, L.M., Meier, J., & Walpole, S. (2005). Learning new words from storybooks: An efficacy study with at-risk kindergarteners. *Language, Speech, and Hearing Services in Schools, 36*, 17–32.

Justice, L.M., Skibbe, L., & Ezell, H. (2006). Using print referencing to promote written language awareness. In T.A. Ukrainetz (Ed.), *Contextualizing language intervention: Scaffolding PreK-12 literacy achievement* (pp. 389–428). Eau Claire, WI: Thinking Publications.

Kaderavek, J.N., & Justice, L.M. (2004). Embedded-explicit emergent literacy intervention II: Goal selection and implementation in early childhood classrooms. *Language, Speech, and Hearing Services in Schools, 35*, 212–228.

Kaderavek, J.N., & Sulzby, E. (1998a, November). *Low versus high orientation toward literacy in children.* Paper presented at the annual convention of the American Speech-Language-Hearing Association, San Antonio, Texas.

Kaderavek, J.N., & Sulzby, E. (1998b). Parent-child joint book reading: An observational protocol for young children. *American Journal of Speech-Language Pathology, 7*, 33–47.

Kaderavek, J.N., & Sulzby, E. (2000). Narrative production by children with and without specific language impairment. *Journal of Speech, Language, and Hearing Research, 43*, 34–49.

Kaderavek, J.N., & Boucher, D.M. (2006). Temperament profiles in children: Implications for academic performance and literacy learning. *Hearsay: Journal of the Ohio Speech-Language-Hearing Association, 18*, 14–20.

Kail, R., & Leonard, L. (1986). *Word-finding abilities in language-impaired children.* Rockville, MD: American Speech-Language-Hearing Association.

Kaiser, A.P., Cai, X., Hancock, T.B., & Foster, E.M. (2002). Teacher-reported behavioral problems and language delays in boys and girls enrolled in Head Start. *Behavioral Disorders, 28*, 23–39.

Kamhi, A.G., & Hinton, L.N. (2000). Explaining individual differences in spelling ability. *Topics in Language Disorders, 20*, 37–49.

Kamhi, A.G., Pollock, K.E., & Harris, J.L. (Eds.) (1996). *Communication development and disorders in African American children: Research, assessment, and intervention.* Baltimore, MD: Paul H. Brookes Publishing Co.

Kan, P.F., & Kohnert, K. (2005). Preschoolers learning Hmong and English: Lexical-semantic skills in L1 and L2. *Journal of Speech, Language, and Hearing Research, 48*, 372–383.

Kaufman, J. (1989). The regular education initiative as Reagan-Bush education policy: A trickle-down theory of education of the hard-to-teach. *Journal of Special Education, 3.*

Kay-Raining Bird, E., Cleave, P.L., & McConnell, L. (2000). Reading and phonological awareness in children with Down syndrome: A longitudinal study. *American Journal of Speech-Language Pathology, 9*, 319–330.

Kayser, H. (1989). Speech and language assessment of Spanish-English-speaking children. *Language, Speech, and Hearing Services in Schools, 20*, 226–244.

Kayser, H. (1998). *Assessment and intervention resources for Hispanic children.* San Diego: Singular Publishing Group/Thomson Learning.

Kayser, H.R. (2002). Bilingual language development and language disorders. In D.E. Battle (Ed.), *Communication disorders in multicultural populations* (3rd ed.) (pp. 205–232). Woburn, MA: Butterworth-Heinemann.

Kayser, H.R. (2004). Biliteracy and second-language learners. *The ASHA Leader, 9*, 4–29.

Kavanagh, J.F. (1991). Preface. In J.F. Kavanagh (Ed.), *The language continuum: From infancy to literacy* (pp. vii–ix). Parkton, MD: York Press.

Kay-Raining Bird, E., Cleave, P., Trudeau, N., Thordardottir, E., Sutton, A., & Thorpe, A. (2005). The language abilities of bilingual children with Down Syndrome. *American Journal of Speech-Language Pathology, 14*, 187–199.

Kayser, H.R. (2004). Biliteracy and second-language learners. *The ASHA Leader, 9*(12), 4–21.

Kearney, C.A., & Drabman, R.S. (1993). The write-say method for improving spelling accuracy in children with learning disabilities. *Journal of Learning Disabilities*, 26, 52–56.

Keeping Families and Children Safe Act of 2003 (Public Law 108-36). Retrieved August 9, 2005, from the National Clearinghouse on Child Abuse and Neglect Information at nccanch.acf.hhs.gov/pubs/factsheets/about.cfm.

Kekelis, L.S. (1992). Peer interactions in childhood: The impact of visual impairment. In S.Z. Sacks, L.S. Kekellis, & R.J. Gaylord-Ross (Eds.), *The development of social skills by blind and visually impaired students* (pp. 13–35). New York: American Foundation for the Blind.

Kekelis, L.S., & Andersen, E. (1984). Family communication styles and language development. *Journal of Visual Impairment and Blindness, 78*, 54–65.

Khan, Z., Roseberry-McKibbin, C., O'Hanlon, L., Roberts, K., Weger, L., & Roy, M. (2005). *A survey of ethnic Pashtuns from Pakistan and Afghanistan.* Paper presented at the annual convention of the American Speech-Language-Hearing Association, San Diego, CA.

Kiernan, B., & Swisher, L. (1990). The initial learning of novel English words: Two single-subject experiments with minority-language children. *Journal of Speech and Hearing Research, 33*, 707–716.

Kim, D., & Hall, J.K. (2002). The role of an interactive book reading program in the development of second language pragmatic competence. *Modern Language Journal, 86*, 332–348.

Klein, H.B., & Moses, N. (1999). *Intervention planning for children with communication disorders: A guide for clinical practicum and professional practice* (2nd ed.). Boston: Allyn & Bacon.

Klin, A., & Volkmar, F.R. (1995). *Asperger's syndrome: Guidelines for treatment and intervention.* Retrieved 5/26/04 from info.med.yale.edu/chldstdy/autism/astreatments.html

Klotz, M.B., & Nealis, L. (2005). *The new IDEA: A summary of significant reforms. National Association of School Psychologists.* Available at nasponline.org.

Knutson, J.F., & Sullivan, P.M. (1993). Communicative disorders as a risk factor in abuse. *Topics in Language Disorders, 13*, 1–15.

Koegel, L.K., Koegel, R.L., Frea, W., & Green-Hopkins, I. (2003). Priming as a method of coordinating educational services for students with autism. *Language, Speech, and Hearing Services in Schools, 34*, 228–235.

Kohnert, K. (2002). Picture naming in early sequential bilinguals: A 1-year follow-up. *Journal of Speech, Language, and Hearing Research, 45,* 759–771.

Kohnert, K. (2004). Processing skills in early sequential bilinguals. In B.A. Goldstein (Ed.), *Bilingual language development and disorders in Spanish-English speakers* (pp. 53–76). Baltimore, MD: Paul H. Brookes Publishing Co.

Kohnert, K., Bates, E., & Hernandez, E. (1999). Balancing bilinguals: Lexical-semantic production and cognitive processing in children. *Journal of Speech-Language-Hearing Research, 42,* 1400–1413.

Kohnert, K., & Derr, A. (2004). Language intervention with bilingual children. In B.A. Goldstein (Ed.), *Bilingual language development and disorders in Spanish-English speakers* (pp. 311–338). Baltimore, MD: Paul H. Brookes Publishing Co.

Kohnert, K., & Windsor, J. (2004). The search for common ground: Part II. Nonlinguistic performance by linguistically diverse learners. *Journal of Speech, Language, and Hearing Research, 47,* 891 903.

Kohnert, K., Yim, D., Nett, K., Kan, P.F., & Duran, L. (2005). Intervention with linguistically diverse preschool children: A focus on developing home languages. *Language, Speech, and Hearing Services in Schools, 36,* 251–263.

Koman, L.A., Smith, B.P., & Shilt, J.S. (2004). Cerebral palsy. *Lancet, 363,* 1619–1631.

Koster, C., Been, P.H., Krikhaar, E.M., Zwarts, F., Diepstra, H.D., & Van Leeuwen, T.H. (2005). Differences at 17 months: Productive language patterns in infants at familial risk for dyslexia and typically developing infants. *Journal of Speech, Language, and Hearing Research, 48,* 426–438.

Kouri, T.A. (2003). Lexical training through modeling and elicitation procedures with late talkers who have specific language impairment and developmental delays. *Journal of Speech, Language, and Hearing Research, 48,* 157–171.

Krashen, S.D. (1992). Bilingual education and second language acquisition theory. In C. Leyba (Ed.), *Schooling and language minority students: A theoretical framework* (pp. 51–79). Los Angeles: California State University.

Kratcoski, A. (1998). Guidelines for using portfolios in assessment and evaluation. *Language, Speech, and Hearing Services in Schools, 29,* 3–10.

Kuder, S.J. (2003). *Teaching students with language and communication disabilities* (2nd ed.). Boston: Allyn & Bacon.

Kumin, L. (2002). Starting out: Speech and language intervention for infants and toddlers with Down syndrome. In W.I. Cohen, L. Nadel, & M.E. Madnic (Eds.), *Down syndrome: Visions for the 21st century* (pp. 395–406). New York: Wiley-Liss, Inc.

Kuster, J.M. (2000). English as a second language: Web sites. *The Asha Leader, 5,* 6.

La Paro, K.M., Justice, L., Skibbe, L.E., & Pianta, R.C. (2004). Relations among maternal, child, and demographic factors and the persistence of preschool language impairment. *American Journal of Speech-Language Pathology, 13,* 291–303.

Lahey, M. (1988). *Language disorders and language development.* New York: Macmillan.

Laing, S.P., & Kamhi, A. (2003). Alternative assessment of language and literacy in culturally and linguistically diverse populations. *Language, Speech, and Hearing Services in Schools, 34,* 44–55.

Landau, B., & Gleitman, L. (1985). *Language and experience: Evidence from the blind child.* Cambridge, MA: Harvard University Press.

Lane, H., & Bahan, B. (1998). Ethics of cochlear implantation in young children: A review and reply from a Deaf-World perspective. *Otolaryngology and Head and Neck Surgery, 119,* 297–313.

Lang, J.S. (2000). Hearing impairment. In E.P. Dodge (Ed.), *The survival guide for school-based speech-language pathologists* (pp. 241–262). San Diego: Singular Publishing Group/Thomson Learning.

Langdon, H.W. (2000). Diversity. In E.P. Dodge (Ed.), *The survival guide for school-based speech-language pathologists* (pp. 367–398). San Diego: Singular/Thomson.

Langdon, H.W., & Cheng, L.L. (2002). *Collaborating with interpreters and translators: A guide for communication disorders professionals.* Eau Claire, WI: Thinking Publications.

Larrivee, L., & Catts, H. (1999). Early reading achievement in children with expressive phonological disorders. *American Journal of Speech-Language Pathology, 8,* 118–128.

Larson, V.L., & McKinley, N. (1995). *Language disorders in older students: Preadolescents and adolescents.* Eau Claire, WI: Thinking Publications.

LaSasso, C., & Mobley, S. (1997). National survey of reading instruction for deaf or hard-of-hearing students in the U.S. *Volta Review, 99,* 31–59.

Laws, G., & Bishop, D.V.M. (2003). A comparison of language abilities in adolescents with Down Syndrome and children with specific language impairment. *Journal of Speech, Language, and Hearing Research, 46*(6), 1324–1339.

Law, J., Garrett, Z., & Nye, C. (2004). The efficacy of treatment for children with developmental speech and language delay/disorder: A meta-analysis. *Journal of Speech, Language, and Hearing Research, 47,* 924–943.

Leonard, L., & Loeb, D. (1998). Government-binding theory and some of its applications: a tutorial. *Journal of Speech and Hearing Research, 31,* 515–524.

Leonard, L.B., Deevy, P., Miller, C.A., Rauf, L., Charest, M., & Kurtz, R. (2003). Surface forms and grammatical functions: Past tense and passive participle use by children with specific language impairment. *Journal of Speech, Language, and Hearing Research, 46*, 43–55.

Lesar, S. (1992). Prenatal cocaine exposure: The challenge to education. In L.M. Rossetti (Ed.), *Developmental problems of drug-exposed infants* (pp. 37–52). San Diego, CA: Singular Publishing Group, Inc.

Leung, B. (1996). Quality assessment practices in a diverse society. *Teaching Exceptional Children, 28*, 42–45.

Lewis, B.A., Freebairn, L.A., & Taylor, H.G. (2000). Follow-up of children with early expressive phonology disorders. *Journal of Learning Disabilities, 33*, 433–444.

Li, S.C. (2003). Biocultural orchestration of developmental plasticity across levels: The interplay of biology and culture in shaping the mind and behavior across the lifespan. *Psychological Bulletin, 129*, 171–194.

Lian, C.H.T., & Abdullah, S. (2001). The education and practice of speech-language pathologists in Malaysia. *American Journal of Speech-Language Pathology, 10*, 3–9.

Linan-Thompson, S., Vaugh, S., Hickman-Davis, P., & Kouzekanani, K. (2003). Effectiveness of supplemental reading instruction for second-grade English language learners with reading difficulties. *Elementary School Journal, 103*, 221–238.

Livingstone, M.S., Rosen, G.D., Drislane, F.W., & Galaburda, A.M. (1991). Physiological and anatomical evidence for a magnocellular defect in developmental dyslexia. *Proceedings of the National Academy of Sciences, 88*, 7943–7947.

Lochman, J.E., & Szczepanski, R.G. (1999). Externalizing conditions. In V.L. Schwean & D.H. Saklofske (Eds.), *Handbook of psychosocial characteristics of exceptional children* (pp. 219–246). New York: Kluwer Academic/Plenum.

Locke, D. (1998). *Increasing multicultural understanding: A comprehensive model* (Multicultural aspects of counseling, Series I: 2nd ed.). Thousand Oaks, CA: Sage.

Long, S. (2005a). Language and children with learning disabilities. In V.A. Reed, *An introduction to children with language disorders* (3rd ed.) (pp. 132–167). Boston: Allyn & Bacon.

Long, S. (2005b). Language and other special populations of children. In V.A. Reed, *An introduction to children with language disorders* (3rd ed.) (pp. 356–383). Boston: Allyn & Bacon.

Lovaas, O. (1987). Behavioral treatment and normal educational and intellectual functioning in young autistic children. *Journal of Counseling and Clinical Psychology, 55*, 3–9.

Lund, N.J., & Duchan, J.F. (1993). *Assessing children's language in naturalistic contexts* (3rd ed.). Englewood Cliffs, NJ: Prentice-Hall.

Luster, T., Bates, L., Vandenbelt, M., & Peck Key, J. (2000). Factors related to successful outcomes among preschool children born to low-income adolescent mothers. *Journal of Marriage and the Family, 62*, 133–146.

Luterman, D. (2001). *Counseling persons with communication disorders and their families* (4th ed.). Austin, TX: Pro-Ed.

Lynch, E.W. (2004a). Conceptual framework: From culture shock to cultural learning. In E.W. Lynch and M.J. Hanson (Eds.), *Developing cross-cultural competence: A guide for working with young children and their families* (pp. 19–40). Baltimore, MD: Paul H. Brookes Publishing Co.

Lynch, E.W. (2004b). Developing cross-cultural competence. In E.W. Lynch and M.J. Hanson (Eds.), *Developing cross-cultural competence: A guide for working with young children and their families* (pp. 1–2). Baltimore, MD: Paul H. Brookes Publishing Co.

Lynch, E.W., & Hanson, M.J. (Eds.) (2004). *Developing cross-cultural competence: A guide for working with children and their families* (3rd ed.). Baltimore, MD: Paul H. Brookes Publishing Co.

Lynch, E.W., & Hanson, M.J. (2004). Children of many songs. In E.W. Lynch and M.J. Hanson (Eds.), *Developing cross-cultural competence: A guide for working with young children and their families* (pp. 449–466). Baltimore, MD: Paul H. Brookes Publishing Co.

Lyon, G.R. (1996). Learning disabilities. *The Future of Children*, Spring, pp. 54–76.

Luterman, D.M. (2001). *Counseling communicatively disordered and their families* (4th ed.). Austin, TX: Pro-Ed.

Lyon, G.R. (1996). Learning disabilities. *The Future of Children,* Spring, pp. 54–76.

Madding, C.C. (1999, April). *Mama y hijo*: The Latino mother-infant dyad. Conference proceedings from the fourth annual communicative disorders multicultural conference, California State University, Fullerton. *The Multicultural Electronic Journal of Communication Disorders, 2*, 1–4.

Madding, C.C. (2002). Socialization practices of Latinos. In A.E. Brice, *The Hispanic child: Speech, language, culture, and education.* Boston: Allyn & Bacon.

Mahecha, N. (2003). Typical and disordered child narration in Spanish-speaking children. In McCabe, A., & Bliss, L.S., Patterns of narrative discourse: A multicultural, lifespan approach (pp. 73–90). Boston: Allyn & Bacon.

Malakoff, M., & Hakuta, K. (1991). Translation skill and metalinguistic awareness in bilinguals. In E. Bialystok (Ed.), *Language processing in bilingual children* (pp. 141–166). New York: Cambridge Press.

Manolson, A. (1992). *It takes two to talk: A parents' guide to helping children communicate.* Toronto, Ontario, Canada: The Hanen Centre.

Marchman, V.A., & Martinez-Sussman, C. (2002). Concurrent validity of caregiver/parent report measures of language for children who are learning both English and Spanish. *Journal of Speech, Language, and Hearing Research, 45,* 983–997.

Marcus, L.M., Garfinkle, A., & Wolery, M. (2001). Issues in early diagnosis and intervention for young children with autism. In E. Schopler, N. Yirmiya, C. Shulman, & L.L. Marcus (Eds.), *The research basis for autism intervention* (pp. 171–182). New York: Kluwer Academic/Plenum Publishers.

Martin, F.N., & Clark, J.G. (2003). *Introduction to audiology* (8th ed.). Boston: Allyn & Bacon.

Martin, S.M., Donovan, S.E., & Senne, M. (2003, November). *The heart of teacher preparation: Inclusion of families through curriculum module development.* Paper presented at the 2003 Teacher Education Division Conference, Biloxi, MS.

Marton, K., & Schwartz, R.G. (2003). Working memory capacity and language processes in children with specific language impairment. *Journal of Speech, Language, and Hearing Research, 46*(5), 1138–1153.

Marshall, C.M., Snowling, M.J., & Bailey, P.J. (2001). Rapid auditory processing and phonological ability in normal readers and readers with dyslexia. *Journal of Speech, Language, and Hearing Research, 44,* 925–940.

Mauer, D.M. (1999). Issues and applications of sensory integration theory and treatment with children with language disorders. *Language, Speech, and Hearing Services in Schools, 30,* 383–392.

McCabe, A. (1997). Developmental and cross-cultural aspects of children's narration. In M. Bamberg (Ed.), *Narrative development: Six approaches* (pp. 137–174). Mahwah, NJ: Erlbaum.

McCabe, A, & Bliss, L.S. (2003). *Patterns of narrative discourse: A multicultural, life span approach.* Boston: Allyn & Bacon.

McCormick, L., & Schiefelbusch, R.L. (1984). *Early language intervention.* Columbus, OH: Merrill/Macmillan.

McCauley, R.J., & Swisher, L. (1984). Use and misuse of norm-referenced tests in clinical assessment: A hypothetical case. *Journal of Speech and Hearing Disorders, 49,* 338–348.

McDevitt, T., & Oreskovich, M. (1993). Beliefs about listening: Perspectives of others and early-childhood teachers. *Child Study Journal, 23,* 153–172.

McEachin, J.J., & Lovaas, O.I. (1993). Long-term outcomes for children with autism who received early intensive behavioral treatment. *American Journal on Mental Retardation, 97,* 359–367.

McGregor, G., & Vogelsberg, R.T. (1998). *Inclusive schooling practices: Pedagogical and research foundations.* Baltimore, MD: Brookes.

McGregor, K.K. (2004). Developmental dependencies between lexical semantics and reading. In C.A. Stone, E.R. Silliman, B.J. Ehren, & K. Apel (Eds.), *Handbook of language and literacy: Development and disorders* (pp. 302–317). New York: The Guilford Press.

McGregor, K.K., & Windsor, J. (1996). Effects of priming on the naming accuracy of preschoolers with word-finding deficits. *Journal of Speech and Hearing Research, 39,* 1048–1058.

McKinney, J.D., Montague, M., & Hocutt, A.M. (1993). *A synthesis of research literature on the assessment and identification of attention deficit disorders.* Coral Gables, FL: Miami Center for Synthesis of Research on Attention Deficit Disorders.

McLaughlin, S. (2006). *Introduction to language development.* San Diego, CA: Singular Publishing Group.

McLoyd, V.C. (1998). Economic disadvantage and child development. *American Psychologist, 53,* 185–204.

McNeilly, L.G., & Coleman, T.J. (2000). Early intervention: Working with children within the context of their families and communities. In T.J. Coleman, *Clinical management of communication disorders in culturally diverse children* (pp. 77–100). Boston: Allyn & Bacon.

McWilliam, R.A., & Scott, S. (2001). A support approach to early intervention: A three-part framework. *Infants and Young Children, 13,* 55–66.

Meece, J.I. (1997). *Child and adolescent development for educators.* New York: McGraw-Hill.

Meltzi, G. (2000). Cultural variations in the construction of personal narratives: Central American and European American mothers' elicitation styles. *Discourse Processes, 30,* 153–177.

Mendez Perez, A. (2000). Mexican-American mothers' perceptions and beliefs about language acquisition in infants and toddlers with disabilities. *Bilingual Research Journal, 24,* 277–294.

Merritt, D.M., & Culatta, B. (1998). *Language intervention in the classroom.* San Diego: Singular Publishing Group, Inc.

Meschyan, G., & Hernandez, A.E. (2004). Cognitive factors in second-language acquisition and literacy learning: A theoretical proposal and a call for research. In C.A. Stone, E.R. Silliman, B.J. Ehren, & K. Apel (Eds.), *Handbook of language and literacy: Development and disorders* (pp. 73–81). New York: The Guilford Press.

Mesibov, G.G., Shea, V., & Adams, L.W. (2001). *Understanding Asperger syndrome and high functioning autism.* New York: Kluwer Academic/Plenum Publishers.

Miller, C.A., Kail, R., Leonard, L.B., & Tomblin, J.B. Speed of processing in children with specific language impairment. *Journal of Speech, Language, and Hearing Research, 44,* 416–433.

Miles, S., & Chapman, R.S. (2002). Narrative content as described by individuals with Down syndrome and typically develop-ing children. *Journal of Speech, Language, and Hearing Research, 45*, 175–189.

Miller, J. (1981). *Assessing language production in children: Experimental procedures*. Baltimore, MD: University Park Press.

Miller, S., Merzenich, M.M., Saunders, G., Jenkins, W.M., & Tallal, P. (1996). Improvements in language abilities with training of children with both attentional and language impairments. *Society for Neuroscience, 23*, 490.

Mirenda, P., & Ianoco, T. (1990). Communication options for persons with severe and profound disabilities: State of the art and future directions. *Journal of the Association for the Severely Handicapped, 15*, 3–21.

Muma, J. (1981). *Language primer*. Lubbock, TX: Natural Child Publisher.

Muma, J. (1998). *Effective speech-language pathology: A cognitive socialization approach*. Mahwah, NJ: Erlbaum.

Moats, L.C., & Lyon, G.R. (1993). Learning disabilities in the United States: Advocacy, science, and the future of the field. *Journal of Learning Disabilities, 26*, 282–294.

Mody, M. (2004). Neurobiological correlates of language and reading impairments. In C.A. Stone, E.R. Silliman, B.J. Ehren, & K. Apel (Eds.), *Handbook of language and literacy: Development and disorders* (pp. 49–72). New York: The Guilford Press.

Moeller, M.P. (2000). Early intervention and language development in children who are deaf and hard of hearing. *Pediatrics, 106*, E43. Retrieved July 13, 2005, from www.pediatrics.org/cgi/content/full/106/3/e43.

Moisset, C.E., Barnard, K.E., Greenberg, M.T., Booth, C.L., & Spicker, S.J. (1990). Environmental influences on early language development: The context of social risk. *Development and Psychopathology, 2*, 127–149.

Mokuau, N., & Tauili'ili, P. (2004). Families with Native Hawaiian and Samoan roots. In E.W. Lynch and M.J. Hanson (Eds.), *Developing cross-cultural competence: A guide for working with young children and their families* (pp. 1–2). Baltimore, MD: Paul H. Brookes Publishing Co.

Mokhemar, M.A. (1999). *The central auditory processing kit*. East Moline, IL: LinguiSystems.

Montgomery, J. (1993). *Special education strategies: Shared goals. What's happening in curriculum and instruction?* Fountain Valley, CA: Foundation Valley School District.

Montgomery, J.W. (1996). Sentence comprehension and working memory in children with specific language impairment. *Topics in Language Disorders, 17*, 19–32.

Montgomery, J. W. (2002). Understanding the language difficulties of children with specific language impairments: Does verbal working memory matter? *American Journal of Speech-Language Pathology, 11*(1), 77–91.

Moog, J. (2002). Changing expectations for children with cochlear implants. *Annals of Otology, Rhinology and Laryngology, Supplement, 189*, 138–142.

Moore-Brown, B.J., & Montgomery, J. (2001). *Making a difference for America's children*. Eau Claire, WI: Thinking Publications.

Morrison, G.S. *Teaching in America* (3rd ed.). Boston: Allyn & Bacon.

Most, T. (2002). The use of repair strategies by children with and without hearing impairment. *Language, Speech, and Hearing Services in Schools, 33*, 112–123.

Murphy, J. (2001). www.nativeamericanculture.about.com/culture/nativeamculture/library/weekly/aa0523ola.htm.

Muscular Dystrophy Campaign (2004). *Introduction—Duchenne muscular dystrophy*. Retrieved 8/9/05 from www.muscular-dystrophy.org.

NICHD Early Child Care Research Network (1999). Chronicity of maternal depressive symptoms, maternal sensitivity, and child functioning at 36 months. *Developmental Psychology, 35*, 1297–1310.

NICHD (2000). *Why children succeed or fail at reading: Research from NICHD's program in learning disabilities*. Available at www.nichd.gov/publications/pubs/readbro.htm

Nakagawa, K., Stafford, M.E., Fisher, T.A., & Matthews, L. (2002). The "city migrant" dilemma: Building community at high-mobility urban schools. *Urban Education, 37*, 96–125.

Nash, M., & Donaldson, M.L. (2005). Word learning in children with vocabulary deficits. *Journal of Speech, Language, and Hearing Research, 48*, 439–458.

Nathan, L., Stackhouse, J., Goulandris, N., & Snowling, M.J. (2004). The development of early literacy skills among children with speech difficulties: A test of the "Critical Age Hypothesis." *Journal of Speech, Language, and Hearing Research, 47*, 377–391.

Nation, K., Clarke, P., Marshall, C.M., & Durand, M. (2004). Hidden language impairments in children: Parallels between poor reading comprehension and specific language impairment? *Journal of Speech, Language, and Hearing Research, 47*(1), 199–211.

National Association of School Psychologists (2002). Position Statement on HIV/AIDS. Retrieved 7/28/05 from www.nasponline.org/information/pospaper_aids.html.

The National Association of State Boards of Education (1992). *Winners all: A call for inclusive schools. The report of the NASBE study group on special education*. Alexandria, VA: The National Association of State Boards of Education.

National Clearing House on Child Abuse and Neglect Information (2003). *Mandatory reporters of child abuse and neglect.* Retrieved June 5, 2003, from www.calib.com/nccanch/statutes/define.cfm.

National Dissemination Center for Children with Disabilities (2004). *Visual impairments: Fact Sheet 13.* Retrieved July 9, 2005, from www.cichcy.org.

National Institute of Allergy and Infectious Diseases (2000). *Pediatric AIDS.* Available at www.niaid.nih.gov/factsheets/pedaids.htm.

National Institute of Mental Health (2004). *Autism spectrum disorders (pervasive developmental disorders).* Retrieved July 15, 2004, from www.nimh.nih.gov.

National Institute of Neurological Disorders and Stroke (2005). *Spina bifida fact sheet.* Retrieved July 11, 2005, from www.ninds.nih.gov.

National Institute on Deafness and Other Communication Disorders (1996). *National strategic research plan: Hearing and hearing impairment.* Bethesda, MD: U.S. Department of Health and Human Services, National Institutes of Health.

National Institute on Deafness and Other Communication Disorders (1999). *Health information: Hearing and balance [On-line].* Available at www.nih.gov/nidcd/health/hb.htm.

National Joint Committee on Learning Disabilities (1997). *Operationalizing the NJCLD definition of learning disabilities for ongoing assessment in schools.* Rockville, MD: Author.

National Organization on Fetal Alcohol Syndrome (2000). *What is fetal alcohol syndrome.* Available at www.nofas.org/stats.htm.

National Reading Panel (2000). Report of the National Reading Panel. *Teaching children to read: An evidence-based assessment of the scientific literature on reading and its implications for reading instruction* (NIH Publication No. 00-4769). Washington, DC: U.S. Government Printing Office.

Neha, V. (2003). Home again: A Native American SLP's experiences teaching in a Navajo reservation school. *The ASHA Leader, 8,* 4–19.

Nehring, W.M. (2000). HIV disease in children. In J.D. Durham & F.R. Lashley (Eds.), *The person living with AIDS: Nursing perspectives* (3rd ed.) (pp. 429–510). New York: Springer Publishing Co.

Nellum-Davis, P., Gentry, B., & Hubbard-Wiley, P. (2002). Clinical practice issues. In D.E. Battle (Ed.), *Communication disorders in multicultural populations* (3rd ed.) (pp. 461–486). Woburn, MA: Butterworth-Heineman.

Nelson, N.W. (1991). Teacher talk and child listening-Fostering a better match. In C. Simon (Ed.), *Communication skills and classroom success. Assessment and therapy methodologies for language and learning disabled students.* Eau Claire, WI: Thinking Publications.

Nelson, N.W. (1998). *Childhood language disorders in context: Infancy through adolescence* (2nd ed.). Boston, MA: Allyn & Bacon.

Nelson, P., Kohnert, K., Sabur, S., & Shaw, D. (2005). Classroom noise and children learning through a second language: Double jeopardy? *Language, Speech, and Hearing Services in Schools, 36,* 219–229.

NICHD (2000). Why children succeed or fail at reading: Research from NICHD's program in learning disabilities. www.nichd.nih.gov/publications/pubs/readbro.htm.

Nickel, R.E. (2000). Human immunodeficiency virus infection. In R.E. Nickel & L.W. Desch (Eds.), *The physician's guide to caring for children with disabilities and chronic conditions* (pp. 391–424). Baltimore, MD: Paul H. Brookes.

Nicolosi, L., Harryman, E., & Krescheck, J. (2004). *Terminology of communication disorders: Speech-language-hearing* (5th ed.). Baltimore: Lippincott Williams & Wilkins.

Niparko, J.K., Cheng, A.K., & Francis, H.W. (2000). Outcomes of cochlear implantation: Assessment of quality of life impact and economic evaluation of the benefits of the cochlear implant in relation to costs. In J.K. Niparko, K.I. Kirk, N.K. Mellon, A.M. Robbins, D.L. Tucci, & B.S. Wilson (Eds.), *Cochlear implants: Principles and practices* (pp. 269–288). Philadelphia: Lippincott, Williams, & Wilkins.

Nippold, M. (1998). *Later language development: The school-age and adolescent years* (2nd ed). Austin, TX: Pro-Ed.

Nippold, M. (1999). Word definition in adolescents as a function of reading proficiency: A research note. *Child Language Teaching and Therapy, 15,* 171–176.

Nippold, M.A., Duthie, J.K., & Larsen, J. (2005). Literacy as a leisure activity: Free-time preferences of older children and younger adolescents. *Language, Speech, and Hearing Services in Schools, 36,* 93–102.

Nippold, M.A., Ward-Lonergan, J.M., & Fanning, J.L. (2005). Persuasive writing in children, adolescents, and adults: A study of syntactic, semantic, and pragmatic development. *Language, Speech, and Hearing Services in Schools, 36,* 125–138.

Nungesser, N.R., & Watkins, R.V. (2005a). Preschool teachers' perceptions and reactions to challenging classroom behavior: Implications for speech-language pathologists. *Language, Speech, and Hearing Services in Schools, 36,* 139–151.

Nungesser, N.R., & Watkins, R.V. (2005b, November). *Peer relations in preschool children with speech and language disorders.* Paper presented at the annual national meeting of the American Speech-Language-Hearing Association, San Diego, CA.

Nuru-Holm, N., & Battle, D.E. (1998). Multicultural aspects of deafness. In D.E. Battle (Ed.), *Communication disorders in multicultural populations* (2nd ed.) (pp. 335–378). Newton, MA: Butterworth-Heineman.

O'Brien, M., & Bi, X. (1995). Language learning in context: teacher and toddler speech in three classroom play areas. *Topics in Early Childhood Special Education, 15*, 148–163.

O'Connor, P.D., Sofo, F., Kenall, L., & Olsen, G. (1990). Reading disabilities and the effects of colored filters. *Journal of Learning Disabilities, 23*, 597–620.

O'Connor, R.E., & Bell, K.M. (2004). Teaching students with a reading disability to read words. In C.A. Stone, E.R. Silliman, B.J. Ehren, & K. Apel (Eds.). *Handbook of language and literacy: Development and disorders* (pp. 481–500). New York: The Guilford Press.

O'Connor, R.E., & Jenkins, J.R. (1999). Prediction of reading disabilities in kindergarten and first grade. *Scientific Studies of Reading, 3*, 159–197.

Oetting, J.B., & McDonald, J.L. (2001). Nonmainstream dialect use and specific language impairment. *Journal of Speech, Language, and Hearing Research, 44*(1), 207–223.

O'Hanlon, L., & Roseberry-McKibbin, C. (2004). Strategies for working with children from low-income backgrounds. *ADVANCE for Speech-Language Pathologists and Audiologists, 14(6)*, 12–20.

Olsen, J.Z. (2003). *Handwriting without tears*. Cabin John, MD: Handwriting Without Tears, Inc.

Olswang, L., Rodriguez, B., & Timler, G. (1998). Recommending intervention for toddlers with specific language learning difficulties: We may not have all the answers, but we know a lot. *American Journal of Speech-Language Pathology, 7*, 23–32.

Olswang, L., & Bain, R. (1991). Intervention issues for toddlers with specific language impairments. *Topics in Language Disorders, 11*, 69–86.

O'Neill-Perozzi, T.M. (2003). Language functioning of residents of family homeless shelters. *American Journal of Speech-Language Pathology, 12*, 229–242.

Ortiz, A.A. (1997). Learning disabilities occurring concomitantly with linguistic differences. *Journal of Learning Disabilities, 30*, 321–332.

Owens, R.E. (2005). *Language development: An introduction* (6th ed.). Boston, MA: Allyn & Bacon.

Owens, R.E. (2002). Mental retardation: Difference and delay. In D.K. Bernstein and E. Tiegermann-Farber, *Language and communication disorders in children* (5th ed.) (pp. 436–509). Boston: Allyn & Bacon.

Owens, R.E. (2004). *Language disorders: A functional approach to assessment and intervention* (4th ed.). Boston: Allyn & Bacon.

Ozonoff, S., Dawson, G., & McPartland, J. (2002). *A parent's guide to Asperger syndrome and high-functioning autism: How to meet the challenges and help your child thrive*. New York: The Guilford Press.

Paglario, C. (2001). Addressing deaf culture in the classroom. *Kappa Delta Pi Record, 37*, 173–179.

Paradis, J. (2005). Grammatical morphology in children learning English as a second language: Implications of similarities with specific language impairment. *Language, Speech, and Hearing Services in Schools, 36*, 172–187.

Paradis, J., & Crago, M. (2000). Tense and temporality: A comparison between children learning a second language and children with SLI. *Journal of Speech, Language, and Hearing Research, 43*, 834–847.

Paradis, J., Crago, M., Genesee, F., & Rice, M. (2003). French-English bilingual children with SLI: How do they compare with their monolingual peers? *Journal of Speech, Language, and Hearing Research, 46*(1), 113–127.

Paris, S.G.(1991). Assessment and remediation of metacognitive aspects of children's reading comprehension. *Topics in Language Disorders*, 12, 32–50.

Park, J., Turnbull, A.P., & Turnbull, H.R. III (2002). Impacts of poverty on quality of life in families of children with disabilities. *Exceptional Children, 68*, 151–170.

Park, K., Shallcross, R., & Anderson, R. (1980). Differences in coverbal behavior between blind and sighted persons during dyadic communication. *Visual Impairment and Blindness, 74*, 142–146.

Parkay, F.W., & Stanford, B.H. (2004). *Becoming a teacher* (6th ed.). Boston: Allyn & Bacon.

Parette, H.P., Huer, M.B., & Wyatt, T.A. (2003/04). Young African American children with disabilities and augmentative and alternative communication issues. In K.L. Freiburg (Ed.), *Annual editions: Educating exceptional children* (15th ed.) (pp. 76–81). Guilford, CT: Dushkin Publishing Group.

Patterson, J.L. (2000). Observed and reported expressive vocabulary and word combinations in bilingual toddlers. *Journal of Speech, Language, and Hearing Research, 43*, 121–128.

Patterson, J.L., & Pearson, B.Z. (2004). Bilingual lexical development: Influences, contexts, and processes. In B.A. Goldstein (Ed.), *Bilingual language development and disorders in Spanish-English speakers* (pp. 77–104). Baltimore, MD: Paul H. Brookes Publishing Co.

Paul, R. (2001). *Language disorders from infancy through adolescence: Assessment and intervention* (2nd ed.). St. Louis, MO: Mosby-Year Book, Inc.

Paul, R., & Smith, R.L. (1993). Narrative skills in 4-year-olds with typical, impaired, and late-developing language. *Journal of Speech and Hearing Research, 36*, 592–598.

Payne, A.C., Whitehurst, G.J., & Angell, A.L. (1994). The role of home literacy environment in the development of language ability in preschool children from low-income families. *Early Childhood Research Quarterly, 9*, 427–440.

Payne, R.K. (2003). *A framework for understanding poverty* (4th ed.). Highlands, TX: Aha! Process, Inc.

Peach, R.K. (2002). From the editor. *American Journal of Speech-Language Pathology, 11*, 322.

Pearson, C.M. (2001). Internationally adopted children: Issues and challenges. *The ASHA Leader, 6*, 4–13.

Pellegrino, L. (2002). Cerebral palsy. In M.L. Batshaw (Ed.), *When your child has a disability* (pp. 275–287). Baltimore, MD: Paul H. Brookes Publishing Co.

Peña, D.C. (2000). Parent involvement: Influencing factors and implications. The *Journal of Educational Research, 94*, 42–54.

Peña, E.D., Iglesias, A., & Lidz, C.S. (2001). Reducing test bias through dynamic assessment of children's word learning ability. *American Journal of Speech-Language Pathology, 10*, 138–154.

Peña, E.D., & Kester, E.S. (2004). Semantic development in Spanish-English bilinguals: Theory, assessment, and intervention. In B.A. Goldstein (Ed.), *Bilingual language development and disorders in Spanish-English speakers* (pp. 105–130). Baltimore, MD: Paul H. Brookes Publishing Co.

Peña-Brooks, A., & Hegde, M.N. (2007). *Assessment and treatment of articulation and phonological disorders in children.* Austin, TX: Pro-Ed.

Peregoy, S.F., & Boyle, O.W. (1997). *Reading, writing, and learning in ESL: A resource book for K-12 teachers* (2nd ed.). New York: Longman Publishers.

Perez-Pereira, M., & Conti-Ramsden, G. (1999). *Language development and social interaction in blind children.* Hove, United Kingdom: Psychology Press.

Podell, S.M. (2004). *An overview of the Irlen method.* Retrieved June 12, 2005, from www.oep.org/Podell1-7an_overview_of_the_irlen_method.htm.

Portes, A., & Rumbaut, R. (2001). *Legacies: The story of the immigrant second generation.* Berkeley, CA: University of California Press.

Prelock, P.A., Beatson, J., Bitner, B., Broder, C., & Ducker, A. (2003). Interdisciplinary assessment of young children with Autism Spectrum Disorder. *Language, Speech, and Hearing Services in Schools, 34*, 194–202.

Preschool Amendments to the Education of the Handicapped Act 20 U.S.C. 1471 *et seq.* (1986).

President's Commission on Excellence in Special Education (2002). *A new era: Revitalizing special education for children and their families.* Washington, DC: Author.

Pressman, H. (1992). Communication disorders and dysphagia in pediatric AIDS. *Asha Magazine*, pp. 45–47.

Pring, L., & Hermelin, B. (2002). Numbers and letters: Exploring an autistic savant's unpractised ability. *Neurocase, 8*, 330–337.

Prizant, B.M. (2004). *Autism spectrum disorders and the SCERTS model: A comprehensive educational approach.* Baltimore, MD: Brookes Publishing House.

Proctor, B., & Dalaker, J. (2002). *Poverty in the United States: 2001, Current population reports*, P60-219. Washington, DC: U.S. Government Printing Office.

Prutting, C.A., & Kirchner, D.M. (1983). Applied pragmatics. In T.M. Gallagher & C.A. Prutting (Eds.), *Pragmatic assessment and intervention issues in language* (pp. 29–64). Austin, TX: Pro-Ed.

Qi, C.H., & Kaiser, A.P. (2004). Problem behaviors of low-income children with language delays: An observation study. *Journal of Speech, Language, and Hearing Research, 47*, 595–609.

Rabidoux, P., & Macdonald, J. (2000). An interactive taxonomy of mothers and children during storybook interactions. *American Journal of Speech-Language Pathology, 9*, 331–344.

Radziewicz, C., & Antonellis, S. (2002). Considerations and implications for habilitation of hearing-impaired children. In D.K. Bernstein & E. Tiegerman-Farber, *Language and communication disorders in children* (5th ed.) (pp. 565–598). Boston: Allyn & Bacon.

Ramirez, J.D., Yuen, S., & Ramey, D. (1991). *Executive summary final report: Longitudinal study of structured English immersion strategy, early-exit and late-exit transitional bilingual education programs for language-minority children.* Submitted to U.S. Department of Education, Washington, D.C.

Redmond, S.M. (2002). The use of rating scales with children who have language impairments. *American Journal of Speech-Language Pathology, 11*, 124–138.

Reed, V.A. (1994). *An introduction to children with language disorders* (2nd ed.). New York: Macmillan College Publishing Company.

Reed, V.A. (2005). *An introduction to children with language disorders* (3rd ed.). Boston: Pearson Education, Inc.

Reed, V.A., & Spicer, L. (2003). The relative importance of selected communication skills for adolescents' interactions with their teachers: High school teachers' opinions. *Language, Speech, and Hearing Services in Schools, 34*, 343–357.

Rees, R.J., & Bellon, M.L. (2002). The acquisition of communication skills by people with brain injury: some comparisons with children with autism. *International Journal of Disability, Development and Education, 49*, 175–189.

Rehabilitation Act of 1973, Public Law 93-112, Section 504, 29 U.S.C. 794 (1973).

Reichle, J. (1991). Developing communicative exchanges. In J. Reichle, J. York, & J. Sigafoos (Eds.), *Implementing augmentative and alternative communication: Strategies for learners with severe disabilities* (pp. 123–156). Baltimore, MD: Paul H. Brookes Publishing Co.

Reid, R., Casta, C.D., Norton, H.J., Anastopolous, A.D., & Temple, E.P. (2001). Using behavior rating scales for ADHD across ethnic groups: The IOWA Conners. *Journal of Emotional and Behavioral Disorders, 9*, 210–218.

Reid, R., Riccio, C.A., Kessler, R.H., DuPaul, G.J., Power, T.J., Anastopolous, A.D., Rogers-Adkinson, D., & Noll, M. (2000). Gender and ethnic differences in ADHD assessed by behavior ratings. *Journal of Emotional and Behavioral Disorders, 8*, 38–48.

Rescorla, L. (1989). The Language Development Survey: A screening tool for delayed language in toddlers. *Journal of Speech and Hearing Disorders, 54*, 587–599.

Rescorla, L. (2002). Language and reading outcomes to age 9 in late-talking toddlers. *Journal of Speech, Language, and Hearing Research, 45*, 360–371.

Rescorla, L. (2005). Age 13 language and reading outcomes in late-talking toddlers. *Journal of Speech, Language, and Hearing Research, 48*, 459–472.

Rescorla, L., & Achenbach, T.M. (2002). Use of the Language Development Survey (LDS) in a national probability sample of children 18 to 35 months old. *Journal of Speech, Language, and Hearing Research, 45*, 733–743.

Rescorla, L., & Alley, A. (2001). Validation of the Language Development Survey (LDS): A parent report tool for identifying language delay in toddlers. *Journal of Speech, Language, and Hearing Research, 44*, 434–445.

Rescorla, L., Berstein Ratner, N., Juscyzk, P., & Jusczyk, A.M. (2005). Concurrent development of the Language Development Survey: Associations with the MacArthur-Bates Communicative Development Inventories: Words and Sentences. *American Journal of Speech-Language Pathology, 14*, 156–163.

Rescorla, L., Dahlsgaard, K., & Roberts, J. (2000). Late-talking toddlers: MUL and IPSyn outcomes at 3;0 and 4;0. *Journal of Child Language, 27*, 643–664.

Restrepo, M.A., & Gutierrez-Clellen, V.F. (2004). Grammatical impairments in Spanish-English bilingual children. In B.A. Goldstein (Ed.), *Bilingual language development and disorders in Spanish-English speakers* (pp. 213–234). Baltimore, MD: Paul H. Brookes Publishing Co.

Restrepo, M.A., & Kruth, K. (2000). Grammatical characteristics of a Spanish-English bilingual child with specific language impairment. *Communication Disorders Quarterly, 21*, 66–76.

Restrepo, M.A., & Silverman, S.W. (2001). Validity of the Spanish Preschool Language Scale-3 for use with bilingual children. *American Journal of Speech-Language Pathology, 10*, 382–393.

Rice, M.L., Hadley, P. & Alexander, A. (1993). Social biases toward children with speech and language impairments: A correlative causal model of language limitation. *Applied Psycholinguistics, 14*, 445–471.

Rice, M.L., Haney, K.R., & Wexler, K. (1998). Family histories of children with SLI who show extended optional infinitives. *Journal of Speech, Language, and Hearing Research, 41*, 419–432.

Rice, M.L., Sell, M.A., & Hadley, P.A. (1991). Social interactions of speech- and language-impaired children. *Journal of Speech and Hearing Research, 34*, 1299–1307.

Rice, M.L., Tomblin, J.B., Hoffman, L., Richman, W.W., & Marquis, J. (2004). Grammatical tense deficits in children with SLI and Nonspecific Language Impairment: Relationships with nonverbal IQ over time. *Journal of Speech, Language, and Hearing Research, 47*, 816–824.

Rice, M.L., & Wexler, K. (1996). Toward tense as a clinical marker of specific language impairment in English-speaking children. *Journal of Speech and Hearing Research, 39*, 1239–1257.

Rivers, K.O., & Hedrick, D.L. (1992). Language and behavioral concerns for drug-exposed infants and toddlers. In L.M. Rossetti (Ed.), *Developmental problems of drug-exposed infants* (pp. 63–71). San Diego, CA: Singular Publishing Group, Inc.

Roberts, J., Jurgens, J., & Burchinal, M. (2005). The role of home literacy practices in preschool children's language and emergent literacy skills. *Journal of Speech, Language, and Hearing Research, 48*, 345–359.

Roberts, J., Pollock, K.E., Krakow, R., Price, J., Fulmer, K.C., & Wang, P.P. (2005). Language development in preschool-age children adopted from China. *Journal of Speech, Language, and Hearing Research, 48*, 93–107.

Robertson, C., & Salter, W. (1997). *The Phonological Awareness Test*. East Moline, IL: LinguiSystems.

Robinson, G.L., Foreman, P.J., & Dear, K.B.G. (1996). The familial incidence of symptoms of scotopic sensitivity/Irlen syndrome. *Perceptual and Motor Skills, 79*, 467–483.

Robinson, N.B., & Robb, M.P. (2002). Early communication assessment and intervention. In D.K. Bernstein & E. Tiegerman-Farber, *Language and communication disorders in children* (5th ed.) (pp. 126–180). Boston: Allyn & Bacon.

Robinson, G.L., & Miles, J. (1987). The use of colored overlays to improve visual processing: A preliminary survey. *The Exceptional Child, 34*, 65–70.

Robinson, J.L., & Acevedo, M.C. (2001). Infant reactivity and reliance on mother during emotion challenges: Prediction of cognition and language skills in a low-income sample. *Child Development, 72*, 402–415.

Rodriguez, B.L., & Olswang, L.B. (2003). Mexican-American and Anglo-American mothers' beliefs and values about child rearing, education, and language impairment. *American Journal of Speech-Language Pathology, 12*, 452–462.

Roseberry-McKibbin, C. (2000). Multicultural matters. *Communication Disorders Quarterly, 21*, 242–245.

Roseberry-McKibbin, C. (2001a). *The source for bilingual children with language disorders.* East Moline, IL: LinguiSystems.

Roseberry-McKibbin, C. (2001b). Serving children from the culture of poverty: Practical strategies for speech-language pathologists. *The ASHA Leader, 6*, 4–16.

Roseberry-McKibbin, C. (2003). *Assessment of bilingual learners: Language difference or language disorder?* Video published by the American Speech-Language-Hearing Association, Rockville, MD.

Roseberry-McKibbin, C. (2008). *Multicultural students with special language needs: Practical strategies for assessment and intervention* (3rd ed.). Oceanside, CA: Academic Communication Associates.

Roseberry-McKibbin, C., & Brice, A. (1998). *Service delivery issues in serving clients from low-income backgrounds.* Paper presented at the annual meeting of the American Speech-Language-Hearing Association, San Antonio, TX.

Roseberry-McKibbin, C., Brice, A., & O'Hanlon, L. (2005). Serving English language learners in public school settings: A national survey. *Language, Speech, and Hearing Services in Schools, 36*, 48–61.

Roseberry-McKibbin, C., & Hegde, M.N. (2006). *Advanced review of speech-language pathology: Preparation for PRAXIS and comprehensive examination* (2nd ed.). Austin, TX: Pro-Ed.

Roseberry-McKibbin, C., Peña, A., Hall, M., & Stubblefield-Smith, S. (1996, November). Health care considerations in serving children from migrant Hispanic families. Paper presented at the annual convention of the American Speech-Language-Hearing Association, Seattle, WA.

Rossetti, L.M. (2001). *Communication intervention birth to three* (2nd ed.). Albany, NY: Singular/Delmar.

Roy, P., & Chiat, S. (2004). A prosodically controlled word and nonword repetition task for 2- to 4-year-olds: Evidence from typically-developing children. *Journal of Speech, Language, and Hearing Research, 47*, 223–234.

Ruiz, N.T., Rueda, R., Figueroa, R.R., & Boothroyd, M. (1995). Bilingual special education teacher's shifting paradigms: Complex responses to educational reform. *Journal of Learning Disabilities, 28*, 622–635.

Ruhl, K.L., Hughes, C.A., & Camarata, S.T. (1992). Analysis of the expressive and receptive language characteristics of emotionally handicapped students served in public school settings. *Journal of Childhood Communication Disorders, 14*, 165–176.

Rvachew, S., Ohberg, A., Grawburg, M., & Heyding, J. (2003). Phonological awareness and phonemic perception in 4-year-old children with delayed expressive phonology skills. *American Journal of Speech-Language Pathology, 12*, 463–471.

Saenz, T.I. (1996). An overview of second language acquisition. In H.W. Langdon & T.I. Saenz (Eds.), *Language assessment and intervention with multicultural students: A guide for speech-language-hearing professionals* (pp. 51–60). Oceanside, CA: Academic Communication Associates.

Saenz, T.I., Huer, M.B., Doan, J.H.D., Heise, M., & Fulford, L. (2001). Delivering clinical services to Vietnamese Americans: Implications for speech-language pathologists. *Communication Disorders Quarterly, 22*, 207–216.

Saint-Laurent, L., & Giasson, J. (2001). Effects of a multicomponent literacy program and of supplemental phonological sessions on at-risk kindergarteners. *Educational Research and Evaluation, 7*, 1–33.

Salas-Provance, M.B., Erickson, J.G., & Reed, J. (2002). Disabilities as viewed by four generations of one Hispanic family. *American Journal of Speech-Language Pathology, 11*, 151–162.

Sanger, D., Moore-Brown, B., Montgomery, J., & Hellerich, S. (2004). Speech-language pathologists' opinions on communication disorders and violence. *Language, Speech, and Hearing Services in Schools, 35*, 16–29.

Santos, R.S., & Chan, S. (2004). Families with Pilipino roots. In E.W. Lynch and M.J. Hanson (Eds.), *Developing cross-cultural competence: A guide for working with young children and their families* (pp. 219–298). Baltimore, MD: Paul H. Brookes Publishing Co.

Sardegna, J., & Otis, T.P. (1991). *The encyclopedia of blindness and vision impairment.* New York: Facts on File.

Saywitz, K.J., Mannarino, A.P., Berliner, L., & Cohen, J.A. (2000). Treatment for sexually abused children and adolescents. *American Psychologist, 55*, 1040–1049.

Schieffelin, B.B., & Ochs, E. (Eds.) (1984). *Language socialization across cultures.* Cambridge: Cambridge University Press.

Schirmer, B. (2000). *Language and literacy development in children who are deaf* (2nd ed.). Boston: Allyn & Bacon.

Schiff-Myers, N. (1992). Considering arrested language development and second language loss in the assessment of second language learners. *Language, Speech, and Hearing Services in Schools, 23*, 28–33.

Schopler, E., Yirmiya, N., Shulman, C., & Marcus, L.M. (2001). *Research basis for autism intervention*. New York: Kluwer Academic/Plenum Publishers.

Schow, R.L., & Nerbonne, M.A. (2002). *Introduction to audiologic rehabilitation* (4th ed.). Boston: Allyn & Bacon.

Schuler, A.L., & Fletcher, E.C. (2002). Making communication meaningful: Cracking the language interaction code. In R.L. Gabriels & D.E. Hill (Eds.), *Autism—from research to individualized practice* (pp. 127–154). London: Jessica Kingsley Publishers.

Schumann, J. (1986). Research on the acculturation model for second language acquisition. *Journal of Multilingual and Multi-cultural Development, 7*, 379–392.

Scott, D.M, (2002). Multicultural aspects of hearing disorders and audiology. In D.E. Battle (Ed.), *Communication disorders in multicultural populations* (3rd ed.). (pp. 335–361), Woburn, MA: Butterworth-Heinemann.

Scott, C.M., & Windsor, J. (2000). General language performance measures in spoken and written narrative and expository discourse of school-age children with learning disabilities. *Journal of Speech, Language, and Hearing Research, 43*, 324–339.

Segers, E., & Verhoeven, L. (2004). Computer-supported phonological awareness intervention for kindergarten children with specific language impairment. *Language, Speech, and Hearing Services in Schools, 35*, 229–239.

Selinker, L. (1972). Interlanguage. *International Review of Applied Linguistics* (IRAL), *X/3*, 31–53.

Seidenberg, P.L. (2002). Understanding learning disabilities. In D.K. Bernstein & E. Tiegerman-Farber, *Language and commu-nication disorders in children* (5th ed.) (pp. 388–435). Boston: Allyn & Bacon.

Semel, E., Wiig, E.H., & Secord, W.A. (2003). *Clinical evaluation of language fundamentals-4*. San Antonio, TX: The Psycho-logical Corporation.

Seung, H.-K., & Chapman, R. (2000). Digit span in individuals with Down syndrome and in typically-developing children: Temporal aspects. *Journal of Speech, Language, and Hearing Research, 43*, 609–620.

Seymour, C.M., & Nober, E.H. (1998). *Introduction to communication disorders: A multicultural approach*. Boston, MA: Butterworth-Heinemann.

Seymour, H.N., Roeper, T.W., deVilliers, J., & deVilliers, P. (2003). *Diagnostic evaluation of language variation*. San Antonio, TX: Psychological Corporation.

Seymour, H.N., & Valles, L. (1998). Language intervention for linguistically different learners. In C.M. Seymour & E.H. Nober (Eds.), *Introduction to communication disorders: A multicultural approach*. Boston, MA: Butterworth-Heinemann.

Sharif, I., Reiber, S., & Ozuah, P. (2002). Exposure to Reach out and Read and vocabulary outcomes in inner city preschoolers. *Journal of the National Medical Association, 94*, 171–177.

Sharifzadeh, V-S. (2004). Families with Middle Eastern roots. In E.W. Lynch and M.J. Hanson (Eds.), *Developing cross-cultural competence: A guide for working with young children and their families* (pp. 1–2). Baltimore, MD: Paul H. Brookes Pub-lishing Co.

Sherman, A. (1994). *Wasting America's future: The Children's Defense Fund report on the cost of child poverty*. Boston: Beacon Press.

Shipley, K.G., & McAfee, J. (2004). *Assessment in speech-language pathology: A resource manual* (2nd ed.). San Diego: Singular/Delmar.

Shipley, K.G., & Roseberry-McKibbin, C. (2006). *Interviewing and counseling in communicative disorders: Principles and procedures* (3rd ed.). Austin, TX: Pro-Ed.

Shriberg, L.D., Paul, R., McSweeney, J.L., Klin, A., Cohen, D.J., & Volkmar, F.R. (2001). Speech and prosody characteris-tics of adolescents and adults with high-functioning autism and Asperger syndrome. *Journal of Speech, Language, and Hearing Research, 44*, 1097–1115.

Shulman, B. (1983). *Pragmatic development chart*. San Francisco: Word-Making Productions.

Sigafoos, J., Drasgow, E., Reichle, J., O'Reilly, M., Green, V.A., & Tait, K. (2004). Tutorial: Teaching communicative rejecting to children with severe disabilities. *American Journal of Speech-Language Pathology, 13*, 31–42.

Sigafoos, J., Woodyatt, G., Keen, D., Tait, K., Tucker, M., Roberts-Pennell, D., & Pittendreigh, N. (2000). Identifying potential com-munication acts in children with developmental and physical disabilities. *Communication Disorders Quarterly, 21*, 77–86.

Silliman, E.R., & Diehl, S.F. (2002). Assessing children with language learning disabilities. In D.K. Bernstein & E. Tiegerman-Farber, *Language and communication disorders in children* (pp. 181–255). Boston: Allyn & Bacon.

Silliman, E.R., Wilkinson, L.C., & Brea-Spahn, M.R. (2004). Policy and practice imperatives for language and literacy learning: Who will be left behind? In C.A. Stone, E.R. Silliman, B.J. Ehren, & K. Apel (Eds.), *Handbook of language and literacy: Development and disorders* (pp. 97–129). New York: The Guilford Press.

Singer, B.D., & Bashir, A.S. (2004). Developmental variations in writing composition skills. In C.A. Stone, E.R. Silliman, B.J. Ehren, & K. Apel (Eds.). *Handbook of language and literacy: Development and disorders* (pp. 559–582). New York: The Guilford Press.

Skinner, B.F. (1957). *Verbal behavior*. Norwalk, CT: Appleton-Century-Crofts.

Skutnabb-Kangas, T., & Toukomaa, P. (1976). *Teaching migrant children's mother tongue and learning the language of the host country in the context of the sociocultural situation of the migrant family*. Helsinki: The Finnish National Commission for UNESCO, 1976.

Smith, K.E., Landry, S.H., & Swank, P.R. (2000). Does the content of mothers' verbal stimulation explain differences in children's development of verbal and nonverbal cognitive skills? *Journal of School Psychology, 38*, 27–49.

Smith, T., Lovaas, N.W., & Lovaas, O.I. (2002). Behaviors of children with high-functioning autism when paired with typically-developing versus delayed peers: A preliminary study. *Behavioral Interventions, 17*, 129–143.

Snow, C., Burns, M.S., & Griffin, P. (Eds.). (1998). *Preventing reading difficulties in young children*. Washington, DC: National Academy Press.

Snowling, M.J. (1996). Developmental dyslexia. In M. Snowling and J. Stackhouse (Eds.), *Dyslexia, speech, and language: A practitioner's handbook* (pp. 111). London: Whurr Publishers.

Snowling, M.J. (2000). *Dyslexia* (2nd ed.). Oxford: Blackwell.

Snowling, M., Bishop, D.V.M., & Stothard, S.E. (2000). Is preschool language impairment a risk factor for dyslexia in adolescence? *Journal of Child Psychology and Psychiatry, 41*, 587–600.

Snyder, L.S., Nathanson, R., & Saywitz, K.J. (1993). Children in court: The role of discourse processing and production. *Topics in Language Disorders, 13*, 39–58.

Snyder, L.E., & Scherer, N. (2004). The development of symbolic play and language in toddlers with cleft palate. *American Journal of Speech-Language Pathology, 13*, 66–80.

Solanto, M.V. (2002). Dopamine dysfunction in AD/HD: Integrating clinical and basic neuroscience research. *Behavioural Brain Research, 130*, 65–71.

Soto, G., Huer, M.B., & Taylor, O. (1997). Multicultural issues. In L.I. Lloyd, D.H. Fuller, & H.H. Arvidson (Eds.), *Augmentative and alternative communication* (pp. 406–413). Boston: Allyn & Bacon.

Southwood, S., & Russell, A.F. (2004). Comparison of conversation, freeplay, and story generation as methods of language sample elicitation. *Journal of Speech, Language, and Hearing Research, 47*, 366–376.

Sparks, S. (1993). *Children of prenatal substance abuse*. San Diego: Singular Publishing Group.

Sparks, S. (2001). Prenatal substance use and its impact on young children. In T. Layton, E. Crais, & L. Watson, *Handbook of early language impairment in children: Nature* (pp. 451–487). Albany, NY: Delmar Publishers.

Speece, D.L., & Cooper, D.H. (2004). Methodological issues in research on language and early literacy from the perspective of early identification and instruction. In C.A. Stone, E.R. Silliman, B.J. Ehren, & K. Apel (Eds.). *Handbook of language and literacy: Development and disorders* (pp. 82–94). New York: The Guilford Press.

Spinal Cord Injury Resource Center (2003). Some questions and answers [online]. Retrieved May 31, 2003, from www.spinalinjury.net/html/_spinal_cord_101.html.

Stach, B.A. (2003). *Comprehensive dictionary of audiology* (2nd ed.). Clifton Park, NY: Delmar Learning.

Stainback, W., & Stainback, S. (1996). *Inclusion: A guide for educators*. Baltimore, MD: Brookes.

Stainback, S., & Stainback, W. (1987). Integration vs. cooperation: A commentary on "Educating children with learning problems: A shared responsibility." *Exceptional Children, 54*, 66–68.

Stainback, W., & Stainback, S. (1984). A rationale for the merger of special and regular education. *Exceptional Children, 51*, 102–111.

Stainback, W., Stainback, S., Stefanich, G., & Alper, S. (1996). Learning in inclusive classrooms: What about the curriculum? In S. Stainback and W. Stainback (Eds.), *Inclusion: A guide for educators* (pp. 209–219). Baltimore, MD: Brookes.

Stanovich, K.E., & Siegel, L.S. (1994). Phenotypic performance profile of children with reading disabilities: A regression-based test of the phonological-core variable-difference model. *Journal of Educational Psychology, 86*, 24–53.

Stein, N.L., & Glenn, C.G. (1975). *An analysis of story comprehension in elementary school children: A test of a schema*. Educational Resources Information Center (ERIC Document Reproduction Service No. ED 121474).

Stone, C.A. (2004). Contemporary approaches to the study of language and literacy development: A call for the integration of perspectives. In C.A. Stone, E.R. Silliman, B.J.Ehren, & Apel, K. (Eds.), *Handbook of language and literacy: Development and disorders* (pp. 3–24). New York: The Guilford Press.

Stothard, S., Snowling, M., Bishop, D.V.M., Chipchase, B., & Kaplan, C. (1998). Language impaired preschoolers: A follow-up into adolescence. *Journal of Speech, Language, and Hearing Research, 41*, 407–418.

Streissguth, A. (1997). Fetal alcohol syndrome in adolescents and adults. *Journal of the American Medical Association, 265*, 1961–1967.

Sue, D.W., & Sue, D. (2003). *Counseling the culturally diverse: Theory and practice* (4th ed.). New York: John Wiley & Sons.

Swanson, L.A., Fey, M.E., Mills, C.E., & Hood, L.S. (2005). Use of narrative-based language intervention with children who have specific language impairment. *American Journal of Speech-Language Pathology, 14*, 131–143.

Swanson, T.J., Hodson, B.W., & Schommer-Aikins, M. (2005). An examination of phonological awareness treatment outcomes for seventh-grade poor readers from a bilingual community. *Language, Speech, and Hearing Services in Schools, 36*, 336–345.

Tabors, P.O. (1997). *One child, two languages: A guide for preschool educators of children learning English as a second language*. Baltimore, MD: Paul H. Brookes Publishing Co.

Tabors, P.O., Snow, C.E., & Dickinson, D.K. (2001). Homes and schools together: Supporting language and early literacy development. In D.K. Dickinson & P.O. Tabors (Eds.), *Beginning literacy with language*. Baltimore, MD: Brookes.

Tager-Flusberg, H. (2005). Putting words together: Morphology and syntax in the preschool years. In J.B. Gleason (Ed.), *The development of language* (6th ed.) (pp. 148–190). Boston: Allyn & Bacon.

Tallal, P. (2005). *Language learning impairment: Integrating research and remediation.* Retrieved 6/4/05 from www.newhorizons.org/neuro.tallal.htm.

Tallal, P., Merzenich, M.M.. Miller, S., & Jenkins, W. (1998). Language learning impairment: Integrating basic science, technology, and remediation. *Experimental Brain Research, 123*, 210–219.

Tallal, P., Miller, S.L., Bedi, G., Byman, G., Wang, X., Nagarajan, S.S., Schreiner, C., Jenkins, W., & Merzenich, M.M. Language comprehension in language-learning impaired children improved with acoustically modified speech. *Science, 5*, 81–84.

Tannen, D. (1990). *You just don't understand: Women and men in conversation.* New York: Ballantine Books.

Taylor, S. (2003). *Disability studies and mental retardation.* Retrieved July 16, 2004, from soeweb.syr.edu/thechp/dsmr.htm.

Teagle, H.F.B., & Moore, J.A. (2002). School-based services for children with cochlear implants. *Language, Speech, and Hearing Services in Schools, 33*, 162–171.

Tepper, T., Hannon, L., & Sandstrom, D. (Eds.) (1999). *International adoption: Challenges and opportunities.* Parent Network for the Post-Institutionalized Child: www.pnpic.org.

Terell, B.Y., & Hale, J.E. (1992). Serving a multicultural population: Different learning styles. *American Journal of Speech-Language Pathology, 1*, 5–8.

Terrell, S.L., & Jackson, R.S. (2002). African Americans in the Americas. In D.E. Battle (Ed.), *Communication disorders in multicultural populations* (3rd ed.) (pp. 113–134). Boston: Butterworth-Heinemann.

Thal, D. & Tobias, S. (1992). Communicative gestures in children with delayed onset of oral expressive vocabulary. *Journal of Speech and Hearing Research, 35*, 1281–1289.

Thal, D.J., O'Hanlon, L., Clemmons, M., & Fralin, L. (1999). Validity of a parent report measure of vocabulary and syntax for preschool children with language impairment. *Journal of Speech, Language, and Hearing Research, 42*, 482–496.

Thal, D., Jackson-Maldonado, D., & Acosta, D. (2000). Validity of a parent-report measure of vocabulary and grammar for Spanish-speaking toddlers. *Journal of Speech, Language, and Hearing Research, 43*, 1087–1100.

Thiemann, K.S., & Goldstein, H. (2004). Effects of peer training and written text cueing on social communication of school-age children with Pervasive Developmental Disorder. *Journal of Speech, Language, and Hearing Research, 47*, 126–144.

Thomas, W.P., & Collier, V.P. (1998). Two languages are better than one. *Educational Leadership, 12/97–1/98*, 23–26.

Thomas, W.P., & Collier, V.P. (2003). *A national study of school effectiveness for language minority students' long-term academic achievement.* Berkeley, CA: Center for Research on Education, Diversity and Excellence and the Office of Educational Research Improvement (ERIC Document Reproduction Service No. ED 475048).

Thomas-Tate, S., Washington, J., & Edwards, J. (2004). Standardized assessment of phonological awareness skills in low-income African American first graders. *American Journal of Speech-Language Pathology, 13*, 182–190.

Thompson, C.A., Craig, H.K., & Washington, J.A. (2004). Variable production of African American English across oracy and literacy contexts. *Language, Speech, and Hearing Services in Schools, 35*, 269–282.

Thorardottir, E.T., & Ellis Weismer, S. (2002). Content mazes and filled pauses in narrative language samples of children with specific language impairment. *Brain and Cognition, 48*, 587–592.

Tiegerman-Farber, E. (2002). Autism spectrum disorders: Learning to communicate. In D.K. Bernstein & E. Tiegerman-Farber, *Language and communication disorders in children* (5th ed.) (pp. 520–564). Boston: Allyn & Bacon.

Tobey, E., Geers, A., Brenner, C., Altuna, D., & Gabbert, G. (2003). Factors associated with development of speech production skills in children implanted by age five. *Ear & Hearing, 24*, 365–465.

Tomblin, J.S., & Buckwalter, P.R. (1998). Heritability of poor language achievement among twins. *Journal of Speech, Language, and Hearing Research, 41*, 188–189.

Tomblin, J.B., Zhang, X., Buckwalter, P., & O'Brien, M. (2003). The stability of primary language disorder: Four years after kindergarten diagnosis. *Journal of Speech, Language, and Hearing Research, 46*, 1283–1296.

Torgeson, J.K., & Bryant, B.R. (1994). *Test of Phonological Awareness.* Austin, TX: Pro-Ed.

Torgeson, J.K., & Mathes, P.G. (2000). *A basic guide to understanding, assessing, and teaching phonological awareness.* Austin, TX: Pro-Ed.

Trickett, P., Aber, J., Carlson, V., & Cicchetti, D. (1991). Relationship of socioeconomic status to the etiology and developmental sequelae of physical child abuse. *Developmental Psychology, 27*, 148–158.

Troia, G.A. (2004). Phonological processing and its influence on literacy learning. In C.A. Stone, E.R. Silliman, B.J. Ehren, & K. Apel (Eds.). *Handbook of language and literacy: Development and disorders* (pp. 271–301). New York: The Guilford Press.

Troster, H., Hecker, W., & Brambring, M. (1993). Early motor development in blind infants. *Journal of Applied Developmental Psychology, 14*, 83–106.

Tur-Kaspa, H., & Dromi, E. (2001). Grammatical deviations in the spoken and written language of Hebrew-speaking children with hearing impairments. *Language, Speech, and Hearing Services in Schools, 32*, 79–89.

Turkstra, L., Ciccia, A., & Seaton, C. (2003). Interactive behaviors in adolescent conversation dyads. *Language, Speech, and Hearing Services in Schools, 34*, 117–127.

Tye-Murray, N. (2004). *Foundations of aural rehabilitation: Children, adults, and their family members* (2nd ed.). Clifton Park, NY: Delmar Learning.

Ukraintez, T.A. (Ed.). (2006). *Contextualized language intervention: Scaffolding PreK-12 literacy achievement*. Eau Claire, WI: Thinking Publications.

Ukrainetz, T., Haroell, S., Walsh, C., & Coyle, C. (2000). A preliminary investigation of dynamic assessment with Native American kindergarteners. *Language, Speech, and Hearing Services in Schools, 31*, 142–154.

United Cerebral Palsy (2001). *Cerebral palsy: Facts and figures*. Retrieved July 11, 2005, from www.ucp.org.

United States Bureau of the Census (2000). *Statistical abstract of the United States, 2000* (120th ed.). Washington, DC: U.S. Department of Commerce.

United States Bureau of the Census (2003). *Percent of people in poverty, by definition of income and selected characteristics, 2002*. Retrieved 5/3/04 from www.census.gov.hhes/poverty/poverty02/r&dtable5.html.

U.S. Department of Education (2001). *23rd annual report to Congress on the implementation of IDEA*. Washington, DC: Author.

U.S. Department of Education (2002). *The No Child Left Behind Act, Title I: Improving the academic achievement of the disadvantaged—Summary of final regulations*. Retrieved June 13, 2005, from www.ed.gov/nclb.

U.S. Department of Health and Human Services, Administration on Children, Youth, and Families (2003a). *12 years of reporting child maltreatment (2001)*. Washington, D.C.: U.S. Government Printing Office.

U.S. Department of Health and Human Services (2003b). *In Focus: The risk and prevention of maltreatment of children with disabilities* (2/01). Retrieved June 5, 2003, from www.calib.com/nccanch/prevention/publications/risk.cfm#scope.

Valdivia, R. (2000). The implications of culture on developmental delay. *ERIC Digest E589*. Retrieved July 17, 2004, from www.ericfacility.net/databases/ERIC_Digest.

Van Bourgondien, M.E., Marcus, L.M., & Schopler, E. (1992). Comparison of DSM-III-R and childhood autism rating scale diagnoses of autism. *Journal of Autism and Developmental Disorders, 22*, 493–506.

Van de Vijer, F. (2000). The nature of bias. In R.H. Dana (Ed.), *Handbook of cross-cultural and multicultural personality assessment* (pp. 87–106). Mahwah, NJ: Lawrence Erlbaum Associates, Inc.

Van Hulle, C.A., Goldsmith, H.H., & Lemery, K.S. (2004). Genetic, environmental, and gender effects on individual differences in toddler expressive language. *Journal of Speech, Language, and Hearing Research, 47*, 904–912.

van Keulen, J.E., Weddington, G.T., & DeBose, C.E. (1998). *Speech, language, and learning and the African American child*. Boston: Allyn & Bacon.

van Kleeck, A. (1994). Potential cultural bias in training parents as conversational partners with their children who have delays in language development. *American Journal of Speech-Language Pathology, 3*, 67–78.

van Kleeck, A. (2004). Fostering preliteracy development via storybook-sharing interactions: The cultural context of mainstream family practices. In C.A. Stone, E.R. Silliman, B.J. Ehren, & K. Apel (Eds.), *Handbook of language and literacy: Development and disorders* (pp. 175–208) New York: The Guilford Press.

van Kleeck, A., Gillam, R.B., Hamilton, L., & McGrath, C. (1997). The relationship between middle-class parents' book-sharing discussions and their preschoolers' abstract language development. *Journal of Speech, Language, and Hearing Research, 40*, 1261–1271.

van Kleeck. A., & Richardson, A. (1989). Language delay in the child. In J.L. Northern (Ed.), *Study guide for the handbook of speech-language pathology and audiology* (pp. 170–177). Philadelphia: B.C. Decker, Inc.

Vaughn, S., Bos, C.S., & Schumm, J.S. (2003). *Teaching exceptional, diverse, and at-risk students in the general education classroom* (3rd ed.). Boston: Allyn & Bacon.

Vaughn, S., Elbaum, B., & Boardman, A.G. (2001). The social functioning of students with learning disabilities: Implications for inclusion. *Exceptionality, 9*, 47–65.

Ventriglia, L. (1982). *Conversations of Miguel and Maria*. Redding, MA: Addison-Wesley.

Vining, C.B. (1999, November). *Navajo perspectives on developmental disabilities*. Paper presented at the annual meeting of the American Speech-Language-Hearing Association, San Francisco, CA.

Vygotsky, L. (1962). Thought and language. Cambridge: MIT Press. (Originally published in 1934.)

Wagner, R., Torgeson, J., & Rashotte, C. (1999). *Comprehensive Test of Phonological Processing*. Austin, TX: Pro-Ed.

Walker, D., Greenwood, C., Hart, B., & Carta, J. (1994). Prediction of school outcomes on early language production and socioeconomic factors. *Child Development, 65*, 606–621.

Wallace, G.L. (1998). Neurogenic disorders in adult and pediatric populations. In D. Battle (Ed.), *Communication disorders in multicultural populations* (2nd ed.) (pp. 309–334). Boston: Butterworth-Heinemann.

Walqui, A. (2000). Contextual factors in second language acquisition. *ERIC Digest, 9/00*. Available at www.cal.org/ericcl/digest/005contextual.html.

Wang, S. (2001, April). *Do child-rearing values in the U.S. and Taiwan echo their cultural values of individualism and collectivism?* Paper presented to the Society for Research in Child Development, Minneapolis, MN.

Washington, J.A., & Craig, H.K. (1999). Performances of at-risk, African American preschoolers on the Peabody Picture Vocabulary Test-III. *Language, Speech, and Hearing Services in Schools, 30*, 75–82.

Wasik, B.H., & Hendrickson, J.S. (2004). Family literacy practices. In C.A. Stone, E.R. Silliman, B.J. Ehren, & K. Apel (Eds.). *Handbook of language and literacy: Development and disorders* (pp. 154–174). New York: The Guilford Press.

Watson, C., & Weitzman, E. (2000). *It takes two to talk: The Hanen Program for Parents*. Toronto, Ontario, Canada: The Hanen Centre.

Wechsler, D. (1991). *Wechsler Intelligence Scale for Children* (4th ed.). San Antonio, TX: Psychological Corporation.

Weiner, C. (2001). *Preparing for success: Meeting the language and learning needs of young children from poverty homes*. Youngtown, AZ: ECL Publications.

Weismer, S., Branch, J., & Miller, J. (1994). A prospective longitudinal study of language development in late talkers. *Journal of Speech and Hearing Research, 37*, 852–867.

Westby, C.E. (1980). Assessment of cognitive and language abilities through play. *Language, Speech, and Hearing Services in Schools, 3*, 154–168.

Westby, C. (2004). A language perspective on executive functioning, metacognition, and self-regulation in reading. In C.A. Stone, E.R. Silliman, B.J. Ehren, & K. Apel (Eds.). *Handbook of language and literacy: Development and disorders* (pp. 398–438). New York: The Guilford Press.

Westby, C. (2006). There's more to passing than knowing the answers: Learning to do school. In T.A. Ukrainetz (Ed.), *Contextualizing language intervention: Scaffolding PreK-12 literacy achievement* (pp. 319–388). Eau Claire, WI: Thinking Publications.

Westby, C., & Cutler, S.K. (1994). Language and ADHD: Understanding the bases and treatment of self-regulatory deficits. *Topics in Language Disorders, 14*, 58–76.

Westby, C., & McKellar, N. (2000). Autism. In E.P. Dodge (Ed.), *The survival guide for school-based speech-language pathologists* (pp. 57–96). San Diego: Singular/Thomson.

Wetherby, A.M., Allen, L., Cleary, J., Kublin, K., & Goldstein, H. (2002). Validity and reliability of the Communication and Symbolic Behavior Scales Developmental Profile with very young children. *Journal of Speech, Language, and Hearing Research, 45*, 1202–1218.

Wetherby, A.M, & Prizant, B. (1992). Profiling young children's communicative competence. In S. Warren & J. Reichle (Eds.), *Causes and effects in communication and language intervention* (pp. 217–253). Baltimore, MD: Brookes.

Wetherby, A.M., & Prizant, B. (1998). *Communicative and symbolic behavior scales*. Itasca, IL: Riverside.

Whiting, P., & Robinson, G.R. (1988). Using Irlen colored lenses for reading: A clinical study. *Australian Educational and Developmental Psychologist, 5*, 7–10.

Williams, K.T. (2001). *Expressive Vocabulary Test*. Circle Pines, MN: American Guidance Service Publishing.

Wilson, W.F., Wilson, J.R., & Coleman, T.J. (2000). Culturally appropriate assessment: Issues and strategies. In T.J. Coleman, *Clinical management of communication disorders in culturally diverse children* (pp. 101–128). Boston: Allyn & Bacon.

Windsor, J., & Kohnert, K. (2004). The search for common ground: Part I. Lexical performance by linguistically diverse learners. *Journal of Speech, Language, and Hearing Research, 47*, 877–890.

Wittmer, D.S., & Honig, A.S. (1991). Convergent or divergent? Teacher questions to three-year old children in day care. *Early Child Development and Care, 68*, 141–147.

Wong Fillmore, L. (1976). *The second time around: Cognitive and social strategies in second language acquisition*. Unpublished doctoral dissertation, Stanford University.

Wong, A.M.-Y., Au, C.W.-S., & Stokes, S.F. (2004). Three measures of language production for Cantonese-speaking school-age children in a story-retelling task. *Journal of Speech, Language, and Hearing Research, 47*, 1164–1178.

Woods, J., & Wetherby, A.M. (2003). Early identification of and intervention for infants and toddlers who are at risk for autism spectrum disorder. *Language, Speech, and Hearing Services in Schools, 34*, 180–193.

Woolfolk, A. (2004). *Educational psychology* (9th ed.). Boston: Allyn & Bacon.

Wechsler, D. (2003). *Wechsler Intelligence Scale for Children* (4th ed.). San Antonio, TX: Psychological Corporation.

Weitzner-Lin, B. (2004). *Communication assessment and intervention with infants and toddlers*. St. Louis, MO: Butterworth-Heinemann.

Weiss, A. (2002). Planning language intervention for young children. In D.K. Bernstein & E. Tiegerman-Farber (Eds.), *Language and communication disorders in children* (5th ed.) (pp. 256–314). Boston: Allyn & Bacon.

Westling, D., & Fox, L. (2000). Teaching students with severe disabilities. Upper Saddle River, NJ: Merrill.

Wetherby, A., & Prizant, B. (1992). Profiling young children's communicative competence. In S. Warren and J. Reichle (Eds.), *Causes and effects in communication and language intervention*. Baltimore, MD: Brookes.

Wiig, E.H., & Semel, E.M. (1975). Productive language abilities in learning disabled adolescents. *Journal of Learning Disabilities, 8*, 578–586.

Wilens, T.E., Biederman, J., & Spencer, T.J. (2002). Attention deficit/hyperactivity disorder across the lifespan. *Annual Review of Medicine, 53*, 113–131.

Willis, W.O. (2004). Families with African American roots. In E.W. Lynch and M.J. Hanson (Eds.), *Developing cross-cultural competence: A guide for working with young children and their families* (pp. 1–2). Baltimore, MD: Paul H. Brookes Publishing Co.

Wilson, F.W., Wilson, J.R., & Coleman, T.J. (2000). *Culturally appropriate assessment: Issues and strategies*. Boston: Allyn & Bacon.

Windsor, J., & Kohnert, K. (2004). The search for common ground: Part I. Lexical performance by linguistically diverse learners. *Journal of Speech, Language, and Hearing Research, 47*, 877–890.

Windsor, J., Scott, C.M., & Street, C.K. (2000). Verb and noun morphology in the spoken and written language of children with language learning disabilities. *Journal of Speech, Language, and Hearing Research, 43*, 1322–1336.

Wolvin, A., & Coakley, C.C. (1988). Listening (3rd ed.). Dubuque, IA: W.C. Brown.

Wong, A.M.-Y., Au, C.W.-S., & Stokes, S.F. (2004). Three measures of language production for Cantonese-speaking school-age children in a story-retelling task. *Journal of Speech-Language-Hearing Research, 47*, 1164–1178.

Wong, B.Y.I., & Berninger, V.W. (2004). Cognitive processes of teachers in implementing composition research in elementary, middle, and high school curriculum. In C.A. Stone, E.R. Silliman, B.J. Ehren, & K. Apel (Eds.). *Handbook of language and literacy: Development and disorders* (pp. 600–626). New York: The Guilford Press.

Wood, F., Felton, R., Flowers, L., & Naylor, C. Neurobehavioral definition of dyslexia. In D.D. Duane & D.B. Gray (Eds.), *The reading brain: The biological basis of dyslexia* (pp. 1–26). Parkton, MD: New York Press.

Woodcock, R.W. (1987). *Woodcock Reading Mastery Test-Revised*. Circle Pines, MN: American Guidance Service.

Woolfolk, A. (2004). *Educational psychology* (9th ed.). Boston: Allyn & Bacon.

Wong Fillmore, L. (1991). When learning a second language means losing the first. *Early Childhood Research Quarterly, 6*, 323–346.

Wright, B.A., Bowen, R.W., & Zecker, S.G. (2000). Nonlinguistic perceptual deficits associated with reading and language disorders. *Current Opinion in Neurobiology, 10*, 482–486.

Wright, H.H., & Newhoff, M. (2001). Narration abilities of children with language-learning disabilities in response to oral and written stimuli. *American Journal of Speech-Language Pathology, 10*, 308–319.

Wyatt, T. (2002). Assessing the communicative abilities of clients from diverse cultural and language backgrounds. In D.E. Battle (Ed.), *Communication disorders in multicultural populations* (3rd ed.) (pp. 415–460). Boston: Butterworth-Heinemann.

Yoder, P., Warren, S., & McCathren, R. (1998). Determining spoken language prognosis in children with developmental disabilities. *American Journal of Speech-Language Pathology, 7*, 77–87.

Yoshinaga-Itano, C. (2003). From screening to early identification and intervention: Discovering predictors to successful outcomes for children with hearing loss. *Journal of Deaf Studies and Deaf Education, 8*, 11–30.

Young, G., & Killen, D. (2002). Receptive and expressive language skills of children with five years of experience using cochlear implants. *Annals of Otology, Rhinology and Laryngology, 111*, 802–810.

Zecker, L.B. (2004). Learning to read and write in two languages: The development of early biliteracy abilities. In C.A. Stone, E.R. Silliman, B.J. Ehren, & K. Apel (Eds.), *Handbook of language and literacy: Development and disorders* (pp. 248–265). New York: The Guilford Press.

Zentella, A.C. (2002). Latina languages and identities. In M. Suarez-Orozco & M.A. Paez (Eds.), *Latinos: Remaking America* (pp. 321–338). Berkeley, CA: University of California Press.

Zimmerman, I.L., & Steiner, V.G., & Pond, R.E. (1993). *Preschool Language Scale-3: Spanish Edition*. San Antonio, TX: Psychological Corporation.

Zimmerman, I.L., Steiner, V.G., & Pond, R.E. (2002). *Preschool Language Scale-4*. San Antonio, TX: Psychological Corporation.

Zuniga, M.E. (2004). Families with Latino roots. In E.W. Lynch and M.J. Hanson (Eds.), *Developing cross-cultural competence: A guide for working with young children and their families* (pp. 179–218). Baltimore, MD: Paul H. Brookes Publishing Co.

Zwolan, T.A. (2002). Cochlear implants. In J. Katz (Ed.), *Handbook of clinical audiology* (5th ed.) (pp. 740–757). Baltimore, MD: Lippincott Williams & Wilkins.

Index